CW01509657

THE LANGUAGE OF BION

THE LANGUAGE OF BION

A Dictionary of Concepts

P. C. Sandler

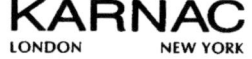
KARNAC
LONDON   NEW YORK

First published in 2005 by
H. Karnac (Books) Ltd.
6 Pembroke Buildings, London NW10 6RE

Copyright © 2005 Paulo Cesar Sandler

The right of Paulo Cesar Sandler to be identified as the author of this work
has been asserted in accordance with §§ 77 and 78 of the Copyright Design
and Patents Act 1988.

All rights reserved. No part of this publication may be reproduced, stored
in a retrieval system, or transmitted, in any form or by any means,
electronic, mechanical, photocopying, recording, or otherwise, without the
prior written permission of the publisher.

British Library Cataloguing in Publication Data

A C.I.P. for this book is available from the British Library

ISBN 1 85575 366 9

Designed and produced by The Studio Publishing Services Ltd,
Exeter EX4 8JN

Printed in Great Britain

10 9 8 7 6 5 4 3 2 1

www.karnacbooks.com

CONTENTS

To Ester, Daniela and Luiz, and to the memory
of my father, Dr Jayme Sandler

ACKNOWLEDGEMENTS

To Francesca Bion, whose fortitude, patience with my limitations, devotion, and caring humanity have constituted a peerless source of inspiration to me during the last twenty-three years. Having benefited from such a generosity and availability since 1981, when I translated *A Memoir of the Future* into Portuguese, this acknowledgement could be seen as trivial. However, its inclusion is much more due to the fact that it is easier to plant a tree, to initiate a business, a marriage, a career, than it is to keep it alive, fit, running, striving and maturing. The help she provided in writing of this dictionary far surpassed that of a gesture. She was able to point out seemingly minor, but serious flaws in my quotations, making the text more readable. This effort and generosity cannot be overestimated, taking into account the hours she spent doing this hard, painstaking work. She granted me the same seriousness and attention to detail that are some of her hallmarks in everything she does. She is the most knowledgeable person I know in the work of her deceased husband, on a level that I have seen in only very few distinguished scholars and scientists.

I would also like to acknowledge a few other people. Mr Oliver Rathbone gave life to this book. Without him, it would not even have the current title, which was his idea, after having discovered its underlying invariance, until then unknown to me: the inspiration in Laplanche and Pontalis's seminal dictionary. I am indebted to his dedicated, serious and patient Publishing Manager, Leena Häkkinen, and her staff.

My daughter Daniela, a knowledgeable scholar in arts and a number of languages, gave her time to proof-read the manuscript, which produced hundreds of corrections. My much loved father, who so prematurely met his fate, was a seasoned analyst keen in the English language. He translated some of Bion's first clinical seminars in Brazil, on the spot; he made me aware of Bion's existence, and also his seminal importance to psychoanalysis. Drs João Carlos Braga, Antonio Sapienza, Jaques Goldstajn, Francisco Claudio Montenegro Castelo, Almerinda Castelo Albuquerque, and Odilon de Mello Franco Filho made stimulating reading of some entries. I am deeply obliged to my son Luiz, due to his unfailing support; and to my wife Ester, without whom I am nothing.

The reader is invited to be escorted in the path that Paulo Cesar Sandler fleshes out in this book. In my view, the author embodies seriousness, subtlety and critical independence in his judgements about Wilfred Bion's instigations and complex contributions. Dr Sandler manages to illuminate the huge labyrinth that characterizes Bion's work and he offers us a whole listing of comprehensive entries in the form of a dictionary.

The dictionary is based on a critical reading that builds up into a genetic–historic study about Bion's ideas. In these entries, the reader can find Bion's affinities and roots in his psychoanalytic ancestors, Freud and Klein. Moreover, the author displays the close relations that these three authors maintain with each other. He also copes with the task of displaying with clarity the differentiations and particularities that characterize Bion's contributions to contemporary psychoanalysis. He does this as a faithful scientist and with devotion to the psychoanalytic method.

I will specifically comment on a single entry in this Foreword: "Dream work alpha". It can serve as a model and an example that illustrates the author's gracefulness in making an exhaustive concept clearer to the reader's mind while incorporating it into Freud's observations. This entry is filtered through bearings in Philosophy and Philosophy of Mathematics and its validation stems from clinical facts. One is invited to read this entry as a valuable sample of the dictionary. In this entry, Dr Sandler presents the reader with excerpts from Bion's texts written from 1959 to 1960, published in *Cogitations* (1992). He outlines a progressive axis that allows one to follow the growing distinction between dream work alpha and the theory of alpha function. The reader is then able to follow the genesis of Bion's proposals on alpha and beta elements, which in their turn will support the psychotic and non-psychotic parts of the personality.

Reading this entry is a rewarding experience. The author invites the reader to accompany him, step by step, in incursions into heuristic irradiations. He deepens our understanding of the Freudian proposal concerning the issue of "dreaming the session". Furthermore, he allows for the difference between the ideogrammatic and symbolic activities proper. The latter is founded in experiencing the depressive position.

During this scrutiny, Dr Sandler ponders the dimensions of space and linking relationships that spring from both the sensuous apprehensible and the psychic reality world. Let us consider an individual, a single person. Some of this individual's modes to feel and know the Universe are indicated—for the author furnishes those unique modes, which compose this individual's paths as well as his plans. One may grasp the psychotic and non-psychotic modes of functioning; they keep close relationship with this individual's store of alpha-elements, as well as the same individual's proficiency in storing them. Alpha-elements are bulwarks, which warrant the fitness of that which separates Unconscious from Conscious. The fitness of this system is understood here as its maintenance, vitality, and lilt.

As he finishes this entry, Dr Sandler emphasizes the "naïve idealist's" functioning, a definition he proposes as matching to Kant's "naïve realist". This is a personality stereotype, crammed with beta-elements. It survives based on his capacity to develop an intense mental activity, the hallmark of which is a prevailing use of projective identification. One may draw an analogy of this kind of personality with an "extruder" of "raw and primitive" thoughts—looking for someone to digest, refine, and think them through.

The reader who consults the entries in this dictionary will find it a work of beautiful, thorough, and professional craftsmanship. To quote just one more example, the entry "Real Psycho-Analysis" hurls the reader into Bion's creative footpaths, which he opened up in his generous Trilogy *A Memoir of the Future* (1975, 1977, 1979). Some interesting questions are raised in this valuable fragment of this text: is there any relationship between real life and psychoanalysis? If one exists, what are the positive aspects of this? What are the limitations of psychoanalysis in the face of emotional turbulence? What is the value of myths and models in the analytic situation? *What is the relationship between feelings of suffering and their use as the basis of experimentation?* Are there any dangers involved in a real analysis? What are they? Dr Sandler fulfills the reader's curiosity and invites him to expand on his ideas.

This is a worthwhile book to consult, and a good companion to a sophisticated psychoanalytic research. A fertile sowing and a safe crop of personal enrichment will reward the reader of this volume.

Antonio Sapienza

Introduction

"There is a scarcity of time; a scarcity of knowledge; scarcity of availability. Therefore choice becomes of fundamental importance—choice of time, theories, and facts observed"

(Bion, 1975)

"P.A. A danger lies in the belief that psycho-analysis is a novel approach to a newly discovered danger. If psycho-analysts had an overall view of the history of the human spirit, they would appreciate the length of that history of murder, failure, envy and deceit"

(Bion, *A Memoir of the Future*, 1979, p. 571)

O TEMPORA, O MORES

... technical term gets worn away and turns into a kind of worn out coin which has lost its value. We should keep these things in good working conditions. [Bion's Brazilian Lectures II, p. 87]

1

ALICE From what I have heard, the complacency and ignorance of psycho-analysts makes it difficult for them to take any adequate steps to perfect either themselves or psycho-analysis. [*A Memoir of the Future*, vol. III, p. 571]

The unconscious is the true psychical reality; **in its innermost nature it is as most unknown to us as the reality of the external world, and it is as incompletely presented by the data of consciousness as is the external world by the communications of our sense organs** [Freud, *The Interpretation of Dreams*, 1900, p.613; Freud's bold]

This book is the result of a conjunction of many factors, chiefly, the constant requests from colleagues, especially Dr Carlos Alberto Gioielli, whom I cannot thank enough. I should also mention candidates of the local institute of psycho-analysis (Sociedade Brasileira de Psicanalise de São Paulo) and students of the post-graduate training course on psycho-analytic therapy of the University of São Paulo. Another factor in the writing of this book can be understood with the aid of the following formulation by Bion:

PRIEST . . . From what I see of psycho-analysts they do not know what religion is; they simply transfer their allegiance from one undisciplined, desire-ridden system of emotions and ideas to another. I have heard psycho-analysts discussing; their discussion itself betrays all the characteristics which I have recognized as pathognomic of religion of a primitive, undisciplined, intellectually unstructured kind. They argue heatedly, adducing national, racial, aesthetic and other emotionally coloured motivations in support of their particular brand of activity.

P.A. I would not deny that we do all these things, but we do in fact continue to question ourselves and our motives in a disciplined manner. We may not succeed; neither do we give up the attempt.

PRIEST I hate to appear to sit in judgement but I have to judge, to appraise such evidence as I have as it touches my private life and my responsibility for my own thoughts and actions. You have as many sects of psycho-analysts as there are in any religion I know. You have as many psycho-analytic "saints" with their individual following of devotees. [1979, 544–5]

The phrase, *"individual following"* brings to light some points to consider. It may reflect—and perhaps in the vast majority of cases it does reflect—idealistic tendencies. Since the eighties it has presented itself as a trend—perhaps more trendy than anything else. It has been named, "readings". Its adepts have jumped on the textualist and post-modernist bandwagons. The basis of the idealism is a religious state of mind, illuminated by Freud: one projects one's omnipotence and omniscience on to a chosen god.

It is doubtful that this attitude has been fully accepted by theologians—an issue raised from time immemorial by the so-called mystic tradition. There is a difference between the attitude of reverence and awe (Bion's terms, used in 1967; *Cogitations*, p. 285) and imitation or projected omnipotence. Bion used this differentiation from 1965. In nominally non-religious organizations the same issue presents itself in a special guise: one reads the work written by an author and replaces the author's meanings with one's own. The religious aspect is marked by the reader's blind fanaticism whose allegiance is to his own idiosyncratic ideas assumed to be reflecting a given author's discoveries. An added complication is when this kind of allegiance is mixed up with writings of authors who also are prey to this tendency. The tendency itself is at least as old as philosophy; at various times through the centuries it has been known as subjectivism, idealism and solipsism. Freud referred to it in his paper, "The question of a *weltanschauung*" (SE, XXIII).

One does not try to assess whether a given concept (and in some cases, a given event) that has been formulated and written in a text has any counterparts in reality. Therefore another factor that contributed to the decision to write this dictionary is the author's observation of the prevalence of an unobserved "idealistic" tendency in the psycho-analytic milieu. By idealism I mean an old omnipotent fallacy: it dictates that the universe and reality itself are products of the human mind. This view proves to be enticing and popular. It is typical of very small children and psychotics stuck in paranoid states. Once installed it seeps faster than water through a rotten wall or through the fingers of a hand trying to hold it.

Bion was fond of John Ruskin and especially of one of his works, *Sesame and Lilies*. He quotes this book in *A Memoir of the Future*. Ruskin cites examples of the damage done when the reader refuses to seek the author's original sense and tries to displace it with his or her own. What is lost to sight is that the personal ways of formulating a reading—an indispensable act—are mistaken by the act of distorting what the author wrote. "Invariance under literacy", as Bion warns in *Transformations*, page 3, cannot guarantee that one will be able to find the author's sense. But it may help if the educated reader attempts to leave aside his prejudices—even if only momentarily.

Apprehension of reality and communication

As psycho-analysts, we are entitled to diminish the interference and bias due to "personal equation" as Freud called it. Not only entitled, but rather obliged, out of an ethical sense of duty, thanks to personal analysis. The uses that Bion makes of the word "imagination" and its counterparts in reality, as well as its function in psycho-analysis, seem to the author to be widely misunderstood. It often serves to leave aside the respect for a given author's meanings.

The author tries his hand at delivering a re-arrangement of Bion's work, in a form that may be more appropriate to our hurried epoch. From old-time *Tractatus* to easy-to-find dictionaries: a tale for our times?

> I am convinced of the strength of the scientific position of psycho-analytic practice (Learning from Experience, p. 77).

There is no possibility of scientific communication without a precise system of notation. This includes—as a matter of necessity—the clearest definitions of concepts, theories and models, as far as possible.

> As an example of an attempt at precise formulation I take alpha-function and two factors, excessive projective identification and excess of bad objects. Suppose that in the course of the analysis these two factors are obtrusive to the exclusion of other factors the analyst has observed. If psycho-analytic theory were rationally organized it should be possible to refer to both these factors by symbols which were part of a system of reference that was applied uniformly and universally. The Kleinian theory of projective identification would be referred to by initials and a page and paragraph reference. Similarly, Freud's view of attention would be replaced by

a reference. This can be done, though clumsily, by reference to page and line of a standard edition even now. Such a statement could lend itself to mere manipulation, more or less ingenious, of symbols according to apparently arbitrary rules. Provided that the analyst preserves a sense of the factual background to which such a formulation refers, there are advantages in the exercise in precision and rigour of thought that is exacted by an attempt to concentrate actual clinical experience so that it may be expressed in such abstract notation. [LE, 38–9]

General principles of the content of this dictionary

The general principles of this re-organization in dictionary form are:

(i)   Faithfulness to the original text.
(ii)   Generalizations.
(iii) Historicity.

(i) Faithfulness to the original text: the definitions included in this dictionary are compiled from Bion's writings. Most of the work is to reunite many ideas scattered in space and time throughout Bion's work. The hostile reader will not err if he is tempted to dismiss this attempt as just a compilation that re-organizes Bion's written work. The sympathetic reader may profit from the attempt—which includes comments about the quotations.

(ii) Generalizations: generalizations that encompass particularities are intrinsic to the scientific ethos. They may express themselves through classificatory systems first devised by Linnaeus and followed by classical and perennial formulations, from Goethe in Botany and the periodical table of elements in Chemistry. These classificatory systems are scientific groupings that try to detect either underlying or overt binding, threading lines. Classification performs the double function of communication and aids the scientist to orient his research; often they illuminated the path to discoveries. In this dictionary, the thread allows the many quotations to cohere into a whole. Each whole forms an Entry.

(iii) Historicity: the entries are developed historically as they appeared in Bion's work. This author observed that Bion's concepts were developed in a way that may be compared to the craft of jewellery. Painstaking, increasingly finer polishing continuously improved them, resulting in transparent luminescence. This gave the impression to many critical onlookers that Bion kept repeating the same old stuff. He agrees with them and even mentioned this aspect in his introduction to *Seven Servants* (a re-print of his four basic books, *Learning from Experience*, *Elements of Psycho-analysis*, *Transformations* and *Attention and Interpretation*), using the comment in his characteristic way with humour. He uses it to learn: the comments brought home to him how little he thinks he knows, and how much he felt he owed to Freud, Rickman and Klein (the two latter being his former analysts).

Sometimes this criticism had hostile overtones. In the opinion of this writer, these readers or audiences perhaps miss the point about the continuous deepening of the concepts. "More of the same" is an expression that could well be applied to oxygen, water and nourishment. One may wonder how fundamental they are and how useful it is if they appear in purified and improved forms.

These principles resulted in entries that (I hope) form a "developing whole"—each entry tries to depict this.

Obscure and difficult?

Freud opened many broad avenues to research. Few analysts ventured to push this research beyond the limits established by the end of Freud's physical life. Bion tackles the task of trying to do this in at least four aspects of Freud's theories: dreams, two principles of mental functioning, Oedipus and the nature of free associations.

This author's comments are meant to clarify some issues. They are built by intertwining Bion's wording (in italics, using semi-colons and with the exact page where they may be found) with this author's wording. This is an attempt to address a fact derived from this author's experience with colleagues around the world for 24 years, namely, that many feel Bion's written work to be "obscure and difficult".

> Is "Sordello" incomprehensible on purpose to make it difficult, or is it Browning's attempt to express what he had to say in the shortest and most comprehensible terms? [AMF, I, 121]

The following comments must be read as an assessment. They are not intended to criticize negatively the difficulties of anyone's reading. This would be a peerless arrogant act indistinguishable from disrespect and inhumanity. The fact must be mentioned because it is behind another driving factor for undertaking the task of writing the dictionary. It seems to this writer that some of the factors involved in this attributed obscurity fall into the following categories:

(i)   Lack of attentive reading, something that has occurred since Freud and was duly emphasized by him (for example, in the latest introductions to *The Interpretation of Dreams*).
(ii)   Lack of analytical experience, here defined as the analyst's personal analysis and experience seeing patients.
(iii) Lack of experience in life itself, which sometimes help the development of concern for life and truth.
(iv)   A constant conjunction of (i), (ii) and (iii).

These difficulties are not new in the history of the psycho-analytic movement. Perhaps they are more usual than not. They are manifested often through feelings of abhorrence when reading valuable, real psycho-analytical written works. This kind of writing touches the reader's innermost aspects in unexpected and unknown ways. Sometimes the reader is led to seek analysis; sometimes he (she) is led to hate analysis right from the start. This fact was well documented by Freud, whose works were regarded as pornographic, Jewish, anti-Jewish, atheistic, progressive, reactionary, Victorian, pan-sexualist, anti-feminist, *romans-à-clef*. As occurs in many specialized fields, especially those that depend on experience, to use Bion's wording again, "*invariances under literacy*" (*Transformations*, p. 3) are necessary but they are not sufficient to allow a real apprehension of attempts at communication. Even in much older disciplines such as music, there are from time to time polemical voices about textualist reading of the score versus a kind of "interpretationist" trend. The problem is: it has to be both. A mathematical system of notation is not easily attainable and perhaps is impossible outside the realm of mathematics.

Lest the reader feel that this assessment from the author is authoritarian, the scientific outlook may help here. There follow some hard-core facts that may illustrate the issue.

Two years ago, a pervasive sense of bewilderment emerged among the twenty-five participants of a seminar. The majority of colleagues who made up the group had been reading the works of Bion for more than ten years; some for thirty years. The seminar was conducted by a colleague who enjoyed a reputation for being a kind of authority on Bion's works. This enshrining was both self- and hetero-attributed. His willingness to assume the role meant that the emotional climate of the group displayed unequivocal signs of the prevalence of one of the basic assumptions of a group (in the classification proposed by Bion in *Experiences in Groups*)—that of the messianic leader. All members of the group had the task of reading the first chapter of *Transformations* prior to the encounter. There was an expositor chosen by this leader of the group.

At the first meeting, the chosen expositor failed to show up on time. After a heavy silence, a member of the group volunteered to contribute and began a summary of the chapter. After a few minutes of exposition some in the group displayed signs of disagreement when the expositor said that the concept of invariants was a built-in, inescapable concept of the theory of transformations. He was put into quarantine. Some displayed incredulity and reacted as if it was non-sense. One said that there was no such thing there; he invoked the words of a local "authority" who had once stated, "Everything in the world was transformations". The discussion heated up and the expositor invited everyone to read the first page of *Transformations*. The "leader" disagreed more strongly than others with the expositor and echoed the view of the majority of members. There was an initial refusal to read the text on the spot.

The expositor, responding to the mounting pressure in none too serene a way, pointed out that the first paragraph of Bion's text already depicted the concept of invariants. The vast majority of the participants, with the possible exception of two, grumbled and then agreed to *read* the text. Some read it. The result was an unwitting confirmation of the "Emperor's new clothes" fable. Some said that Bion did not know what he was writing; some said that the point had no importance whatsoever. They continued with their prejudiced reading.

In light of the experience of this writer, there are two observations to be made: (i) this particular kind of reading of *Transformations* proves to be popular. It adapts Bion's text to the acknowledgedly flawed dictum of Lavoisier; it seems enticing to some readers who are prone to over-simplification; (ii) the basic pattern of this experience repeated itself many times in different contexts for more than twenty years, even though many of them were devoid of the hostile personal tone. Some more sympathetic audiences in post-graduate courses at the University and among candidates of the local institute of psycho-analysis where this author has been teaching for the last fifteen years profited from the experience of observation of the prevalent forms of misunderstanding and mis-reading: denials, splits and transformations into the contrary of what was written. The bewilderment proved to be useful to them: how many times does one do this with patients?

Therefore the statements this author makes in the entries and the definitions of the terms are always backed by Bion's writings, from which the definitions derive. The entries have the privilege of hindsight; that is, they try to follow the evolution of the concepts throughout Bion's entire work.

When Bion wrote *Learning from Experience* he felt the need to state that *"The methods in this book are not definitive. Even when I have been aware that they are inadequate I have often not been able to better them. I have found myself in a similar position to the scientist who continues to employ a theory that he knows to be faulty because a better one has not been discovered to replace it"* (LE, last page of the Introduction, item 9). This definitely puts his attempts into the realm of science. He would repeat this often, even in the sub-title of one of his books, *Attention and Interpretation*.

Therefore, an effort towards a kind of standardization and precision in expressing Bion's concepts is not undue. This author can find no way other than to use Bion's own terms. In adding an Index to *Attention and Interpretation* he states, *"like the rest of the book,* (the Index) *is the outcome of an attempt at precision. The failure of the attempt will be clear; what may not be clear is the following dilemma: 'precision' is too often a distortion of the reality, 'imprecision' too often indistinguishable from confusion"* (AI, 131).

The extensive inclusion of Bion's texts is an attempt further to enable the reader to reach his or her own conclusions. It is to be hoped that they will serve as an enticing invitation, "Please now go and taste the original in its wholeness". All quotations are accompanied by the exact work and page of Bion's writings. The book is designed to provide a quick guide, provided that the potential reader does not confuse an attempt at speed with superficiality. The entries are meant to spare the reader the work of having to track down the scattered references and their development in Bion's work.

To paraphrase Bion, in his Introduction to *Learning from Experience*: this dictionary is **not** designed to be read straight through once. Each paragraph, each entry (in many cases divided into subtitles) is designed to function as a checking point and to be checked, in the hope that it will dispel the idea that Bion was obscure. Even a single entry is not designed to be read straight through, unless the reader prefers to do this. The entries and comments are designed to be the object of minute thought. The canonical or idolatrous reader will feel, not without reason, that this dictionary's mode of presentation may run against Bion's mode of presentation. The author thinks that there is no use dealing with Bion's works as if there is a "Saint Bion" to be followed and imitated. Imitation is the offspring of fear and rivalry. The helpless little child has no other means of survival; but if it is maintained in adulthood, its outcome is destructive and it shares with hallucination the quality of "unreal-ness". The analytical movement has had enough of imitators, repeaters, mimicry and aping. Bion's stature has always enticed this kind of follower, a fact he lamented and that has been emphasized by acknowledged authors such as Ignacio Matte-Blanco, James Grotstein and André Green. In connection with this, this author thinks that no student of Bion's work—or the work of any great author—qualifies as a self-appointed minister of his scriptures.

The experience of obscurity and difficulty in reading Bion's writings is not something that the present writer is able to share with many readers. At first it was the cause of considerable anxiety, something that happens when the individual finds himself out of tune with the herd. (A fact emphasized by Bion in *A Memoir of the Future*, Book III. Please refer to the entry in this dictionary, "Establishment".) This did not diminish this author's sympathy towards the difficulties observed in others. Quite the contrary, it is just another factor that motivated the present attempt. In trying to examine the origin of the sense of clarity that Bion's writings always had on this author, some hypotheses surfaced, all of them linked to practice:

(i) Eleven years of continuous psychiatric practice in a traditional mental hospital dealing with so-called psychotics on a daily basis. The experience included "intensive psychotherapy" using Frieda Fromm-Reichmann and John Rosen's methods; also, work in the psychiatric emergency care service, 24 or 48 hour shifts. There was a sense of personal guilt when reading Bion's *Second Thoughts* for the first time, regret for not having had them at hand when first dealing with the patients in the hospital.

(ii) Nine years in a community mental health centre.

(iii) Last, but first in importance, fifteen years of analysis deeply influenced by the contributions of Freud, Klein and Bion.

After at least ten years of trying to convey the clarity and usefulness of his works in talks with colleagues; after having written an Introductory book to *A Memoir of the Future* together with the translation of the Trilogy into the Portuguese language, this writer realized that perhaps it would be wiser to keep private the sense of clarity that pervaded his own reading. Too many older and experienced people felt the books to be obscure; Bion himself felt the need to warn the reader about this. For sure, this was because of reactions he witnessed against his writings.

Very early on this author became aware that some of those reactions were rabid. That is, there are at least two kinds of people who feel Bion's writings to be obscure: some are sincerely interested but give up reading, and some are hostile. Making part of the hostile critics who felt Bion's work obscure, one person who was trying to be politically influential in the psycho-analytic establishment once wrote that the book *Transformations* is "fascinating" and "contradictory". This person, paradigmatically, did not bother to illustrate this easy use of rhetoric with hard facts. That is, this person did not display evidence of any single part that could be seen as fascinating or contradictory. Also, no one of these critics asks if reality is simple, clear and easy—the same, for psycho-analysis, dreams, life itself. Or, as if all of these are given to us as a gift, easily. If Bion's—or Freud's—work has anything to do with reality as it is, from what kind of stuff were those works made? Is Bion's work more difficult than any worthwhile work? Many times the obvious and the simple is the most difficult.

Anyone who nourishes interest, love of truth, analytical experience (personal analysis and seeing patients in real analysis) and a faultless attention to the minute detail of his writings can apprehend Bion's work. This personal opinion may be mistaken, but no one could level against this writer the accusation that this statement is not born of experience.

The compilation was made *after* approximately twenty years of continuous study of his works. This study comprises:

(i)   Attending clinical and theoretical seminars at the local Institute when I was a candidate, with senior colleagues who had personal contact with Bion; one of them, who also supervised some cases, had an analysis with Bion.

(ii) Conducting seminars since this author was accepted as a professor of the local institute of psycho-analysis (1987); teaching a regular post-graduate course about the work of Bion, since 1998—perhaps the first such course to have been delivered in the academic milieu, world-wide.

(iii) Writing approximately twenty published papers about Bion's work, since 1983—two of them were awarded prizes at Brazilian Congresses of Psycho-analysis; three of them try to expand his theories of mental functions, basic assumptions in a group, and links. Also, the Brazilian version of the majority of Bion's books (including the first foreign-language version of *A Memoir of the Future*).

The entries, despite the fact that they respect historicity and underlying threads, were built mainly by using the author's free-associations at the moment of writing, coupled with annotations made throughout the years. The phenomenon is akin to that which happens when the analyst exercises his free floating attention with a patient. He or she is able to recall in a dream-like state the memoirs of his experiences with that patient, of sessions with him; he or she is able to have the tools, on the spur of the moment, of myths, forgotten personal experiences and so on. They flow spontaneously to his or her mind. Any writer has this method at his disposal. This means that the compilation is not the result of the currently adopted approach, namely, that of resorting to computerized methods of "reading". The computer was used here just as a word processor.

General principles of this dictionary

(A) Formal principles

How to resist the temptation to reproduce exhaustively all the parts that deal with the topics chosen? Some headings were expanded in this way, namely, those that were considered to embrace polemic topics, in the sense that they are subject to gross misunderstandings. The reader will also find some quotations being used in more than one entry.

This method of repetition is linked to a teaching experience which shows that it functions better in texts whose intention is to serve as a primer to the neophyte. Eugene Delacroix believed that in many instances what the so-called geniuses did, or do, is to present (old) buried truths in a formulation that must make sense to their contemporaries; Bacon also said something similar; Freud and Bion perhaps did this.

Therefore one faces a question of language; this is the sense of the word "neophyte"—of a new language. New languages are learned, even though not exclusively, by repetition and sedimentation. Bion dwells on this in the way an infant learns to turn the word "Daddy" into the unconscious, in *Learning from Experience*. Bion himself, as Franz Schubert before him, was often accused of repeating the themes either in the same piece or in different variations. He reached the point of registering this in the introduction to *Seven Servants* already mentioned above.

To the reader who cannot grasp the sense the first time, the "repetition method" can serve well. To the readers who are acquainted with Bion's work it may give the impression of an old friend revisited.

(B) Concepts

As far as possible in psychiatry, in psycho-analysis, and consequently in Bion's contribution, no effort was spared to elicit the inner quality (or nature) that some of the entries seem to possess, namely, the quality of a concept. Bion was very cautious not to attribute the status of scientific concepts to his contributions hastily. In this text, we start from the principle that when a verbal formulation can depict its counterpart in reality, it qualifies to be treated as a concept. To some readers, the verbal formulation does not convey just this counterpart; it also brings with it, immaterially, the very reality it tries to depict. Obviously it will depend on the reader's experience to intuit that which the words strive to convey (but are doomed to fail). For this reason alone *"invariances under literacy"* are not enough. Freud and Bion stated that psycho-analytic works should be read by psycho-analysts, which presumes the analyst's analysis to be as extensive and profound as possible. In this sense, many concepts of Bion's work, as happens with all successful and valid psycho-analytical concepts, originate from his experiences of life: the bestial, murderous and violent behaviour of so-called human beings and their accompanying sublime and lovely counterparts. He suffered from them in two wars, as a soldier; his physical loss of his first wife; his second chance of a real analysis with two gifted and sincere analysts and above all, a dedicated wife. As did Freud with Oedipus and Klein with *Envy and Gratitude*, Bion made the best of a bad job: suffering turned into contributions to psycho-analysis.

The numinous realm and the ethos of psycho-analysis

This dictionary is **not** intended to be a "reading" in the post-structuralist and post-modernist sense. Phrases such as "according to Bion", "according to Freud" raise some problems. Is there any possibility in science other than to be "according to reality"? Even though reality or truth is not something one can understand, know, preview, master, own or see, one may intuit it. One may nourish faith that it exists. One may use it and apprehend it—albeit momentarily in fleeting glimpses. One may be "at-one" with it, using Bion's verbal formulation. He states—not devoid of humour—in *Transformations* that reality is not something that can be known in the same sense that one cannot sing potatoes. One may plant potatoes, peel them, cook them, eat them. Nevertheless, their ultimate reality, the immaterial invariance that makes a potato a potato and nothing else—"potatoeness"—cannot be known. It can be intuited, it exists, but what is left to us human beings is to use it, to take advantage or disadvantage of its manifestations.

Freud, Bion, Klein, Winnicott, Einstein, Shakespeare, Bach or whoever it be, was or shall be, were able to formulate verbally, mathematically, or musically, *that* which has a counterpart in reality. We can no more than suddenly, eternal as long as it lasts, have a transient, fleeting glimpse of "it" in an intuitive way. The great authors in science and art made formulations that fleetingly apprehended some emanations of reality. In this resides also the possibility of a "real analysis", a term coined by Bion. In the analytic setting the "great author" is the analytic couple.

The task of this present writer was greatly facilitated by the extreme precision with which, in the vast majority of cases, Bion formulates his concepts. This is accompanied by a remarkable consistency in the way they are used throughout his entire work. Among one hundred entries that depict concepts, this author spotted just two cases of lack of precision. Therefore it is hoped that the phrases "extreme precision" and "remarkable consistency" will not appear laudatory, but a fair depiction of the real situation. The same applies to the quotation of origins of his statements and terms. A "vast majority" includes the very few exceptions. It seems that some of them were due to faulty literary revision. As a writer and translator myself, I must say that that experience shows that despite all efforts of reviewers and the pain involved in such a strenuous task, many publishing houses turn it into a frustrating task. In the end, when a batch of brand-new shiny covers reach the bookshelves of bookstores, some errors that the author or the translator or the reviewer corrected are still there. Sometimes, a fresh crop of errors displays its unwelcome face. The concepts are coherently used in the same way throughout the books; in just four instances they are put differently.

The four inconsistencies are linked to the definition of the term, "conception"; to the definition of alpha-function; to the definition of the process of transformations, and one odd attribution to alpha-function. Where his possible intellectual forebears are concerned, Bion leaves aside the precise quotation of their names at just three points of his work (among hundreds).

The dictionary includes misuses and misconceptions of his terms. A word must be added about the origins of at least two of them. Perhaps no other work in psycho-analysis, with the possible exception of those of Freud, Klein and Winnicott, was, and continues to be, subjected to attacks from contemporaries, as does that of Bion. These attacks show idolization and misunderstanding; more often then not, a conjunction of both. Rabid criticism also means idolization, even if it is hidden from sight. They provoke precocious dismissal. Even though he is in good company, this state of affairs does not help analysts or patients.

The sources of the misconceptions are depicted in the specific entries. Broadly speaking, they originate from two main problems: (i) Bion's use of borrowed terms; (ii) the reader's analytic experience.

(i) Bion points out that *he borrows some terms from other disciplines.* He preferred not to resort too much to neologisms and, even less, to indulge in jargon. He makes this preference clear in *A Memoir of the Future*, for example, Book II, pages 228, 231, 234. He intentionally does this to profit from the penumbra of associations of some already-existing terms. He usually emphasizes when a specific term is already endowed with some known and widely-accepted meaning and connotation. He wants the reader to be reminded of them. For example, "transformations and invariances", "hallucinosis". Sometimes he uses the term giving specific warnings that the reader must see that the term is used differently in his work. For example, the non-hyphenated term "preconception". And sometimes he creates new terms just to avoid any associations with existing ones, such as "O", "α" and "β". Finally, sometimes he stresses some meanings that the term allows and sticks only with them, such as "hyperbole". Unfortunately, it seems that many do not pay attention to those warnings and explanations of the use of the term in his work and this leads to confusion. Again he is in good company: in the preface of the 10th edition of *The Interpretation of Dreams* Freud commented that people were not really reading it. The disciplines that furnished terms and conceptions for Bion are science, mathematics, physics, art and the mystic tradition (mainly the Jewish-Christian Cabbala). The use of those borrowed terms with the specific purpose of facilitating communication seems to have been debased. Some readers cannot see that the use of terms does not mean that Bion used or transplanted models from other sciences. As late as 1975 he warned: "*Relativity is relationship, transference, the psycho-analytic term and its corresponding approximate realization. Mathematics, science as known hitherto, can provide no model.*

Religion, music, painting, as these terms are understood, fail me. Sooner or later we reach a point where there is nothing to be done except—if there is any exception—to wait (AMF, I, 61).

(ii) In 1970 he was still trying to make it clear that he hoped that *practising* psycho-analysts would realize that to read *about* psycho-analysis differs from *practising it*. He *"could only represent"* the prac-tice *"by words and verbal formulations designed for a different task"* (AI, Introduction). This means that Bion counted on the personal analy-sis of the reader, and his or her analytical experience. The lack of analytic practice makes the reader blind to the value of Bion's heavy use of analogy. *"The psycho-analytical approach, though valuable in having extended the conscious by the unconscious, has been vitiated by the failure to understand the practical application of doubt by the failure to understand the function of 'breast', 'mouth', 'penis', 'vagina', 'container', 'contained', as analogies. Even if I write it, the sensuous domi-nance of penis, vagina, mouth, anus, obscures the element signified by analogy.* (AMF, I, 70–71).

Those who cannot go beyond sensuously-apprehensible appear-ances, cannot grasp the fact that mystic tradition, as well as mathe-matics, art and philosophy, were *earlier modes that expressed human attempts to approach human nature and the mind's functioning.* They tried to serve mankind before the obtrusion of science and psycho-analytic science. The present author cannot dwell on this now, having tried to display the issue in a whole series of books and some papers. It concerns the negative realm of the noumena.

This aspect is one of Bion's contributions to human knowledge. He followed Freud's hint; *Transformations, Attention and Interpret-ation,* and *A Memoir of the Future* represent the climax of his attempts. Bion used to say that people such as Shakespeare were great analysts before there appeared a Freud to think the thought without a thinker, "psycho-analysis". In *Transformations,* he plainly states that Plato was a patron of Melanie Klein's internal object (p. 138). But a failure to grasp the real, albeit immaterial and non-sensuously apprehensi-ble stuff of the unconscious, whose negative nature shares the fea-tures of the noumena, seems to persist. The down-to-earth reader takes Bion's words as if they were used in their artistic, religious, mathematical or neo-positivist senses *per se;* as if he were an artist, religious man, mathematician or neo-positivist trying to impinge art, religion, mathematics or neo-positivism on to psycho-analysis.

These readers fail to see the analogy. Bion's reverence and awe before the unknown equals that of Plato, Kant, Diderot, Goethe, Keats, Freud, Einstein, Heisenberg, to quote a few. Many do not hesitate to state that Bion was: (i) crazy, deteriorated, senile (for example, Joseph, 2002); (ii) incomprehensible, non-psycho-analytic (for example, the chairman of the IPAC's panel on schizophrenia in Edinburgh, 1961 is reputed to have said, "This is not psycho-analysis any more!" while throwing away his manuscript containing the study, "A theory of thinking", just after its public presentation; Bicudo, 1996); or that the concept of thought without a thinker has no psycho-analytical value (Segal, 1989); (iii) just a theoretician whose work had no clinical application (Joseph, 1980); (iv) that Bion had a poor grasp of Freud's work (Sandler, 1992). Bion himself addressed those critics in some parts of his work (for example, *Cogitations*, p. 377).

Some entries display the chronological evolution of the concepts. For the sake of clarity, on the occasions that an improved, later definition is available, it is given at once.

Few theories

A final word on the nature of the concepts. With the exception of a theory of thinking, of the theory of container and contained and that which he provisionally named metatheory, Bion did not make new theories in psycho-analysis. He expanded existing theories in order to have them fit the empirical (clinical) data better. He also made many theories of observation for the practising psycho-analyst.

There are some concepts that seem to the author not sufficiently developed by Bion. They have been omitted from the dictionary. For example: "vogue" (C, 374). The choice was to include that which Bion wrote in a clear way. As a consequence the attempt does not include personal ideas or interpretation of what Bion was saying or meant or intended to say. In the opinion of this writer. this is at best an exercise in imagination. It often ranges from frivolity to preposterousness. It does not mean, either, that the comments do not include the experience and opinion of this particular writer; the intention is, Ruskin-like, that they do not prevail over the writing.

Many entries were illuminated, especially as regards Bion's fore-bears, through the use of his personal copies of the great authors' works. He used to write in the margins of the books he read, from Plato to Popper. Due to the indescribably generous help provided by Francesca Bion, who sent this writer facsimiles of some of these pages throughout the years after having perused her library to meet my requests, and granted me access to it, the statements made in the entries relating to these origins can be safely regarded as going beyond the status of hypotheses.

Is this list of entries complete? This writer would be indebted to the reader who may eventually find missing definitions and concepts from Bion's work; otherwise, this dictionary and future students will be condemned to bear the burden of this writer's limitations.

That this volume can be at least minimally useful and can serve as an invitation to further readings of Bion's writings is my wish to you, dear reader.

Conventions:

EG *Experiences in Groups*, Heinemann Medical Books, 1961.
ST *Second Thoughts*, Heinemann Medical Books, 1967 and reprinted by Karnac Books.
LE *Learning from Experience*, Heinemann Medical Books, 1962 and reprinted by Karnac Books.
EP *Elements of Psycho-Analysis*, Heinemann Medical Books, 1963 and reprinted by Karnac Books.
T *Transformations*, Heinemann Medical Books, 1965 and reprinted by Karnac Books.
AI *Attention and Interpretation*, Tavistock Publications, 1970 and reprinted by Karnac Books.
BLI *Brazilian Lectures, I*, Imago Editora, 1974.
BLII *Brazilian Lectures, II*, Imago Editora, 1975.
AMF *A Memoir of the Future*, Imago Editora, 1975, 1977 and Clunie Press, 1979 and reprinted by Karnac Books,1991.
CSOW *Clinical Seminars and Other Works*, Karnac, 1994.
BNYSP *Bion in New York and São Paulo*, Clunie Press, 1979.
C *Cogitation*, Karnac Books, 1997.
TLWE *The Long Week-End*, Fleetwood Press, 1982 and reprinted by Karnac Books,1991.

AMSR *All My Sins Remembered*, Fleetwood Press, 1985 and reprinted by Karnac Books.
WM *War Memoirs*, Karnac Books, 1997.

In brackets: The first number refers to the page of the editions mentioned above and the second number refers to the itemized paragraphs, when available.

Except when indicated, the bold and italics are by Bion himself. When applicable, the concepts contain:

📖 *suggested further readings.*

🕒 *evolution of the concept within Bion's work.*

&⟨ *suggested clarifications or extensions by other authors starting from Bion.*

Usefulness indications of uses when they are not often seen in the literature.

The entries direct the reader to two types of cross-references:

1. Recommended—the entries are mutually complementary and the reading of both (or more) is a must.
2. Suggested—the entries are mutually enriching and the reading of both (or more) augments the reader's scope.

A

Absolute truth: An imaginary, lying entity created by paranoid states. It has at least three factors:

(i)   An attempt to deal with the animate with methods that are fairly successful in dealing with the inanimate. It is an offshoot of a state of mind that tries to turn dynamic situations into static ones. The static state seems to the "beholder" to be one that is "amenable" to be owned, in phantasy.

(ii) An attempt to replace the discrimination of true and false (or reality and hallucination) with moral values, to dictate how things, events or people should be.

(iii) Primary envy, primary narcissism and disregard for truth and love.

The "beholder" abhors movement, transient evolution, development and reality. "How" is replaced by "ought to", "have to". Autism and "independence" are some of its perceptible manifestations.

Suggested cross-references: Analytic view, Atonement, Becoming, Common sense, Compassion, Correlation, Disturbed personality, Enforced splitting, O, Jargon, Lies, Manipulations of

Symbols, Mystic, Philosophy, Real psycho-analysis, Reality Sensuous and Psychic, Sense of Truth, Thinking, Truth, Truth-Function, Ultra-sensuous, Unknowable, Unknown.

Ad hoc theorising Please refer to the entries, Manipulations of symbols and Multiplicity of theories.

Alpha (α) An early concept that was discharged in favour of the concept of α-function. It was also used as a shorthand notation for dream-work-α In consequence, it is part of the development of this theory. Please refer to the entries, α-function and dream-work-α.

It was used almost exclusively as a heading for papers written during the year of 1959. Curiously, after sixteen years it would resurface, in isolated form, in 1975 (AMF, I, 59).

Alpha-elements Hypothetical elements belonging to an observational model. The model tries to deal with an unknown chain of events. The chain itself can be known through manifestations of its beginning and ending situations. Sensory stimuli are the beginning; manifestations of the psychic realm linked to the stimuli are the end. How is it that sensory stimuli are transformed, in order to get access to the inner mental realm? The mysterious pathway of such a transformation remains unknown; only the transformation itself is acknowledged.

Alpha-elements are defined as the end-product of the action of alpha-function in ultimate reality, the things-in-themselves, which are apprehensible as inner or outer sensory stimuli. Bion called the latter, beta-elements (q.v.).

Bion names the model that depicts that such a transformation has occurred alpha-function (q.v.). The process itself remains unknown. One can grasp the meaning of the function using the words, "traduction" or "translation". It seems to this author that a precise term may be borrowed from physics and neurophysiology: "transduction". Microphones, loudspeakers, Meister and Paccini corpuscles are transducers. Alpha-function "transforms" Beta-elements—raw sensory impressions—into alpha-elements. Alpha-elements are the transduced products of this operation that could be named, "betalphalization". Therefore, alpha-elements are transduced beta-elements.

In a second phase, hypothetical Alpha-elements are "put into use". They can be regarded as elementary immaterial particles, building blocks, amenable to be used to dream, to think, to store in the memory.

Usefulness: The mystery lingers on. How is it that sensuous impressions can ever gain the status of psychically useful inputs? Bion does not resolve the problem, which borders one of the most mysterious secrets of life itself. It has to do with no less than the transition from inanimate to animate. The most gifted authors from time immemorial tackled the same issue. This was the research of the ancient writers of myths, and of the Bible; Plato, Kant, Goethe, Freud, Dobzhansky, Schrödinger and a list too long to mention made attempts to deal with the issue.

To ask how this occurs equals asking, what is life? Many times the answer—if it exists at all—is represented by flights into religion. Bion's scheme of an alpha-function and alpha-elements is restricted to a specific path, namely, from non-mental to mental. In Freud's terms, from material to psychic reality.

Bion started critically from Freud's suggestions of consciousness as the sense organ for the perception of psychic quality. He also started from Freud's theory of instincts. It provides a practical working model for the practising analyst. The analyst who profits from this theory is armed with a tool that enables him to detect some inanimate features in the analysand's discourse that usually passes for "normal". Also, it provides a fresh approach to the dream work made when the person is awake.

&; Parthenope Bion Talamo, at the unofficial second meeting of "Bion's Readers Around the World", organized by Thalia Vergopoulo at the IPAC, San Francisco, 1995, compared the alpha-elements to "LEGO"™ blocks.

Antonino Ferro suggested the existence of narrative derivatives of alpha-elements, as seen in the clinical material (1999).

Suggested cross-references: Alpha Function, Bizarre Elements, Dream-Work-α, K

Alpha-element oedipal pre-conception An inborn pre-conception of Oedipus. This apparently cumbersome term is shorthand for a precise definition in Bion's work. It encircles the most profound mystery of mankind, that of procreation, first studied in its psychic sense by Freud. It is a synthetic unification of Freud and Klein:

Analysts need . . . to consider that the Oedipal material may possibly be evidence for primitive apparatus of pre-conception and therefore possessing a significance additional to its significance in classical theory. I am postulating a precursor of the Oedipal situation not in the sense that such a term may have in Melanie Klein's discussion of *Early Phases of the Oedipus Complex*, but as something that belongs to the ego as part of its apparatus for contact with reality. In short I postulate an aelement version of a private Oedipus myth which is the means, the pre-conception, by virtue of which the infant is able to establish contact with parents as they exist in the world of reality. The mating of this a-element Oedipal preconception with the realization of the actual parents gives rise to the conception of parents. [EP, 93]

Procreation is one of the bridges from inanimate to animate.

Suggested cross-references: Alpha-Elements, Alpha-function, Concept, Conception, Pre-conception.

Alpha-function A mental function that transforms sensuously apprehensible stimuli into elements useful for thinking, dreaming, memory.

But there are no sense-data directly related to psychic quality, as there are sense-data directly related to concrete objects. [LE, 53]

The unconscious is the true psychical reality; in its innermost nature it is as much unknown to us as the reality of the external world, and it is as incompletely presented by the data of consciousness as is the external world by the communications of our sense organs. [Freud, 1900, p.613; Freud's italics]

The theory of functions and alpha-function are not a part of psychoanalytic theory. They are working tools for the practising psychoanalyst to ease problems of thinking about something that is unknown. [LE, 89]

We do not know what is concerned in the transformation from inanimate to animate though we know, or think we know, something of the change from animate to inanimate. [AMF, I, 129]

The verbal formulation "alpha-function" refers to a model that developed into a theory. It was created by Bion around 1960 and first published in 1961. It was an attempt to deal with a puzzling question: how do sensory stimuli achieve the status of psychic facts? Conversely, why in some cases do they not achieve it?

In order to realize what this function is all about, one should keep in mind:

1. The concept of function, borrowed from Euclidean geometry. A simple formulation is: a given variable **functions** in some given way *vis-à-vis* another given variable. The two have a relationship with each other.
2. Alpha-function is a model that tries to deal with a cognitive issue, namely, the apprehension of reality.
3. The "port of entry" of reality into us is the sensuous apparatus.
4. Freud's model of consciousness as the sensuous organ for the apprehension of psychic quality (Freud, 1900).

The theory of alpha-function has a philosophical (Kantian) and a biological (neurophysiological) foundation.

It is linked to Kant's work in the sense that it deals with phenomenal manifestations (sensuous impressions, which Bion names beta-elements). It is linked to neurophysiology to the extent that it bridges the Autonomic Nervous System (the receptors and transducers of the sensory apparatus) with the Central Nervous System. The study of this passageway had been neglected hitherto.

Bion's model of alpha-function purports to describe the fact that human beings' ANS takes raw sensuous apprehensible facts and then couples with the CNS in order to translate them into something else. This "something" is not just a "thing"; it has an immaterial nature. In brief, we human beings are able to "de-sense-fy" the stimuli that comes from exterior reality and from inner reality. Bion uses the terms "translate" and "transform". One may borrow from physics and from neurophysiology and use the term "transducer". Transducers are devices that transform one kind of energy into another, without debasing the invariances conveyed by them. For example, a microphone and a loudspeaker are transducers. The former transforms a mechanically conducted form of energy— sound—into electric energy; the latter does the obverse. The human body's corpuscles of Meissner and Paccini do the same.

The stimuli are things-in-themselves. This means that alpha-function allows for a recognizance that one cannot have a direct contact with ultimate reality. Things-in-themselves are called, in the frame of the theory of alpha-function, "beta-elements" (q.v.). When one is not able to "de-sense-fy" the things-in-themselves, either stemming from the sense apparatus or inner feelings, one is pervaded by sensations of "ownership" with regard to absolute truth. In this case, beta-elements remain undigested.

☉ In his first published definition, Bion still did not posit the "existence" of beta-elements:

"I have described . . . the use of a concept of alpha-function as a working tool in the analysis of disturbances of thought. It seemed convenient to suppose an alpha-function to convert sense data into alpha-elements and thus provide the psyche with the material for dream thoughts and hence the capacity to wake up or go to sleep, to be conscious or unconscious" (ST, 115). To study the development of the definition of α function as well as that of β-elements, please refer to the entries, β-elements; Dream-work-α.

One can state that alpha-function is a "de-sense-fying" function of the mind.

This definition includes particulars that would be greatly expanded in the ensuing four years: the sense data would be seen as phenomena betraying the thing-in-itself, which would be called beta-elements (in 1962) and thereafter, "O" (1965). The dream-thoughts would be seen as an ongoing daytime activity. Concepts such as contact barrier (q.v.) would be created to deal with consciousness and its relationship with the unconscious. The particulars of the theory were to be expanded and polished like jewels; meanwhile the definition itself remained unchanged (EP, 4).

A second definition of it appeared one year later. It augments the scope of the theory that was created to deal with patients with disturbances of thought. It was in 1962 that its more general character was fully recognized:

Alpha-function operates on the sense impressions, whatever they are, and the emotions, whatever they are, of which the patient is aware. In so far as alpha-function is successful alpha elements are produced and these elements are suited to storage and the requirements of dream thoughts. [LE, 6]

This broader range of application coincided with Bion's growing awareness that a permanent underlying layer of psychosis permeates the so-called "normal" personality. It also coincides with Bion's movement towards revising his concepts of cure and pathology. They were made more explicit in 1967—in the Commentary to *Second Thoughts*. In 1970 they reached a more mature form—with a critical view on using ideas of cure derived from medical goals as a model to analysts—in *Attention and Interpretation*.

An analogy with the functioning of the digestive system was put forward in the second, expanded definition of Alpha-function. If mind can "process", "digest", beta-elements, they are transformed into "something else" that was called "alpha-elements" (q.v.).

Alpha-elements can be used to think, to store in memory and to dream. Alpha-function abstracts the "concreteness" of sensory impressions. Conversely, beta-elements are only suitable for projective identification. The similarity between the metabolism of a meal is striking. Alpha-elements can be compared with glycogen being stored in the liver, or ATP. Beta-elements can be compared with faeces. Both are by-products of a process that transforms raw material into nourishment and faeces.

Alpha-elements are postulated to be present in infant life—if and when a good enough mother is capable of "reverie" (q.v.). The exercising of reverie is a kind of temporary borrowing. Infants, so to say, "borrow" from their mothers' alpha-function. Therefore the mother detoxifies the child's beta-elements; they are returned to the infant in a digested form. "Reverie" refers to an ability of mothers to contain their own anxieties of annihilation. A continuous exposure to someone who does this may allow learning that such a state—not to become unstructured, fragmented before anxiety—may be achieved.

Some personalities have a low capacity to tolerate frustration and the pain associated with it. This capacity seems to be innate. The first frustration to be coped with seems to be the absence of the idealized breast. There is no possibility of abstracting immaterial qualities from a breast. The baby who does this is enabled to use warmth, solace and understanding. Conversely, these personalities cannot apprehend more than, or cannot go beyond the concrete breast, nipple and milk. An enforced splitting ensues (q.v.)

The concept appeared first under the somewhat vague denomination of α It was then, perhaps, too attached to the theory of dreams. In this epoch it was called dream-work-α. When Bion was more at peace with Freud's theory of consciousness, as well as when he was more able to use his findings with psychotics, it acquired its status of a mental function. Please refer to this specific entry, dream-work-α.

The first time that a published paper mentions α function was placed by Francesca Bion in *Cogitations* as in about January or February 1960 (C, 120). In her own introduction to this book, she describes her careful, quasi-Sherlockian methods used to determine the dates when Bion's undated papers were written. When translating *Cogitations* into Portuguese, the author gathered data linked to the content of the studies. Actually, this data strongly suggested that this paper belongs to a later time. Francesca Bion agreed—for the inception of this theory as a final replacement of dream-work-α occurred at a later time, as can be gathered from the contents of all the papers printed in *Cogitations*. It more probably took two years to be elaborated; in the Brazilian version, with Mrs. Bion's authorization, the paper was duly moved to a later ordinal position in the book.

The concept of α-function was to be revived in *A Memoir of the Future*. The possibility of emerging from states of non-integration and disintegration evolve to the use of dreams. From there, to real thinking in a dialogical form held by imaginary characters. They can be seen as Bion's part-objects according to his own life experiences. The latter perform the function of ß-elements. The books are a product of Bion's (and the reader's) alpha-function.

Misuses and misconceptions: Many readers mistake alpha-function for thinking itself; and many mistake it for dreaming itself. Perhaps this confusion arises from a persistent difficulty, namely, reading phrases of Bion's texts excised from the whole.

Those readers seem to lose sight of the fact that the model of alpha-function is just a model. It exists in the reality that human minds can construe models. Alpha-function is a model purporting to describe immaterial functions of the human mind. **It does not exist concretely**. It purports to describe a fact that is a prelude both to thinking and dreaming. It refers to a kind of permeable boundary or filter that transforms the unthinkable into building blocks for thinking and/or dreaming and remembering.

Bion's preparatory papers about alpha-function (1959–60) display his doubts in discerning thinking, dreaming and hallucinating. He named alpha-function differently then, calling it "dream-work-alpha". In due course he gave up this term; this was possible when he separated alpha from dreams. Those papers were released only in 1992; some readers dismiss the chronology and the fact that Bion revamped the theory. To quote Bion as if he had written exclusively about dream-work-alpha equals quoting Freud as a supporter of trauma theory. This would restrict his work to pre-1900.

The terms alpha and beta were used in a way that tried to get precision into communication. Bion tried to emulate the mathematical sense of notation (rather than mathematics proper). Like mathematical unknowns, they had no previous meanings and should be left unsaturated. Anyway, as occurred with Freud's models, they are often taken as existent-in-themselves, as entities. Bion left many warnings about this. One of them, issued at the end of his life, reads:

> P.A. These primitive elements of thought are difficult to represent by any verbal formulation, because we have to rely on language that was elaborated for other purposes. When I tried to employ meaningless terms—alpha and beta were typical—I found that "concepts without intuition which are empty and intuitions without conceptions which are blind" rapidly became "black holes into which turbulence had seeped and empty concepts flooded with riotous meaning". [AMF, II, 229]

Another misuse is not specific to this theory. It plagues the grasping of theories in psycho-analysis in general. It may be a manifestation of the mythical prohibition of knowledge. Perhaps it is ironical that one concretizes a theory that was planned to mark the "de-concretizing" or "de-sense-fying" ability of mind (Sandler, 1997a). Many other theories have met this fate.

Another misunderstanding is due to a split reading coupled with a posture of "being more royal than the king". Namely, some readers refuse to define the concept. The "split reading" seems to be aided by item 7, page 3 of *Learning from Experience*:

> The term alpha-function is, intentionally, devoid of meaning
> ... Since the object of this meaningless term is to provide

psycho-analytic investigation with a counterpart of the mathematician's variable, an unknown that can be invested with a value when its use has helped to determine what that value is, it is important that it should not be prematurely used to convey meanings, for the premature meanings may be precisely those that it is essential to exclude. [LE, 3]

This paragraph clearly refers to the use of the concept **in analytical practice**, rather than to the definition of the concept itself. For this concept forms a theory, and a theory is just a model. Theories are attempts to present realities—but they are not realities in themselves, as Bion writes in the Introduction to *Learning from Experience*. Any scientist and practising analyst should know this.

Just after writing the text quoted above, Bion sets out the "area of investigation" to be covered by the theory. The pre-condition for using the theory effectively is to know what a mathematical variable is all about. An unknown in mathematics is just this: an unknown, whose value may or may be not determined. Nevertheless, the theory that introduces the concept of variables or the unknown is not vague or indefinite. Bion stresses the issue again and again, for example, on page 38 of *Learning from Experience*. Therefore, those who refuse to define the function mistake the theory with its use.

&ʒ Roger Money Kyrle's papers "Cognitive development" and "The aim of psycho-analysis" (1968 and 1970, IJPA) can be seen as the earliest investigation of some issues linked to alpha-function. He can be regarded as the first to expand Bion's work.

Imprecision There are exceedingly few places where one is able to spot a lack of precision in Bion's writings. Up to now the author has been able to spot only four of them.

The definition of alpha-function is given precisely in all parts of his work with the possible exception of two. The student can see that in the beginning of chapter 14 (LE). Instead of using the term "sense impressions", Bion uses the term "emotional experience". Perhaps this is not exactly an error; as late as 1965 Bion felt that there were no conditions for discriminating between feelings—which he definitely puts, in the very definition of alpha-function, as belonging to the sensuous realm—and emotions. He sees "feelings" as internal sense impressions.

Also, in *Attention and Interpretation*, page 11, in synthesizing his earlier contributions about a model of "mental space", Bion states that "*In thought I include all that is primitive, including alpha-elements as I have so far described them*". In all his previous descriptions alpha-elements were the raw material that eventually could be used to think. They were never regarded as thinking or thoughts. If taken separately, this text becomes somewhat imprecise; it may give rise to misunderstandings.

Usefulness The mystery lingers on. How is it that sensuous impressions can ever gain the status of psychically useful inputs? The fact is that they do; this fact is inferred and constitutes Freud's first steps towards psycho-analysis. It is the basis of his elaboration of the concept of psychic reality.

Bion does not set himself to solve the problem, which borders one of the most mysterious secrets of life itself. It is about no less than the transition from inanimate to animate. The most gifted authors of mankind from time immemorial have been trying to tackle the issue—at least since the epoch of the writers of the myths, of the Bible, and then Plato, Shakespeare, Kant, Goethe, Freud, Dobzhansky, Schrödinger and a list too long to mention.

It is necessary to add these authors' readers to the list; the unsung onlookers of all epochs tried equally to tackle the same issue. In order to do this they listened to myths, to music, to philosophers and mystics, flocked to theatres, and read written works.

To ask how this occurs equals asking, what is life? Many times the person who feels that he (she) has the answer—if it exists at all—takes flight into religion and belief. Bion's scheme of an alpha-function and alpha-elements is restricted to scrutinizing the path from non-mental to mental.

It is a theory purposely limited. It was devised to be a non-explanatory theory; it is just an observational theory. This limited theory of Bion's at least provides a practical working model for the practising analyst. The analyst who profits from his theory is enabled to detect some inanimate features in the analysand's discourse that usually pass for "normal". Also, it provides a fresh approach to the daytime dream work.

As regards the usefulness of a theory, Bion recommended often that one should not discharge a useful theory, albeit in some aspects it could well be flawed, when no other that proved to be better was available (for example, T, 4). This seemed to be his own path. He was at first critical of Freud, but afterwards accepted Freud's suggestions about consciousness as the sense organ for the perception of psychic quality; ditto, for Freud's theory of instincts. But it is exactly his non-destructive criticism coupled with his final acceptance of both Freud's theories that led him to formulate the theory of alpha-function.

Suggested cross-references: Alpha Elements, Bizarre Elements, Dream-Work-α, Mind, Minus, Reversal of Alpha-Function, Thoughts without a Thinker

Analogy: Bion resorted to analogies, metaphors and aphorisms. He wrote in a way that seems to hark back to the great French writers of the Renaissance and Enlightenment, as well as English thinkers of the Enlightenment. Freud did the same in order to depict the mental realm, which is ultimately ineffable and unknowable.

In fact, any scientific model is an analogy. It belongs to the "correspondence" sense of science, as established by Spinoza and Kant. That is, science tries to construe models that have a correspondent, or counterpart, in reality. Kant called the models "schemes".

Bion was worried about the future of psycho-analysis because of the effects of the establishment. This tends to crystallize the achievement of knowledge, or knowing, in the form of an ossified final knowledge. It seems that the psycho-analytic movement has a tendency to miss the point in taking the analogy as the thing-in-itself. The analogic value of a model or theory is lost; the concrete sense of the analogy prevails.

One of the main analogies used by Bion is mathematical. Please refer to the entry, "Mathematization of psycho-analysis". This matters both scientifically and during a session. To lose sight of what the meaning of an analogy is implies losing sight of the very reality that the analogies strive to depict.

The issue at stake is the fact that we perceive phenomena and intuit noumena; analogies belong to the realm of phenomena. This is the same one that characterizes, according to Kant, the "naive realist"—one who believes that one is able to apprehend reality through the exclusive use of one's five basic senses—and that reality is that which is apprehended by the senses.

The psycho-analytical approach, though valuable in having extended the conscious by the unconscious, has been vitiated by the failure to understand the practical application of doubt by the failure to understand the function of "breast", "mouth", "penis", "vagina", "container", "contained", as analogies. Even if I write it, the sensuous dominance of penis, vagina, mouth, anus, obscures the element signified by analogy. . . [AMF, I, 70–1]

Suggested cross-references: Atonement, Analytical view, Mathematization of Psycho-analysis, Models, Real Psycho-analysis, Thoughts-without-a-thinker.

Analytic view

. . . we regard analytic procedure as essential if people are to understand what beliefs they hold and by which they are held. [AMF, II, 332]

It is difficult to conceive of an analysis having a satisfactory outcome without the analysand's becoming reconciled to, or at one with, himself. [AI, 34]

In psycho-analytic methodology the criterion cannot be whether a particular usage is right or wrong, meaningful or verifiable, but whether it does, or does not, promote development. [LE, Introduction, 3]

An explorer's knowledge of instruments must be such that he can use them in situations of stress. The analyst must use instruments that are altered by the circumstances they are devised to study. [T, 75]

This entry is a depiction of some views about a frequently asked question: "What is psycho-analysis?" Bion addresses it throughout all his written work.

P.A. I try to demonstrate the qualities of the individual. Whether they are assets or liabilities he can then decide for himself. [AMF, III, 541]

The hope is that psycho-analysis brings into view thoughts and actions and feelings of which the individual may not be aware and so cannot control. If he can be aware of them he may, or may not, decide—albeit unconsciously—to change them. [AMF, III, 509–10]

In New York, 1977

The analytic procedure is an attempt to introduce the patient to who he is, because whether he likes it or not that is a marriage which is going to last as long as he lives. [BNYSP, 40]

P.A. I have great respect for the individual. Do you think that is wrong?

FIFTY YEARS No, but it is not in keeping with the growth of the Herd. I can see P.A. will be in serious trouble if the Herd develops faster than he does

P.A. If the development of the Herd is incompatible with that of the individual, either the individual will perish, or the Herd will be destroyed by the individual who is not allowed to fulfil himself. . . Some of us think that the development of the individual needs careful supervision. [AMF, III, 461]

The ethos of psycho-analysis

These formulations summarize the ethos of psycho-analysis. The texts depict the clinical situation and its philosophical origins, namely, the highest goals of the Enlightenment, which were continued in part by some offshoots of the Romantic Movement. The defence of the individual being and his caring development has been the ethos of psycho-analysis since Freud discovered it.

In other words, there is a lack of subservience to authority; there is freedom, defence of the individual; the use of science and medicine as methods developed to help suffering individuals. This unslavish state includes the recognizance of the unconscious and attempts at knowing something about its functioning and manifestations. To know, albeit imperfectly, something about some of the manifestations of the unconscious is a way of not being enslaved by them. It is more than a philosophical recognizance; it is a practical application of it at the service of suffering individuals, in a novel and basic way.

To display the ethos of psycho-analysis means also trying to discriminate psycho-analysis from anything else. There is a need to recognize what it is—and what it is not. In other terms, what are its "qualities"; in the same sense that Shakespeare, through Hamlet, looked for real actors and asked them, "*Come, give us the taste of your quality*" (*Hamlet*, II, ii, 408). Both Hamlet and patients in need of analysis are looking for truth.

It would not be an exaggeration to state that Bion spent a great deal of his psycho-analytic life, first and foremost, in trying to assess what an analyst does intra-session: "*It seems absurd that a psycho-analyst should be unable to assess the quality of his work*" (AI, 62).

The issues that Bion emphasizes are:

(i)   human interest, or in his own terms, concern for life and truth (C, 125, 247);

(ii) becoming who one really is;

(iii) detailed, attentive scrutiny of what is taking place in the here and now of the session;

(iv) problems of communication of that which is observed (either to the patient, which implies in the use of colloquial language, models and myths);

(v)   obstacles to observation, which implies certain problems of perception and cognition;

(vi) the immaterial nature of underlying patterns that call to be intuited.

Broadly speaking, the analytic view is concerned with a "*matter of interest*", as a former analysand of Bion's, Kenneth Sanders, puts it. Or, compassion and truth (C, 125). It is an amiable, growth-promoting, life-oriented interest in the individual being, in the wake of the achievements of the Enlightenment and Romantic movements. Analysis is a collaboration that "*should be healing*" rather than "*wounding*" (T, 25).

"*Psycho-analysis is concerned with love as an aspect of mental devel-opment and the analyst must consider the maturity of love and 'greatness' in relation to maturity*" (T, 74). The analytic view includes a capacity for "*mature compassion*" (T, 143).

The issue of development is mentioned often: "*. . . the analyst is concerned with development of the personality*" (T, 169); "*We consider the attempt to improve humans both worthwhile and urgent*" (AMF, III, 528).

In less colloquial terms, Bion's statements do not differ from Freud's last proposals on analysis as a method of investigation of the mind with therapeutic implications.

> The task confronting the analyst is to bring intuition and reason to bear on an emotional experience between two people (of whom he is one) in such a way that not only he but also the analysand gains an understanding of the analysand's response to that emotional situation, and does so through an appreciation of the evidence to which the analyst is drawing attention in the course of his interpretations. It is not enough for the analyst to be convinced that there is evidence for the truth of his interpretations; he must have enough evidence available to afford the analysand the opportunity of being persuaded, by his reason, of the cogency of the interpretation. [C, 91]

There is no trace of an authoritarian or pedagogical posture. The patient's function is not only stated as seminal in the process of insight, which would be a truism. Instead, there is a description of how or why it is seminal.

> . . . psycho-analysts do not aim to run the patient's life but to enable him to run it according to his lights and therefore to know what his lights are. [T, 37]

> P. A. You need not be sheep. We do not aspire to be leaders or shepherds; we hope to introduce the person to his "real" self. Although we do not claim to be successful, the experience shows how powerful is the urge of the individual to be led—to believe in some god or good shepherd. [AMF, II, 266]

Bion's posture would remain essentially unaltered throughout his work, albeit improved in some technical details. Compare these quotations with the last phrases of the character "Myself", in volume I, *A Memoir of the Future*, which is reproduced below in this same entry. It depicts the act of obscuring something in order to make this same something clear (pages 202–4).

The analytic view concerns *"what is taking place"* (T, 7). It corresponds to Freud's "here and now"; its goal is the achievement of insight into the truth about oneself. An analysis is conceived as a living, unrepeatable life experience impossible to obtain anywhere else. This experience always includes paradox.

We may now consider further the relationship of rudimentary consciousness to psychic quality. The emotions fulfil a similar function for the psyche to that of the senses in relation to objects in space and time. That is to say the counterpart of commonsense view in private knowledge is the common emotional view; a sense of truth is experienced if the view of an object which is hated can be conjoined to a view of the same object when it is loved and the conjunction confirms that the object experienced by different emotions is the same object. A correlation is established.

A similar correlation, made possible by bringing conscious and unconscious to bear on the phenomena of the consulting room, gives to psycho-analytic objects a reality that is quite unmistakeable though their very existence has been disputed. [ST, 119]

One example, where one may vouch for a humanistic and caring approach, can be seen when Bion was investigating the dream, dreaming during the session, fears of dreaming, presence of cruelly annihilating superego and the possibility of a "dream-work-α":

The starvation of the psyche of all elements needed for growth and development gives extreme urgency to the patient's inability to dream. But this activity is extra-sessional and impregnated with the dangers incidental to a restored super-ego. The fear of this conflicts with the necessity to restore the capacity to dream, for the fear is of nothing less than annihilation. Consequently the patient...needs to restrict these attempts to sessions. Then, and only then, is he sure of the external aid that the presence of the analyst affords. It is this that leads to the events I have already described in which the patient strives to dream in the session. [C, 97–8]

This means that analysis will perhaps continue to be a subject that is disparaged by people who have never experienced it. The experience of analysis precludes any learning that does not come from experiencing it. It does not differ from any practical endeavour.

The analytic view needs to be put into action in the way the analyst expresses himself. He "should not express himself in any terms other than those used by an adult; theoretically this excludes certain categories (notably column 2) [please refer to specific entry, Grid-column 2; in brief, this category expresses statements that are lies] . . . the analyst is under an obligation to speak with as little ambiguity as possible, in fact his aims are limited by the analysand who is free to receive *interpretations in whatever way he chooses . . .The analyst is not free except in the sense that when the patient comes to him for analysis he is obliged to speak in a way which would not be tolerable in any other frame of reference and then only from a particular vertex. The patient's response would also be intolerable if there were no psycho-analytic indulgence to excuse it, or, if it were not for a psycho-analytic vertex"* (T, 145).

Bion tries to classify the material that comes as the final views construed by the patient after receiving any stimulus, in order to construe that which he must tell the patient. He names the original stimulus or experience as "O", ultimate reality (q.v.) and the "material" (which also comprises an immaterial dimension), the final products of the transformations effected by the patient in "O", as Tpβ (q.v.).

> The problem of classifying the material is complicated because it contains elements of all three: T, Tpα and Tpβ. It is a matter of consequence because the decision depends on what is most convenient for the analyst . . . The problem is to reformulate Tpβ in conversational, but precise, English. [T, 26]

Like Freud and other authors such as Reik, for Bion psychoanalysis is impossible without regard for truth, "*. . . healthy mental growth seems to depend on truth as the living organism depends on food* [T, 38]

Correct interpretation

Regard for truth implies absence of lies: thus the correct interpretation must be free of lies. A correct interpretation, being an approximation to the patient's truth-O, a pursuit of truth-O, depends on the evolution of the unknown. It admits no authority and, much less, official speakers. The analytic couple has an opportunity to assess, or to glimpse in a transient way, parts of it. It stems from the nonspoken, the negative or numinous realm. This has a seminal significance for the work of the analyst concerning what he will or will not say, of his choice of issues, of the rationality or lack of it that is involved:

> Nobody need think the true thought: it awaits the advent of the thinker who achieves significance through the true thought. The lie

and its thinker are inseparable . . . The only thoughts to which the thinker is absolutely essential are lies . . . Whether the thoughts are entertained or not is of significance to the thinker but not to the truth. If entertained, they are conducive to mental health; if not, they initiate disturbance . . . Since the analyst's concern is with the evolved elements of O and their formulation, formulations can be judged by considering how necessary his existence is to the thoughts he expresses. The more his interpretation can be judged as showing how necessary *his* knowledge, *his* experience, *his* character are to the thought as formulated , the more reason there is to suppose that the interpretation is psycho-analytically worthless, that is, alien to the domain O. [AI, 103 and 105]

In Bion's terms, an analytic interpretation must illuminate a relationship that concerns knowledge (or in other terms, apprehension of reality or truth) and must necessarily be far from lies. Bion's terms focused for many years on one of the links or relationships as specific to the analytic view as well as, in the negative sense, as something to be avoided. Namely, the K link, which means "knowledge" (q.v.), is specific to the analytic view. In the negative sense, the links H and L and column 2 are specific in terms of being avoided or subjected to a discipline to diminish their influence. In any case they shall not prevail (q.v.):

The peculiarity of a psycho-analytic session, that aspect of it which establishes that it is a psycho-analysis and could be nothing else, lies in the use by the analyst of all material to illuminate a K relationship. . . the analyst is restricted to interpretations that are an expression of a K relationship with the patient. They must not be expressions of L or H. [EP, 69–70]

Bion changed his view a few years later; even though K has to do with psycho-analysis, it is still not enough. Analysis belongs ultimately to the numinous realm and transcends knowledge:

Formulations of the events of analysis made in the course of analysis must possess value different from the formulations made extra-sessionally. Their value therapeutically is greater if they are conducive to transformations in O, less if conducive to transformations in K . . . The analyst must focus his attention on O, the unknown and unknowable. The success of psycho-analysis depends on the maintenance of a psycho-analytic point of view; the point of view is the psycho-analytic vertex; the psycho-analytic vertex is O. With this the analyst cannot be identified: he must *be* it. [AI, 26–7]

The symbol "O" (q.v.) stands for the noumena, truth. To be identified with it means either collusion or pretensions to knowing absolute truth.

The issue of truth and sincerity obtrudes in the language that the analyst must use too:

ALICE Punning is a very low form of life.

P.A. Life fundamentally is really "low life"—cock-roaches, and "bloody cunt" and swimming in a sea of amniotic fluid and meconium, and now psycho-analysis. Even the fetus is involved with *non-fetus*. One cone intersects another cone. Here the eyes of each of us can be described as sweeping out an area of space more or less cone-shaped. But these cones intersect other cones whose focal origin is different. These points of intersection could be pictorially depicted by resorting to geometrical figures. That is an over-simplification which, as Robin said, is complex enough to make any further description redundant. However, I do not see why the universe in which we live should oblige us by being comprehensible to us mere human beings. This is true of our own bodies and minds in which we have to live. Even if we don't trouble with the "universe", the *not-us*, we find that merely trying to know who "I" am involves an intolerable amount of discovery of what we have never been able to tolerate and which, as likely as not, we are right not to tolerate . . .

ROLAND You remind me—Britannia reminds me—of the mother who on her death-bed collected her children because she wished to confess that she had never loved her husband, their father, and had been constantly unfaithful and promiscuous. The eldest, recovering first from the stupefying information, announced, "Well, I don't know about you other bastards, but I'm going to the movies", and they all fucked off.

ALICE Very amusing. I regret that my facial muscles do not express my entertainment.

ROBIN I expect you are not perceiving how amused you are at being not-amused.

ALICE Though I said it was "very amusing" I did not expect you to believe I meant just that.

P.A. Though you do not call it psycho-analysis, you interpret naturally and expect others to interpret your behaviour, including the language you talk. These diagnoses, interpretations, are intrusions, outrages perhaps, on your privacy—our privacy.

ALICE If you are right that seems to me to be one more reason for behaving in a reasonably civil manner.

P.A. Certainly. But in reality, as far as I am capable of perceiving reality or truth, the more I am aware that reality is not civilized or reasonable or considerate of our feelings or ideas. This applies to you and me; we are not polite, civilized, considerate *only*. So, in so far as we achieve "civilized" character, our capacity for lying, murdering, robbing, being in *rude health*, "fusts in us unused", as Milton puts it.

ALICE Milton certainly did not mean what you say he meant.

P.A. I am ready to believe that Milton did not mean to mean that. It requires, at least, considerable training to achieve any idea now of what Milton meant—or Nietzsche, or Newton, or any other great figure of the past. In the present we do not have to bother because there are not perceived to be any great figures. In fact we are learning to regard them as figments or our imaginations.

ROLAND I remember the fashion for "Father Figures"; the mental landscape was such that one could not see one's genetic father the air was so thick with Father Figures.

ROBIN I smell a Father Figure; I see him in the Air; I will nip him in the Bud.

ROLAND Call me Buddy—so much more friendly.

P.A. Technical terms are not safe from de-value-ation; hence my resort to spelling out the word in a hope that the return to that childhood learning difficulty might re-inforce my communication. Must we keep our technical terms in constant repair? The bloody cunt which is *not* anything to do with anatomical sex, not masculine, not feminine, not haematology, not religion but could be said to be sacred, has nevertheless an almost universal—western at least—comprehensibility. It made Alice angry; even articulate. It degrades the user almost as much as the recipient.

ALICE Then why use it?

P.A. I am not advocating or deprecating its use. Since it is there it seems wise to acknowledge or respect its presence as one should respect any other fact, whether we like it or not.

ROBIN I can see Alice's point—why go out of your way to look for the unpleasant?

P.A. If it were only a matter of pleasant or unpleasant that would depend on the character or person, and on his or her likes or dislikes. I suggest it also involves *is* or *is not*. If it *is* then the individual should respect the *is-ness* or *is-not-ness* of it. *You* think these "things" are so rare that it is perverse to go out of our way to find them. I say they are so universal that it is perverse to make great mental detours to avoid being aware.

ROBIN But who uses language like that?

P.A. I do, for one. So do you. So does Alice.

ALICE I beg your pardon—I don't . . .

P.A. But you said "fucking bastard" a little while back; you reacted as to the manner born to Roland saying "bloody cunt". If it were a foreign language I would say you must have been born to it, lived it, loved it as your very own favourite language. I agree with you that you spoke to it as if you had forgotten it and didn't want to be reminded of it. [AMF, III, pp. 490–93]

The issue of Truth in analysis is not exactly an "issue". It has a meaning that approximates it to the social usage to the extent that it is an ethical posture. Truth in analysis concerns self-knowledge: "*. . . self-knowledge is an aim of psycho-analytic procedure. . .*" (EP, 91).

Psycho-analysis brought home the fact that truth is not a theoretical problem of the philosopher of science: "*. . . the psycho-analyst is concerned* **practically** *with a problem that the philosopher approaches* **theoretically**" (AI, 97).

Psycho-analytic procedure pre-supposes that the welfare of the patient demands a constant supply of truth as inevitably as his physical survival demands food. It further presupposes that discovery of the truth about himself is a precondition of an ability to learn the truth, or at least to seek it in his relationship with himself and others. It is supposed at first that he cannot discover the truth about himself without assistance from the analyst and others. [C, 99]

I assume that the permanently therapeutic effect of a psycho-analy-sis, if any, depends on the extent to which the analysand has been able to use the experience to see one aspect of his life, namely himself as he is. It is the function of the psycho-analyst to use the experience of such facilities for contact as the patient is able to extend to him, to elucidate the truth about the patient's personality and mental characteristics, and to exhibit them to the patient in a way that makes it possible for him to entertain a reasonable convic-tion that the statements (propositions) made about himself repre-sent facts.

It follows that a psycho-analysis is a joint activity of analyst and analysand to determine the truth; that being so, the two are engaged—no matter how imperfectly—on what is in intention a scientific activity. [C, 114]

If we—as Bion did—start from Freud, we will pay attention to his coining of the term "psychic reality" vis-à-vis material reality, both being different forms of the same reality—a fact often over-looked. We must consider that psycho-analysis has Platonic-Kantian-Hegelian roots. That is, it deals in practice with the noumena, the "absolute" and its negative, immaterial nature. Psychic reality, which corresponds to the numinous realm, remains ultimately unknowable for our consciousness, if we regard it, as Freud and Bion did, as the sense organ for the apprehension of psychic quality. It is the same case with material reality, which remains ultimately unknowable to the senses.

What must be perceived and expressed underlies the phenome-nal realm. We analysts look for **underlying, immaterial patterns**: *"The interpretation given the patient is a formulation intended to display an underlying pattern"* (ST, 131). The underlying pattern is uncon-scious: *"The psycho-analyst tries to help the patient to transform that part of an emotional experience of which he is unconscious into an emotional experience of which he is conscious"* (T, 32).

The search for underlying patterns would remain for the rest of Bion's professional life:

I put forward, herewith, a theory of ψ with a recently proliferated sense organ known as the "end", in which various functions, usually associated with psycho-analysis (the Oedipus situation, aggression, rivalry) are supposed to be observed (on the model of forms of dis-order, dis-ease, sex, fear, love). In reality they are patterns, configurations, insignificant in themselves but, if delineated, indicative of an *underlying* reality by their perturbations, regroupings, shifts in pattern and colour; they reflect a category and kind that the human mind cannot formulate or conjecture in their presence. [C, 121–2]

The detection of those patterns is dependent on analytically trained intuition (T, 49); there are immaterial constant conjunctions that can be perceived and confer meaning to something. Bion proposes some terms borrowed from mathematics to depict what composes the underlying patterns: selected facts and invariances.

Another ever-present feature underlying appearances is emotion:

> Superficially, an analytic session may appear boring, or featureless, alarming, or devoid of interest, good or bad. The analyst, seeing beyond the superficial, is aware that he is in the presence of intense emotion; there should be no occasion on which this is not apparent to him. The intense experience is ineffable but once known cannot be mistaken . . . if such a contact is maintained the analyst can devote himself to evaluating and interpreting the central experience and, if he sees fit, the superficialities in which it is embedded. [T, 74]

Bion states that all psycho-analysts would agree that "*correct analysis*" demands that the analyst's verbal formulations obey a need, namely, to "*formulate what the patient's behaviour reveals; conversely, that the analyst's judgement should be embodied in an interpretation and not in an emotional discharge (e.g. counter-transference or acting out.*" (T, 35).

This is the march into the unknown, the exploration into the *unbewußt*, which means "not-known" in German. It is usually translated as "unconscious". Freud, Klein, Bion and Winnicott practised it: the continuous *becoming* that elicits who the patient in reality is, unknowingly.

The numinous or negative nature of the ever-evolving psychic reality dictates that the analytic view is obtained intra-session through the scrutiny of that which one is *not* but one thinks one is.

> The supreme importance of transference lies in its use in the practice of psycho-analysis. It is available for observation by analysands

and analysts. In this respect it is unique—that is its strength and its weakness; its strength, because two people have a "fact" available to both and therefore open for discussion by both; its weakness, because it is ineffable and cannot be discussed by anyone else. The failure to recognize this simple fact has led to confusion. [C, 353]

One may add that this demands not only concern for life and truth, but also an ability or willingness to tolerate paradoxes. Patients come but their willingness to be analysed cannot be taken for granted:

> Psycho-analysis tells you nothing; it is an instrument, like the blind man's stick, that extends the power to gather information. The analyst uses it to gather a *selected* kind of information: the analysand uses it to gather material that he can use (1) for purposes of imitation, (2) to learn the analyst's philosophy, (3) to learn how to conduct his life in a socially acceptable manner, and (4) to become acquainted with his Self. Although it is true that it is not his intention to satisfy (1), (2) and (3), or any other desire other than (4), it is impossible to make any statement that gratifies only (4) because the lack of precision of spontaneous English speech. The analyst can try not to pollute his interpretation on the one hand, or to speak as if he were a living computer, stranger to human heartedness, or the life that the rest of our human companions are familiar with as members of our universe. Certain words and phrases appear to be necessary for the communication of "happenings" recurring in that part of human experience with which I am most familiar, and which happens also to be that part of my life that is my profession—what, for the lack of power to describe adequately, I call "mental suffering". [C, 361]

Also, it is paradoxically an amiable and dangerous activity: "*An analyst is not doing his job if he investigates something because it is pleasurable or profitable . . . anyone who is not afraid when he is engaged on psycho-analysis is either not doing his job or is unfitted for it*" (AMF, III, 516–7).

Perhaps the analytic view and its consequent analytic posture are better illuminated in Bion's late works. Modifying his earlier attempts at clarity and concision through the use of mathematical and philosophical models, his clearer formulations about the analytical view appear in *A Memoir of the Future*through verbal formulations more akin to theatrical and poetical prose.

One may read there a practical application of the fine perception that Bion had regarding the "negative", that is, the numinous realm and its relationship with insight and the psycho-analytic interpretation. The negative realm of the noumena was first described by Plato; insights about it, despite strong denials from Aristotle, Descartes and many others, re-emerged with Hamann, Kant (who delimited it more precisely), Maimon, Von Herder, Goethe, Fiche and Hegel (who perhaps was the first to name it as the "negative").

Freud gave practical use to it, with his formulation of psychic reality, of the unconscious and of the Id. Bion, after Freud and Klein, was able to focus his research on the Id as the pure analytical posture. In this sense, more than thirty years after Bion having written it, it seems that very few authors worldwide could apprehend the profoundly psycho-analytical ethos of A *Memoir of the Future*, in terms of the unconscious and of the Id. One of them, albeit belatedly, is André Green (2002). Not coincidentally, he is one of the very few authors that Bion quotes explicitly in the Trilogy, side by side with Freud, Money-Kyrle, Strachey, Rickman and Klein.

The texts of the Trilogy are self-explanatory, but to be grasped they require analytic experience and a discipline over theoretical prejudices about how one ought to write psycho-analytical texts.

BION I don't understand.

MYSELF Perhaps I can illustrate by an example from something you *do* know. Imagine a piece of sculpture which is easier to comprehend if the structure is intended to act as a trap for light. The meaning is revealed by the pattern formed by the light thus trapped—not by the structure, the carved work itself. I suggest that if I could learn how to talk to you in such a way that my words "trapped" the meaning which they neither do nor could express, I could communicate to you in a way that is not at present possible.

BION Like the "rests" in a musical composition?

MYSELF A musician would certainly not deny the importance of those parts of a composition in which no notes were sounding, but more has to be done than can be achieved in existent art and its well-established procedure of silences, pauses, blank spaces, rests. The "art" of conversation, as carried on as part of the conversational intercourse of psycho-analysis, requires and demands an extension in the realm of non-conversation . . .

I have suggested a "trick" by which one could manipulate things which have no meaning by the use of sounds like "α" and "β". These are sounds analogous, as Kant said, to "thoughts without concepts", but the principle, and a reality approximating to it, is also extensible to words in common use. The realizations which approximate to words such as "memory" and "desire" are opaque. The "thing-in-itself", impregnated with opacity, itself becomes opaque: the O, of which "memory" and "desire" is the verbal counterpart, is opaque. I suggest this quality of opacity inheres in many O's and their verbal counterparts, and the phenomena which it is usually supposed to express. If, by experiment, we discovered the verbal forms, we could also discover the thoughts to which the observation applied specifically. Thus we achieve a situation in which these could be used deliberately to obscure specific thoughts.

BION Is there anything new in this? You must often have heard, as I have, people say they don't know what you are talking about and that you are being deliberately obscure.

MYSELF They are flattering me. I am suggesting an aim, an ambition, which, if I could achieve, would enable me to be deliberately and *precisely* obscure; in which I could use certain words which could activate precisely and instantaneously, in the mind of the listener, a thought or train of thought that came between him and the thoughts and ideas already accessible and available to him.

ROSEMARY Oh, my God! [AMF, I, 189–191]

Is this the most colloquially written illumination of the realm of "minus", in the sense that it is constantly conjoined with the realm of "plus"? In philosophical terms, it displays the Hegelian realm of the "negative", which must, anyway, as Freud showed, remain linked to the material reality, namely, the instinctual endowment.

This realm can also be seen as the Platonic realm, or the numinous realm later described by Kant, which was later on mapped by Freud in his investigation of psychic reality. Its insight is a conjoint work of analyst and analysand. Let us follow with Bion. His next step seems to follow a hint by Freud, when he realized the hallucinatory realm of transference. (Freud, 1912) This is a need for an immersion in psychic reality and in hallucination (slave of pleasure or desire and avoidance of pain) which also is part of psychic reality.

Or, as the author proposed elsewhere (Sandler, 1997), psychic non-reality, an inseparable companion of psychic reality, in the same sense that the production of nourishing chemical products (such as ATP, adenosine tri-phosphate) is inseparable from the production of faeces, or the storage of oxygen in the blood cells is inseparable from the production of carbon dioxide.

> P.A. My problem is the relationship when two minds, persons, characters, meet. Freud drew attention to one aspect of that relationship which he called "transference". I think he meant that when a man meets his analyst he transfers to him characteristics which were probably once consciously , and not unreasonably, thought to inhere in some member of the parental family. These characteristics are inappropriate when felt about a stranger—the analyst.
>
> PAUL Why the analyst? Why not other people?
>
> P.A. The analyst is typical of these "other people". In analysis these characteristic "transfers" can be discussed.
>
> ROBIN *Only* by the patient?
>
> P.A. No; the analyst also reacts to the patient. But in so far as he is unconscious of it, it is known as the counter-transference. You can read all about this in the literature, or better still, find out for yourself by having a psycho-analysis. I do not want to go into that because here, at best, we can only "talk about it"—not experience it. [AMF, II. 249–50]

To talk about analysis means a splitting of material reality from psychic reality (as defined by Freud in chapter VII of *The Interpretation of Dreams*). To experience analysis means to live both material reality and psychic reality, or "reality sensuous and psychic" as Bion puts it in *Attention and Interpretation*.

In 1975, he recommended, as an invitation to attaining the analytical view, that analysts should try to avoid formalism, or rational, clever manipulations of symbols, as well as "investigations in psycho-analysis":

> SHERLOCK The simple part of it has been dealt with by Watson. You heard that fellow Bion? Nobody has ever heard of him or of

Psycho-analysis. He thinks it is real, but that his colleagues are engaged in an activity which is only a more or less ingenious manipulation of symbols. There is something in what he says. There is a failure to understand that any definition must deny a previous truth as well as carry an unsaturated component. [AMF, I, 92]

... The most profound method known to us of investigation—psycho-analysis—is unlikely to do more that scratch the surface. [BLI, 52]

MYSELF The practical point is—no further investigation of psycho-analysis, but the psyche it betrays. *That* needs to be investigated through the medium of *mental* patterns; *that* which is indicated is *not* a symptom; *that* is not a cause of the symptom; *that* is not a disease or *any*thing subordinate. Psycho-analysis itself is just a stripe on the coat of the tiger. Ultimately it may meet the Tiger—The Thing Itself—O. [AMF, I, 112]

In his short papers, "Evidence" (1976) and "Emotional turbulence" (1977), Bion first adumbrated his hypothesis on the risk of the whole of psycho-analysis becoming "*a vast paramnesia intended to fill the void of our ignorance*". In 1979 he would summarize the whole issue:

ROLAND Yes; but is there any evidence for a mind at all? It has no colour, smell, or any other sensuous counterpart. Why should not the whole of psycho-analysis be just a vast, towering Babel of paramnesias to fill the gap where our ignorance ought to be? [AMF, III, 540]

Bion tried to endow psycho-analysis with the scientifically sound foundation that Freud tried to attain. With his observational theories, Bion looked for evidence and ways to refute interpretations. Freud established them in "Constructions in analysis"; they were based on the patient's reactions before the analyst's interpretations, in terms of free associations.

Bion's attempts at refutations appear in *Elements of Psycho-Analysis and Transformations*; during his last phase of courtship with his own modified form of neo-positivism. He observed the "truth value" of verbal statements made in sessions, through a precise formulation of the vertexes under which both analyst and analysand's verbal statements were made. Refutations can be seen as scientific "devil's advocates". If an interpretation can survive the refutation, it may undergo a development, or correction.

> P.A. I do not think that Freud or any psycho-analyst would welcome such an extension; it is typical of the devaluation to which the language we use is subjected. I am prepared to entertain the possibility that any cloud-capp'd tow'rs of human imaginative structures may disappear like the insubstantial vision of a dream. I do not have any difficulty in thinking that the human race itself might disappear in a puff of smoke. Suppose the sun were to flicker as a prelude to its disintegration, would any human survive? This world is only a grain of cosmic dust and our sun an ordinary star— so the astronomers tell us. We know of no other world to which we could fly as a new home.
>
> ROBIN On the other hand it would be extraordinary if amongst the many millions of solar systems there were not some other accident similar to that which produced "homo-sapiens".
>
> ROLAND A fat lot of use that would be to us.
>
> P.A. In the meantime we should remain true to our nature and endeavour to make the best of ourselves.
>
> ROLAND Is P.A. also among the moralists? I thought you people prided yourselves on being above that.
>
> P.A. I am not aware that we pride ourselves or deprecate ourselves on account of our being ordinary members of the human race. Like my fellows I would be gratified if I discovered that I was in some way excellent; in fact I have found no evidence of my "excellence"as a psycho-analyst.
>
> ALICE Your colleagues think highly of you.
>
> P.A. Some do, luckily; I am not unappreciative of the fact, but it tells me more of the generosity and affection of my colleagues than of *my* merits. I think we could discuss something of greater interest than me and my qualities and defects."

Concerning the too often overlooked issue of the analyst's prejudices, disguised as morals:

> ROLAND Doesn't your working day consist in discussing the qualities and defects of others?

P.A. I try to demonstrate the qualities of the individual. Whether they are assets or liabilities he can then decide for himself. [AMF, III, 540–41]

The analytic view must entertain a critical appraisal of the concept of cure. Freud demonstrated the universality of the neuroses; Klein, the same for the psychosis; and Bion sees the curative model in a critical way (q.v.).

One of the deadliest enemies of the analytic view is the use of jargon (q.v.), which enables a pre-patterned mode of non-thinking that passes for real thinking. Jargon is a clothing to feelings of "already known". In contrast, the analytic view enables one to march into the unknown. Bion simply rescues Freud, who once wrote that we must tell the patient that which he *does not know*:

PAUL Timidity is a fact of our nature. We cling to anything which gives us the chance of saying "Thus far and no further". Any discovery is followed by a closure. The remainder of our thoughts and endeavours is devoted to consolidating the system to prevent the intrusion of yet another thought. [AMF, II, 265]

🕲 Bion saw the necessity of keeping his analytic view in the emotional tempest created by the so-called psychotics and borderlines (a fashionable term in the sixties) who were predominantly narcissistic, coupled with disturbances of thought. They resorted to projective identification in order to turn analysis into a game of emotional responses instead of a march towards knowledge. The development of this necessity came when Bion, after Klein, observed how the universality of the psychotic nuclei functions, with a seminal paper on the psychotic and the non-psychotic personalities (1956).

This meant that the phenomena he observed in so-called psychotics were present, albeit in a modified form, more subtle and in the guise of hallucinosis, in so-called "normal" or "neurotic" patients—and vice-versa. The subtleties of the presentation of the psychotic phenomena dictated that the analytic view could be even more difficult to attain and to keep. This problem would occupy the rest of his life as a practitioner.

First he tried to ensure the truth-value of the analyst's statements through the Grid (q.v.). He came to state that the analyst must avoid statements belonging to categories of column 2—lies. Truth became the criterion; *Elements of Psycho-Analysis* and *Transformations* mark his attempts inspired by the neo-positivists such as Carnap, who also attempted to establish the truth-value of scientific statements (see entries Grid, and Transformations and Invariances).

But he abandoned this; he resorted to other traditions of apprehension of reality as it is, in order to keep the analytic view, that of the so-called mystics (both the Lurianic movement and the Christian Cabbala). At this moment he states that the numinous realm, which he calls "O", must be the compass of the analyst; to analyse equals the "pursuit of truth-O", of becoming, of turning transformations in K into transformations in O. In order to do this one must eschew memory, desire and understanding.

This would mark his work *Attention and Interpretation*, which can be seen as his great attempt towards attaining the analytical view under a commonsensical vertex. The analytic view is closely related to the analyst's ability to dream the patient's material (refer to specific entry under this heading). The "trained intuition", already adumbrated in Transformations, is seen as the analytic tool.

Pain

The analytic view always deals with pain. Intuition is linked to pain to the extent that it composes a kind of analytical ethics:

> The emotion to which attention is drawn should be obvious to the analyst, but unobserved by the patient; an emotion that is obvious to the patient is usually *painfully* obvious and avoidance of unnecessary pain must be one aim in the exercise of analytic intuition. Since the analyst's capacity for intuition should enable him to demonstrate an emotion before it has become *painfully* obvious it would help if our search for the elements of emotions was directed to making intuitive deductions easier. [EP, 74]

An analytic view cannot be achieved if one tries to avoid pain, which is inimical to the unknown. Conversely, to avoid pain is the ally of desire, as Freud observed. Explanations are one of the tools for avoiding pain—in illusion, hallucination and delusion.

Pain cannot be absent from the personality. An analysis must be painful, not because there is necessarily any value in pain, but because an analysis in which pain in not observed and discussed cannot be regarded as dealing with one of the central reasons for the patient's presence. The importance of pain can be dismissed as a secondary quality, something that is to disappear when conflicts are resolved; indeed most patients would take this view. Furthermore it can be supported by the fact that successful analysis does lead to diminution of suffering: nevertheless it obscures the need, more obvious in some cases than in others, for the analytic experience to increase the patient's *capacity* for suffering even though patient and analyst may hope to decrease pain itself. The analogy with physical medicine is exact; to destroy a capacity for physical pain would be a disaster in any situation other than one in which an even greater disaster—namely death itself—is certain. [EP, 61–2]

To deal with pain in analysis is fundamental to achieving the analytical view. It requires the notion of reversible perspective (q.v.)—a special use of projective identification in order to render a dynamic situation static.

The work of the analyst is to restore dynamic to a static situation and so make development possible . . . the patient manoeuvres so that the analyst's interpretations are agreed; they thus become the outward sign of a static situation . . . In reversible perspective acceptance by the analyst of the possibility of an impairment of capacity for pain can help avoidance of errors that might lead to disaster. If the problem is not dealt with the patient's capacity to maintain a static situation may give way to an experience of pain so intense that a psychotic breakdown is the result. [EP, 60 and 62]

A good-humoured paper of this time was kept unknown but was published posthumously by his dedicated wife; its title is "Predictive psycho-analysis and predictive psychopathology: a fable for our time" (*Cogitations*) This paper subsumes and synthesizes his warnings about the loss of the analytic view, the dangers that encircled the psycho-analytic movement as a social fact, the attacks the members of the movement made against the analytic view and many expressions of the death instinct. His Trilogy *A Memoir of the Future* would cap all those attempts and integrate them in a novel form of presentation, where poetry and much more of the mystics are included in order to show how the analytic view may and must be maintained during the sessions.

The analytic view is precluded if the professional tries to replace the need to develop an analytically trained intuition with pre-patterned theories, explanations: *"The erudite can see that a description is by Freud, or Melanie Klein, but remain blind to the thing described"* (AMF, I, 5). Those explanations usually function as pain relievers.

Binocular vision and correlation

The analytic view demands an ability to make a couple, or marriage. The concept of container and contained works during the here and now of the analytic session; binocular vision (q.v.) provides the confrontation of at least two vertexes, allowing the formation of a commonsensical view. Kant's criticism re-emerges in the analytic session; the confrontation—in the sense of *vis-à-vis*—is the condition for growth. This contrasts with autism. Or, in other words, the idea that there is such a thing as "total independence". This is perhaps the most profound basis of hallucinosis (q.v.) hitherto observed. Correlation, relationships between objects allow for emotional experiences; they cannot be conceived of in isolation from a relationship (LE, 42). *". . . I assume that correlation is a necessary part of confrontation and that confrontation is a necessary part of analysis"* (AI, 93).

The improvement of the analysis includes the "circular argument" (q.v.). It is a concept destined to gauge the effectiveness of an interpretation given by an analyst *vis-à-vis* the patient's statements. The "correct interpretation" (q.v.) must be such that one avoids restricting it to "knowing about" but reaches "becoming" (q.v.).

The analytic view would receive a lasting expansion when the concept of $♀♂$, container/contained, was introduced. It would integrate Oedipus and the sexual component in the here-and-now of the evolving session. Refer to the entry, container/contained.

The personal equation

That an analytic view is only achieved through personal analysis is beyond any doubt in Bion's work. There are many mentions and even recommendations that an analyst should look for the best analysis he can. The same sense is conveyed when he warns that his books are to be read by practising analysts.

Freud was the first to coin the expression "personal equation" and the possibilities for dealing with it; it encircles the interference of the observer in the object observed in terms of gauging them and disciplining them—up to a point (1925, "On negation", SE, XIX; 1938, "An outline of psycho-analysis", SE, XXIII). Ferenczi would return to the issue (1928, "The elasticity of the psycho-analytic method") but it seems that up to 1965 no other analysts would emphasize this factor that is fundamental to an analytical view.

> The first requisite for the use of a theory is proper conditions for observation. The most important of these is psycho-analysis of the observer to ensure that he has reduced to a minimum his own inner tensions and resistances which otherwise obstruct his views of facts by making correlation of conscious and unconscious impossible. The next step is for the analyst to bring his attention to bear. Darwin pointed out that judgement obstructs observation. The psycho-analyst however must intervene with interpretations and this involves the exercise of judgement. A state of reverie conducive to alpha-function, obtrusion of the selected fact, and model-making together with an armoury limited to a few essential theories ensure that a harsh break in observation of the kind Darwin had in mind becomes less likely; interpretations can occur to the analyst with the minimum disturbance of observation" [LE, 86–7]

> I shall ignore disturbance produced by the analyst's personality or aspects of it. The existence of such disturbance is well known and its recognition is the basis for analytic acceptance of the need for analysts to be analysed and the many studies of counter-transference. While other scientific disciplines recognize the personal equation, or the factor of personal error, no science other than psycho-analysis has insisted on such a profound and prolonged investigation of its nature and ramifications ... I shall assume an ideal analyst and that Ta α and Ta β are not distorted by turbulence—though turbulence and its sources are part of O" [T, 48]

Usefulness It may sound disposable and pleonastic to state the possible usefulness of such a concept. In simpler terms, to establish the analytic view is to establish the borders between psycho-analysis and anything else. The pursuit of such an improvement is the basic reason for the existence of the analyst's own analysis (the so-called training analysis). This effort was made first by Freud himself in many well-known papers. Thereafter some distinguished and experienced analysts such as Karl Menninger tried to establish a theory of technique, and others such as Reik tried to establish the purely analytic posture; in the nineties, the outstanding attempts of André Green. Many others tried to transplant other models to analysis; even though I do not do justice in this text both to all involved and the many ways they tried to do it. For example, James Strachey's attempt was through a careful translation of Freud, Winnicott tried to warn Klein about politics interfering in science, Clifford-Scott and Wisdom in respect to the clinical posture, and many "good enough" analysts in more isolated countries—I refer to the attempts at a purely analytic posture.

An analytic view would enable one to attain a specific success, an **analytic** success. This is in entire agreement with Freud: "*If analysis has been successful in restoring the personality of the patient he will approximate to being the person he was when his development became compromised*" (T, 143). Judgement does not belong to analytic practice, except when a judgmental posture is part of the patient's personality.

What is at stake here? The possibility of making analysis a real, truthful and useful activity for patients in the first place, and analysts and mankind. In the long run, it means survival or oblivion.

&; Bion tried to unearth Freud's pure psycho-analysis. On the basis of his work in the Trilogy, it can be said that he avoided by every means two kinds of splitting, which the author named elsewhere the "naïve realistic" and the "naïve idealistic". "Naïve realism" is the concretization that favoured and still favours material reality. It was initiated with Broca's and Penfield's highly speculative schemata fitting rationally with Freud's models of mind, and returned in the guise of the more recent "neuro-psycho-analytic", "neuro-scientific" and positivistic minded research. "Naïve idealism" comprises the disordered flights of imagination that plagued the psycho-analytic movement from its inception. The famous warning of Freud, namely, "that sometimes a cigar is just a cigar" addresses this issue. Since the late seventies "naïve idealism" manifests itself in textualist, semantic, post-modernistic trends and many other kinds of "evidenceless", improbable, brainy, paramnesic manipulations of symbols and imaginary causal chains framed in quasi-psycho-analytical wording. It is a characteristic of written works from the thirties to the seventies. Such writing imagines a disembodied mind (Sandler, 2001, b, c)

Suggested cross-references: Atonement, Becoming, Circular Argument, Compassion, Container/Contained, Cure, Disaster, Disturbed personality, Dream the patient's material, Dream-work-α, Intuition; Jargon, Judgmental values, Mind, "O", Principle of Uncertainty, Real analysis, Thoughts without a thinker, Truth, Ultra-sensuous.

Animate and inanimate: Already in his earlier papers Bion had noticed that people try to deal with the animate with methods that are appropriate to the inanimate realm. He observed people who could not go to sleep or be wide awake; who could not dream or think; their state could neither be described in terms of being alive nor dead.

Having killed, from the violence of their emotions, the living aspect of the breast (love solace, understanding), the truthful nature of the breast was denied and split off; all that remained was the concrete milk (LE, 10). The issue is important not only from a theoretical point of view. It may discriminate between real analysis and imitative practices. This may explain the present tribulations of the psycho-analytic movement, which was not able to profit, as a whole, from Bion's attempts to rescue Freud and Klein's contributions, which are not concrete. The psycho-analytical movement is lost in the search for concrete, neurological, inanimate or social causes and solutions. In this sense the psycho-analytical movement functions just like patients. For, during analysis, the patient cannot deal with interpretation without a craving for love that remains unsatisfied; it "*turns into overweening and misdirected greed*" (LE, 11).

The patient tries to force the analyst to furnish concrete cure, solutions, answers, wisdom, counsel, and more and more interpretations that are swallowed as if they were truth-in-themselves or things-in-themselves, with no working through. The patient "*does not feel he is having interpretations for that would involve an ability to establish with the analyst the counterpart of an infant's relationship with a breast that provides material wisdom and love. But he feels able only to establish the counterpart of a relationship in which such sustenance can be had as inanimate objects can provide; he can have analytic interpretations that he feels to be either flatus or contributions remarkable for what they are not rather than for what they are"* (LE, 11–12).

The issue has consequences for science and epistemology. Bion borrowed formulations from the philosopher. The object of study of psycho-analysis and of philosophy is sometimes the same, namely, the human mind. Bion stressed the fundamental difference between the philosopher's and the analyst's tasks; namely, the practical objectives of the analyst.

With regard to science, there are difficulties for the positivistic-minded person who mistakes science for that which Kant called "naïve realism". The problem obtruded and carried on obtruding with Darwin and Einstein in the fields of biology and physics. It emerged with full force with Freud in the field of medicine.

To the same extent that Freud's discoveries are misunderstood, forgotten and debased, the issue obtrudes again *within* the psycho-analytic movement:

> The scientist whose investigations include the stuff of life itself finds himself in a situation that has a parallel in that of the patients I am describing. The breakdown in the patient's equipment for thinking leads to dominance of a mental life in which his universe is populated by inanimate objects. The inability of even the most advanced human beings to make use of thoughts, because the capacity to think is rudimentary in all of us, means that the field for investigation, all investigation being ultimately scientific, is limited, by human inadequacy, to those phenomena that have the characteristic of the inanimate. We assume that the psychotic limitation is due to an illness: but that that of the scientist is not. It appears that our rudimentary equipment for "thinking" thoughts is adequate when the problems are associated with the inanimate, but not when the object for investigation is the phenomenon of life itself. Confronted with the complexities of the human mind the analyst must be circumspect in following even accepted scientific method; its weakness may be closer to the weakness of psychotic thinking than superficial scrutiny would admit. [LE, 14]

One may see that Bion was circumspect in criticizing directly that which he names, "accepted scientific method". Max Planck faced the fierce opposition of Ernst Mach in the same way that Freud faced the opposition of the medical establishment. More of the same, with Klein, who faced the opposition of the self-entitled "Freudian" establishment. Bion's work faced the opposition of many parts of the psycho-analytic establishment during the eighties—this fact had already crept in during the attempts to co-opt him during the sixties, as well as in the attempt to exclude him in the ensuing years. Green mentioned the last occurrence in his book review of *Cogitations* in the IJPA [1992]

Learning and Experience was written around 1960–61. One may consult the various chapters on "Scientific Method" published in *Cogitations*, which date from 1959. They were preparatory studies to that text. During 1964–65, in *Transformations*, Bion would put the issue in a slightly different manner—with regard to the human equipment for knowing reality. That which is animate came to be equated with the immaterial realm of psychic reality.

In order to get a model for discussing the situation, Bion resorted to Kant's terminology: noumena and phenomena. Bion now more confidently puts the phenomena into the realm of the concrete, sensuously apprehensible facts. They can be seen as emanations of ultimate reality: the latter (including psychic reality) is a negative realm. Once one had attained a glimpse of its existence, there is no need to search, to prove, or to multiply the concrete formulations of it:

> It can be represented by terms such as ultimate reality or truth. The most, and the least that the individual person can do is to be it. Being identified with it is a measure of distance from it. The beauty of a rose is a phenomenon betraying the ugliness of O just as ugliness betrays or reveals the existence of O . . . O, representing the unknowable ultimate reality can be represented by any formulation of a transformation—such as "unknowable ultimate reality" which I have just formulated. It may therefore seem unnecessary to multiply representations of it; indeed from the psycho-analytical vertex that is true. But I wish to make it clear that my reason for saying O is unknowable is not that I consider human capacity unequal to the task . . . [T, 139–40]

Truth may be the most synthetic formulation that marks that which belongs to the immaterial, animate reality. The animate is ineffable. The inanimate can equally express truth and untruth. The inanimate can be put into words.

Arrogance: Bion observed that a triadic behavioral conjunction appears when one feels prevented from making projective identification. The person may feel that he is prevented. It can actually be prevented. The triad is made of arrogance, stupidity and curiosity. Clinically, every time that a psychotic personality cannot function through projective identifications, he or she resorts to this triad or to a variation of it in which one or two of each of these behaviours prevails (ST, 86, 92).

   Suggested cross-references: Curiosity, Stupidity, Projective Identification.

Atonement, at-one-ment:

> P.A. I do not think we could tolerate our work—painful as it often is for both us and our patients—without compassion (AMF, III, 522).

> The central postulate is that atonement with ultimate reality, or O, as I have called it to avoid involvement with as existing association, is essential to harmonious mental growth. [ST, 145]

An observational concept belonging to the realm of the psychoanalytic posture, psycho-analytical view (q.v.) and formulations in the decisive moment of the here and now of the session. It borrows a term from the mystic tradition (especially from the Jewish and Christian Cabbala, as well as from some of the Reform postures). This is done in order to depict a mental state. It is a tool for attaining "real psycho-analysis" (q.v.). To grasp the meaning of the concept one must have an idea of that which Bion named "O", a quasi-mathematical notation for the realm of the noumena, the unconscious, the id (q.v.). Bion proposed the symbol "O" to denote *"ultimate reality, absolute truth, the godhead, the infinite, the thing-in-itself"*.

At-one-ment is a verbal (written) indication describing situations that are experientially alive and truthful, with no taints of lies. It formulates an evolving ultimate reality during the here and now of the session. It is not a tool to *know* one's own psychic reality, but *to apprehend* it in a transient way. A given reality as it evolves and becomes amenable to be formulated under a series of guises: literary, musical, among others. This is done, partially, as a glimpse. At-one-ment is a passageway to insight.

It is not a tool for knowing psychic reality due to the fact that psychic reality, as any form in which that reality eventually may present itself, *"is not something which lends itself to being known. It is impossible to know reality for the same reason that makes it impossible to sing potatoes; they may be grown, or pulled, or eaten, but not sung. Reality has to be 'been': there should be a transitive verb 'to be' expressly for use with the term 'reality'"* (T, 148).

Reality-O, or "truth-O" (AI, 29) is the leitmotiv of analytic pursuit (AI, 29). It can "become", but it cannot be "known" (AI, 26). The analyst "becomes O" (AI, 27), being expressions of O, the emotional experience as experienced by the analysand and analyst, towards the reality of the patient as he or she really is.

In so far as the analyst becomes O he is able to know the events that are evolutions of O" (AI, 27). Therefore the experience of atonement or at-one-ment cannot be described. It can be lived. It is not a matter of mere feelings—that Bion ascribes as appertaining to the realm of inner sense impressions. As a preparation for the concept of atonement, he paves the way: *". . . people exist who are so intolerant of pain or frustration (or in whom pain and frustration is so intolerable) that they feel the pain but will not suffer it and so cannot be said to discover it"* (AI, 9).

This quotation allows the introduction of a factor of at-one-ment: pain and its dialectical pair, nourishment. Bion had previously illuminated this in *Transformations*.

This was one of his first forays into the observation of methods to make approximations to "O". The tolerance of frustration and pain allows experience of the "No-(something)", or the negative by means of which reality as it is emerges. From the renouncing of achieving whatever it is, there emerges the truth or reality-O of that which was the object of nourishment of that which was regarded as nourishment. I'm proposing to differentiate nourishment, which includes frustration, from fulfilment or satisfaction (see below on atonement and satisfaction).

To qualify O for inclusion amongst the column 1 categories by defining its definitory qualities I list the following negatives: Its existence as indwelling in an individual person or in God or Devil;

it is not good or evil; it cannot be known, loved or hated. It can be represented by terms such as ultimate reality or truth. The most, and the least that the individual person can do is to be it. Being identified with it is a measure of distance from it. The beauty of a rose is a phenomenon betraying the ugliness of O just as ugliness betrays or reveals the existence of O. [T, 139–140]

The experience of "to be at-one" is strictly linked to the moment of the analytic interpretation. It is not an act of knowing but of being: "*Formulations of the events of analysis made in the course of analysis must possess value different from that of formulations made extra-sessionally. Their value therapeutically is greater if they are conducive to transformations in O; less if conducive to transformations in K . . . the analyst must focus his attention on O, the unknown and unknowable. The success of psycho-analysis depends on the maintenance of a psycho-analytic point of view; the point-of-view is the psycho-analytic vertex; the psycho-analytic vertex is O. With this the analyst cannot be identified: he must be it . . . the psycho-analyst can know what the patient says, does, and appears to be, but cannot know the O of which the patient is an evolution: he can only 'be' it . . . the interpretation is an actual event in an evolution of O that is common to analyst and analysand*" (AI, 26, 27).

"To be" and "become" depends on having regard to truth: "*There can be no genuine outcome that is based on falsity. Therefore the outcome depends on the closeness with which the interpretative appraisal approximates to truth*" (AI, 28).

The state of at-one-ment is described thus: "*To put it in more popular terms, I would say the more 'real' the psycho-analyst is the more he can be at one with the reality of the patient*". This experience is real, but it does not rely on split factual, concrete, and sensuously apprehensible situations such as the universe of the patient's discourse, statements and the like: "*Conversely, the more he [the analyst] depends on actual events the more he relies on thinking that depends on a background of sense impression*" (AI, 28) The already known, or the tendency to state "*thus far and no further*" (AMF, II, 265) precludes the at-one-ment: "*The impulse to be rid of painful stimuli gives the 'content' of the memory an unsatisfactory quality when one is engaged in the pursuit of truth O . . . an analyst with such a mind is one who is incapable of learning because he is satisfied*" (AI, 29).

"O" stands for the absolute truth in and of any object; "*it is assumed that this cannot be known by any human being; it can be known about, its presence can be recognized and felt, but it cannot be known. It is possible to be at one with it. That it exists is an essential postulate of science but it cannot be scientifically discovered. No psycho-analytic discovery is possible without recognition of its existence, at-one-ment with it and evolution*"(AI, 30).

Atonement and truth

"*It may be wondered what state of mind is welcome if desires and memories are not. A term that would express approximately what I need to express is 'faith'—faith that there is an ultimate reality and truth—the unknown, unknowable, 'formless infinite'*" (AI, 31). The issue is not the particular truth(s); even less "the truth"; but truth itself. There is a hope that truth is strong and shall prevail. Faith, here, is faith in the existence of truth and reality.

Atonement and interpretation

> The interpretation should be such that the transition from *knowing about* reality to *becoming real* is furthered . . . The interpretations that effect the transition from knowing about O to becoming O are those establishing . . . the material through which the argument circulates. [T, 153]

Bion examines the properties of the number "one" and at the same time he states that mystics are people who seem to have had some kind of contact with O. They rest in a capacity to tolerate paradoxes, as in the example of St John of the Cross, whose descriptions of "repellent" qualities "*may be an unconscious tribute to his identification of absolute real evil with absolute real good*" (T, 139). Isaac Singer describes the same in many of his novels, such as in *The Moskat Family*. The main character, Asa Herschel, discovers that the Jewish people's Messiah is Hitler.

In 1967 Bion resorts to Wordsworth to express the posture:

> If psycho-analysts can abandon themselves to analysis in the psycho-analytical sessions, they are in a position when recollecting the experience in tranquillity [this is Wordsworth's wording to

convey his "sense of poetry"; Wordsworth, (1798, p.171)] to discern their experience as part of a greater whole. Once that is achieved, the way is open for the discovery of configurations revealing yet other and deeper groups of theory. But the discoverer must be prepared to find that he has started another round of group oscillations. Persecution⇔Depression. [Cogitations, 285]

The practical point is—no further investigation of psycho-analysis, but the psyche it betrays. *That* needs to be investigated through the medium of *mental* patterns; *that* which is indicated is *not* a symptom; *that* is not a cause of the symptom; *that* is not a disease or *any*thing subordinate. Psycho-analysis itself is just a stripe on the coat of the tiger. Ultimately it may meet the Tiger—The Thing Itself—O. [AMF, I, 112]

Atonement and science

The failure to apprehend the use of analogy may hamper the realization of the scientific nature of atonement; and by extension, of psycho-analysis:

The scientific approach, associated with a background of sense impressions, for example the presence of the psycho-analyst and his patient in the same room, may be regarded as having a base. In so far as it is associated with the ultimate reality of the personality, O, it is baseless. This does not mean that the psycho-analytic method is unscientific, but that the term "science", as it has been commonly used hitherto to describe an attitude to objects of sense, is not adequate to represent an approach to those realities with which "psycho-analytical science" has to deal. Not is it adequate to represent that aspect of the human personality that is concerned with the unknown and ultimately unknowable—with O.

The criticism applies to every vertex, be it musical, religious, aesthetic, political; all are inadequate when related to O because, with the possible exception of the religion of the mystic, these and similar vertices are not adapted to the sensually baseless. The realities with which psycho-analysts deals, for example, fear, panic, love, anxiety, passion, have no sensuous background, though there is a sensuous background (respiratory rate, pain, touch, etc.) that is often identified with them and then treated, supposedly scientifically. What is required is not a base for psycho-analysis and its theories but a science that is not restricted by its genesis in knowledge and sensuous background. It must be a science of at-one-ment. It must have a mathematics of at-one-ment, not identification. There can be no geometry of "similar", "identical", "equal"; only of analogy. [AI, 88–9]

Atonement is linked to dream-work; refer to the entry "Dream the patient's material".

Misuses and misconceptions: Bion makes explicit that he borrows some terms from other disciplines. Sometimes he does this intentionally to profit from the penumbra of associations of the terms.

Many of the terms he borrowed already had known, widely-accepted meaning and connotation. He wants the reader to be reminded of them. For example, "transformations and invariances", "hallucinosis". Sometimes he uses the term giving specific warnings that the reader must see that the term is used differently in his work when compared with the common usage. For example, the non-hyphenated term "preconception" (q.v.). Sometimes he creates new terms to avoid any associations with existing terms such as "O" and "α". Finally, sometimes he stresses some meanings already ingrained in a given term and sticks with them, such as "hyperbole".

Does lack of attention to these warnings and explanations of the use of a term arouse confusion and polemic? Do prejudices hamper the full realization of Bion's use of terms derived from mystic experience, such as faith and atonement?

The use of a known term facilitates communication without resorting to neologisms. Concrete-minded people cannot grasp the fact that the mystic tradition, as well as art and philosophy, were early human attempts to approach human nature and mind's functioning before the obtrusion of science and psycho-analysis. Some of the mystic's insights gained durability, to the extent that they were truthful, quite independent of time and the forms in which they were first couched and then conveyed. Does the concrete-minded reader take these words literally as if Bion had used them in their religious sense, or with religious purposes? Was he trying to impinge religion on psycho-analysis?

Bion did not attack religion—nor did Freud. This statement runs contrary to the current prevailing (religious) belief that attributes to

Freud an anti-religious posture. This belief turns the psycho-analytic movement into another form of religion. It would suffice to read with real attention that which Freud says about religion in "The question of a *Weltanschauung*".

Bion had described the religious states of mind that characterize human mindlessness:

> . . . I wonder how many plausible theories have been used and bewildered the human race. I would like to know. I am not sure of the ease with which "plausible" theories are produced. In this context of "plausible theories" about which we are talking, the plausible theory, or "convincing interpretation", may be hard to come by. It can be plausible and false. Witness the idea that "the sun rises"—what trouble that has caused! We do not know the cost in suffering associated with the belief in a Christian God, or the god of Abraham's Ur, or Hitler's Germany, or peyotism—or god of any kind. [AMF, I, 172]

And the danger that religious states of mind represented a real capacity for faith or belief that truth exists:

> BION If all else fails you could rage, as I too can, against yourself, your youth or your age, your strength or your weakness. It is one of the uses you can make of God—if you can believe in God.
>
> ROBIN Well, can't you?
>
> BION Which god are you referring to?
>
> ROBIN Allah Akbar!
>
> BION I don't think you are being serious. I shall use psycho-analytic licence to take jokes seriously. To start with, you show you are aware that you have a choice.
>
> ROBIN You think of me as joking. It would not be so easy to suppose that, if I were in fact a member of a Muslim culture. Nor would you suppose that you could "choose" to take it seriously "because" you are a member of a psycho-analytic group. You would be compelled to take it seriously. It has nothing to do with being a member of a particular group, profession or culture, but that particular "culture" has a great deal to do with some underlying, unobserved, constant conjunction of beliefs; an actual God of which the various religious formulations are only approximations to the underlying configuration of facts.

BION You are asking me to suppose that there is a "thing-in-itself", noumenon, Godhead, which, using Kant's terminology for my purposes, becomes "manifest" as a phenomenon; "God" as contrasted with "Godhead", "finity" as contrasted with "infinity"; "won", as Milton says, "from the void and formless infinite"; a geometrical, Euclidean figure, a triangle with sides of 2, 4 and 5 units, as contrasted with an algebraical deductive system. But a rational fact gives no scope for "belief". Belief itself is destroyed if it is transformed to find a "reason" for belief. [AMF, I, 179–80]

Bion respected the contributions that some people who were nourished by religious tradition gave to mankind. He differentiated between the mystic tradition and bigotry. The dialogues between the characters "Priest" (first called "Paul") and "P.A." in volumes II and III of *A Memoir of the Future* plainly shows this. Please refer to the entry, "Science versus Religion".

All the references to St John of the Cross, John Ruysbroeck (in *Transformations*), Isaac Luria (after Georg Scholem, in *Attention and Interpretation*), the Bhagavad Gita (especially *A Memoir of the Future*, I, p. 69, 79, 140, 147; II, 333; *Cogitations*, p. 371), Israel's God (*A Memoir of the Future*, I, p. 80) and Christ (*A Memoir of the Future*, I, p. 140) indicates his way: a respect for the wisdom contained in mystic tradition, outside of religious rites or submission.

Bion's reverence and awe before the unknown equals that of Einstein, Freud and Heisenberg, to quote a few. On this basis some have accused Bion of being a deteriorated man, gaga. They try to base their accusation, in part, on Bion resorting to these models (for example, Meltzer, 1981; Segal, 1989; Joseph, 2002). The fact was reported, albeit talking about religion rather than mystics, by Joan and Neville Symington. Do they fail to see the analogic value of models (q.v.) in psycho-analysis?

Bion tried to use other models, such as mathematical notation. Also, he tried to formulate the analytic experience in more colloquial terms. In this he was influenced by the British Romantic poets, such as Wordsworth.

Analytic communication was degenerating into jargon (q.v.) and controversy (q.v.). But to be colloquial is not enough: there is the issue that analysis includes, and is, an emotional experience. Therefore Bion uses some terms that are derived from realms that take emotional experiences into consideration. The religious realm is one of them. Words such as intuition, mystics, faith, were brought to the fore.

> If the psycho-analytical situation is accurately intuited—I prefer this term to "observed" or "heard" or "seen" as it does not carry the penumbra of sensuous association—the psycho-analyst finds that ordinary conversational English is surprisingly adequate for the formulation of his interpretation. Further, the emotional situation serves to make the interpretation comprehensible to the analysand although resistances require some modification of this statement as too optimistic. [ST, 134]

The verbal formulation "atonement" derives from religious experience. Taking into account the scarcity of better terms, made more scarce after the way that the psycho-analytical movement debased the original psycho-analytical formulations of Freud and Klein, it is no wonder that one resorts to verbal formulation derived from other realms. They are no indications of Bion's alleged mystic religiosity. As concerns O, *"the religious mystics have probably approximated most closely to expression of experience of it"* (AI, 30). The key here may be that one must differentiate mysticism from the mystic tradition.

If one reads it in a respectfully Ruskinian way, one will notice "expression of experience". This definitely encircles the issue as a matter of verbal formulation, of analogic expression intended to communicate something. This something is the ability to apprehend reality. One may verify this when Bion specifically quotes the so-called mystics.

> Verbal expressions intended to represent the ultimate object often appear to be contradictory within themselves, but there is a surprising degree of agreement, despite differences of background, time and space, in the descriptions offered by mystics who feel they have experienced the ultimate reality. Sometimes the agreement seems close even when, as with Milton, the individual seems to know of it rather than to have experienced it.
>
> The rising world of waters dark and deep
>
> Won from the void and formless infinite" [Milton, Paradise Lost, Book 3]

... The process of binding is a part of the procedure by which something is "won from the void and formless infinite"; it is K and must be distinguished from the process by which O is "become."'
[T, 151]

This is not a question restricted to theoretical issues:

The psycho-analyst accepts the reality of reverence and awe, the possibility of a disturbance in the individual which makes atonement and, therefore, an expression of reverence and awe impossible. The central postulate is that atonement with ultimate reality, or O, as I have called it to avoid involvement with as existing association, is essential to harmonious mental growth. It follows that interpretation involves elucidation of evidence touching atonement, and not evidence only of the continuing operation of immature relationship with a father ... Disturbance in capacity for atonement is associated with megalomaniac attitudes. [ST, 145]

Atonement is incompatible with greed, fantasies of satisfaction, idolization, or religious "contact with God" as a father or an omnipotent incarnate God.

Suggested cross-references: Analytic View, Correct Interpretation, Dream the Patient's Material, O, Real Analysis, Religion versus science, Thoughts without a thinker, Transformations in O, Ultra-sensuous.

B

Basic assumptions: In dealing with small groups, Bion observed some expressions of the paranoid–schizoid position. They corresponded to a kind of prejudice that shaped the outcome of the group's functioning, in a specific sense: these assumptions precluded the formation and/or development of a work group.

Bion, influenced by his analysis and further collaboration with John Rickman, who in turn profited from Klein's work, was enabled to exercise that which he would later name the "analytically trained intuition" (q.v.).

The author has proposed elsewhere to specify the exercise of "analytically trained intuition" as belonging to the posture of psycho-analytic "participating observation". Bion used it in group settings. Psycho-analysis is a "two-body psychology" in the terms coined by Rickman; therefore it qualifies to be seen as a group setting. Moreover, in the fullest sense of the Aristotelian dictum, "man is a political animal", there is no humanity in isolation or *in abstractio*. Psycho-analytically speaking this would correspond—at its best—to autism, depression or masturbation. Conversely, the sense of solitude (Alves, 1989) differs from the sense of loneliness. In the sense of solitude, the person is with him/herself. Therefore even if we consider a single person, when he or she realizes the existence of his or her mental life, this "whole entity", a single person, can also be regarded as something endowed with a "two-ness" (Bion, 1977) Aristotle perceived this and wrote about the *nous*—the mind thinking about itself. Therefore, these group functions and modes of functioning also occur in a single mind, in terms of introjected objects.

In his early studies, Bion's analytic intuition allowed the detection of three underlying modes of organization/disorganization of groups, which he named "basic assumptions" of a group:

i.   *Fight/flight*: the group splits itself in mutual destruction of its members; the aggression is often overt and there is a hostile search for and choice of culprits.

ii. *Pairing*: the fragmentation consists of the members forming pairs that would bring forth a saviour; those pairs have a "Homo" nature. The members of the group, frozen in the paranoid–schizoid position, cling to each other due to features they attribute to each other that are felt (invariably in a hallucinatory way) to be similar or identical.

iii. *Messianic or dependence*: the group agglutinates itself around a leader felt to be a saviour, a superior being. Those attributes are hallucinated products of shared projective identifications of the members of the group, who feel they are able to divest (in a phantastic way) themselves of their self-responsibility. Mind itself is extruded, in phantasy, and "placed" into another person, the "saviour". This messianic leader is felt as *the* —and not only *a*—source of wisdom, authority and knowledge.

The three basic assumptions occur many times in succession; sometimes the pairing group paves the way to the messianic group; sometimes flight/fight groups are a prelude to the pairing group. The messianic group can lead to renewed fight/flights. The cycles follow on in a kind of feed-back with no possibility of change. The group can die, starved of truth; it cannot nourish itself through work, because it forms no work group, just "basic assumptions groups". Therefore the self-feeding cycles are characterized by a primitive (emotionally speaking) destructive intra-group relationship, almost wholly based on hallucination and delusion. This contrasts with work-groups, who can change and make thrusts into the unknown.

The psychotic nature of the three basic assumptions was clear in Bion's original writings in the forties. Thanks to his later advancement in grasping of the facts of the herd, especially after his books, *Transformations, Attention and Interpretation* and *A Memoir of the Future*, we can now see that the three underlying modes of functioning are the stuff of hallucinosis.

It is its hallucinated character that hampers or precludes the formation of "work groups", whose existence is dependent on regard to truth. *"The assumption underlying loyalty to the K link is that the personality of analyst and analysand can survive the loss of its protective coat of lies, subterfuge, evasion and hallucination and may even be fortified and enriched by the loss. It is an assumption strongly disputed by the psychotic and a fortiori by the group, which relies on psychotic mechanisms for its coherence and sense of well being"* (T, 129).

Bion hoped that further observation could lead to the description of basic assumptions other than these three. The possibility of a more mature functioning corresponds to the diminishing allegiance to the basic assumptions.

Synonymy: Basic groups (not often used).

&; Some later authors have tried to describe other basic assumptions. The extent that they succeed will depend on a more effective replication or refutation of clinical observations. In 1974, P. Turquet stated that there is a fourth basic assumption, *"oneness"*: *"a mental activity in which members seek to join in a powerful union with an omnipotent force, unobtainably high, to surrender self for passive participation, and thereby feel existence, well-being, and wholeness . . . the group member is there to be lost in oceanic feelings of unity or, if the oneness is personified, to be a part of a salvationist inclusion"* (Turquet, 1974, pp. 357, 360).

Starting from Turquet, W. Gordon Lawrence, Alastair Bain, and Lawrence Gould named a fifth basic assumption group, *"Me-Ness"*. According to them, this fifth basic assumption is the opposite of Turquet's "One-Ness". It consists of an anti-group group mentality. The authors *"do not want to explain away baM (basic assumption Me-Ness) in terms of individual narcissism, as can be found in analysands and patients, because we are focusing on baM (basic assumption*

Me-Ness) *as a cultural phenomenon"*. They hypothesize that this basic assumption is becoming *"more salient in industrialized cultures"*; an individualist tendency that they detect in different ages of western civilization (Lawrence, Bain & Gould, 1996, p. 28).

The discussion of those authors' ideas is not within the scope of this dictionary. Anyway, only to hint at possible discussions that could strengthen their contributions, as far as my grasp of their writing goes, it is not clear to what extent they are depicting manifest phenomenal expressions of Bion's "messianic leader" and/or "dependence" basic assumption.

The author observed phenomena that allowed for the possibility of the existence of a sixth "basic assumption", which was provisionally to be named "Hallucinosis of Exclusion/Appertaining" (Sandler, 2001). A quasi-symbolic notation may be, Groups {"**A**" and "**Outside A**"}. I suppose that people hallucinate that they belong to a given group (or subgroup within a group) and/or hallucinate that they are excluded from the given group they aspire to be part of. The very group is a product of the mind and has no counterpart in reality, its "materialness" notwithstanding. This sixth assumption has a psychotic and a non-psychotic nature: the latter is to be found in the Oedipus situation. There is a possibility of existence of "natural groups" that *may* qualify to be endowed with realness. They were adumbrated by Durkheim: he observed two kinds of "solidarities" that cohere people in groups: "mechanic" and "organic". The latter can foster a real "inclusion attitude" towards, and in its members. It is a matter of interest (Sanders, 1986).

There are some differences between my hypothesis and the ideas of these authors. Firstly, I deal with it as a hypothesis to be discussed. Secondly, they make a sociological study drawn from analogies of some socio-economic and political facts that may now be dated. Thirdly, their experience is drawn primarily from their *"roles as consultants to and directors of . . . working conferences"* about group relations and education *"in addition to"* their *"practices as social scientists, organizational consultants, psycho-analysts, and university teachers"*, and mine is drawn from clinical psycho-analysis proper, as well as an active involvement in community psychiatry and in the observation of movements within some psycho-analytic institutions.

Become, becoming:

> ROSEMARY . . . I feel I am "becoming" it even if I do not, and never shall, "understand" what I am "becoming" or "being".

> BION In short, "being" something is different from "understanding" it. Love is the ultimate which is "become", not understood.

> ALICE (looking at Rosemary) I have "become" something and this, if I could say it, would depend on my saying, "I love". [AMF, I, 183]

This term is defined in the entries "At-one-ment", "Transformations in O", "Transformations in psycho-analysis". Refer to these specific entries.

The verbal formulation, "becoming", is an early attempt by Bion (1965) that pays respect to the severe constraints imposed both by sensuously apprehensible and sense-based methods of verbal communication. It refers to the communication in the analytical setting and among psycho-analysts. Words both convey and disguise meaning.

Terms such as "to know oneself" are seen in *Transformations, Attention and Interpretation* and *A Memoir of the Future* as belonging to the realm of philosophy. Analysis is a practical, living experience: *"Herein lies one advantage that the psycho-analyst possesses over the philosopher; his statements can be related to realizations and realizations to a psycho-analytic theory"* (T, 44).

In order to emphasize this with its built-in ever changing nature, Bion resorts to the term, "becoming". In *A Memoir of the Future* there are three fictitious characters who are named, "Bion", "Myself" and "Psycho-analyst", who may be seen as steps towards becoming who one is. In the last volume they are called Somites, Body, Psyche, Mind, Soma, Term, Boy, and various ages (Eleven, Twenty-One, Thirty-two, Fifty, up to Seventy-Eight).

All of them correspond to Bion's memories of his own learning from experience. They may be regarded as fictional expressions of his part-objects, reflecting his own trajectory in life. To a certain extent they are manifestations of himself, the man and the professional. There are many parts of the text that offer opportunities to see the integration and the disintegration of a whole life, being lived in a moment—the moment one "becomes". Life, after all, only exists in the moment it is being lived. Facts are "presented".

Becoming may be seen as a continuous process during a life-cycle. It is becoming who one is in reality; a marriage of an internal couple. This couple is made up of the person and its true self.

A *Memoir of the Future* offers many formulations of "becoming"; the books themselves are a "becoming-in-themselves". They are not amenable to being understood, but rather as "becoming-evoking" devices. For example:

BION You do not regard them as historically distributed?

MYSELF I do, but not exclusively. In fact, I would find it helpful to borrow from a schizophrenic patient a capacity for a transference relationship which was alternatively penetrating and planar; deep and confused, or superficial and of great "spread", like a monomolecular film. At the same time these states, though apparently mutually exclusive, are reconciled and co-existent—like wave motion and quanta, objects in a pattern conforming to a Poisson distribution displayed on two planes—one temporal, one spatial—at right angles to each other. Seen from the temporal plane the other "transference" spreads monomolecular-wise: seen from the vertex of the spatial plane, the "transference" is penetrating.

BION I don't think I understand. You mean that from an historical vertex events are distributed sequentially one after another in what we call time, but that is possible to regard them, by ignoring the temporal vertex, as distributed in space, not time?

MYSELF Yes, but then two views are obtained, one which is very narrow and extremely penetrating, the other very broad and spread out without depth or penetration.

ALICE So what? Is this any different from what I and my girl friends have always known? Our boy friends are all the same—either for ever pawing us about though it's clear it doesn't mean a thing, or "poking" us, having what they call sex, which doesn't mean a thing either.

BION Or both—and calling it schizophrenia.

MYSELF And that means nothing whether it is spread out over the whole of psychiatry or concentrated to apply to a particular, specific "thing" or "person".

MAN You could say the same about "psycho-analysis" or "sex" or "hate" or any other verbalization.

MYSELF Or "feelings" or names of feelings. They don't mean a thing. Or, as Kant said, "concepts without intuition are empty and intuitions without concepts are blind".

BION I know the quotation to which you refer, of course, but—is *that* what he meant?

MYSELF I have no idea what he meant, but I am using *his* "concepts" to match with *my* "intuitions", because in this way I can bring together a concept and an intuition, making it possible to feel that *I* know what *I* mean. If I could also juxtapose you and myself, the two together would be meaningful.

ROSEMARY You certainly sound as if you get on very well. So well indeed that I almost wondered if you were not the same person.

BION & MYSELF (together) So do I. [AMF, I, 193–4]

Belief: Refer to Analytic View, Facts, O, Psycho-analytic paramnesias, Science versus Religion, Scientific Method, Sense of Truth.

Beta-elements

In the model of alpha-function (q.v.) this quasi-mathematical symbol, "beta-elements", sometimes written as β-elements, stands for things-in-themselves, when they are felt to be such by the beholder.

They are suitable for projective identification but not for thinking. They constitute the raw material that is amenable to be sensuously apprehended and decoded into elements suitable for thinking, dreaming and remembering, called alpha-elements (q.v.).

⊕ They were first defined in 1960, as objects that are felt by the infant in its earliest phases of development as dead and non-existent—due to the fact that before the inception of the reality principle, "*objects are felt to be alive and to possess character and personality presumably indistinguishable from the infant's own ... the real and the alive are indistinguishable; if an object is real to the infant, then it is alive; if it is dead, it does not exist*".

Bion wanted to discuss objects in a pre-verbal state that are not felt as alive due to being, so to speak, "extinguished" by the infant's rage. "*If the object is wished dead, it is dead. It therefore has become non-existent, and its characteristics are different from those of the real, live, existing object; the existing object is alive, real and benevolent*". Bion proposes *"to call the real, alive objects α-elements; the dead, unreal objects I shall call β-elements"* (all quotations, C, 133).

He calls both primitive objects proto-objects; *"It is therefore, in so far as it [the infant] feels pleasure, surrounded by these proto-real objects felt to be real and alive. But should pain supervene, then it is surrounded by dead objects destroyed by its hate, which, since it cannot tolerate pain, are non-existent"* (C, 133–4).

The β-elements seem to constitute the bulk of the infant's mental life as well as the stuff of the psychotic functioning, when they remain in an "undigested" state. Why undigested? Because if the intolerance of these objects is prevalent, the infant attacks the mental apparatus, which continuously receives sensuously apprehensible stimuli that inform the baby that the objects felt as dead are still there.

> The existence of the real objects can be denied, but the sense impressions persist . . . The next stage, imposed by yet more powerful intolerance, is the destruction of the apparatus that is responsible for the transformation of the sense impressions into material suitable for waking unconscious thought—a dream thought. This destruction contributes to the feeling that "things", not words or ideas, are inside. [C, 134]

The reader can see in this quotation that Bion defines β-elements in conjunction with the earliest definitions of α-function (which was not called such at this time) that is attacked and cannot function.

The infant depends on the mother's alpha-function to digest its beta-elements, and the adult may revert alpha-elements into a special kind of beta (c.f. bizarre elements). The adult may never transform them into alpha-elements.

Bion defined α-function more precisely, and, still considering the possibility of the non-functioning of α-function, he improves the definition of beta-elements:

> If alpha-function is disturbed, and therefore inoperative, the sense impressions of which the patient is aware and the emotions which he is experiencing remain unchanged. I shall call them beta-elements. In contrast with the alpha-elements the beta-elements are not felt to be phenomena but things-in-themselves. The emotions likewise are objects of sense. [LE, 6]

To "own" and to "know" ultimate reality or take phenomena as if they were ultimate reality is the mental state of a person whose beta-elements remain undigested. Kant named it "naïve realism"; psychiatrically speaking, it corresponds to deluded states of omniscient grandeur. In due time, Bion associated this state to splitting of material from psychic reality (especially in chapters IV, V and VI of *Learning from Experience*), which he called, "forced splitting" (q.v.).

Beta-elements, therefore, must be regarded under two different vertexes. From the point of view of the person, he or she may have feelings of owning absolute truth. Or he (or she) may in fact be deluded, displaying paranoid features. There is an invariance that permeates beta-elements and bizarre objects, in so far as they share the characteristics of beta-elements: *"the moral component"* (T, 64). From the point of view of the scientist they are realities-in-themselves whose manifestations can be apprehended through the living being's sensuous apparatus.

> I therefore suggest provisionally that the β-element categories of the grid should not be dismissed off-hand as non-existent, but should be thought of, in the domain of expressions of feeling, as related to phantasies that are felt to be indistinguishable from facts. [EP, 97]

The analyst must take care not to fall on either side. One must not display contempt towards delusional manifestations in the theoretical sense, that is, as grid categories to guide him. Also, one must not fall into the witchcraft apprentice's syndrome of hyper-valuing the patient's productions as if they were truth in themselves, in a distorted, idealistic view of Freud's notion of unconscious phantasies and Klein's extensions of it.

Misuses and misconceptions: Beta-elements are often seen as pathological. This view is a persistent distortion that encircles the understanding of many psycho-analytic theories. Their primitive, basic nature is again denied when people talk of a "beta-function", something that Bion never defined. If it existed, it would have a teleological or religious outlook. For the beholder would entertain the idea that he knew how ultimate reality was created, originated and maintained.

Suggested cross-references: Absolute truth, Alpha function, Alpha-elements, Bizarre elements, Dream-work-α, K.

Beta screen: Bion defined a "beta screen" when he was faced with patients who had some disturbances of thought and were unable to sleep or to wake, to be either conscious or unconscious. The ensuing mental confusion, elicited through unsuccessful interpretations both under Freud and Klein's vertexes, was also visible through out-pourings that resembled dreams. The outpourings were disjointed phrases and images, or were something that resembled one who feigned dreaming; outpourings that evidenced presence of halluci-nations or the patient hallucinated he (or she) was dreaming. All of this seemed to prevent the emergence of the depressive position in an emotional experience with the analyst, of murderous nature.

This state precludes the formation of a "contact barrier" (q.v.). Beta-screen is a special kind of device that replaces contact barrier. It is formed from beta-elements rather than alpha-elements; there-fore the patient is unable to separate conscious from unconscious. The purpose is to preclude the consciousness of the analyst; the analyst, when confronted with a patient whose beta screen is func-tioning, sees himself with "*a plethora of interpretations*", based on common places. Usually those interpretations are collusive or made of reassurances of the patient's goodness. "*The beta-screen . . . has a quality enabling it to evoke the kind of response the patient desires, or, alternatively, a response from the analyst which is heavily charged with counter-transference*" (LE, 23).

The beta-screen replaces the contact-barrier (q.v.) in a "*living process*" (LE, 24) that can be seen in analysis. "*Thanks to the beta-screen the psychotic patient has a capacity for evoking emotions in the analyst; his associations . . . evoke interpretations . . . which are less related to his need for psycho-analytic interpretation than to his need to produce an emotional involvement*" (LE, 24).

Bion warns that this has nothing to do with counter-transference.

Misuses and misinterpretations: Usually in this part of the work of Bion it is seen as if patients could provoke certain reactions in the analyst. Probably the reader mistakes the expression "*evoking emotions in the analyst*" with "*provoking acting-out*". The emotions that are evoked—depending on the analyst's personal analysis—are subjected to scrutiny. It is this scrutiny that matters, in furnish-ing the analytic vertex to the analyst. He must detect the emotions evoked in order to realize the function of the beta-screen; namely, to create an emotional climate "*less related to his need for psycho-*

analytical interpretation than to his need to produce an emotional involvement". Readers who do not consider this are prone to take the beta screen as an endorsement of the already existing distortion of Melanie Klein's concept of projective identification, a distortion that tries to divest it of its phantastic character. This tendency tries to extract the analyst's self-responsibility and tries to put this very same analyst's responsibility for his own shortcomings or lack of personal analysis into the patient.

Binocular vision: Although the binocular vision *model* pervades the whole of Bion's work from 1944 (a group's "Basic assumptions" are binocular), its first *explicit definition* dates from 1962, when it was linked to Bion's observation of psychotics with thought disturbances (LE, 54). For example, the obese patient who sheltered a greedy, skinny inner self; or the shy, pale patient who was unable to blush sensuously. The bulk of clinical observations that form the empirical basis of the concept appeared in *Cogitations*. They seem to correspond with intra-session data obtained from 1959 to 1960. The clinical data suggested to Bion the need to amend—rather than reject—a specific aspect of Freud's theory of consciousness as a sensuous organ for the perception of psychic quality. He found that the Pleasure/Displeasure principle and the Reality principle were to be regarded as genetically non-sequential, *simultaneous* events: *"the conscious and the unconscious thus constantly produced together do function as if they were binocular therefore capable of correlation and self-regard. Because of the manner of its genesis, impartial register of psychic quality of the self is precluded: the 'view' of one part by the other is, as it were, 'monocular'"* (LE, 54) . . . *"The model is formed by the exercise of a capacity similar to that which is in evidence when the two eyes operate in binocular vision to correlate two views of the same object. The use in psycho-analysis of conscious and unconscious in viewing a psycho-analytical object is analogous to the use of the two eyes in ocular observation of an object sensible to sight"* ([LE, 86). *"The analyst is therefore in the position of one, who, thanks to the power of 'binocular' perception and consequent correlation that possession of a capacity for conscious and unconscious thought confers, is able to form models and abstractions that serve in elucidating the patient's inability to do the same"* (LE, 104, n. 19. 2.1). The possibility of making a correlation seems to depend on the existence of a difference of vertices (AI, 93).

Philosophical origins

Bion was able to integrate seemingly different but in fact mutually complementary philosophical achievements from Locke, Hume and Kant (Sandler, 1997b). "Binocular" refers to obtaining a discrete image through the constant conjunction (Hume, 1748) of two images by the two human eyes or two sets of lenses, along an imaginary longitudinal axis. The revival and improvement of Aristotle's concept of "common sense" (Locke, 1690) allowed the establishment of a fundamental epistemological method of apprehension of reality, brought to psycho-analysis by Freud and Bion. It is constructed from pairs, or counterpoints. For example, in a dark room one has the tactile impression of fur. A second sense, hearing, informs us that a "meow" is present too (C, 10). The overall perception, and consequently the apprehension of reality, is enhanced. This reality to be apprehended is beyond the spectrum covered by the human sense apparatus; it is the realm of noumena (Kant, 1781), or psychic reality, latent contents in Freud's terms, the psycho-analytic realm (Freud, 1900).

Psycho-analytical roots

In an innovative way, Bion integrated Klein's observations on splitting processes with Freud's theory of the unconscious, specifically concerning their effect in the area of perception (both of the analyst and analysand) and of thinking. He disclosed what Freud himself had already prefigured: the coexistence of the conscious with the unconscious through a dynamic functional in-between, the **contact barrier** (c.v.).

Some Implications The *model* is an epistemological tool to be used in the psycho-analytical session. It provides a way to enlighten previously existent, but hitherto unobserved, clinical facts. Whether it is a concept or a personal way of dealing with clinical matters is open to debate. In my experience it sheds light on some general epistemological issues, to the extent that it can constitute a step forward from what is called "dialectics" in philosophy. Rather than dealing with a pair of competing opposites, under the aegis of Death instincts, it elucidates by operating with a creative couple, taking into account the product of the antithetical pair: Oedipus

(Sandler, 1997b). Regarding *"correlation and self-regard"*, "binocular vision" is an unattainable ideal mode of functioning that makes allowances for neither conscious nor unconscious predominance. The correlation and self-regard refers to the levels of psychic functioning but also refers to a capacity for self-apprehension of one's own self. In other words, to apprehend whom one really is. It paves the way to awareness of whatever it is, up to a point. Binocular vision allows insight; the patient and the analyst are a binocular. When functioning intra-psychically, binocular vision means learning from experience and self-observation. It cannot be done without the help of others; in the first instance, from mother.

"Monocular", in contrast, refers to the "view" that one system, either conscious or unconscious, "holds" of the other. "Binocular" thus applies to integration, while "monocular" refers to splitting in cognitive processes (the realm of perception) as well as in thought processes. In clinical practice this model helps to elicit the latent content from the unfolding conscious material, not unlike a musical counterpoint. By way of correlation and contrast it highlights the patient's inability to bring to bear his/her own binocular vision. The model generated further clarifications of notions that had been lurking in Freud's original insights: *"nothing can be conscious without having been unconscious"* (C, 71; LE, 8). Any analytic session displays a dream-like nature, so far unobserved; through binocular vision the analyst may *"dream the session"* (C, 38, 39, 43). The patient's consciously verbalized material is akin to the manifest dream content, and can be dealt with as such.

I suggest that "binocular vision" helps the analyst to tolerate paradoxes without rushing into an attempt to solve them (Sandler, 1997b, 2000a,b, 2001a,b,c). In psychic reality it expresses a basic fact of human life as it is: the fundamental "supremely creative couple" (Klein, 1932; Money-Kyrle, 1968). A baby is "monocularly" hungry; a breast provides a "second view". A good (or bad) breast is the experiential binocular outcome of a matching non-sensuous pair, i.e. mother-baby. Binocular vision provides two points of view susceptible to being integrated, through common sense, into a kind of "son" or "daughter". This is a transient act dependent on the data then available; a living process, bound to develop. A bad breast can be seen as the former "binocular outcome" of the matching of a mouth and a nipple. Now it is the "monocular" component on standby, waiting to be matched with yet another counterpoint provided by a further experience. The "former bad breast" can turn into a good breast; or lead to a more integrated view, in a ceaseless cycle of matching pairs. The marriage of two points of view produces a third that is neither the first nor the second, which creates something new and, thus, unknown. This can be observed in *all* areas of human activity: the formation of thought processes; the mother-baby relationship; the creative sexual couple; the perception of reality; the marriage between an artist and his/her media, a psycho-analyst and his/her patient's conscious/unconscious material. The unknown, new "product" of binocular vision is, respectively, the apprehension of thoughts without a thinker, maternal love for a son or a daughter, "percepts" of facts; a work of art, an insight in an analytical session and so on. This insight is the product of the meeting of the person with him/herself: an elementary "two-ness", the internal basic group.

As always occurs in Bion's strictly scientific and analytic outlook, there is no judgmental value involved. The useful, but risky, use of binocular vision, coupled with the alleviating but dangerous prevalence of monocular vision, or of one vertex, is depicted in the approaching end of his life in many parts of *A Memoir of the Future*. For example, the talks in Book III, between pre-natal somites and post-natal boys, grown ups and old personalities that are parts of himself. A compacted whole that depicts the analyst at work, limitations of analysis and of the human being who practises it and the observational theory of binocular vision is offered in Book I. This includes Dodgsonian mathematics and the place of dreaming and alpha-function:

> And what seductions, treasures remain to be unveiled, concealed (though betrayed) by Memory and its binocular, Desire?. . . the range is microscopic from one vertex, and yet too enormous to be likely to be bridged by anything so trifling, so trivial as the products of the human animal. Even so stupendous (on one scale of measurement) a mind as that of Pascal, when face to face with what he and others cooperatively can reveal in the domain of the space of visual capacity alone, was only able to arouse fear and cravings for omnipotent power. Ces espaces infinies m'effraient. Newton's vertex, whether employed in the religious or the scientific domain, cost him the disintegration of his mind. Henry IV, limiting himself

to the ambition to possess Paris, could do so because its cost appeared to correspond to the smallness of his ambitions—a Mass "only". He, like Pascal and Newton, made his vertex "binocular", but with one eye relatively blind. Nelson, a man of action like Henry IV, could achieve his ambitions so long as he used an eye that was "blind" for purposes of "not" seeing (which is different from "seeing"; that activity he left to the "better" half . . . The revelatory instrument, if used, could be employed by the object scrutinized to look at the scrutineer in the other sense (direction). The poet or genius can look at the scientist or genius, and the revelations, as at the opposite ends of the telescope, are too large and too small to be tolerable or even to be recognizably related. It is felt to be the "fault" of the instrument that brings such different objects together. But it might be the "fault" of the objects for being so different—or is it the human animal that has to "use" its accumulations of facts, that it has not the experience that would enable it to "understand" what it sees, blind or sightful? Time I went to sleep. Excuse me . . . (Exit to α. [AMF, I, 55–7]

Suggested cross-references: Atonement, Analytic View, Constant Conjunction, Invariances, and Selected Fact.

"Bionian":

P.A. We are all scandalized by bigotry. We are none of us bigot-generators; that is, we none of us admit to being the spring from whom bigotry flows. As a result we do not recognize those of our offspring of whose characters we disapprove. [AMF, II, 228]

A term much used after Bion's death, corresponding to the phenomena that he described as the ways the group deals with the mystic.

The counterpart in reality to which this term refers, corresponds to a group's shared hallucination. Out of despair, there is a pervasive feeling in the group that the group itself or some of its members have found a saviour.

The same had happened with Freud, who prohibited the use of the term "Freudian" (see Jones' biography of Freud). Klein experienced the same thing; she became perplexed when she heard people saying "Kleinians". According to Bion (AMF, II, 259), she was warned about the impossibility of doing anything to counter her group's deluded functioning.

Bion left some remarks on idolization in some talks between the characters P.A. and Priest (AMF, II and III). At the end of his life— scarcely two months before he met his fate—he left a testimony that leaves no margin for doubt:

> Comparing my own personal experience with the history of psycho-analysis, and even the history of human thought that I have tried to sketch out roughly, it does seem to be rather ridiculous that one finds oneself in a position of being supposed to be in that line of succession, instead of just one of the units in it. It is still more ridiculous that one is expected to participate in a sort of competition for precedence as to who is top. Top of what? Where does it come in this history? Where does psycho-analysis itself come? What is the dispute about? What is this dispute in which one is supposed to be interested? I am always hearing—as I have always done—that I am a Kleinian, that I am crazy. Is it possible to be interested in that sort of dispute? I find it very difficult to see how this could possibly be relevant against the background of the struggle of the human being to emerge from barbarism and a purely animal existence, to something one could call a civilized society. [C, 377]

His remarks on wars among psycho-analysts (AMF, II, 273) are relevant to the idea of "-ians" of any kind. One may also enjoy or hate his descriptions of the behaviour of groups of analysts (C, 303, on a typical "scientific meeting" and 327, on candidates of the institutes).

Taking into account that Bion makes at least two references to Dr Samuel Johnson on truth, one is reminded of other ideas of this outstanding Englishman of the Enlightenment. Namely, the latter's remarks on Nationalism. He thought that it constitutes the "last refuge of the scoundrel". All "-isms" and "-ians" in the psycho-analytic movement can be regarded as aping reflections of the macro-social fact, "Nationalism", in the micro-cosmos of the psycho-analytic establishments. Both share the nature of hallucination (q.v.)—perceptions devoid of an object in reality.

> ROBIN At least we have so far avoided forming ourselves into an Institution with a doctrine and a uniform—not even a mental uniform.

> P.A. So far. I have been surprised to find that even *my* name has been bandied about. I used to think Melanie Klein was a bit

optimistic and unrealistic—though sincere—in deploring the idea that people would call themselves Kleinian. Freud was alert to the danger that many would want to climb under the umbrella of "psycho-analysis", but I did not expect to find myself included amongst the brightly, but rapidly fading, coloured ephemera of spiritual refreshment. [AMF, II, 259]

He had more to warn about himself as analyst, placing in subtle, colloquial ways the widespread tendency to nurture narcissism and paranoid nuclei, with its concomitant abhorrence of analysis:

P.A. I am not aware that we pride ourselves or deprecate ourselves on account of our being ordinary members of the human race. Like my fellows I would be gratified if I discovered that I was in some way excellent; in fact I have found no evidence of my "excellence" as a psycho-analyst.

ALICE Your colleagues think highly of you.

P.A. Some do, luckily; I am not unappreciative of the fact, but it tells me more of the generosity and affection of my colleagues than of *my* merits. [AMF, III, 540–41]

Suggested cross-reference: Kleinian.
📖 "Why we cannot call ourselves Bionians", by Parthenope Bion Talamo.

Bizarre objects: Bion first described bizarre objects when he studied schizophrenic thought (q.v.) (ST, 39). He observed that in the same sense that the infant phantasizes sadistic attacks on the nourishing breast, psychotics direct such attacks to its apparatus of perception. Taking into account that Bion accepted Freud's hypothesis about consciousness—as a sense organ for perception of psychic reality—these attacks result in damages to consciousness. Bion integrated Freud and Klein's contributions. In this case, he was able to observe that the apparatus used to achieve conscious awareness of internal and external reality is dealt with as an undesired fragment. Therefore it is phantastically expelled from the personality. The apparatus is felt as if it were an "expel-able" fragment. As such, its fate is to be lodged outside.

Deprived of conscious awareness, the patient *"achieves a state which is felt to be neither alive nor dead"* (ST, 38). These three situations, namely, an attack on the breast, on the perceptual apparatus up to its ejection, and the ensuing mental confusion about death and life creates a proneness to deal with the animate with methods that would be more successful if applied to the inanimate.

> In the patient's phantasy the expelled particles of ego lead to an independent and uncontrolled existence outside the personality, but either containing or contained by external objects, where they exercise their functions as if the ordeal to which they have been subjected had served only to increase their number and to provoke their hostility to the psyche that ejected them. In consequence the patient feels himself to be surrounded by bizarre objects . . .

> each particle is felt to consist of a real external object which is encapsulated in a piece of personality that has engulfed it. The character of this complete particle will depend partly on the character of the real object, say a gramophone, and partly on the character of the particle of personality that engulfs it. If the piece of the personality is concerned with sight, the gramophone when played is felt to be watching the patient. If with hearing, then the gramophone when played is felt to be listening to the patient. The object . . . suffuses and controls the piece of personality that engulfs it: to that extent the particle itself is felt to have become a thing. [ST, 39–40]

Therefore, to grasp the concept of bizarre object one must, as Bion did, tolerate a paradox, here expressed simultaneously as to engulf/be engulfed, that occurs between the phantastically expelled fragment of personality and the hallucinated factual object "findable" in external reality.

This object "carries", in the feelings of the beholder, real parts of this same beholder's personality. It has a concrete, factual existence. Due to these two factors, its real nature—that of an hallucination— is often overlooked. For hallucination is a perception devoid of the object. In this case it seems that there is an object; in fact there is not, but to realize this, one must grasp Klein/Bion's illumination quoted above.

Further investigation (in "On hallucination") allowed an even more summarized formulation: ". . . *the patient felt he was surrounded by bizarre objects compounded partly of real objects and partly of fragments of the personality*" (ST, 81). Bion now defines the bizarre objects. This formulation adumbrates a novel kind of psycho-analytic writing, resorting to quasi-poetical metaphors:

> The patient now moves, not in a world of dreams, but not in a world of objects which are ordinarily the furniture of dreams. These objects, primitive yet complex, partake of qualities which in the non-psychotic are peculiar to matter, anal objects, senses, ideas, superego, and the remaining qualities of personality [ST, 40]

To grasp this concept, as others in analysis, one must bear firmly in mind that all of this is phantastic. It is felt as *if it were real. The person under the sway of this kind of mental functioning undergoes a real impoverishment or distortion in the area of thought.*

> ... The reversal of alpha-function did in fact affect the ego and therefore did not produce a simple return to beta-elements, but objects which differ in important respects from the original beta-elements which had no tincture of the personality adhering to them. The beta-element differs from the bizarre object in that the bizarre object is beta-element plus ego and superego traces. [LE, 25]

> This split, enforced by starvation and fear of death through starvation on the one hand, and by love and the fear of associated murderous envy and hate on the other, produces a mental state in which the patient greedily pursues every form of material comfort; he is at once insatiable and implacable in his pursuit of satiation. Since this state originates in a need to be rid of the emotional complications of awareness of life, and a relationship with live objects, the patient appears to be incapable of gratitude or concern either for himself or others. This state involves destruction of his concern for truth. Since these mechanisms fail to rid the patient of his pains, which he feels to be due to lack of something, his pursuit of a cure takes the form of a search for a lost object and ends in increased dependence on material comfort; quantity must be the governing consideration, not quality. He feels surrounded by bizarre objects, so that even the material comforts are bad and unable to satisfy his needs. [LE, 11]

The interpretations are likewise swallowed as inanimate bizarre objects. They are taken at their face value and appearance. The patient increasingly demands more and more of them because they are taken for what they are not, so that they are destroyed in the bud; they carry no wisdom or love. The latter are animate features. The patient "*uses an equipment suited for contact with the inanimate to establish contact with himself*"; confusion ensues when he becomes aware that he is alive. When the production of bizarre objects is prevalent, there is a search-for-concreteness, but there is always a neurotic part of the personality functioning too: "*the patient does ultimately grasp some of the meaning of what is said to him*" (LE, 12). The enforced splitting creates a situation where material reality prevails at the expense of psychic reality. It differs from states that are "idealistic", hallucinated and deluded, where the flights into imagination seem to be less amenable to being dealt with through psycho-analysis.

The bizarre object partakes of the features of hallucination; it is a building block of delusions, which are clusters of hallucinations linked by rational constructs where reason is a slave of memory (in neurotics) and desire (in psychotics). Bizarre objects have often had a built-in feature: "*something analogous to a capacity of judgement*" (ST, 81). This is easily seen if one remembers that the situations that are well known in analysis as fetishism and collectionism are founded by bizarre objects. They are usually accompanied by guilt or a kind of financial sense of profit.

Finally, Bion correlates cure and explanations to the analyst's constructions (in Freud's sense of the term), to bizarre objects. "*It appeared to me, during this period of the analysis . . . that some of his delusions were attempts at employing bizarre objects in the service of thera-peutic intuition*" (ST, 82). In this we see that the "pathological" vertex was being dispensed with. Bion was already taking Freud's posture about symptoms to its last consequences. Freud regarded symptoms, or that which was hitherto regarded as "illness", as a kind of court of last-resort, a last attempt towards an equilibrium or homeostasis that had health itself as its goal.

⊘ The area encompassed by bizarre objects was expanded with Bion's increased realization about the lack of utility of the "pathol-ogy" vertex. His view that the psychotic personality and the non-psychotic personality operated in tandem continuously is an expression of his change.

Thanks to Bion's contributions one may state today that bizarre objects are the hallucination of everyday life. They form the social fabric of most human "non-mutual" relations, of inanimate interests, of the hypocrisy of social life. Bion would characterize bizarre objects and the permanent underlying layer of hallucinosis when establishing the concepts of alpha-function, beta-elements and transformations (q.v.).

Bizarre objects appear in an illustrated and vivid form in the Trilogy *A Memoir of the Future*. Consumerism, fetishism, fanaticism, and politicking may be activities in which the basic tool is bizarre objects. In all of Bion's work, there is an invariance that permeates beta-elements and bizarre objects, in so far as they share the characteristics of beta-elements: *"the moral component"* (T, 64).

&; The author once suggested that the realm of bizarre objects could be expanded if one could detect seemingly comprehensible beta-elements (Sandler, 1990,1997). In this view, collectionism and fashion may be regarded as composed of bizarre objects. Also, in a session of analysis, there can be prejudiced shared values—even a shared language that remains unchecked would belong to this area.

Breast, good and bad: Bion starts from Freud and especially from Klein concerning the basic function performed by the relationship of the infant with the breast. Namely, how it contributes to shaping of the personality (or mind, psyche, character, whatever name one may prefer to give to it). The word "basic" is used here in the sense of something necessary, inescapable and fundamental.

Unpublished (or posthumously published) theory

Bion displayed a distinct preference for developing observational theories for the psycho-analyst's use, rather than for creating new theories to add to the already huge apparatus available. One of the few exceptions, which would remain unpublished during his lifetime, was a paper entitled "Metatheory". It was an attempt to describe *scientifically*some elementary basics of psycho-analysis. One of its terms is "Breast". Like "penis", "splitting" and "violent emotions" it was devised as a *"class of interpretations"* (C, 253).

Bion seems to have attempted to formulate a stopgap when a fully scientific theory and method were not available in psychoanalysis: *"I propose to improvise temporary solutions of our problems by these short interjections of metatheory between the discussions of successive elements of theory"* (C, 254). The *"interpretation breast"* is made in conjunction with the *"interpretation penis"* (refer to the entry, Penis).

He treats the "name given to the word 'breast'", as a hypothesis, following Hume's view *"that a hypothesis is the expression of a subjective sense that certain associations are constantly conjoined, and is not a representation corresponding to an actuality"*. Breast is a condensation *"into the verbal counterpart of a visual image. . ."* (C, 250). Breast is not treated as a symbol nor as a thing-in-itself; it is *"a definitory hypothesis that can be used by the analyst to provide the patient with the selected fact that he cannot find for himself"* (C, 251).

The theory that was published during his lifetime

Bion scrutinizes the role of the infant-mother relationship as a function in the formation and development of thought processes. The inception of consciousness and all processes of cognition and contact with inner and outer reality are seen under this vertex. Bion values in a hitherto unavailable manner the function of the emotional experiences (q.v.) as seen in relationships. He offers a way out of the excessive and violent valuing of feelings, affects and so on. This overvaluing is visible in patients and professionals alike. They take feelings, affects and emotions as things-in-themselves, which would be amenable to be studied per se. Academic psychology and superficial psychology already do this.

The way out appears with the aid of Descartes, albeit in a negative sense. One may refer to the entries under the headings on "Thinking" in this dictionary. In the present entry we will examine more minutely, as Bion did, how things occur. There he described *what* the things were that occurred; now we will follow him to see *how* they occur.

There are soft-humanist and paradisiacal phantasies that marked and still mark strong tendencies of the psycho-analytic movement. These tendencies ape the paradisiacal phantasies stemming from the Principle of Nirvana, as Freud called it. In other terms, hate directed to the principle of reality or hate of truth, as Bion puts it. These tendencies form an ideological cosmology and shape the understanding of psycho-analytic theories that already exist and obviously form a specific kind of theory too. The views on cure, mothering and the good breast can be influenced by the Nirvana principle, which may prevail in the mind of the professional.

Bion reverses this tendency. He proposes to examine the hypothesis that what really matters is not the good breast, or more precisely, the breast that is felt as good, in the sense that Klein described it. Quite the contrary, what allows the inception of thinking processes and symbol formation—first and foremost, the symbolization of the breast itself—is its un-materialization or "psychic-ization", with the experiencing of the no-breast (see also the entry, Circle, Point, Line). One gets an idea of a real breast through the absent, frustrating breast, rather than through the positive, "satisfying" concrete breast:

> This breast is an object the infant needs to supply it with milk and good internal objects. I do not attribute to the infant an awareness of this need; but I do attribute to the infant an awareness of a need not satisfied. We can say the infant feels frustrated if we assume the existence of some apparatus with which frustration can be experienced. Freud's concept of consciousness as that of "a sense organ for the perception of psychical qualities", provides such apparatus.
>
> . . . We can see that the bad, that is to say wanted but absent, breast is much more likely to become recognized as an idea than the good breast which is associated with what a philosopher would call a thing-in-itself or a thing-in-actuality, in that the sense of a good breast depends on the existence of milk the infant has in fact taken. The good breast and the bad breast, the one being associated with the actual milk that satisfies hunger and the other with the non-existence of that milk, must have a difference in psychical quality . . . Let us suppose the infant to have fed but to be feeling unloved . . . It if it is correct to suppose that the central question rests on discrimination of psychical quality and if consciousness is legitimately regarded as the sense-organ of psychical quality it is difficult to see how consciousness comes into existence . . . We must assume that the good breast and the bad breast are emotional experiences. [LE, 34–35]

Metatheory

Is the baby aware of the necessity of milk as well as of good objects? Or is it race, biology-dependent? This necessity simply is; in a

certain sense, it is the thing-in-itself that cannot be known consciously. Is it life itself, or is it the instinctual basis of life itself? The
sheer factuality by means of which this necessity manifests itself
may correspond to the unknowable mystery of life. The breast is a
source of the maintenance of life. Conversely, if a necessity is not to
be satisfied, to use Bion's wording, a negative feeling towards the
good breast may ensue. The absent breast is equated to the bad
breast. If the bad breast can be tolerated, this allows for the inception of the thought, "breast". Or the bad breast **cannot** be tolerated
and this ignites hallucination akin to the Paradise described in
Genesis, an autistic or religious state.

A great many of Bion's efforts were devoted to elaborating theories of observation in psycho-analysis, destined to enhance the
scientific validity of the psycho-analytical method. Nevertheless,
Bion once used the term "breast" as part of one of his rare attempts
at a theory in psycho-analysis.

It must be noticed that he uses the *term* to do it; the term and the
theory must not be confused with their counterparts in reality. It is
advisable to take into account that the term "breast" already has a
long history in the psycho-analytical movement; it has acquired a
strong appeal for analysts. This fact determines that the term
embodies a sizable penumbra of associations around it.

Bion called his attempt at a comprehensive theory of psycho-
analysis, metatheory. It was an attempt to add precision to the then
existing theories in psycho-analysis. This attempt was probably
made between 1962 and 1964; Francesca Bion made it public in
1992. It seems to precede Bion's theory of Transformations.

In this theory, the term "breast" is used to mark a constant conjunction—Bion uses Hume's terms, that is, facts felt as reuniting in a
subjective sense; or as a condensation—here Bion uses Freud's terms.

Indeed, Bion uses the term "breast" as a means for the analyst
to provide a selected fact (q.v.) to the patient who cannot obtain it
for himself, in the here and now of the session. The term "breast"
seems to fulfil a function of knowledge to the infant, to the analytic
couple in the here and now of the session and to the analyst as a
valid theory (formulated by Klein, after Freud) It conveys, albeit
imperfectly, its counterpart in reality *as it is*.

The reality here, of the "breast" being the selected fact and
furnishing a selected fact, is seen as the ever-evolving event,

life-like, sharing with the numinous realm some of the living mysteries of life itself. In advancing the theory of the breast, Bion uses all his earlier theories of thinking, formation of concepts, and the nourishing effect of the breast in helping to cope with the first and foremost fact of life; a frustration-ridden, ever-evolving fact— life itself.

Why is such a word used? In what sense is it illuminating to employ a term with such a penumbra of associations (many of which are physical, concrete, primitive and sensuous) to provide a definitory hypothesis, functioning as a selected fact, for the situation in analysis which, on the face of it, bears no resemblance to the historical meaning of the breast? The situation in the analysis that requires the use of the term, "breast", requires it precisely because it has become so divorced from the penumbra of associations adhering to breast that it bears superficially no resemblance to them. It requires it because breast, if the interpretation is correct, is a hypothesis in the Humean sense which fixes a constellation of associations that are constantly conjoined but have lost their connection with the material expressed by the free associations of the analysis, these last having become conjoined with material now alienated from, or never in contact with, the penumbra of associations of breast. The juxtaposition, by interpretation of breast, to the events of the analysis can be seen to resemble, as I have already said, a provision by the analyst of a selected fact that the patient cannot find for himself, but there are also important differences. The selected fact is a discovery made by the patient or individual and is the tool by which he ensures the constant progression, the very essence of learning and therefore of growing. This is represented by the sequence: paranoid–schizoid position, selected fact (precipitating coherence of the elements of the paranoid–schizoid position) ushering in the depressive position, which then instantaneously reveals yet vaster areas of hitherto unrelated elements belonging to domains of the paranoid–schizoid position which were previously unrevealed and unsuspected—a revelation that contributes to the depression peculiar to the depressive position. The *selected fact* then is an essential element in a process of discovery. The *interpretation*—employing definitory hypothesis, such as breast, which have many resemblances to, and in some respects are identical with, the selected fact—is concerned not with the *discovery* so much as with *repair*. [C, 252–3]

Suggested cross-references: Pre-conception, Conception, Saturation, Psycho-analytical objects, Elements of psycho-analysis, Penis.

C

Caesura: An event that simultaneously unites and disunites.

Bion took a few broad avenues opened by Freud and developed them, namely, Freud's theories of dreams, thinking and instincts. More often than not, analysts did not realize them as broad; instead, much like Shakespeare, who would often put some of his immortal insights in the words reserved for seemingly minor characters, Bion realized the full potential ensconced in seemingly minor observations made by Freud, which can be regarded as casual, made "en passant".

The concept of caesura is one of them. In Freud's work it was a penetrating observation. It was elevated to the status of a concept by Bion. As an annex to his paper delivered in 1977, "Emotional turbulence", which Bion called, "On a quotation by Freud", he uses the concept; perhaps thanks to his emphasis Freud's observation is well known today.

It deals with a paradox; Bion, as Freud before him, does not try to resolve the paradox. He tries to apprehend it and to use it. The paradox is the caesura itself. Caesura marks something that embodies simultaneously something that flows continually, and at the same time, because of its "formidable" sensuously apprehensible appearances, it seems to undergo a total change. There are changes, but they are not all-encompassing as they seem to be. Again and again, outward appearances are deceiving; after all, beauty is more than skin deep. The same underlying truth functions in PS⇔D; in the two principles of mental functioning; in the interplay between conscious and unconscious; reality sensuous and psychic; container and contained. This "truth" can be apprehended if one tolerates a paradox.

The concept of caesura is well-suited for displaying some of the difficulties in communicating real psycho-analysis in written form. Also, it displays some difficulties intrinsic to actually doing real analysis in the analytical setting, to the extent it depends on verbal formulations. Verbal formulations are almost impervious to expressing the tolerance of paradoxes that is needed to make analysis and to live life as it is.

The concept can be seen as the mode of functioning of the contact barrier (q.v.) and of transformations and invariances (q.v.). Freud's now classical example dealt with the perception of the formidable continuities between pre-natal and post-natal life. This perception can be hampered if and when one mesmerizes oneself with the "formidable caesura of birth". Bion would expand the concept in the essay "Caesura"—also from 1977.

Again in 1977, in *A Memoir of the Future*'s dialogues, there is a specific one between the fictitious-real characters "Paul" (who stands for a priest); "Roland" (the foolhardy common man who acts out instead of thinking); "Alice" (a weak but sensitive woman), and "P.A." (who stands for a psycho-analyst). The characters may be regarded as part-objects of Bion, subsuming his life experiences. In this dialogue, which is in the form of free association, one of the characters, "P.A.", makes a kind of ironic exhortation, inspired by John Ruskin. Namely, that some people "of course had read the classics". The character "Roland" says, "Touché", signalling that he had not read them properly but had got the message to go and read them. The free associations follow on, centring in a most clear definition of caesura:

> PAUL I don't know why, but you reminded me of a cartoon which I once saw in the *New Yorker* in which a duellist, having just delivered a mortal stroke, says "Touché".

ROLAND I saw a horrible photograph of a duel between two people armed with sabres in which one had decapitated his opponent in one stroke. I was not really claiming to have been so completely separated from my nervous system, or the seat of my intelligence.

ALICE You often talk as if, because I am a woman, I can't ever have had an intelligence from which to be separated.

P.A. Perhaps that is because he has never been completely separated from his primordial mind and is still dominated by the belief that as a woman has not got a penis she cannot have a capacity for masculine thinking.

ALICE Does the caesura connect or separate? He often behaves as if he were not a male sexual animal.

ROLAND That's not fair! You're behaving like a female sexual animal and I can hardly be blamed if I am cautious—sometimes.

PAUL This is not an occasion for display of matrimonial experience. But if I say so, it will be assumed that I and my nominally saintly predecessor are opposed to sex. The biological creator does not appear to be on good terms with the creator of morals. Verbal intercourse is not granted the freedom that sociologically we are supposed to have.

P. A. Freedom often seems to be driven "underground"—or should I say "subterrane"?

ALICE Please yourself; but suppose both the dictator and liberator go underground and meet there.

P.A. I shall avail myself of your permission to say "infra-conceptual".

PAUL Well, *that* is horrible enough to escape durability as an artistic expression. The world of thought shrinks its boundaries in inverse proportion to the length of the verbal weapons it uses; the shorter the "bayonet" the wider the empire it sways. [AMF, II, 248–9]

Thanks to splitting and concretization we usually think in terms of the mind/body conundrum. Hence Paul's first phrase in the dialogue. "Day life experiences" would constitute P.A.'s talk on the classics. As happens with free associations, in a way not unlike that of a *bricolage*, the cartoon of the American weekly magazine furnishes the form, the "carcass" that clothes and thus expresses his thinking. It is meaningful that it is reserved to a "Priest" to assume the careful posture of trying "not to put asunder that which God reunited". The cartoon's duellist kills—the factual actuality, the concrete, material existence ceases to be. Life's immaterial nature is not separable from material survival; in the cartoon it may express a kind of gentleman-like aplomb that would sound ridiculous and misplaced if life itself is at stake; "Touché". The common man, "Roland", takes the clue: he remarks on how difficult it is **not** to separate mind and body.

"Alice" enters into the debate. This debate may be seen, up to that point, as a "male" affair. Or, in other terms, the caesura between male and female "*cannot be stable*" (AMF, I, 196). Her contribution seems to be enlivening, as only females can be with male issues. It is now that analysis comes to the fore: the envy of the breast, the contempt towards women, displays its face. The dialogue goes on, displaying the caesura as an event that is characterized by simultaneous union and dis-union. Its earliest roots—Freud's three essays on sexuality—are resumed in "P.A.'s intervention: "*Perhaps that is because he has never been completely separated from his primordial mind and is still dominated by the belief that as a woman has not got a penis she cannot have a capacity for masculine thinking.*"

"Alice" goes on, making the issue explicit: "*Does the caesura connect or separate? He often behaves as if he were not a male sexual animal*". Now we enter into the area of two-person relationships: female and male and the mystery that encircles (pro)creation.

"Paul", the "Priest", intervenes now and quotes Christ, warning about super-ego and morals. "P.A." supposes that freedom—sexual freedom, mental freedom—is a manifestation of psychic reality. It is more than skin deep. "*Freedom often seems to be driven 'underground'—or should I say 'subterrane'.*" Freud, after all, suggested that the unconscious and the id were "deep". "Alice" is now able to furnish a kind of social counterpart of the apparent split between the dictator and liberator. In reality this is a caesura: both meet in the "underground", meaning, in their minds. It is a well-known fact that the worst dictators thought highly of themselves. They thought they were just liberators (or benefactors, etc.). Significantly, both leftists and rightists buy their weapons from the same vendors.

"Priest", the mystic, is a character more prone to have glimpses of the "infinite", the invariance, the transcendence. Transcendence is that which gives the immaterial "substance" to formulations that prove to be valuable. They are valuable if the meaning that they convey is truthfully real. But to be so, they must be immaterial. They must transcend the factual form or formulation; the shell, the phenomenon. "Priest" (sometimes Bion called this character "Paul") seems to be more able to warn about the limitations of verbal formulations to express "O". His warning begins with an admonition towards the character "P.A.". Namely, that his attempts at scientific formulations lack elegance. The caesura proceeds to splitting when it is not tolerated.

Misuses and misconceptions: Despite the clarity of Bion's text, it seems to many readers that it is just the sensuous bombardment of changing appearances that counts. Usually the concept is taken as if it simply meant a break, an interruption. Its double, paradoxical nature of inner [continuity] ⇔ [sensuously] apprehensible break is thus denied.

📖 Parthenope Bion Talamo attempted a clinical application of the concept.

&; The author proposes to name the basic psycho-analytic posture "tolerance of paradoxes".

Catastrophic change, catastrophe: Broadly speaking, the term catastrophe is used by Bion to depict a sudden perturbation or change in a given real or hallucinated status quo. This perturbation leads to the destruction of the status quo. It marks a resistance to growth, especially as regards experiencing the depressive position.

It was gradually endowed with the qualities of a concept, which was developed throughout the whole of Bion's work. It does not depict an external world event. Therefore one must avoid using the term as if it were a commonplace—which it is in common language. Many times Bion uses terms with the same meaning they have in common language, but this has exceptions and "catastrophe" is one of them. The term must not be debased, as it is if it is mistaken for trauma. Many times Bion wants the reader to be reminded of the common usage, but the sense of the phrase must convey something more. This is the case here, for it is used to depict a mental configuration. There is no causality implicated.

It is more easily seen in certified psychotics; this was Bion's pathway to eliciting the existence of this particular configuration. Nevertheless, even if it must be seen as a psychotic state, it is not confined to the province of certified psychotics. It is detectable in everyday occurrences and in dreams. It marks a resistance to growth.

⊕ It was outlined from the time of Bion's first papers; its final formulation and illumination appears in *A Memoir of the Future, The Long-Week End and War Memoirs*.

In *A Memoir of the Future* the concept of catastrophic change can be regarded as the one of underlying selected facts that characterizes the whole Trilogy. Many of the multiple descriptions of these changes are linked to at least two of Bion's experiences: war and disillusion, namely, the loss of his fellows-in-arms; the loss of confidence in politicians and officials. For example, after his return from war his mother became unable to address him with the previously customary treatment ("Dear"). In *The Long Week End*, the catastrophic change appears as the aftermath of Bion's posture with his daughter Parthenope as a baby, and his first wife Betty's pregnancy (TLWE, II). It was subsumed by a quotation from Shakespeare's Hamlet: "Nymph, in thy orisons, be all my sins remembered". In *War Memoirs*, it is depicted in Bion's quasi-suicidal reaction when under heavy fire in precarious shelters (WM, 94 and 106). In brief, catastrophic change, or changes that are felt as catastrophic, are wholly dependent on working-through of the depressive position.

As with any really useful psycho-analytic concept, it has a foot in the possibilities that outstanding analysts had to work through some of their life experiences, as representative samples of the human mind. For example, Oedipus and Freud's personal experiences with his mother and father; Manic states, Envy/Greed and Melanie Klein's experiences with her progeny.

Catastrophic change can be regarded as a resistance to natural change, which is felt by some people as catastrophic. The "habit to habits" seems to express reactions against change. Its basis is a kind of constitution of the personality whose motto could be *"Thus far and no further"* (AMF, II, 237); when clung to it equals autism. To deny it construes a catastrophe; to face it risks another kind of catastrophe—at least in the eyes of the beholder.

The feeling that a catastrophe had occurred is linked to cravings for pleasure, intolerance of frustration and, above all, intolerance of the absence of meaning of phenomena. Meaninglessness is felt as intolerable. Ultimately, facts of life such as hate, slaughter and death itself are felt as impossible to face and to deal with: "... *the patient's intolerance of meaninglessness is not interpreted: he will pour out a flood of words so that he can evoke a response indicating that a meaning exists either in his own behaviour or in that of the analyst. Since the first requisite for the discovery of the meaning of any conjunction depends on the ability to admit that phenomena may have no meaning, an inability to admit that they have no meaning stifles the possibility of curiosity at the outset*" (T, 81). The perspective of a catastrophic change is present when the analyst faces psychotic strata of his own personality which were not worked through.

This term tries to encircle a complex emotional experience as a reaction before some kinds of stimuli. This reaction may be realistic or not. In any case it conveys a sense of catastrophe. This sense of catastrophe may obtrude as a premonition, as a hallucinated reaction or as a realistic reaction.

Catastrophic change is linked to attempts to deny some facts, namely:

(i)   Natural change.
(ii) The unknown and uncontrollable nature of emotional reality as it is.
(iii) Violent inception of feared inner truths.
(iv) Peculiarities of reaction to external sudden, unexpected, denied and/or violent stimuli. They may provoke—to many people—a situation that the person is left *"naked, incongruous, alien, without a point of reference that made sense"* (AMF, I, 27).

The violence may either be real or not. As examples of change, Bion quotes apparently changing behaviour that is easily apprehended by the senses. This is the case of a psychotic breakdown as it is seen in classical psychiatry. This kind of change is described in *Transformations*. The change shelters the un-change: psychosis was already present in the pre-catastrophic phase as psycho-somatic complains; in the post-catastrophic phase it reveals itself by a changed outward appearance, as autism.

Another kind of change is that of facts external to us. They form a very broad range: from stellar movements that provoke the extinction of beings that were developed during trillions of years, to social events such as that depicted in the opening chapters of *A Memoir of the Future*—the invasion of an "English Farm". Modelled after the attempts of the Nazi invasion of the British Islands, it states explicitly, *"True, there was defeat, but this was on a scale of defeat so disastrous that it would be necessary to suppose that something analogous to the Norman Conquest had taken place"* (AMF, I, 27).

Nevertheless the change produced is not necessarily catastrophic, as a matter of fact. This sense is conveyed by the colloquial meaning of the word, but the development of the concept gradually brought it near to the intrapsychic situation. It occurred after Bion had proposed the theory of container and contained (1962). It came to mean a catastrophe to a container that will be destroyed by the contained. Birth and death are this kind of event; it can be linked to growth.

Points of view

It is necessary to observe the point of view under which the term is used:

(i) It can be the point of view dictated by judgmental values; the change will be feared. It always implies that change—any change—is wrong due to the pain involved. It is pain before the unknown when omniscience prevails, but it is not restricted to that. Changes are unavoidable when a situation of loss exists. To the greedy and omnipotent characters this is a seemingly unbearable fact.

(ii) It can be an observational point of view: there is an appreciation of the event quite independently of the pain involved or any judgmental value.

Therefore it is always *felt* as catastrophic by the individual who fears change and growth, who fears contact with his or her psychic reality as it is. If it shelters hate, the patient's reaction resembles depression; if it shelters love, the patient may become persecuted. *"Mental evolution or growth is catastrophic and timeless"* (AI, 108). This is seen in the most basic human achievements. It was first observed in certified psychotics:

> From the patient's point of view the achievement of verbal thought has been a most unhappy event. Verbal thought is so interwoven with catastrophe and the painful emotion of depression that the patient, resorting to projective identification, splits it off and pushes it into the analyst. The results are again unhappy for the patient; lack of this capacity is now felt by him to be the same thing as being insane. On the other hand, reassumption of this capacity seems to him to be inseparable from depression and awareness, on a reality level this time, that he is "insane". This fact tends to give reality to the patient's phantasies of the catastrophic results that would accrue were he to risk re-introjection of his capacity for verbal thought . . . The analyst's problem is the patient's dread, now quite manifest, of attempting a psycho-analytic understanding of what they mean for him, partly because the patient now understands that psycho-analysis demands from him that very verbal thought which he dreads. [ST, 32]

In a group, catastrophic change is seen as such when a basic assumption must be abandoned. The group nourishes these feelings of abhorrence towards change in a particularly marked way:

> The assumption underlying loyalty to the K link is that the personality of analyst and analysand can survive the loss of its protective coat of lies, subterfuge, evasion and hallucination and may even be fortified and enriched by the loss. It is an assumption strongly disputed by the psychotic and a fortiori by the group, which relies on psychotic mechanisms for its coherence and sense of well being. [T, 129]

Clinical situation

In *Transformations*, pages 8, 9 and 10, Bion describes the psychotic breakdown of a patient and its accompanying set of acted-out events. Those events occur in tandem with the patient's skilful manipulation of feelings and emotions destined to provoke some emotional states in the encircling milieu—which includes the analyst. The patient performs this through projective identifications destined to rid him of certain feelings. It will depend on the analyst's ability to maintain an analytical posture whether or not this fact constitutes a problem.

Part of these appearances is constituted by the analysand's emotionally charged behaviour. He or she performs a role, namely, the role of a fool. To be fooled by outward appearances was something that Freud did not do. Not to be fooled by the violent imposition of them will determine the outcome.

The analyst, Ulysses-like, should become impervious to the siren of propaganda. In a certain sense if he or she divests himself of memory, desire and understanding, he or she becomes immune to the make-believe situations the patient tries to impose. This is especially true of the situations that are presented as catastrophic.

The analyst bestows names that make psycho-analytic sense to some events; for example, physical pains and even illnesses, or hypochondriacal symptoms. The analyst does not take them at their face value when he or she can see that these names reflect the state of the patient's internal objects. If this recognition is possible, a more adequate name can be attributed to them.

The patient, his or her relatives, friends and also the doctor who made the referral, are prone to resort to acting-out: "*impending lawsuits, mental hospitals, certification, and other contingencies apparently appropriate to the change in circumstances, are really hypochondriacal pains and other evidences of internal objects in a guise appropriate to their new status as external objects*" (T, 9).

Bion describes the ensuing catastrophe: it is catastrophic **to the maintenance of analysis,** which necessarily includes self-containment, insight and some degree of contact with one's psychic reality in a responsible way. This is replaced by a mounting crisis involving people other than the analytic pair. The crisis is an extrapolation of the limits of the analytic consulting room: "*It is catastrophic in the restricted sense of an event producing a subversion of the order or system of things; it is catastrophic in the sense that it is accompanied by feelings of disaster in the participants; it is catastrophic in the sense that it is sudden and violent in an almost physical way . . . there are three features to which I wish to draw attention: subversion of the system, invariance (q.v.), and violence (q.v.)*" (T, 8).

I would stress the word "feelings", which must be taken in its exact sense. To feel is not necessarily "to be". The same issue is the crux of a problem with Melanie Klein's writings on projective identification.

The pre- and post-catastrophic moments

A fundamental difference is the emotion that is or is not easily apprehended by the senses. Hypochondriacal elements may lack ideational counterparts of violence. This can be seen as theoretical:

> Analysis in the pre-catastrophic stage is to be distinguished from the post-catastrophic stage by the following superficial characteristics: it is unemotional, theoretical, and devoid of any marked outward change. Hypochondriacal symptoms are prominent. The material lends itself to interpretations based on Kleinian theories of projective identification and internal and external objects. Violence is confined to phenomena experienced by psycho-analytical insight: it is, as it were, *theoretical* violence. The patient talks as if his behaviour, outwardly amenable, was causing great destruction because of its violence. The analyst gives interpretations, when they appear to be appropriate to the material, drawing attention to the features that are supposed by the patient to be violent.
>
> In the post-catastrophic stage, by contrast, the violence is patent, but the ideational counterpart, previously evident, appears to be lacking. Emotion is obvious and is aroused in the analyst. Hypochondriacal elements are less obtrusive. The emotional experience does not have to be conjectured because it is apparent. [T, 8–9]

The discrimination calls for a clinical search for invariances in the domain represented by theories of projective identifications and internal/external objects (q.v.): "... *the analyst must search the material for invariants to the pre- and post-catastrophic stages ... restating this in terms of the clinical material, he must see, and demonstrate, that certain apparently external emotionally-charged events are in fact the same events as those which appeared in the pre-catastrophic stage under the names, bestowed by the patient, of pains in the knee, legs, abdomen, ears, etc., and, by the analyst, of internal objects*" (T,9).

One may see that by catastrophe is meant an event where violence intervenes. Truth emerges when one focuses on "*the invariants or the objects in which invariance is to be detected*". A main invariance is violence itself. From the pre- to the post-catastrophic, "*the change is violent . . . and the new phase is one on which violent feelings are violently expressed"*.

Violence was there in the pre-catastrophic moment, albeit in a non-sensible form. There were violent feelings, but they were not violently expressed. Truth is robust and will prevail: it emerges in the post-catastrophic moment. One faces a fact that is not only one's feelings but also one's violence. Violence is not a feeling; it is a fact. It can be a violence of emotions, for example. Facing the violence one shelters may be felt as catastrophic: the truth of one's violent feelings or violence of feeling (C, 249).

The encircling milieu's response may be catastrophic when doctors, relatives, law officers and psychiatrists become good containers for the patient's projective identification. The phrase "good containers" may give the impression of a misprint. If the reader is surprised or disagrees, this can be due to simplified read-ings of Melanie Klein's concepts that currently prevail—such as a direct transposition from her descriptions that apply to mothers of little babies. In that particular instance, mothers accept, as part of their motherly function, their babies' projective identification as a means of communication. The problem is, the doctors, relatives, law officers and psychiatrists, are not mothers of little babies any more—even though a mother can be involved in this mêlée. The situation is described in an adult setting:

> . . . the patient's state of violent emotion sets up reactions in the analyst and others related to the patient in such a way that *they also tend to be dominated by their over-stimulated internal objects* thus producing a wide externalization of internal objects. [T, 9; my italics]

This is the catastrophe: due to a kind of generalized, crossed projective identification among all involved there is an overall crisis of responsibility. All involved try to get rid of painful stimuli. The encircling milieu uses the stimulus provided by the patient to become "dominated by" its own "over-stimulated objects" too. The analyst has to rely solely on his own analysis. He risks being the object of the hate of the group to the exact extent that he persists in maintaining his analytic posture.

Bion warns that even though the analyst *"hardly"* can concern himself with the cultural background against which analytic work must be done, *"the culture may concern him"*. Today (2005) this sounds a foresight. If only his warnings could be heard, perhaps the psycho-analytical movement would not face the problematical issues it now faces.

In the end, the change that is feared is the creative birth of whatever it is. There is a fear that the contained will destroy its container, or vice versa, and this is the catastrophe to be avoided. This also can mean that a baby or a thought cannot be born (AI, 95).

Bion's clinical example is that of the stammerer, who tries unsuccessfully *"to contain him"* (AI, 94); earlier he suggested that the stammerer evacuated (did not contain) awareness itself (C, 77). The stammerer offers an example of a catastrophe in the sense that he is *"so overwhelmed by emotion that he stammers and becomes incoherent"*. There is a rift between meaning and its expression, between emotion and its expression. *"If the man remained coherent, this could correspond to an overwhelming of the content by the container: his speech would in this case be so restrained that it could not express his feelings. But suppose he expressed himself 'perfectly': one could then imagine that his emotions had served to develop his ability for well-chosen speech and that his capacity for speech had helped his emotional development"* (AI, 95–6).

The example of the stammerer is an illustration of the failure of a "parasitic" relationship between container and contained. Container and contained produced a third object—incoherence—which makes both expression and its means impossible; this would be a catastrophic change.

His final works emphasize that the change is felt as catastrophic to the extent the individual has a lessened or lesser tolerance to the unknown. In 1971, he writes that it *"... seems reasonable to suppose that our somewhat insignificant speciality, psycho-analysis, has already exhausted its impetus and is ready to disappear into limbo, either because it is a burden too great for us, as we are, to carry, or because it is one more exploration destined to display a blind alley, or because it arouses or will arouse fear of the unknown to a point where the protective mechanisms of the noösphere compel it to destroy the invading ideas for fear that they will cause a catastrophe in which the noösphere disintegrates into the no-amorph. This catastrophic change could be brought about by advances in astronomy, physics, religion, or indeed any domain for which there may as yet be no name. The principles of psychical growth are not known"* (C, 319–20).

The invasion of the "English Farm" in the first chapter of *A Memoir of the Future* and the denial of change by the characters seems to provide a more vivid expression of the fear of change that characterizes a catastrophe. Closing a cycle, it may be considered that "English Farm" was also the bitter, sarcastic name given to the no-man's land of the fields of Flanders in the First World War. That is, the place where Bion met one of his own catastrophic changes: from adolescent delusions of grandeur to impossibly fast and precocious facing of reality.

Often the perspective of abandonment of the hallucination system or the allegiance to hallucinosis is felt as catastrophic. The issue is explored more in *Transformations*, pp. 130ff; also, chapter eleven, p. 147, on the belief that a *"curtain of illusions"* could have protective powers.

Less obvious are the changes linked to Bion's two analyses and his relationship with his second wife. Still less obvious was the co-option that was an attempt to bring an end to Bion's proposals of change. According to him the British Psycho-Analytical Society offered him a succession of prestigious administrative posts that menaced his creative activity—and avoided the BPS's potential changes that were felt to be potentially catastrophic. His moving to Los Angeles seemed to offer this opportunity of catastrophic change to himself and to this society; this was also refused.

The catastrophic change can be produced by experiencing real free associations and dreaming:

P.A. One of your prophets, Isaiah, who was the kind of person to whom you religious people pay attention—forgive me if I don't know what your brand of religion is—

PRIEST (bows slightly) I am flattered. May I congratulate you on your discriminatory integrity in not having "labelled" me with a particular "brand" of religion .

P.A. Let us leave out the introductory courtesies. I was referring to Isaiah who describes his contact with the Lord in matter-of-fact terms, precisely dated. Of course, we cannot know what happened, but we may have opinions. My object is not to discuss that past experience but to illustrate the unlimited possibilities when you say, "a queer dream"; possibilities which are limited in this discussion only by my ignorance. The *experience* is not "limited" by "finite" considerations of our capacity though our "discussion" of it is.

PRIEST I dreamed of an explosion of vast, tremendous and majestic proportions. It was terrifying. It was black as night; not night that I might understand in the solar system, but dark night of the soul—

P.A. As described by Saint John of the Cross perhaps?

PRIEST I am not Saint John of the Cross, nor yet Isaiah; that itself contributes to the sense of queerness that it should be *my* dream.

P.A. I am familiar with reports of terrifying experiences described in terms of varying inadequacy—as you have just been doing. We are both aware of the awe-ful experience. Many are not; they fear "going mad", some indescribable disaster, "break-down"; they may express themselves by bringing about disaster. We psycho-analysts think you do not know what a dream is; the dream itself is a pictorial representation, verbally expressed, of what happened. What actually happened when you "dreamed" we do not know. All of us are intolerant of the unknown and strive instantaneously to feel it is explicable, familiar—as "explosion" is to you and me. The event itself is suspect *because* it is explicable in terms of physics, chemistry, psycho-analysis, and other *pre*-conceived experience. The "conception" is an event which has become "conceivable", the "conceivable" it has become is no longer the genetic experience. Pre-conception, conception, birth—what a shock it must have been to know that a woman has a baby! How absurd to suppose that it could have any connection with sexual intercourse! I have found those who think it ridiculous that a woman could initiate an idea or have a thought worthy of consideration. [AMF, II, 381–2]

Misuses and misunderstandings: As far as this author's observation goes, the majority of misunderstandings encircling the usage of this concept are due to an over-simplification. It debases the concept into a cause-effect relationship (q.v.)—something that Bion always avoided. Perhaps it must be remembered that cause-effect formulations are disposable tools used as provisional steps. Many try to use it in its easier-to-grasp commonplace usage, that is, as if it could be equated to trauma. This posture disparages the psycho-dynamic nature of psycho-analysis itself. Also, the oversimplification is apparent when the phenomenon is seen as if the word simply reproduced the sense of the word that became a social common place. For a comparison between catastrophic change and emotional turbulence, please refer to that entry.

Suggested cross-references: Commensal, Container/ Contained, Controversy, Parasitic, Symbiotic, Emotional Turbulence, Transformation in Hallucinosis.

Cause (cause-effect): Bion remained critical of simplistic, positivistic cause-effect linear relationships throughout his work, from the beginning (one may consider *Experiences in Groups* as one of his earlier works). His general view of causes is that of an idea that is false—but despite this it can be useful in certain conditions, as a step to further knowledge. He considers the patient's building of causes, the analyst's use of it and the theoretical status of causes.

Bion does not dwell on philosophical considerations but he leaves no doubt about the works of philosophers who influenced him. He seems to take for granted the reader's familiarity with the work of Hume, Kant, Bradley, Braithwaite and Prichard.

In the earlier phases of his work, Bion's approach to the so-called traumatic and war neuroses clearly challenged the non-critical or hypocritical acceptance of external causes of a soldier's disability. This cause was and still is socially understood as corresponding exclusively to unfavourable external conditions. Bion and Rickman's approach to the wounded soldiers at Northfield produced almost immediate practical results: the soldiers were put back to work, albeit light tasks, in a comparatively short time compared with customary practice.

In a posthumously published paper that is undated but seems to belong to the years when he was developing the ideas that would be reunited in *Learning from Experience*, as is clear from its content, Bion dwells on causes and selected facts. Certainly the paper was written after his seminal study on psychotic and non-psychotic personalities.

He seems to have been reviewing critically the concept of cause. Hume's influence on him is apparent. He tries to discern selected facts and causes and at the same time he tries to verify the similarities between them. His psycho-analytical (meaning, clinical) approach ties the cause and the selected fact to psychosis and neurosis in an original way. He states all the time that both appertain to the realm of belief. There is a remarkable tolerance to paradoxes, as one can see from the text:

> The cause and the selected fact are alike in that they are both ideas that have the power of being associated with an emotional experience that at one moment gives rise to a sense of creative synthesis *and* awareness of still un-synthesized discrete objects. [C, 275]

To sum up, there are two uses of the idea of cause: (i) one may use it with an awareness of its limitations, as a provisional tool to enable the thinker or researcher to further investigate; (ii) one may use it as a truth-in-itself, an unquestionable belief; it is the manifestation of intolerance to the unknown and denial of that which is ultimately unknowable.

The use of an idea known to be false can be useful to the extent that one is aware of its falsity. An example often quoted by Bion is the idea that the sun rises. In some parts of his work (as in "The cause and the selected fact", in *Cogitations*) this example is used to display the usefulness of a false idea; in later works the same idea is used to display the damage it made to knowledge (*A Memoir of the Future*):

> I am not sure of the ease with which "plausible" theories are produced. In this context of "plausible theories" about which we are talking, the plausible theory (or "convincing interpretation") may be hard to come by. It can be plausible and false. Witness the idea that "the sun rises—what trouble that has caused!" [AMF, I, 172]

Some ideas and emotional experiences give rise to the sense that a creative synthesis or integration—in Klein's terms, the integration of the whole object—is possible, as well as awareness of discrete objects. Ideas—and this includes the idea of cause and the idea of a selected fact—belong to the realm of something that does not necessarily exist in the sense that it does not necessarily have a counterpart in reality. The idea furnishes a sense. This sense is what matters: the sense allows for an emotional experience in transition, that of creation, synthesis and awareness of singleness—the idea—and coupling—with reality itself.

The idea of cause may include the resistance to change and to growth, a manifestation of life and death instincts:

Every emotional experience of knowledge gained is at the same time an emotional experience of ignorance unilluminated. The sense of creative success with its accompanying elation is therefore inseparable from a sense of failure to synthesize the discrete objects, the elementary particles, which are revealed by the success. [C, 275]

Or as Bion puts it later: any solution to a question opens a space for still more questions. Bion was fond of André Green's quotation of Blanchot's aphorism, *"La réponse est le malheur de la question"*. The issue is, to tolerate or not to tolerate the unknown, the march of life, the absence of final answers. This view of cause differs from the positivistic view.

"Dominance of the life instincts carries with it the continued repetition of this experience. In extreme form, fear of this experience can lead to repudiation of the life instincts, and the reinforcement of the death instincts that are idealized and libidinized" (C, 275). Which is to say, to cling to causes as if they were final, instead of experiencing the detection of provisional causes, is a manifestation of the prevalence of death instincts. This includes rationality and logic.

The Kantian sense of cause—that is, the succession of phenomena in time—is elicited when Bion differentiates the cause from the selected fact: *"The selected fact relates to synthesis of objects felt to be contemporaneous or without any time component. The selected fact thus differs from the cause that relates to the synthesis of objects scattered in time and therefore with a time component"* (C, 275).

The psychotic use of cause is characterized by the attribution of realizations in the material realm:

Though cause has no realization corresponding to the concept, the patient regards cause as having an existence as a thing in itself, not independent of thought but as a part of his personality possessing independence in the sense that he cannot control it ... There is therefore no possibility of his feeling that he has discerned the link that brings phenomena together, and therefore cannot have the emotional experience that the non-psychotic personality recognizes under the name of "cause". His experience is quite otherwise: he feels that various objects have cohered; they are felt to have done so voluntarily, and independently of his volition [or in Bion's previous terms, and as any experienced psychiatrist, anthropologist or a person who takes care of children knows, the primitive mind attributes animate qualities to inanimate objects]; yet since the objects are part of his personality, he is responsible for their voluntary and independent concatenation. (C, 276).

Causes and the arrow of time

In many fields an enthroning of causation theories occurred. Some of them abandoned the idea. Development, growth, usefulness or lack of it brings the issue of causation again and again. What about examining the evolution of time? Causes are seen, in the Kantian scheme that Bion adopts, as successions of certain events in time—as growth also is. What does promote growth? What are the causes of it? In discussing the intolerance of frustration, intolerance of the no-breast, Bion hypothesizes that the obtrusion of mathematical thinking occurred in the form of the point, as reflecting the tolerance of the no-thing:

> Why, then, to revert to the point and line, do these visual images lead in one case to the efflorescence of mathematics and in the other to mental sterility? And is it certain that "mental sterility" is a correct assessment? The question implies the validity of a theory of causation which I consider misleading and liable to give rise to constructions that are basically false; if it is fallacious we may discard it for one as fallacious—which may be true of the formulation, by Heisenberg [Heisenberg, W.: *Physics and Philosophy*], of the problem of multiple causation. Both views have proved of value in the development of science, but developments of physics by the Copenhagen school appear to have made the theory irrelevant. If so, the logical step would be to bother no longer with causation or its counterpart—results. In psycho-analysis it is difficult to avoid feeling that a gap is left by its disappearance and that the gap should be filled. Over a wide range of our problems no difficulty is caused by regarding the theory of causation as fallacious but useful. When it comes to problems presented by disturbances in thought the difficulty cannot be met in this way ... The proposed chain of causation can then be seen as a *rationalization* of the sense of persecution. Furthermore, if the patient is capable of seeing that his proposed chain of causation is nonsensical he may use it to deny the persecution and thus evade any explanation that would reveal the depression that he dreads. [T, 56–7]

Bion's interest in searching for factors in the platonic realm, that is, in the unconscious or the numinous realm, and his empirical approach, led him naturally to the Humean notion of causality:

"*Hume's objection to a theory of causation supposes that since neither a hammer nor a nail can feel force it is not correct to speak of a nail being forced into position by the hammer, the term 'force' being properly applicable only to the sense-experience of a human being who exerts force or on whom it is exerted. He supposes therefore that to speak of force as an external reality is a projection of human feeling . . . I think Hume's argument has validity for psycho-analysis . . . It follows from the theory of transformations that whenever I see one element of the equation O, Tp α, Tp β + L, or H or K, the others must be present. But I shall **not** assume that one causes the other, though for convenience I may (as I have already done when I used the phrase 'because of the hatred', etc. p. 68)*" (T, 64–9). [On page 68, Bion writes: "*The patient entertains a transformation (Tp β) (it might be of a loved object) because of the hatred he feels for the person O of the analyst*".] For a detailed discussion of Humean causality, one may consult Hempel (1962) and Ruben (1993).

Hume observed that there are psychological needs that led human beings to "find" causes in constant conjunction of observed facts. If we use Kant's puzzled view, we may state that Bion was not afraid to immerse himself in the "shame of philosophy". Namely, that in psychology one should look for the root of the idea of causes as well as the origin of the search for causes. Using a graphical device he often resorted to, he created a quasi-mathematical, short-hand graphical symbol to help the student of the issue. He hyphenated the term. Hence, "psycho-logical", in order to enhance the fact that reason is a slave of passion. That is, the mind creates causes in a rational way. Rational stems from mathematics and meant originally to extract roots; philosophically it had debased itself in the search for essences; and causes are regarded as essences, having been used by St. Thomas Aquinas to serve some interests of the Roman Catholic Church.

Even though it may be said that Bion used the Kantian concept of cause (a succession of phenomena in time) he used it from clinical observation, rather than from philosophical brooding:

Patients * show that the resolution of a problem appears to present less difficulty if it can be regarded as belonging to a moral domain;

causation, responsibility and therefore a controlling force (as opposed to helplessness) provide a framework within which omnipotence reigns. [* Bion's Footnote: And not only patients. The group is dominated by morality—I include of course the negative sense that shows as rebellion against morality—and this contributed to the atmosphere of hostility to individual thought on which Freud remarked"]. [T, 64]

One must be prepared to find it an everyday occurrence. People use it as a commonplace way of (non)thinking that passes for real thinking. This can be seen in phrases such as that reproduced above, in which Bion warned: *"But I shall **not** assume that one causes the other, though for convenience I may (as I have already done when I used the phrase 'because of the hatred)'"*.

The cause-effect reasoning is typical of schizophrenic thinking. It builds rational schemata relied on in causes. Freud, as did Kant before him, intuited the fallacies and pitfalls of pure reason. Freud called it "rationalization", a fact he first observed in Schreber's case. In other words, rational schemata of cause and effects are psychotic phenomena. Any experienced psychiatrist can vouch for that. The psychotic paranoid delusion is endowed with an internal logic that is rationally impeccable.

Causes are devices intended to disburden the personality of self-responsibility. Reasoning along the cause-effect schemata precludes the psycho-analytic view (q.v.). Networks of relationships, meanings and functions cannot be elicited by the mind that believes in causes: *"A proper use of the oedipal elements is obscured by a tendency to allow the narrative form of the myth to impose a cause-and-effect outlook on the investigator"* (T, 96).

There seems to be confusion between causes and the act of naming a constant conjunction:

The name, in its function of binding a constant conjunction, partakes of the nature of a definition; it commences by being significant, but meaningless, till experience gives it accumulations of meaning; it derives negative force both by virtue of its genesis as part of thought and by the necessary logic of its coming into existence precisely because the constant conjunction it binds is *not* any of the previous and already named constant conjunctions. Dislike of it is therefore derived from its genesis and from fear of the implications of its "use". [Fn: Cf. Aristotle and definition. Topics, VI, 4, 141b, 21.] As naming and definition are inescapable this contributes to dislike of the unknown and the challenge it presents to the learner. The intensity of the dislike depends on other factors. As what point the dislike of the unknown and its impact on the development of procedures which are a part of finding out must be regarded as pathological is an academic question; it is decided for the analyst whenever there is evidence of a desire to learn and an inability to do so. In such a situation primitive levels of thought are stimulated to discover the "cause" of the obstruction. [Fn: Cf. Hume, D: Enquiries Concerning Human Understanding. Q 43–45.]. Evidence of the employment of a theory of causation is evidence of the operation of a theory that is not adequate. I shall consider the genesis of a theory of causation and its use with the aid of the grid and its two axes. Appearance in a given situation—inquiry obstructed either by analyst or patient—must be assessed on the category in the grid to which it should be relegated. If it appears to belong to column 2 categories the presumption of a pathological origin will be strong. If it belongs to column 4 it is evidence, especially in a K link such as an analysis ought to be, for something compatible with healthy growth. [T, 63–4]

The belief in causes differs from using them as steps towards the illumination of functional relationships. It is a way of formulating something to be investigated. One may be aware of their false nature. It is the bizarre objects of the pseudo-scientist. The issue in science is to establish some relationships between objects in order to elicit their respective functions. Religion in its turn looks for "why?" Science looks for "how".

Cause and morals

Invariant to beta-elements and bizarre objects, in so far as they share the characteristics of beta-elements, is the moral component of such objects. The moral component is inseparable from feelings of guilt and responsibility and from a sense that the *link* between one such object and another, and between these objects and the personality, is moral causation. The theory of causation, in a scientific sense in so far as it has one, is therefore an instance of carrying over from a moral domain an idea (for want of a better word) into a domain in which its original penumbra of moral association is inappropriate.

The observation of constant conjunction of phenomena whose conjunction or coherence has not been previously observed, and therefore the whole process of Ps⇔D interaction, definition and search for meaning that is to be attached to the conjunction, can be destroyed by the strength of a sense of causation and its moral implications. [T, 64]

In 1967, reviewing his clinical study "Attacks on linking", Bion would put the issue in a more explicit way:

I regard the idea of causation, implicit throughout the paper, as erroneous; it will limit the perspicacity of the analyst if he allows this element in Attacks on Linking to obtrude. The "causal link" has apparent validity only with events associated closely in space and time. The fallacious nature of reasoning based on the idea of "causes" is clearly argued in Heisenberg, *Physics and Philosophy*, Allen & Unwin, 1958, p. 81, in terms which should evoke an understanding response in any psycho-analyst. Provided the psycho-analyst does not allow himself to be beguiled into searching for, and proposing, except in conversational terms, "causes", the paper may stimulate enquiries of his own. The discovery of a "cause" relates more to the peace of mind of the discoverer than to the object of his research. [ST, 163]

⬚ Pages 56–59 of *Transformations* offers a comprehensive and detailed scrutiny of causation; even though it is fallacious, it is useful, because its detection allows the analyst to track the patients' use of it. A patient can use a nonsensical theory of causation in order to *"deny the persecution and thus evade any explanation that would reveal the depression that he dreads"* (T, 57). Therefore, one must separate the epistemological use of a criticism of causation theories and a directive, authoritarian view that can infiltrate during an analysis when the analyst observes the patient using such a "device". To believe in causes points *"to a conflict between omniscience on the one hand and inquiry on the other. Further steps will show that the logical causal approach produces a circular argument"* (T, 58).

&⟩ The author of this text has tried to show elsewhere how Bion's experiences as a tank commander seem to have enabled him to acquire a non-authoritarian view on this specific "cause", "war trauma" (in Pines and Lipgar, 2002).

Circle, point, line: Bion used the developments of mathematics over centuries as an analogic **model** to scrutinize the development of thinking processes and some of its disturbances. The disturbance being, in some aspects, a necessary step to the processes of development. This entry intends to synthesize the use of one of these mathematical analogies. Bion proposes regarding mathematics as an early attempt by mankind to deal with psychosis. Mathematics as well as geometry seems to be implied in the inception of thought processes.

He starts from two main contributions:

(i)   That of Freud, mainly as regards the disturbances of contact with reality as it is, when the pleasure/displeasure principle prevails. Freud's inference that some babies hallucinate a breast when the breast is not physically available is a root of Bion's observations.

(ii) That of Klein, as an outgrowth from Freud, as regards the prevalence of greed and envy, which fuels feelings of frustration in the relationships of the baby with the first reality that is endowed with features of the animate—the mother's breast. This is a task to be tackled during post-natal life. Other observations by Klein relating to the characteristics of the "paranoid–schizoid position", mainly the tendency to equate, rather than to symbolize, and projective identification, are the other roots of Bion's observations.

From these main guidelines Bion proceeds to examine minutely the emotional development that is consequent to specific ways of dealing and not-dealing with frustration. These ways are, at the inception of post-natal life, exclusively dependent on how each person experiences the absence of the breast; or, in other words, the way that frustration is felt.

It is a kind of prototype of all further feelings of frustration. They assume, throughout a life cycle, increasingly complicated forms. Bion proposes the terminology "no-breast" to describe the experiencing of the absent breast. This terminology already borrows an arithmetical model, that of negative numbers, derived from the theory of numbers.

Bion examines the outcome of innate or acquired excessive intolerance of frustration. This outcome corresponds to that which was known since pre-psycho-analytical days, and amended by Freud and Klein's contributions, such as psychosis. Bion observes clinically that the excessively intolerant being, so-called psychotic, cannot put up with the no-breast. He (she) equates the no-breast with noughtness. Or, to use some synonyms Bion proposes, the No-thing is equated with noughtness. In still other terms, the extent that each individual tolerates or does not tolerate the negative, frustration—in the first place, the no-breast—will determine that psychotic mechanisms predominate.

Bion proposes to regard geometry (as a development of mathematics) with its conceptions of point, circle, line, as a manifestation that indicates the existence of tolerance of frustration. *The point refers to the place where the breast was.*

The first time that Bion appealed to the history and philosophy of mathematics is in his now classical paper from 1961, "A theory of thinking". There is an intimate relationship between primitive emotions and the ability to develop mathematical thinking. This was reflected by a well-known fact: children with emotional difficulties have notorious difficulty in learning mathematics.

The relationship between an ability to abstract and to reach the reality beyond, and the fitness of the apparatus to think, was and is well known. One may say that "to abstract" is an ability to extract a real, albeit immaterial, quality or existence out of concreteness. In other terms, to borrow from Aristotle, an ability to "go beyond physics". From this, Bion relates the development of mathematical thought, as expressed in the ability of the mathematician and the geometer to deal with issues that became known as numbers and the theory of numbers—among many other mathematical developments. His paper on thinking uses Gotlob Frege's theory of numbers.

> Mathematical elements, namely straight lines, points, circles and something corresponding to what later becomes known by the names of numbers, derive from realizations of two-ness as in breast and infant, two eyes, two feet and so on. If intolerance of frustration is not too great modification becomes the governing aim. Development of mathematical elements, or mathematical objects as Aristotle calls them, is analogous to the development of conceptions. [ST, 113]

During the ensuing two years Bion would deal more with the development of concepts and conceptions in general (q.v.)—and comparatively less with the primitive formation of specific conceptions such as the breast and the intolerance of the no-breast. The development of a more detailed study was, so to say, postponed. Meanwhile he continued using mathematical models drawn from Aristotle's metaphysics and meta-mathematics, in the suggestions of "psycho-analytical object" and "elements of psycho-analysis" (q.v.).

He would return to his own suggestion contained in the text quoted above. In *Transformations*, p. 2, he warns: the descriptions of Euclidean geometry are too *"closely wedded to marks on paper"*. This was unhelpful to the onlooker or student who tried *not* to apprehend geometry as a thing-in-itself, or the symbols of the Euclidean system of notation as things-in-themselves. Perhaps the difficulty is not entirely due to Euclid's contributions, but it may rather be due to centuries of concretized misuse. It is true that when many children learn Euclid's geometry, they often fail to grasp its ethos. Many feel the whole issue to be useless and boring. Was this the case with the ancient Greeks? Probably not: one may be reminded that they were studied by grown-up people. Is infancy an age not well-suited for learning these concepts? Or the issue is, as some mathematicians interested in pedagogy put it during the sixties, the way mathematics is taught.

The mathematician was able to dispense with the "concreteness" of his objects. Therefore he was able to think about and use those objects in their absence. This fact seems to have intrigued Bion. As an experienced clinician, he observed that one of the foundations of psychosis was a difficulty in doing exactly that which the mathematician seemed able to do. Moreover, even a not too profound study of the history of mathematical concepts displays how this mathematician's ability was improved, as mathematics developed. Mathematics grew in a way that seems well suited to express the emotional growth from psychosis to neurosis (using Freud's definition of both, in his classic paper, "Neurosis and psychosis"). Or, in more descriptive terms, the "journey" from almost absolute lack of tolerance of frustration to a more marked degree of tolerance to it. This means an ability to postpone an imperial satisfaction of desire. Primary narcissism and primary envy establish the limit of such a journey.

Bion would expand this in *A Memoir of the Future*. For example, the following dialogue depicts the evolution of mathematics from "visual" Euclidean geometry to "mental" Cartesian algebraic models. A man of action who has difficulties in thinking (Robin) contrasts with the more perceptive female who is intuitive (Rosemary) as well as with a servant (Tom) who learned by experience. The use of this dialogic form seems to add a good-humoured, if subtle and serious humane tone to the issue:

TOM He means it as a mental aid to insight; as a circle or a line or a triangle aids Euclid, or Thales before him.

DOCTOR These corporeal aids become limitations; the asset becomes a liability. The anatomical and physiological structure is an asset to the baby who grows to be mobile.

P.A. Becomes "auto-mobile" in short.

TOM But Euclidean geometry, aided by space, geo-metric space, grows so powerfully that in a couple of thousand years it becomes irked by its visual frame. At this point the demands of the mind are imprisoned in the corporeal structure.

DOCTOR Enter the fairy prince to release the sleeping beauty.

P.A. Namely? I think you should introduce the characters as they come on the stage.

TOM Cartesian Co-ordinates.

ALICE What a pretty name.

ROSEMARY Mr Robin ma'am.

ALICE Hello Robin. We were just thinking of Cartesian Co-ordinates

ROBIN Good Heavens! I hope you aren't suggesting that I should use those. I would have my farm overrun with co-ordinates—they would grow much faster than the seeds of thought would germinate in my mind. [AMF, II, 224]

Or, in a more abridged way, coining a metaphor: *"The mind that is too heavy a load for the sensuous beast to carry"* (AMF, I, 38).

The reference to this part of the history of mathematics appears in *Transformations* and in *A Memoir of the Future*. It seems to have been inspired by Alfred North Whitehead's history of mathematics.

Both Whitehead and Bion point out that algebraic calculus frees mathematics from the sensuous limitations of pictorial, concrete representations. The issue is that of formulation. When it is necessary to make "public" a given insight, verbal, artistic, musical and scientific formulations are also a matter of necessity. The same issue is at stake with a patient who must make his emotional experience "public". Also, with the analyst who must "publicize" his findings either to his patient or to his colleagues. Mathematical notation seemed to have been successful in overcoming the psychotic allegiance to satisfaction of desire, to the extent that this satisfaction is precluded when the concrete object must be dispensed with.

Bion dwells on psycho-analytic communication: *"the difficulty of the 'public' to grasp that an analogy is an attempt to vulgarize a relationship and **not** the objects related. The psycho-analytical approach, though valuable in having extended the conscious by the unconscious, has been vitiated by the failure to understand the practical application of doubt, by the failure to understand the function of 'breast', 'mouth', 'penis', 'vagina', 'container', 'contained', as analogies. Even if I write it, the sensuous dominance of penis, vagina, mouth, anus, obscures the element signified by analogy . . ."* (AMF, I, 70–71).

This entry is limited to quoting parts of the Trilogy *A Memoir of the Future* that seem to this writer to develop an earlier attempt by Bion in *Transformations*. Unlike the latter, even though he used mathematical models, in the Trilogy it is done in a way that resorts more to history and concepts and less to quasi-mathematical formulations. It seems to this writer that for the reader who feels uneasy with the use of quasi-mathematical symbols, to rely on *A Memoir* may facilitate the apprehension of Bion's earlier attempts.

Anyway, before trying this dialogic, quasi-artistic way, Bion had already resorted to conventional, verbal formulations, even when he used mathematical analogies: *"The point and straight line have to be described by the totality of **relationships** which these objects have to other objects"* (T, 2). One gathers that the important part here is not the mathematical analogy but the analogy used to introduce the issue of relationships. That, after, all is what mathematics is all about. Earlier, in making use of the model of relationships, he defined that *"An emotional experience cannot be conceived of in isolation from a relationship"* (LE, 42).

His next analogy is with music, in two ways. In one of them he warns that to some people, the little black marks in a pentagram can be seen just as that, black marks. In contrast, an experienced musician can "extract" music from them (AMF, I). In the other he returns to the realm of the minus field, retaking the lead first introduced in *Learning from Experience*—his model now depicts the value of pauses in a musical score and in music itself.

He uses these analogies to talk about the breast, thinking, and the experience of the no-breast: *"The state of mind I have described is represented for me by a model—that of an adult who **violently** maintains an exclusively primitive omnipotent?helpless state. The model by which I represent **his** vision of **me** is that of an absent breast, the place or position, that I, the breast, **ought** to occupy but do not. The 'ought' expresses **moral** violence and omnipotence. The visual image of me can be represented by what a geometer might call a point, a musician the staccato mark in a musical score"* (T, 53).

In other words, the lack of tolerance of frustration of the no-breast leads to omnipotent claims; the place where the breast used to be is abhorred. Absence is abhorred. Denial of wish fulfilment is felt as absence and equally abhorred. In some cases, real necessities that demand to be satisfied cannot be so; the reaction may be equally violent. There ensues no realization of the point; the point is equated with frustration; this is irreducible. *"In the illustration the problem centres on the fact that the absent breast, the no-breast', differs from the breast. If this is accepted, the "no-breast" can be represented by the visual image of the point"* (T, 54).

This seems to be fundamental to grasping Bion's mathematical model as an aid to thinking about intolerance of frustration. **The point is used as a visual representation of the "no-breast".** This is not mathematics, even though it can be seen as a representation of an emotional experience borrowed from, and inspired by geometry.

Bion includes in the text some discussions between Plato, the Pythagoreans, Euclid and Archimedes. This discussion centres on the inadequacies of representing the point as a perforation. The ancient Greeks argued whether it was to be called a shmeton or a stigma (σημετον or (στιγμη): *"I shall have reason to quote illustrations that strengthen the impression of the sexual component in the mathematical investigation ..."* (T, 55–6). Bion also quotes Aristotle's seemingly rational discussions about the indivisibility of the line. The point is indivisible; how could a junction of points be divisible?

This serves as an attempt to illuminate the origins of mathematics itself. Bion proposes to regard mathematics as a primitive way to deal with psychosis, for psychosis in the adult ensues when intolerance of frustration is too great. *"I have sought to show that geometrical constructions related to, and strove originally to represent, biological realities such as emotions . . . mathematical space may represent emotion, anxiety of psychotic intensity, or repose also of psychotic intensity—a repose more psychiatrically described as stupor. In every case the emotion is to be a part of a progression, breast ? emotion (or place where the breast was) ? place where emotion was"* (T, 105).

". . . tolerance of frustration involves awareness of the presence or absence of objects, and of what a developing personality later comes to know as 'time' and (as I have described the 'position' where the breast used to be) 'space'" (T, 54, 55). In other words: Kant's "a priori" are not possible at all if intolerance to frustration is too great. Kant proposed to regard space and time as two innate a priori categories in human understanding—or mind as we may call it today.

If the patient tolerates the "point", meaning, the no-breast, he may make visual images of it; the same applies to the line. The process is akin to dreaming; the patient can *"think them, that is, use thoughts in accordance with rules which are acceptable to, and understandable by, others* (T, 56). This produces *"the efflorescence of mathematics"* (T, 57), here understood as a capacity to think. A divergent course, expressed by the inability to make visual images out of intolerance to frustration and abhorrence of the experience of the no-breast *"leads . . . to mental sterility"* (T, 57). Even though Bion uses the phrase, "leads to", he warns that there is no causation involved here, causation itself being related to the issue of not tolerating frustration conjoined with other factors, such as a harsh super-ego (please refer to the entry "Cause").

The analyst who deals with disturbances of thought also deals with the difficulties with the no-breast; *"The appearance in psychoanalysis of black-heads, spots, dots, staccato marks in musical scores, points, etc., can all be represented by the geometer's point; similarly the variety of supposedly phallic symbols can be represented by the geometer's line"*. Now, *". . . certain patients, who believe others do the same"* use the point and the line *"as if they or their signs were things"*.

This seems to be a fundamental issue. The model of points and lines seems to help the fundamental underlying issue in that which the author proposes to call the "sense-fy-ing" and "concretizing" tendencies of mind. These tendencies prevail in those who feel they cannot tolerate frustration. If the patient hears or feels that there emerged a "point" or a "dot" either said or seen by himself or by the analyst or whoever it is, *"however it is signified or represented"*, he (or she) concludes that the utterance or the visual image *"marks the place where the breast (or penis) was . . . this 'place' seems to be invested by the patient with characteristics that less disturbed people might attribute to an object they would call a ghost. The point (.) and the term point are taken as sensible manifestations of the 'no breast' . . . 'the place where the breast was' having many of the characteristics of a breast that is hostile because it no longer exists . . . It is in this way that a certain class of patient 'concludes' that a thought is a thing . . . such a view contrasts with that which enables a mathematician to use a point, however represented, to elaborate a geometric system. Similarly, it contrasts with the ordinary view of the word 'breast' or 'point' that enables it to be used to elaborate anatomical or physiological or artistic or aesthetic (in the philosophical sense) systems"* (all previous quotations, T, 76, 77; my bold).

The patient becomes "backward looking", prone to function by making transference in Freud's sense of the term. It is an unending search for *"what has been lost"*. This contrasts with a capacity to march into the unknown, which Bion calls *"ordinary view"*. This capacity leads to mathematics, science, and commonsensical life, which is *"forward looking and relating to what can be found"*. Perhaps Freud's study on mourning and melancholia as well as Klein's study on the depressive position, are the forerunners of Bion's research. Bion expands these contributions specifically to the processes of thought involved. He thought that the history of geometry could help to apprehend the problem; it seems that it helped him and he had put it at the disposal of the psycho-analytic movement.

The geometrical elaboration proceeds as follows: commencing with a point, line or any more complex figure such as those associated with the theorem of Pythagoras, the proposition is read off the figure, that is to say, it seems to be regarded as self-evident from the nature of the figure. Inspection of the figure may be followed by a formulation in terms other than pictorial. Plutarch gives a fanciful and oedipal description of the 3, 4, 5 triangle. [T, 78]

It must be emphasized that in the text quoted above, when one takes a *"geometrical elaboration"* that *"proceeds as follows: commencing with a point, line or any more complex figure"*, it must **not** be regarded as a concrete object despite the sensuous apprehension that is the first step in this proceeding, and despite the imagery that is kept in mind. Otherwise, it would not be possible to apprehend what is conveyed by the growing complexities *"such as those associated with the theorem of Pythagoras"*. Identically, it would not be possible to realize that *"the proposition is read off the figure"*, nor to apprehend something that *"seems to be regarded as self-evident from the nature of the figure"* In other words, to grow mathematically may be, and may have been ontogenetically, a counterpart of growing from psychosis to neurosis, or from part-objects to Oedipus, or from material to psychic reality. Bion is not mathematicizing psycho-analysis but rather he is using the history of mathematics as a model.

The problem also belongs to the area of communication. This communication is needed in at least two realms: the intrapsychic communication one must perform with oneself; the communication with others. Mathematicians can communicate with themselves and with other mathematicians through their systems of non-visual and non-verbal symbols. Should we analysts be enabled to do the same? And what can be said of a patient with his (her) analyst? What can be said about words, which also are symbols? After all, they are in many instances invested with a myriad—Bion calls it, "penumbra"—of associations. Is it valid to look for more precise methods of communication? Where was Bion led when he resorted to the aid of the concepts of points and lines?

I have described the point or line as an object indistinguishable from the place where the breast or penis was. Owing to the difficulty of being sure what the patient is experiencing I resort to a variety of descriptions, each of which is unsatisfactory. The spot, for example, seems to be part conscience, part breast, part faeces, destroyed, non-existent yet present, cruel and malignant. The inadequacy of description or categorization as thought at all has led me to the term β-element as a method of representing it. *The spoken word seems significant only because it is invisible and intangible; the visual image is similarly significant because it is inaudible. Every word represents what it is not—a "no-thing", to be distinguished from "nothing".* [T, 78–79, my italics]

In other words, Bion's resorting to mathematical analogies led him to the realm of minus—Kant's numinous realm, or Freud's unconscious realm. The importance of this to the genesis of the thinking processes and the capacity to dream cannot be over-stressed. Plato, Kant, Freud and now Bion show that the unconscious apprehension of reality **as it is** has a necessary preliminary step. Namely, to tolerate what **it is not**, that which is not what we wish it to be. The wish is important, but is not to be fulfilled. Every meaning springs from the tolerance of the no-meaning; all communication springs from tolerance of that which is not communicated; all light springs from tolerance of periods of no-light. Midas-like, the alternative is "nothing": an endless, greedy search for concrete, material things that try to deny the existence of the no-thing.

Let us turn to the circle:

The thought, represented by a word or other sign, may, when it is significant as a no-thing, be represented by a point (.). The point may then represent the position where the breast was, or may even *be* the no-breast. The same is true of the line, whether it is represented by the word line or a mark made on the ground or on paper. The circle, useful to some personalities as a visual image of "inside and outside", is to other personalities, notably the psychotic, evidence that no such a dividing membrane exists.

Intolerance of a no-thing, taken together with the conviction that any other object capable of a representative function is, by virtue of what the sane personality regards as its representative function, not a representation at all but a no-thing itself, precludes the possibility of words, circles, points and lines being used in the furtherance of learning from experience. They become a provocation to substitute the thing for the no-thing, and the thing itself as an instrument to take the place of representations when representations are a necessity as they are in the realm of thinking. Thus actual murder is to be sought instead of the thought represented by the word "murder", an actual breast or penis rather than the thought represented by those words, and so on until quite complex actions and real objects are elaborated as part of acting-out. Such procedures do not produce the results ordinarily achieved by thought, but contribute to states approximating to stupor, fear of stupor, hallucinosis, fear of hallucinosis, megalomania and fear of megalomania. [T, 82]

The concept of the circle is a step forward to the extent that it expresses the capacity of the mind to tolerate paradoxes without hasty attempts to solve them. (This writer proposed elsewhere, based on Freud, Klein, Bion, and Winnicott's achievements, that a discipline of tolerating paradoxes marks the analytic posture.)

The association of the circle with "in and out" contributes to the difficulty of understanding the concepts of the line that cuts a circle in points that are conjugate complex. The difficulty arises from the supposition that the line that does so lies "outside" the circle; as opposed to the line that cuts it in two points, whose roots are real and distinct, and is supposed to lie "inside" the circle. The difficulty is diminished if there is no intolerance of the no-thing to contend with and therefore no opposition to a term of which the meaning is undetermined.

The simple example I have taken of the straight line that may cut a circle in two points that are (i) real and distinct, or (ii) real and coincident (if the line is a tangent), or (iii) conjugate complex (if the line lies entirely "outside the circle') poses a problem that the mathematician has been able to solve by taking a mathematical point of view, but I use it to illustrate the nature of the psychological problem. I shall state this as follows: in the domain of thought where a straight line can be regarded as lying within, or touching, or wholly outside, a circle, a transformation has been effected whereby certain characteristics, lending themselves to mathematical manipulation, have been manipulated mathematically to adumbrate and then solve a mathematical problem. The residual characteristics however retain their problem, un-named (un-bound) and so uninvestigated. *Hallucinosis is a domain, analogous to that of mathematics, in which a solution is sought.* [T, 83]

The reader may consult the entry "Hallucinosis". In brief, a state where hallucinations and delusions can appear albeit the rest of the personality—or ego functions—are comparatively fit. Again, the intolerance of the no-thing, of frustration, can be seen as the anti-scientific (or anti-musical, or anti-analytic) function of the mind that functions under the aegis of death instincts. The obverse is to nourish regard for the principle of reality (or truth).

> The mathematical problem resembles a psycho-analytic problem in that it is necessary that the solution should have a wide degree of applicability and acceptance and so avoid the need to apply different arguments to different cases when the different cases appear to have essentially the same configuration. Any analyst will recognize the confusion that is caused, or at best the sense of dissatisfaction that prevails, when a discussion by members makes it quite clear that the configuration of the case is apprehended by all, but the arguments formulated in its elucidation vary from member to member and from case to case. It is essential that such a state of affairs should be made unnecessary if progress is to take place. The search must be for formulations that represent the essential similarity of the configurations, recognized by all who deal with them, and thus to make unnecessary the ad hoc nature of so many psycho-analytic theories. [T, 83–4]

Vertex

The importance of points, lines and circles starts from the tolerance/intolerance of the breast and proceeds to the development of vertexes. The point is the origin of vertexes. The latter are amenable to be dealt with as **senses**, or, to use a term borrowed from physics: a vector. Each one of the basic five human senses can be regarded as one vertex: we have a visual vertex, an aural vertex, a smell vertex, and so on. Bion deals with the mental counterparts of some vertexes, as the reproductive system, which is *"related to premonitions (q.v.) of pleasure and pain"* (T, 91).

The various vertexes, stemming from points—the no-breast and the place where the breast used to be, originally—generate multifarious, perhaps infinite, possibilities. This fact has consequences for an analysis. In order to facilitate the presentation of the issue we will resort to the supremacy of the visual vertex. The infinite possibilities are available both to hallucinatory production as well as to dream work. In the former the infinite has a meaning, that of a greedy, chaotic production of everything that equals nothing; in the latter the seemingly infinite possibilities converge on truth, or infinity: *"The point/line may be transformed by central projection from any one of a number of vertices, or it may be transformed by parallel projection by a single point at infinity"* (T, 91). Both are parallel developments. The supremacy of the visual vertex occurs in any mind and contributes to the construing of dreams into visual images—a fact that deeply impressed both Freud and Bion.

At this time Bion began his efforts to stress the importance of putting colloquial language at the service of analysis, as Freud did. It had definite advantages over the use of jargon, which prevailed at that time. But at the same time he thought that mathematical notation should confer precision to communication. This precision seemed to be such that the use of colloquial language could never even aspire to offer.

Bion uses colloquial terms such as hot-point, clouds, in order to depict his visual images when seeing a patient (chapter nine, *Transformations*). Simultaneously he points out the limitations of using this kind of terminology, *vis-à-vis* the use of concepts derived from mathematics:

> The combination of terms such as "hot-point" with other terms such as "cloud" and "probability" denied the model any variety of applicability but restricted its usefulness to one context. Terms such as "probability" and "cloud" are not homogeneous. Can they be replaced by signs that are? Yes: if they are replaced by points. [T, 121]

Misuses and misconceptions: In trying to elucidate Bion's use of mathematical analogies, the author bows to the fact that they were grossly misunderstood. The failure to grasp the value of analogy seems to be a hallmark of the psycho-analytic movement. Bion's warnings about this failure and his attempts to avoid it suffered the same fate.

> P.A. We are all scandalized by bigotry. We are none of us bigot-generators; that is, we none of us admit to being the spring from whom bigotry flows. As a result we do not recognize those of our offspring of whose characters we disapprove. Indeed, Melanie Klein discovered that primitive, infantile omnipotence was characterized by fantasies of splitting off undesired features and then evacuating them.
>
> ROLAND I am sure you don't mean that children *think* like that?
>
> P.A. It would be inaccurate and misleading to say so. That is why Melanie Klein called them "omnipotent phantasies". But although

I found her verbalization illuminating, with the passage of time and further investigation which her discoveries made possible, her formulations were debased and became inadequate. These primitive elements of thought are difficult to represent by any verbal formulation, because we have to rely on language that was elaborated later for other purposes. When I tried to employ meaningless terms—alpha and beta were typical—I found that "concepts without intuition which are empty and intuitions without concepts which are blind" rapidly became "black holes into which turbulence had seeped and empty concepts flooded with riotous meaning". [AMF, II, 228–9]

The mathematical analogy was subjected to an oversimplification; Bion's appeal to the history and philosophy of mathematics was seen as if he was appealing to mathematics-in-itself. His writings that use mathematical models are usually quoted—with the possible exception of Matte-Blanco—as a "proof" of a so-called "attempt of Bion to mathematize" psycho-analysis.

These readings ignore or dismiss phrases such as: "*I hope that in time the base will be laid for a mathematical approach to biology, founded on the biological origins of mathematics, and not on an attempt to fasten on biology a mathematical structure which owes its existence to the mathematician's ability to find realizations, that approximate to his constructs, amongst the characteristics of the inanimate*" (T, 105).

This can be compared with his clinical studies on psychosis and schizophrenic thinking, where he states that some patients deal with the animate realm through measures that would be successful if applied to the inanimate.

Intolerance of a no-thing, taken together with the conviction that any object capable of representative function is, by virtue of what the sane personality regards as its representative function, not a representation at all but a no-thing itself, precludes the possibility of words, circles, point and lines being used in the furtherance of learning from experience. They become a provocation to substitute the thing for the no-thing, and the thing itself as an instrument to take the place of representations when representations are a necessity as they are in the realm of thinking. [T, 82]

The rules governing points and lines which have been elaborated by geometers may be reconsidered by reference back to the emotional phenomena that were replaced by "the place (or space) where the mental phenomena were". Such a procedure would establish an abstract deductive system based on a geometric foundation with intuitive psycho-analytic theory as its concrete realization. [T, 121]

It seems that the difficulties in profiting from Bion's analogies started from the first public presentation of a paper that contained such a proposition ("A theory of thinking"). A common reaction is, "why would an analyst talk about maths in an analytic paper?" Also, the absence of psycho-analytic jargon did not appeal to some readers. Bion himself commented on the idea that a book that does not mention Oedipus or repression or any known theory is considered as non psycho-analytical. The question, if made under the aegis of scientific curiosity, may lead to development; if made under the aegis of already existent ideas, it leads to decay.

Deep-seated motives illuminate the objection. They may be related to the same kind of intolerance to frustration that Bion tried to encircle with his analogy. The reader who "finds" him(her)self in this situation could still resort to his experiences of life or with patients to get some help; in some cases, the difficulty cannot be addressed outside the realm of the analyst's personal analysis.

Recommended cross-references: Function, Hyperbole, Mathematization of Psycho-analysis.

Suggested cross-references: Hallucination, No-breast, Frustration.

📖 On the expanding of the theory of numbers and Euclidean geometry: *A Memoir of the Future*, volume I p. 71–72.

There are books written by professional physicists and mathematicians as primers for young mathematicians and for the interested layman. They may be useful for grasping Bion's background. His forebears are Aristotle, Euclid, Albert Einstein, Werner Heisenberg, Alfred North Whitehead, Bertrand Russell. Other authors also wrote primers that may interest: A. Eddington, Roger Penrose, Stephen Hawking, Paul Davies, among others.

Circular argument A concept destined to gauge the effectiveness of an interpretation given by an analyst *vis-à-vis* the patient's statements. The "correct interpretation" (q.v.) must be such that one avoids restricting it to "knowing about". It must reach a state that Bion describes as "becoming" (q.v.). The circular argument is the stuff that an analytic session is made of.

The concept of circular argument seems to demand a grasp of previous concepts formulated by Bion. All these concepts are reviewed in this dictionary. The concept of "circular argument" embodies a concise summary of these concepts.

"Circular argument" reunites the following concepts that Bion formulated in his book *Transformations*: O, ultimate reality, becoming, incarnation, reminders of ultimate reality as well as the Grid categories; also, ideas of causation, the theory of Forms according to Plato, deity according to Jewish and Christian Cabbala, the theory of incarnation, Freud's practical use of the idea of the unconscious, the two principles of mental functioning, Klein's theory of evacuation and projective identification, Bion's theories of concretization and hyperbole.

It is necessary to have in mind some basic, intuitive concepts from mathematics and physics. In doing this we may well be following that which this writer presumes was Bion's pathway. This can be done through using colloquial language and common sense.

One may start from elementary geometry: the idea of a circle and the idea that it has a diameter. The diameter of the circle is infinitely variable (quantity). The concept, variation of diameter, is qualitative. A visual, dynamic view of a circle according to its variations in diameter displays an enlarging or contracting circumference.

If one keeps this enlarging and contracting figure in mind, one may now proceed with the aid of Bion's formulation, which **refers to an interpretation given by an analyst**:

> The interpretation should be such that the transition from *knowing about* reality to *becoming real* is furthered. This transition depends on matching the analysand's statement with an interpretation which is such that the circular argument remains circular but has an adequate diameter. If it is too small the circular argument becomes a point; if too great it becomes a straight line. The point and straight line together with numbers are representatives of states of mind which are primitive and unassociated with mature experience. The profitable circular argument depends on a sufficiency of experience to provide an orbit in which to circulate. To re-state this in terms of greater sophistication, the analytic experience must consist of

knowing and being successively many elementary statements, discerning their orbital or circular or spherical relationship and establishing the statements which are complementary. The interpretations that effect the transition from knowing about O to becoming O are those establishing complementarity; all others are concerned with establishing the material through which the argument circulates.

The transition from "knowing about" to "becoming" O can be seen as a particular instance of the development of the conception from the pre-conception (row E from row D) (q.v. Grid). [T, 153]

The phrase, "*The point and straight line together with numbers are representatives of states of mind which are primitive and unassociated with mature experience. The profitable circular argument*" summarizes the proposition of the psychic function of representations and abstractions such as points and lines and numbers. This occupies a good deal of the book, *Transformations*.

Mathematics is seen as an early attempt to deal with psychosis, during the pre-psycho-analytic era—which constitutes almost the whole of the history of mankind.

The terms orbital, circular, spherical, pertain to the actual experience of the analytic session. Sometimes we analysts furnish hints to our patients that are "orbital" to the patient's O. The concept of "*complementarity*" is seminal. It demands elaboration of the relationship between breast and mouth, baby and mother, femininity and masculinity. In Bion's later terms (1970), it is a commensal relationship (q.v.) between container and contained (q.v.). The "*elementary statements*" are the building blocks of a session, the experience of conversing and talking.

The diameter of the circle in a circular argument marks the possibility of having a real talk with the patients. The American Indians encircle through diminishing increments of diameter, the area that allows them to get nearer a Mustang until they can mount it. The process may take years.

The complexity of a statement whether made by analyst or analysand imposes a choice on the analyst: he must decide what dimension of the patient's statement he is to interpret and in what terms he will interpret it. To a great extent the choice is already determined by the analyst's personality and historical development and with those factors I do not intend to deal; I am concerned more with the immediate circumstances and those factors which are under the analyst's conscious control. He must beware of interpretations for no better reason that that the interpretation is one he can make. He cannot "win" it "from the void and formless infinite" of the analysand's personality, but only from the elements of the statement that the analysand won from his own "void and formless infinite". Nothing is to be gained from telling the patient what he already knows unless what he "knows is being used to exclude what he "is" (K opposed to O). Such an interpretation is part of the circular argument of which the "diameter" is too great. How is the "diameter" to be measured? If the interpretation is made mainly because it is available it is a column 2 statement intended to prevent "turbulence" in the analyst. The abstruse interpretation relates to desire in the analyst, a wish to feel that he can see further than his analysand or some other who serves as a rival. It belongs to the domain of hyperbole. Too small and too large diameters indicate defence against and projection of hyperbole: defence is against hyperbole originated by the analysand. [T, 166–7]

Suggested cross-references: Analytic View, Atonement, Correct Interpretation and Hyperbole.

📖 The author proposed an extension of Bion's theory of thinking that integrates the digestive and reproductive models into a model of complementarity of analyst and patient, in terms of exercising femininity and masculinity (in *W. R. Bion between Past and Future*, ed. Parthenope Bion Talamo, Silvio Merciai and Franco Borgogno. London: Karnac Books 2001).

Classical analysis: Please refer to the entries, Classical Theory, −K

Classical theory: Bion's use of the term defines the traditional guidelines to analysis. The sense conveyed by the word "classic" in the work of Bion is that of a perennial, transcendent form discovered as a constant conjunction, selected fact or invariance. It expresses an ultimately unknowable fact (or counterpart) in psychic reality as it is. These formulations had, have and will have *"durability and extensibility"* (AI, Introduction, page 1). This was a permanent concern of Bion. He puts it in terms of the lasting effects of a real analysis (see specific entry). How can analysis turn into a "classic" in each analysand's life?

Bion sees his own contributions to the theories of Freud and Klein as "additional". These contributions were given to (i) the theory of dreams, (ii) the free interchange between conscious and unconscious, (iii) the free interchange between paranoid–schizoid and depressive position, (iv) pre-conceptions of Oedipus and the breast. They are not meant to replace Freud or Klein's theories. The differentiation between Bion's contributions and those of the classic authors is caused by the requirements of scientific communication.

How does she come to waste all her treasures like this? . . . Does she not know what the value of her gifts is—the education, the health, her beauty, our beauty? Does she not know that we were Penelope's suitors? That Homer celebrated us? That we died even before there was a poet to confer immortality upon us? Ronsard knew of us when we were beautiful?. . .

"But tell me who you are; I shall wrestle with you from dawn to dusk, from dusk to dawn, from O to God, from God to science; from science to God; from security to the infinite that is man's infinity; from the infinite confines of stupidity, from stupor to the bigotry of certitude; from infinite hate to infinite love; from infinite coldness, indifference of the absolute, to the intolerable infinitude of absolute love. Show me." "No". "Show me".

"Because of your importunity I will lift the veil. I will not give you sight, but I will give you insight so your greatest will be able to see me in a glass darkly, me in whom there is no shadow cast by turning. You will pay as even your greatest had to pay—"from that time on the balance of his mind was disturbed". He was condemned to live imprisoned in everlasting sanity."

"Who are you?"

"I am compassion."

"Who are you?"

"I am your maid—but even then you did not see."

"Open my eyes."

"No—I sent the prophets but you would not listen."

"Open my ears."

"I sent you Bach."

"He had perfect pitch."

"He tempered the clavier well."

"Send me a better one."

"No. I sent you Mozart."

"You took him back too soon."

"I sent you Beethoven."

"He was flawed."

"You flawed him; you would not look at the flaws I made." [AMF, I, 34–5]

Poetic and religious expressions have made possible a degree of public-ation in that formulations exist which have achieved durability and extensibility. To say the same thing differently, the carrying power of the statement has been extended in time and space. Vixere fortes ante Agamemnona multi and "Not marble, nor the guilded monuments/Of princes, shall outlive this powerful rhyme" . . . [AI, Introduction, pages 1 and 2]

The reference to the Greeks includes a real wife, Penelope, menaced by sexual beasts disguised as suitors. The reference to Ronsard concerns his appreciation of women. Newton, according to Lord Keynes and some historians, lost his sanity when he was on the verge of making new discoveries; he turned religious and almost killed himself in a mysterious fire. Bion became impressed with these facts, which he also records in *Transformations* (T, 156). The text brings a sharp differentiation between the transcendence of truth and beauty, as expressed in the classics, and the feeling of the absolute, be it love or hate, which are fused in those paranoid and narcissistic states. This links with Christ "seen in a glass darkly, a reference to St Paul".

Or, still: *"What part of England or Shakespeare was it that forged the England that is eternal and will be for ever England?"* (AMF, I, 43).

The issue of classics is subsumed by the idea that psycho-analysis was a thought without a thinker until there appeared a Freud to think it.

Misuses and misunderstandings: Many use Bion's comments about classical theory as if he was against it. To mark differences and to make expansions differs from ideas of superiority.

The same situation occurred with certain interpretations of Einstein's extensions of Newton's theories. Lest any doubts remain about the sense of the word "classics" in the work of Bion, they can be dispelled by *A Memoir of the Future*. The newness is never separated from the transcendence of truth itself. The issue matters to the extent it touches creation, procreation, beauty, femininity ("Truth is beauty, beauty truth", in the words of Keats, a poet of whom Bion was very fond).

> If psycho-analytical intuition does not provide a stamping ground for wild asses, where is a zoo to be found to preserve the species? Conversely, if the environment is tolerant, what is to happen to the "great hunters" who lie unrevealed or reburied? [AMF, I, 5]

Commensal: Bion introduces this term, borrowed from biology, in *Learning from Experience*, page 90. The term can be seen as an extension of his theory of links; and indeed it depends on that, as well as on the theory of container/contained. Soon after having introduced the concept of container and contained (q.v.) he reconsiders the K link (q.v.) under the vertex of the container and the contained. Or, more precisely, he considers that K is a factor of (therefore it is subordinate to) the function container and contained. It is just at this moment that he defines "commensal":

> In K, L and H being factors and therefore subordinate, ? is projected into ? and abstraction, of a type that I shall use the term commensal to describe, follows. By commensal I mean ?and ?are dependent on each other for mutual benefit and without harm to either. In terms of a model the mother derives benefit and achieves mental growth from the experience: the infant likewise abstracts benefit and achieves growth. [LE, 90–91]

The phenomena that present themselves in material reality have a biological nature. They also have an immaterial counterpart in psychic reality. These counterparts are amenable to being dealt with psycho-analytically. The model of a commensal relationship is a way to put these facts into an integrative trans-disciplinary, multi-level approach. It detects invariances common to different modes of observation. "Commensal" seems to be one of them. There are some impediments to establishing a commensal relationship, among them, envy (LE, 96). Eight years later, the definition was presented in a more developed form: *"By commensal I mean a relationship in which two objects share a third to the advantage of all three"* (AI, 95).

Suggested cross-references: Container/Contained, Parasitic, Symbiotic.

Common sense: Bion used this term to indicate that more than one point of view must be used in order to increment apprehension of reality and facts **as they are**. *"As a criterion for what constitutes a sensible experience I propose common sense in the meaning that I have given it elsewhere, namely some 'sense' that is common to more than one sense. I shall consider an object to be sensible to psycho-analytical scrutiny if, and only if, it fulfils conditions analogous to the conditions that are fulfilled when a physical object's presence is confirmed by the evidence of two or more senses . . . The correlation thus established entitles one to claim the term 'common sense' to characterize one's view that a given object is a stone: and that the view that it is a stone is common to one's senses and therefore a common sense view"* (EP, 10–11).

The term has social implications: *"I propose that we may now say that common sense is a term commonly employed to cover experiences in which the speaker feels that his contemporaries, individuals whom he knows, would without hesitation hold the view he has put forward in common with each other. Common sense, the highest common factor of sense, so to speak, would support his view of what the senses convey"* (C, 10).

The senses are the port of entry of all stimuli, whatever they are. Their conjoint action and integration is provided by the central nervous system. The earlier denomination of the impressions conveyed by the sensuous apparatus was, "sensible experiences". The term was created by philosophers. Common sense is a very old concept that has a history which mixes with the history of science; it was first defined by Aristotle; Spinoza, Descartes, Bacon and Locke used it to define the basic tenets of science; "empiricism" was founded with the basis of knowledge acquired by the use of senses. Hume and Kant's criticism of that which the latter named "naïve realism", served also to improve its uses, as can be seen in the work of modern scientists such as Planck and Einstein, and epistemologists such as Bradley, Braithwaite, Prichard, Russell (please refer to the entries, Scientific Method, Scientific Deductive System).

In Scientific Method (C, 10) Bion furnishes a good humoured example of common sense: "*I may cite the experience in which a tactile impression of, say, fur—sudden and unpredicted—gives rise to the idea of an animal, which then has to be confirmed or refuted visually; and so, it is hoped, the common-sense view is achieved*". The matching of two different senses—touch and sight—allows a more precise idea of reality.

Two senses are needed. The meaning of the term "sense" is of direction. The physicist called it vector. Later Bion introduced the term vertex. Therefore it is necessary to have at least two vertexes in order to get a commonsensical view, or an approach to reality. This forms the basis of scientific inquiry. "*It follows that the scientific law is closely related to, and an epitome of, experience*" (C, 8).

Let us figure out that more than two senses are used. Add to this a repetition of the experience throughout a period of time. In a certain way, four days a week, year after year, may allow the formation of a commonsensical view of a specific mind **as it is** (C, 10).

Common sense was an early way to regard reality as synonymous with truth, and to see the situation in terms of an instinctual basic need of the human being: "*The failure to bring about this conjunction of sense-data, and therefore of a commonsense view induces a mental state of debility in the patient as if starvation of truth was somehow analogous to alimentary starvation*" (ST, 119).

> Logic, common sense, induction, deduction are terms that often represent mechanisms for bringing an intuition within reach of a realization should one exist. [T, 109–10]

A senseless realm?

Is it possible to use the concept of common sense, which is restricted to the use of senses, in other realms? Is there any realm which is beyond the senses? This area is covered in another entry in this dictionary; please refer to the entry "Ultra sensuous". With the narrower focus on common sense, it may be useful to remember that many are prone to consider psychic reality as a sense-less realm. It was defined by Freud in *The Interpretation of Dreams* as an immaterial form of existence. Is the word "immaterial" expressing a realm that is independent of the senses? Many also tend to see consciousness as a non-sensible realm.

A careful scrutiny of Freud's definitions of psychic reality and consciousness in *The Interpretation of Dreams* may throw some light on the issue. They continue to be the only definitions available, one hundred years later.

The "sense-less" view would be unwarranted if one remembers that psychic reality has a built-in characteristic of some senses (vectors). They are given by the instincts and their psychic representatives, unconscious phantasies. The immaterial form of existence (to use Freud's words), psychic reality, is different from the other form of existence, material reality. Also, the sensuous apparatus is just a differentiated "brain". They are just forms; the existence is a discrete one—ultimately unknowable and ineffable. Psychic reality, so to say, has a "foot" in material reality, given by the instincts, which are of biological origin. Conversely, material reality has a "hand" in shaping psychic reality, also via instincts and the sensuous apparatus. Therefore, our search for Freud's definition led us, again, to common sense. It is given by the internal—instinctual—senses that each guide one's life and above all, by the common sense obtained through the paradoxical matching of material and psychic reality. Both, constantly conjoined, furnish common sense.

Consciousness is seen by Freud as a sense organ, which apprehends psychic qualities. Thus it would not be seen, psycho-analytically speaking, as "sense-less". And what about feelings? They can be regarded—and Bion effectively regards them as such—as internal sense impressions. We say, "I feel cold"; but we also say "I feel hate". Bion quotes an example of a person who is entitled to state that a stone can feel heat, for its temperature varies if the external temperature varies too.

Do emotional experiences, links, relationships lie outside the range of the sensuous apparatus? Certainly anxiety and depression have no colour or smell, as Bion writes in the Commentary to *Second Thoughts and in Attention and Interpretation*. But have they any sense? Again, how can we conceive them without the port of entry, the senses?

In fact it seems that there are events that are not sensuously apprehensible, at least by the human sensual apparatus. They are dealt with in the entry "ultra-sensuous". There are many instances when the use of the senses is impossible; how can we get a commonsensical grasp of a given reality in those cases? For example, there are instances when there are no mechanical, optical or other inanimate devices that can help, such as telescopes, smoke drums and the like (as Bion says in *Attention and Interpretation and A Memoir of the Future*).

> There is nothing new in the criticism of lack of objectivity in psycho-analysis, and I am not proposing to waste time on it . . . in order to convey to the reader an impression of the psycho-analytical experience (which cannot in fact be seen or smelled or heard, for one is not listening to what the *patient* thinks he is saying), a description is given in terms of what *can* be sensuously experienced. No wonder psycho-analytical interpretations give rise to scepticism.
>
> Although no one doubts the reality of, say anxiety, it cannot be sensuously apprehended. [ST, 132]

Our search seems to indicate that the concept of common sense is applicable to psycho-analysis, up to a point. It is relevant to analysis concerning the communication of the patient with himself, with his analyst, of the analyst with the patient, and among analysts. It is relevant as a method that is necessary but not sufficient for apprehending reality.

Common sense and the correct interpretation

Common sense being a basic scientific tool to apprehend reality with less error, Bion, at the time that he was interested in neo-positivism, tried to construe commonsensical ways to verify the truth-value of analytic interpretation. He devised the conjunction of three senses, which he named dimensions. From these dimensions the analyst could draw different vertexes: the dimensions of senses, of passion and of myth (EP, 11).

Bion seemed to be an intuitive person with an uncanny ability to grasp the messages conveyed by patients who resorted to seemingly irrational talk and seemingly minor acting-out. In a paper published posthumously, Bion shows a psycho-analytic application of the concept. He differentiates between a kind of "lost common sense" that characterizes the patient under a superficial view and another kind of "common sense", non-rational, which emerges when analysis happens (C, 9).

This shows that Bion was prone to make use of the concept of common sense—provided it could be cleansed from its macro-social applications. The latter are put at the service of the group's well-being. When this occurs, common sense can be mistaken with good sense—the tool of hallucinosis. Good sense is the product of common sense mixed with judgmental values. Good sense relies on logic; it tames wild thoughts. Good sense is seen as the right sense; from there, it proceeds to being the only sense. The "neurological sense" of the word as well as its dual nature is lost.

At the end of his life, Bion would leave a clear warning about this alternative:

> . . . & EPILOGUE
> . . . FUGUE
> . . . DONA ES REQUIEM
> . . . MANY

All my life I have been imprisoned, frustrated, dogged by common-sense, reason, memories, desires and—greatest bug-bear of all—understanding and being understood. This is an attempt to express my rebellion, to say "Good-bye" to all that. It is my wish, I now realize doomed to failure, to write a book unspoiled by any tincture of common-sense, reason, etc. (see above). So, although I would write, "Abandon Hope all ye who expect to find any facts—scientific, aesthetic or religious—in this book", I cannot claim to have succeeded. All these will, I fear, be seen to have left their traces, vestiges, ghosts hidden within these words; even sanity, like "cheerfulness", will creep in. However successful my attempt, there would always be the risk that the book "became" acceptable, respectable, honoured and unread. "Why write then?" you may ask. To prevent someone who KNOWS from filling the empty space—but I fear I am being "reasonable", that great Ape. Wishing you all a Happy Lunacy and a Relativistic Fission . . . [AMF, III, 578]

Pepe Romero, the great guitar player, reports a good humoured comment from Joaquin Rodrigo a few months before the composer's death: "See, Pepito, I will go and you will visit me. We will enjoy a good 'Puro' [cigar], looking at all those guitar players so busy with all this score and fingers stuff . . . we will have good laughter!" (History Channel, 2003).

Misuses and misconceptions: There are two frequent confusions: to mistake common sense with "good sense" and "common place". The former confusion was discussed above; common sense, even though it can indicate a shared vision of whatever it is in a group, cannot be mistaken for good sense, which is a socially elected judgmental value.

The latter confusion seems to have arisen from the work of an outstanding thinker: Gaston Bachelard. He proposed an ideological view of Kant's criticism of "naïve realism": the idea that the universe and facts can be adequately apprehended by the sensual apparatus. That ideology underrated dismissively something that was labelled "British empiricism". He mistook the concept of common sense with the popular, socially shared view of facts. Bachelard was aware that the popular view is usually based on the sensuously apprehensible appearances of things. That view could be named, "commonplace". It seems that in dating, "sociologising" and "ideologising" the issue, Bachelard initiated a gross misunderstanding that confused common sense with commonplace.

Recommended cross-references: Analytical view, Binocular view, Establishment, Scientific deductive system, Scientific method, Sense of truth, Truth.

Communication: Please refer to the entries, Correlation, Controversy, Realistic Projective Identification.

Compassion:

> P.A. I do not think we could tolerate our work—painful as it often is for both us and our patients—without compassion. [AMF, III, 522]

The words compassion and passion (q.v.) are used by Bion in some seminal texts. Nevertheless, they did not attain the status of concepts. Bion uses the word "compassion" in its vernacular, colloquial sense. It was brought to the consideration of the practising analyst from Bion's experience with psychosis. It has to do with the limits, limitations and predicaments of the analytic method in the treatment of certain patients, namely, those who harbour excessive envy and narcissism, resulting in rivalry and willing abeyance to the "rules of hallucinosis" (q.v.). The rules of hallucinosis are expressed by two tendencies: to be "the top" and to act out instead of thinking:

> When the presenting problem in analysis is the hallucinations of the patient a crux has been reached. In addition to the problem that the patient is attempting to solve by transformation in hallucinosis is the secondary problem presented by his method of solution. This secondary problem appears in analysis as a conflict between the method employed by the analyst and the method employed by the patient. The conflict can be described as a disagreement on the respective virtues of a transformation in hallucinosis and a transformation in psycho-analysis. The disagreement is coloured by the patient's feeling that the disagreement between patient and analyst is a disagreement between rivals and that is concerns rival methods of approach. When it has been made clear the disagreement still continues but it becomes endo-psychic: the rival methods struggle for supremacy within the patient . . .

> The "rules" according to which he manipulates these elements are: (i) He needs no analyst because he provides the material for his own cure and knows how to obtain the cure for it . . . (iv) The relationship between the contestants is designed to prove the superiority of the patient and hallucinosis over the analyst and psycho-analysis . . . Following those "rules" certain anomalies arise: any benefit achieved as a result of analytic cure is vitiated by its being indistinguishable from "defect" of the analysand. Any victory of the analysand is vitiated by perpetuating the painful status quo. The painful element is due to the obtrusion of the analyst—"the analyst's fault" . . . all his interpretations are psycho-analytic elements designed to prove the superiority of himself and psycho-analysis. In so far as he is guilty of (i) his actions as a psycho-analyst are "acting-out"; and of (ii) his actions as a psycho-analyst are acts (as opposed to acting-out) and are expressions of a capacity for compassion. But a capacity for compassion is a source of admiration and therefore envy in an analysand who feels incapable of mature compassion. [T, 142–3]

It must be emphasized that the analysand feels incapable of mature compassion. As Bion pointed out often (just as Freud and Klein did), feelings may or may not be realistic. To mistake "to feel" with "to be" seems to be a persistent habit in the psycho-analytic movement. It is especially remarkable when the professional faces persons who floridly display florid manifestations of florid feelings. Is it a kind of "witchcraft apprenticeship" that precludes going more than skin deep? Which means, precludes the adoption of the psycho-analytic vertex. Even though "to feel" may be employed to denote a kind of intuitive hunch, I propose to leave narrow its semantic field in psycho-analysis in the sense Freud, Klein and Bion used it.

Feelings, through their links with hallucination, are more often than not unrealistic. The exercise of a pseudo-compassion may lead to some non-analytic aftermaths: (i) collusion; (ii) reassurance; (iii) despising of the patient's real potential; (iv) corny pseudo-psycho-analysis; (iv) psycho-babble; (v) false humanity, soft-humanism. The analyst will be entrapped in the same unending circle of a raging nothingness based on created feelings to which the patient was prey.

Bion, very early in his work, quotes Freud in his paper "Neurosis and psychosis" (1924). Based on his experience with psychotics, Bion makes a closer scrutiny of the statement, "... *the* ... *ego in the service of the id, withdraws itself from a part of reality*" (Freud, quoted by Bion, ST, 45).

He proposes "*two modifications in Freud's description*". He does this in order "*to bring it into closer relation with the facts. I do not think, at least as touches those patients likely to be met in analytic practice, that the ego is ever wholly withdrawn from reality*" (ST, 46), One may argue that Freud—and Bion quotes him—also made allowances for "*insufficient knowledge*" and warned that he would describe the processes "*very cursorily*". *Freud also leaves a door open when writing,* "parts of reality". *That is, the patient withdraws from parts of reality and does not withdraw from other parts of reality. Even though it is clear that for those parts from which the patient withdraws the withdrawal is complete. What does this mean?*

It means that Bion had constant touch with, and was constantly monitoring both the more mature and the more primitive aspect of personality. He did not embark on the easy choice of condemning people to illness. Perhaps this is compassion, because it leads to confidence in the hard work to be done and being careful with appearances of cure or appearances of worsening states when there is the realization of insanity (ST, 33; T, 8). He had earlier warned against reassuring patients and pointed out the necessity not to be crushed by the patient and his family's acting-out (ST, 44; T, 8). Later (1965) this view would be the origin of the concept of catastrophic change (T, chapter 1). And later still (1967), he would speak about detachment, or the necessity to limit confusion between patient and analyst: *"The psycho-analyst must be capable of more detachment than others because he cannot be a psycho-analyst and dissociate himself from the state of mind he is supposed to analyse"* (ST, 146).

In any case, a way out from being seduced by ideas of pathology or total madness is to use an analytical vertex. That is, what is at stake is a relationship between analyst and analysand who seem to be rivals, but the true rivalry is originated by an intrapsychic conflict of rival methods within the analysand's mind.

> It follows that it is a matter of difficulty for the analyst to conduct himself in such a manner that his association with the analysand is beneficial to the analysand, The exercise, in the patient's view, is the establishment of rivalry, envy and hate over compassion, complementation and generosity. The crux to which I referred is found in the character of the co-operation between two people and not in the problem for which the co-operation is required. The nature of the co-operation may be determined by the disturbances in the personality of the patient, but the situation may be presumed to be amenable to psycho-analysis; it differs form the situation produced by the inborn disposition of the patient. If analysis has been successful in restoring the personality of the patient he will approximate to being the person he was when his development became compromised. [T, 143]

A seminal preparatory paper that depicts how to deal psychoanalytically with the idea of compassion was published posthumously. It illuminates some issues linked with compassion as well as some issues linked to "reported feelings". This seems to be important in nourishing hallucination and belief, and in the "witchcraft apprenticeship syndrome" that befalls the practising professional who is caught unaware in an environment full of feelings. One risks collusion with the analysand's feelings instead of analysing them. If real, analysis occurs, it often displays their belonging to the realm of hallucination. Conversely, no compassion but rather counter-transference and collusion are possible in this context of undetected hallucination. This can be linked to a hidden, unconscious under-estimation by the analyst of the patient's abilities. Disguised as patience, forbearance and "humanity", a lenient or indulgent activity in fact means lack of compassion.

Bion proposes to differentiate compassion as a sense from compassion as an impulse. Even though compassion can be expressed as a feeling, *it appertains to the realm of instincts and nature.* Bion's paper is very short from a visual point of view, but it brings forth seminal concepts: among them, the idea of primary narcissism and primary envy and their influence in the outcome of an analysis. It seems to have served as a motto to his whole work thereafter.

Compassion and Truth

1.   Compassion and truth are both senses of man.
2.   Compassion is a feeling that he needs to express; it is an impulse he must experience in his feelings for others.
3.   Compassion is likewise something that he needs to feel in the attitude of others towards him.
6.   Truth and compassion are also qualities pertaining to the relationship that a man establishes with people and things.
7.   A man may feel he lacks a capacity for love.
8.   A man may lack capacity for love.
10.   He may in fact lack such a capacity.
11.   The lack may be primary or secondary, and may diminish truth and love, or both.
12.   Primary lack is inborn and cannot be remedied, yet some of the consequences may be modified analytically.
13.   Secondary lack may be due to fear or hate or envy or love. Even love can inhibit love. [C, 125]

A serious clinical situation is that of rivalry aroused by a compassionate analyst. In those cases the focus must not be the problem presented as content. Conversely, the sadistic professional uses the truth he observes but has little respect for truth; he creates unnecessary suffering (e.g., guilt) in the analysand; the high-brow or intellectualized analyst acts to impinge feelings into the patient as if he was an ad-man. In all there is a definite lack of compassion.

Summing up:

(i)   Compassion must not be mistaken with feelings and much less with overt demonstrations of them.

(ii) Compassion is an innate ability bound to ignite aspects of envy and greed. This is a built-in paradox of psycho-analytic practice and entails real dangers to the honest and gifted professional.

Concept: In "A theory of thinking" (1961), Bion establishes a theory about the **genetic development** of thought processes. This theory would be expanded clinically and detailed in *Elements of Psycho-Analysis* (1963). The basic tenets would remain unchanged. Bion classifies thoughts according to the *"nature of their developmental history"*: pre-conceptions, conceptions (which in that paper are synonymous with thoughts) and concepts.

In 1961 he defined concepts as *"fixed conceptions or thoughts"*. And why are concepts fixed? Because they were *"named"*. Bion would soon change this somewhat loose and imprecise definition. It was replaced by the view that even concepts can be unsaturated. It was later to be amended by the idea that they **must** be unsaturated, in order to avoid ideas of having attained absolute truth. But the concept of "O" and a broader use of Plato and Kant's formulations were still in the future.

The concept of saturation (q.v.) and lack of it were already implicit in the concepts of pre-conception and conception, to the extent that they were dependent on frustration and tolerance of it.

Concepts and science

In 1963 he would assign an important, if perhaps overlooked, function to concepts: *"The concept is derived from the conception by a process designed to render it free from those elements that would unfit it to be a tool in the elucidation or expression of truth"* (EP, 24). In other words, the concept belongs to the realm of scientific formulations. Oedipus as well as e=mc^2 may qualify as concepts.

Concepts can be used as compounds of a scientific deductive system. It *"means a combination of concepts in hypotheses and systems of hypothesis so that they are logically related to each other. The logical relation of one concept with another and of one hypothesis with another enhances the meaning of each concept and hypothesis thus linked and expresses a meaning that the concepts and hypotheses and links do not individually possess . . . the meaning of the whole may be said to be greater than the meaning of the sum of the parts"* (EP, 24).

This is conveyed with another concept, that of saturation. Bion again changes his former definition of concepts as fixed thoughts: *"A capacity for negative growth is needed partly to revivify a formulation that has lost meaning. . . . perhaps most important of all to achieve naiveté of outlook when a problem is so overlaid by experience that its outlines have become blurred and possible solutions obscure"* (EP, 85–86).

The A–H axis of the Grid depicts the evolution that characterizes the formation of a concept. It is the genetic axis, which involves growth that depends on particularization, generalization, and successive saturation. The cycle renews itself after a concept is created: a concept can be used as a new pre-conception, in a renewed cycle. Later he would call these cycles, "transformations". The pre-conception was given the formula of a constant (ψ) that combines itself with an unsaturated element (ξ).

Suggested cross-references: Pre-conception, Conception.

Conception: Because of inborn pre-conceptions the baby searches and eventually finds realizations in the outer world. This finding is essential to survival. When a pre-conception finds a realization, a conception is born. Conception is the outcome of a mating between a pre-conception and its realization.

☯ In "A theory of thinking" (1961), Bion published a compacted, completely summarized version of a lengthy series of observations and their elaboration stemming from his experience with patients suffering from severe disturbances of cognitive and thought processes. This experience spanned from the late forties to the early sixties. Part of it, from the late fifties, was published in 1992 by his dedicated wife Francesca, in *Cogitations*. It comprises the clinical papers and his attempts to correlate the psychotic's tribulations in dealing with reality with the philosopher's vicissitudes when he tackled the same task.

The final summary that Bion achieved to convey his elaboration in the form of a short paper ("A theory of thinking") is seemingly theoretical. Nevertheless it is embedded with the clinical ethos. Its clinical usefulness is recognizable to the reader with analytical experience. Its philosophical bearings are to be found in the work of Plato, Hume and Kant. Through living experiences with people who could not form concepts, Bion gave a practical application to that which was hitherto known as a philosophical problem.

The Kantian concept that Bion uses is that of "pre-conceptions" (q.v.). It corresponds to a priori knowledge quite independent of pure reason or dogma. The human being seems to be endowed with inborn notions that Kant proposed to call, "a priori". Bion hypothesizes that due to inborn pre-conceptions the baby searches and eventually finds realizations in the outer world. This finding is essential to survival. When a pre-conception finds a realization, a conception is born.

> The conception is initiated by the conjunction of a pre-conception with a realization ... When the pre-conception is brought into contact with a realization that approximates to it, the mental outcome is a conception. Put in another way, the pre-conception (the inborn expectation of a breast, the a priori knowledge of a breast, the "empty thought') when the infant is brought into contact with the breast itself, mates with awareness of the realization and is synchronous with the development of a conception ... Conceptions therefore will be expected to be constantly conjoined with an emotional experience of satisfaction. [ST, 111]

Satisfaction: fulfilling?

The issue of "satisfaction" seems to demand consideration in the light of the totality of Bion's work. "Emotional experience" was then a fumbling concept; even in 1965 Bion still warned about the impossibility that he felt to define with more precision emotions, affects, and emotional experiences. Even though his research enabled us to do this, the concept must be seen in the context of his time. This context demands a sharp differentiation between feelings of satisfaction and real satisfaction.

> Conceptions, that is to say the outcome of a mating between a pre-conception and its realization, repeat in a more complex form the history of pre-conception. A conception does not necessarily meet a realization that approximates sufficiently closely to satisfy. If frustration can be tolerated the mating of conception and realizations whether negative or positive initiates procedures necessary to learning by experience. [ST, 113]

Bion's growing perception of the importance of the "No" stemmed from his experience with people who seemed to be unable to tolerate this "No". "No" may be regarded as shorthand for frustration. Two years later, when devising the Grid (q.v.) the definition of conception was enriched by findings previously unavailable such as the psycho-analytical object (q.v.) and the issue of saturation. Therefore the concept was modified accordingly; it may be regarded "*as a variable that has been replaced by a constant. If we represent the pre-conception by $\psi(\xi)$ with (ξ) as the unsaturated element, then from the real-ization with which the pre-conception mates there is derived that which replaces (ξ) by a constant. The conception can however then be employed as a pre-conception in that it can express an expectation*" (EP, 24).

The emphasis in the cycle of pre-conceptions and their way to conceptions was now seen not exactly as illuminating the whole process of thinking, but rather as a part of it: the "genetic" part of it. The processes seemed much more complex due to Bion's acceptance (at the beginning, a bit critical and perhaps reluctantly) of Freud's proposal of consciousness as the sense organ for the perception of psychic quality. He integrated the models of Kant into those of Freud.

From then on, the Grid (q.v.), or "Idea" as he called it, the whole process, the genetics of thinking, was enriched by Sylvester and Cayley's concept of transformations and invariances. The saturation of a conception and its use as a new pre-conception would be used in broader terms: cycles of transformations (q.v.) Immobilizing in conceptions is a manifestation of death instincts; it is the refusal to go further into PS. PS shelters experiences of disarray, disorder, persecution, fear, helplessness. In brief, the human condition.

The conception lies within the conscious (secondary process) domain. Bion's latest view on it can be gauged by examples such as:

> All of us are intolerant of the unknown and strive instantaneously to feel it explicable, familiar—as "explosion" is to you and me. The event itself is suspect *because* it is explicable in terms of physics, chemistry, psycho-analysis, and other *pre*-conceived experience. The "conception" is an event which has become "conceivable"; the "conceivable" it has become is no longer the genetic experience. Pre-conception, conception, birth—what a shock it must have been to know that a woman has a baby! How absurd to suppose that it could have any connection with sexual intercourse! I have found

those who think it ridiculous that a woman could initiate an idea or have a thought worthy of consideration. [AMF, II, 382]

Bion posited the existence of two innate pre-conceptions and therefore, conceptions: that of the breast and that of Oedipus:

I postulate an α-element version of a private Oedipus myth which is the means, the pre-conception, by virtue of which the infant is able to establish contact with the parents as they exist in the world of reality. The mating of this α-element Oedipal pre-conception with the realization of the actual parents gives rise to the conception of parents. [EP, 93]

Misuses and misunderstandings: Bion's writing requires careful scrutiny; the emphasis is in the awareness of realization rather than in an alleged whole satisfaction of the pre-conception. In terms of the evolution of Bion's theory, it may be useful to be reminded that during this epoch he was—from clinical experience—paving the way to grasp the movement between conscious and unconscious (c.f. contact barrier). This point—awareness, perception of reality and its vicissitudes—is fundamental. If it is not taken into consideration it will give a distorted reading of Bion's contribution.

Is the distortion of leaving aside the issue of awareness of a given reality—the term that Bion used is "realization"—a reproduction of an earlier distortion of Freud's theory from which these contributions of Bion originated? Perhaps the problem is the **idea** of satisfaction. Is there any realization that approximates to it? Or is it a word that just expresses a hallucination? Many readers think that the whole issue is to satisfy the pre-conception. Bion's text indicates an utterly different situation. When an *"awareness of realization"* occurs, there also occurs—*"synchronous"*—the *"development of a conception"*.

There is a catch here. The following phrase associates conceptions with an expectation (namely, of *"an emotional experience of satisfaction"*) in a constant conjunction. One may fail to grasp that Bion writes about conscious feelings, about a constant conjunction in the strictest Humean sense; and finally, about *"an emotional experience of satisfaction"* that differs fundamentally from factual fulfilment. Many readings transform Bion's observation as if it depicted the actual fulfilment.

The rationale underlying this is a kind of reading and apprehension of psycho-analysis that displays many a reader's ideology or *Weltanschauung*. What is at stake is the very old human allegiance to the pleasure/displeasure principle. Freud's concept of instincts and the act of looking for their satisfaction seems to be one of the first distortions of this kind that was made. The goals of instincts have been persistently mistaken for a search for fulfilment of desire. The philosophically informed reader would be trained to avoid this pitfall; Hume's constant conjunction meets a psycho-logical need of the observer.

Imprecision There are exceedingly few places where one is able to spot any lack of precision in Bion's writings. Up to now this writer has been able to spot just four. One of them is with the definition of conception. All definitions are given precisely and are used in the same sense throughout his work. Nevertheless, one may see that in *Learning from Experience*, page 91, one of the imprecise formulations occurs. There Bion states that the conception is "*that which results when a pre-conception mates with the appropriate sense impressions*". At this point he was just defining container and contained (q.v.) and it seems that the concept of realization is confused here with the concept of sense impressions. Sense impressions are a most primitive form that harbour realizations, but they are not realizations.

Also, sense impressions are the raw data used to form alpha-elements, after the digestion of sense impressions by alpha-function. The reader may realize the confusion if he compares this specific definition with both earlier and latest parts of Bion's work. In all of them he uses the same basic definition, that dates from 1963 (reproduced above) and 1965 (see page 40 of *Transformations*). It seems safe to consider that:

1) This definition is not used anywhere else in his work.
2) It does not fit precisely either into the concept of alpha function or into the theory of the genetic evolution of thinking. In the first case, alpha function refers to taking in of the sense impressions and in the second, there's a string of events, namely, pre-conceptions mating with realizations rather than with sense impressions, as this phrase states, leading to conceptions.

One may well leave it aside and adopt the one that is consistently repeated throughout his earlier and later writings.

Suggested Cross-references: Catastrophic change, Concepts, Container/contained, Controversy, Myth, Pre-conceptions; Psychoanalytical objects; Reverie; Transformations.

Confrontation: Intrapsychically and in the relationships one maintains with other people, how can we cope with different views without turning them into conflict but into respect for the differences involved? Biologically this expresses itself in the reality of sexual reproduction, male and female. Oedipus, newness, unknown and the prevalence of life are one possible outcome. Disruption, impossibility of marriages and extinction of life are their contrapuntal matching pairs, which marks another possible outcome.

Confrontation may mean, *"vis-à-vis"*, to be in front of whatever it be. Socrates' maieutics and Kant's criticism seem to be earlier manifestations of confrontation; psycho-analysis one of its later forms. Manifest and latent contents, the two principles of mental functioning, PS and D seem to be basic formulations of this basic confrontation. The analysand confronts the analyst with that which is unknown to both; the analyst confronts the patient with that which the patient had himself turned into unknown to him.

Is it true to state that confrontation, in the sense of a difference of vertexes, is the stuff that real analysis (q.v.) and real life is made of? The difference must be tolerated; false compliance or war are signs of intolerance to it. For the insecure or seductive professional, confrontation is ever seen as the mark of rude conflict and is actively avoided. No search for truth is possible in this case.

> ... there must be a difference of vertex to make correlation possible. It must ultimately take place in the individual. (For the moment I assume that correlation is a necessary part of confrontation and that confrontation is a necessary part of analysis). Schizophrenic defences are mobilized against confrontation: violence makes confrontation impossible because both sides of a confrontation are annihilated. [AI, 93]

One may remember that there is no growth without a contrary force.

Suggested cross-reference: Controversy.

Constant conjunction: A term that Bion borrows from Hume, with no modification. Hume observed that some facts can be observed as constantly conjoined, but this conjunction may have no counterpart in reality. There are flaws in observation, especially when the constant conjunction or association is seen as having causal effects. He states that the constant conjunction is drawn from the observer's psychological necessity, convenience or belief.

Kant felt that Hume's observation is the scandal of philosophy. At first he attacked his forebear but in due time (in the "Prolegomena") he stated that he owed his greatest moves to Hume. Bion stated that reason is the slave of passion, and therefore reason is psycho-logically necessary (T, 73). This also corresponds to Hume's awareness, perhaps the first in Western philosophy since Plato, that the observer interferes with the object observed.

Contact barrier: An active and living filter that regulates the relationship between the conscious and unconscious. It both links **and** separates the conscious and the unconscious.

℘ More often than not the work of Bion comes from the work of Freud. Here he uses a term that Freud coined in the *Project*.

The psycho-analytic establishment usually regards this term as exclusively mirroring Freud's foresight about the neuronal synapses. It is a way to use Freud's contribution with an emphasis on material reality. Bion does not follow this lead from the psycho-analytic establishment. Without detracting from it he uses the same term as a model for describing the relationship between the conscious and unconscious.

In studying patients with severe disorders of thought, he realized a weakness in Freud's theory of consciousness for dealing with those patients. Freud's theory of consciousness states that the unconscious precedes the conscious, in terms of succession in time.

Bion observes in psychosis an intermingling of unconscious with conscious, suggesting that they function simultaneously on psychotic levels (please see the entry, Beta-screen). This is the first weakness that Bion sees in Freud's theory. It is important to state, as Bion states explicitly, that weakness does not imply falsity. Bion does state that Freud's theory is true, not false. [LE, 54]

Also, Freud's theory of consciousness as the sense organ of psychic quality seems to make no allowances for registers of psychic quality that are not *"impartial"* (LE, 54). Thus terms such as primary and secondary processes would be unsatisfactory. Bion's proposal of a contact-barrier allows for simultaneity of both—conscious and unconscious, primary and secondary with no primacy at all.

Those patients have an inability to dream and therefore an inability to sleep or wake, to be either conscious or unconscious. Therefore, one may see that Bion was taking Freud's theory of unconscious and of conscious to its extreme. The timelessness of the unconscious is at stake in Freud and is rescued in Bion's theory. Was Bion "out-Freuding" Freud?

There would be no time succession between conscious and unconscious, but a kind of filter that allows a movement to and fro between the two instances. This filter is called "contact barrier". It is a paradoxical concept, as it both links and separates. Therefore one may say that we deal with a monistic unit [conscious and unconscious]. Or, in other words, the concept of contact barrier makes clear that the situation is simultaneously conscious with unconscious **and** conscious separated from the unconscious. This concept may be considered as an ancestor of that of caesura (q.v.)

"The term contact-barrier emphasizes the establishment of contact between conscious and unconscious and the selective passage of elements from one to the other. On the nature of the contact-barrier will depend the change of elements from conscious to unconscious and vice-versa" (LE, 17). The concept of contact barrier is part of the theory of alpha-function, in which *"the powers of censorship and resistance are essential to differentiation of conscious and unconscious and help to maintain the discrimination between the two"* (LE, 16).

After examining the function of the dream, helping to *"explain the tenacity with which the dream, as represented in classical theory, defends itself against the attempt to make the unconscious conscious"* (LE, 16), Bion transfers what he said about the *"establishment of conscious and unconscious and a barrier between them a supposed entity"* that he designates, a "contact barrier".

A man talking to a friend converts the sense impressions of his emotional experience into alpha-elements, thus becoming capable of dream thoughts and therefore of undisturbed consciousness of the facts whether the facts are the events in which he participates or his feelings about these events or both. He is able to remain "asleep" or unconscious of certain elements that cannot penetrate the barrier presented by his "dream". Thanks to the "dream" he can continue uninterruptedly to be awake, that is, awake to the fact that he is talking to a friend, but asleep to elements which, if they could penetrate the barrier of his "dreams", would lead to domination of his mind by what are ordinarily unconscious ideas and emotions.

The dream makes a barrier against mental phenomena which might overwhelm the patient's awareness that he is talking to a friend, and, at the same time, makes it impossible for awareness that he is talking to a friend to overwhelm his phantasies ... the ability to "dream" preserves the personality from what is virtually a psychotic state. [LE, 15, 16]

The contact-barrier "is made" of "alpha-elements". Therefore the soundness of "alpha-function" (q.v.) is seminal in the formation of the contact-barrier. It *"may be expected to manifest itself clinically— if indeed it is manifest at all—as something that resembles dream. As we have seen the contact barrier permits a relationship and preservation of belief in is as an event in actuality, subject to the laws of nature, without having that view submerged by emotions and phantasies originating endo-psychically. Reciprocally it preserves emotions with endo-psychic origin from being overwhelmed by the realistic view. The contact barrier is there- fore responsible for the preservation of the distinction between conscious and unconscious and for its inception. The unconscious is thus preserved"* (LE, 26–7).

Suggested cross-references: Alpha-function, Alpha-elements, Beta-elements and Beta-screen, Dream the session.

Container/contained: This double term contains a paradox: some- thing that contains and something that is contained perform the functions of containing, and being contained *vis-à-vis* each other.

It is derived from Melanie Klein's theory of projective identifi- cation and maintains a close kinship with it. It defines both a func- tion of the personality and an "element of psycho-analysis" (q.v.). It is a form of relationship from the inception of life that allows emotional growth and growth of thinking processes. It is the process through which accrual of meaning is obtained; therefore container/contained is equated to thinking itself. It represents the most developed form of Bion's theory of thinking, which took approximately nine years to achieve. The deepest and most secret mysteries of human life are explored within this theory.

Emotions and thought processes

For many years there was a loosely-stated relationship between emotional and intellectual growth. Freud, Klein and Winnicott made it clear that this relationship did exist. Spitz and Bowlby began to display the proofs of this relationship, in specific "privation settings". Montessori's methods as well the Summerhill experiment were early attempts to give a practical form to it. It may be thought that among pre-psycho-analytic contributions Rudolf Steiner's ideas and Piaget's studies were also some forms that expressed awareness of this link. Bion's theory furnished insight about *how* this relationship functions at its inception. Emotional and intellectual growth are put into terms of the relationship between the infant and the breast in its most minute features. It does not state the relationship as a matter of principle, postulate or imaginary construct of an authority.

Growth

Container/contained forms a theory of psycho-analysis, one of the few that Bion formulated. It is *"the essential feature of Melanie Klein's conception of projective identification"* (EP, 3). Bion, together but independently from Rosenfeld, had earlier observed the communicative function of projective identification. Now he displayed another function of this mechanism—relating growth and learning. Bion uses a quasi-mathematical symbol derived from genetics to denote the evolving relationship between container and contained: $\female \male$ *"Growing $\female \male$ provides the basis of an apparatus for learning from experience"* (LE, 92).

☉ Bion began to work with the idea of a container, developing from Klein's observations about the result of processes of denial, splitting and projective identification. It seems, as he indicates later, that his experiences in war also provided him with an experiential background that gave sense to Klein's observations; more specifically, the idea of a warring army containing the enemies. As late as 1970 he would use the metaphor in the clinical depiction of the container and containment: *". . . a man speaking of an emotional experience in which he was closely involved began to stammer badly as the memory became increasingly vivid to him. The aspects of the model that are significant are these: the man was trying to contain his experience in a form of words; he was trying to contain himself, as one sometimes says of someone about to lose control of himself; he was trying to 'contain' his emotions within a form of words, as one might speak of a general attempting to 'contain' enemy forces within a given zone"* (AI, 94).

This first use of the term dates from 1955–56, in "Development of schizophrenic thought" and "Differentiation between the psychotic and non-psychotic personality". It deals with the fact that expelled fragments of personality exert a function of containment. The patient feels he is able to expel parts of his ego that were attacked. Why were they attacked? Because they *"would make him aware of the reality he hates"* (ST, 47)—the reality of his fear, pain, and sadism; also, the pain that the human condition inflicts on infantile omnipotence. He feels that those fragments are spread around him, put into objects or people. To put this into terms of hate towards reality, so clearly expressed, means that Klein's illumination about projective identification received an emphasis from Bion: the epistemological aspect.

The *"patient experiences a failure in his capacity for perception. All his sense impressions appear to have suffered mutilation of a kind which would be appropriate had they been attacked as the breast is felt to be attacked in the sadistic phantasies of the infant. The patient feels imprisoned in the state of mind he has achieved and unable to escape from it because he feels he lacks the apparatus of awareness of reality, which is both the key to escape and the freedom itself to which he would escape. This sense of imprisonment is intensified by the menacing presence of the expelled fragments within whose planetary movements he is contained . . .*

> In the patient's phantasy the expelled particles of ego lead to an independent and uncontrolled existence outside the personality, but either containing or contained by external objects, where they exercise their functions as if the ordeal to which they have been subjected has served only to increase their number and to provoke their hostility to the psyche that ejected them. [ST, 39]

Therefore something exists that is felt as meriting to be expelled as undesirable, hostile, potentially annihilating. It would later be named, in *Transformations*, *"nameless dread"*, and in *A Memoir of the Future*, *"sub-thalamic fear"*. This "something" struggles to find an adequate container. But this something is mind itself, full of fear and hostility. At this point in Bion's work, it is already clear that such a containment should be made originally by the breast in the sense that it can either refuse or agree to receive those phantasies. The refusal heightens the predicament. As often happens with psycho-analysis, those findings were first seen in severely disturbed patients. Later it was realized that those phenomena emerge in any person; they are typical of the newborn, and encircle its relationship with the breast.

The lack of capacity to contain those fragments of ego jeopardize at the outset all the features of the personality *"which should one day provide the foundation for intuitive understanding of himself and others"* (ST, 47). Bion furthers the description. It is not just some unwanted parts of the ego that are expelled, but also those functions of the ego that provide contact with reality. Namely, consciousness of sense impressions, attention, memory, judgement, thought. They *"have brought against them, in such inchoate forms as they may possess at the outset of life, the sadistic splitting eviscerating attacks that lead to their being minutely fragmented and then expelled from the personality to penetrate, or encyst, the objects"* (ST, 47).

Bion would make the definition more explicit some years later (1962), in *Learning from Experience*. The concept of container and contained is now given as a new theory in psycho-analysis. This is a remarkable difference if compared with most of Bion's contributions to psycho-analysis. He uses his earlier clinical findings, amended by an important aspect, namely, that of "saturation". This amendment seems to allow him to see that those issues encompass something beyond pathology.

In scientific terms, Bion has an acute awareness of the nature of theory, that is, of a model (after Kant, who called it "scheme"; Sandler, 1999):

5.   Melanie Klein has described an aspect of projective identification concerned with the modification of infantile fears; the infant projects a part of its psyche, namely its bad feelings, into a good breast. Thence in due course they are removed and re-introjected.

During their sojourn in the good breast they are felt to have been modified in such a way that the object that is re-introjected has become tolerable to the infant's psyche.

6. From the above theory I shall abstract for use as a model the idea of a container into which an object is projected and the object that can be projected into the container: the latter I shall designate by the term contained. The unsatisfactory nature of both terms points the need for further abstraction.

7. Container and contained are susceptible of conjunction and permeation by emotion. Thus conjoined or permeated or both they change in a manner usually described as growth. When disjoined or denuded of emotion they diminish in vitality, that is, approximate to inanimate objects. Both container and contained are models of abstract representations of psycho-analytic realizations. [LE, 90]

Bion relies on Klein's seminal paper from 1946 and refines the study of paranoid–schizoid mechanisms.

His next step was to resort to quasi-mathematical symbols. The first attempt was to use well-known symbols drawn from biology: *"I shall use the sign* ♀ *for the abstraction representing the container and* ♂ *for the contained"* (LE, 90).

The borrowing of the symbols hitherto used by the geneticist denotes natural facts that can be depicted verbally: penetration, lodging, insemination, growing and experience. At the same time it divests the situation of the pleasure principle. It conveys the natural, biological nature of the mind. Bion states that ♂ has a power of *"penetrability"* in *"elements* ♀*"* (LE, 93).

It also brings with it the indication that container and the contained are amenable to being dealt with as functions. As is explained in the entry "functions and factors" of this dictionary, the idea of function presumes that something or someone functions. It is a dynamic activity: *"The activity that I have here described as shared by two individuals becomes introjected by the infant so that the* ♀♂ *apparatus becomes installed in the infant . . . a model is provided by the idea of the infant who explores an object by putting it into his mouth. What talking was originally done by the mother, possibly a rudimentary designatory function, is replaced by the infant's own baby talk"* (LE, 91).

The theory of container and contained is part of the theory of alpha-function (q.v.) and had a model in the area of thinking: the mating of a pre-conception with a realization (that has as its origin, sense impressions) to produce a conception. As stated above, the model is represented by ♀♂.

The container and contained, the mating of pre-conceptions and realizations, in their repetition (LE, 91, item 14) *"promotes growth in ♀♂"*. Bion would later assume a *"benign operation"* of ♀♂ (EP, 33). This benign operation is in 1963 seen as an evolution in genetic terms of the lettered axis in the Grid. *"The benignity or otherwise of change effected by the mechanism ♀ ♂ depends on the nature of the dynamic link L, H or K"*.

The growth is not necessarily "good" or constructive, for there are no judgmental values in analysis. For example, a container/contained link can evolve in the minus sense: *"the infant feels fear that it is dying, and projects its feelings of fear into the breast together with envy and hate of the undisturbed breast. Envy precludes a commensal relationship. The breast in K would moderate the fear component in the fear of dying that had been projected into it and the infant in due course would re-introject a new tolerable and consequently growth-stimulating part of its personality. In −K the breast is felt enviously to remove the good or valuable element in the fear of dying and force the worthless residue back into the infant. The infant who started with a fear he was dying ends up by containing a nameless dread"* (LE, 96). The growth of this process is inextricably associated with violence of emotion. Its increased sophistication is conveyed *"by saying that the will to live, that is necessary before there can be a fear of dying, is a part of the goodness that the envious breast has removed"* (LE, 97). (To see the definition of "commensal" see below, in "the quality of the link between container and contained"; also, the specific entry, "commensal".)

The possibility of a −(♀ ♂) (minus container contained) is expanded. It possesses a growing morality. There emerges a *"super-superego"* that asserts the moral superiority of undoing and unlearning and the advantages of *"finding fault with everything"*. *"The most important characteristic is its hatred of any new development in the personality as if the new development were a rival to be destroyed. The emergence therefore of any tendency to search for the truth, to establish contact with reality and in short to be scientific in no matter how rudimentary a fashion is met by destructive attacks on the tendency and the reassertion of the 'moral' superiority. This implies an assertion of what in sophisticated terms would be called a moral law and a moral system superior to scientific law and a scientific system*" (LE, 98). This is growth, even though it occurs in a reversed form. Socially the issue appears in a peaceful or destructive use of nuclear energy, or consumerism.

In fact in some cases it seems that the person feels that his mind is unbearable, especially when there is a defusion of life and death instincts: "*The mind is too heavy a load for the sensuous beast to carry. I am the thought without a thinker and the abstract thought which has destroyed its thinker Newtonwise, the container that loves its content to destruction; the content that explodes its possessive container*" (AMF, I, 38). The reference to Newton was that, according to Lord Keynes and some historians, he lost his sanity when he was on the verge of making new discoveries. He turned to religion and almost killed himself in a mysterious fire. Bion became impressed with this comment, which was recorded in *Transformations* (T, 156).

The perverse growth in the realm of minus is made more explicit when Bion formulates transformations in hallucinosis (q.v.) "*The ability of 0 [meaning, zero] to increase thus by parthenogenesis corresponds to the characteristics of greed which is also able to grow and flourish exceedingly by supplying itself with unrestricted supplies of nothing*" (T, 134). The final result seems to be, "*a raging inferno of greedy non-existence*". Bion would expand the issue considerably in many parts of *A Memoir of the Future*. See for example the entry "Controversy" in this dictionary and the first five chapters of vol. I, *The Dream*, of a swelling experience of nothingness in the false marriage of "Alice" and "Roland".

The annotations of Bion's copy of Freud's *The Future of an Illusion* illustrate the issue. It faces truth quite independently of the pain involved in this act: "*Too much of the thinking about psycho-analysis precludes the possibility of regarding as good a theory that would destroy the individual or the group. Yet there will never be a scientific scrutiny of analytical theories until it includes critical appraisal of a theory that by its very soundness could lead to a destruction of mental stability, e.g., a theory that increased memory and desire to a point where they rendered sanity impossible*" (C, 378).

An often overlooked observation seems to have been made clear in *A Memoir of the Future*—see for example chapters 12 and 23 in volume I, also the "liberation" of the character "Rosemary"; also, the "marriage" of the characters "Rosemary" and "Man" in volume

II chapters 1 to 5. The observation here is that the paranoid–schizoid phenomena are as fundamental to thinking as the depressive phenomena are; Bion rescues the analytical posture. He followed Freud's footsteps concerning the death instincts, life instincts and their fusion and defusion. He did the same with Klein's elucidation of the paranoid–schizoid and depressive position; it is an eternal tandem-like movement. At the same time he also integrates Freud and Klein into a unified theory of thinking. This new evaluation of PS⇔D is not a praise of folly (such as many do when they praise the "imaginaire"). Much less would it be a eulogy of ⇨D two different forms of denying the advancement into the unknown that this idea represents.

In *Elements of Psycho-Analysis* Bion would propose that ♀♂ qualifies for that which he calls an "element of psycho-analysis". This implies that it is an elementary particle of the psyche itself. *"It is a representation of an element that could be called a dynamic relationship between container and contained."* Bion was gradually rescuing the dynamic ethos of Freud's conception of psycho-analysis. It seems that it was at this time—especially after Melanie Klein's death—that analysis was becoming progressively static, imprisoned in manipulations of symbols. Theories were subjected to learning by heart; therefore they were applied mechanistically, both as *a priori* and *ad hoc* patterns. In consequence they were gradually denuded of their stuff—of life itself.

Learning, thinking and sexuality

Still in *Elements of Psycho-Analysis*, ♀♂ his, so to say, "upgraded" to the status of thinking itself, where it concerns construing of meaning: "I propose provisionally to represent the apparatus for thinking by the sign ♀♂. The material, so to speak, out of which this apparatus is manufactured is I . . . We must now consider I in its ♀♂ operation, an operation usually spoken of in ordinary conversation as thinking. From the point of view of meaning thinking . . ." (EP, 31). "I" stands for Idea—it is the growth of thinking processes as well as its backward movement and can be "seen" through the Grid.

Tolerating doubt and the unknown is the essence of a succession of ♀♂ in a loosely connected and "perforated" reticulum. (Bion borrows the concept of reticulum from Elliott Jaques) In other words, thinking is regarded as a thrust into the unknown, rather than a "deposit" of logic and rationality.

He proposes a graphic symbol, a mixture of maths and biology, to represent the growing container: ♀^{n}: *"Learning depends on the capacity for* ♀^{n} *to remain integrated and yet lose rigidity"* (LE, 93). One may visualize it through some models drawn from its counterparts in external reality. Their concrete aspect may facilitate the apprehension of ♀^{n}: a uterus with a growing foetus, a theoretical system that accepts new empirical data. *"This is the foundation of the state of mind of the individual who can retain his knowledge and experience and yet be prepared to reconstrue past experiences in a manner that enables him to be receptive of a new idea"* (LE, 93).

That which commenced primitively as *"preconceptions probably related to feeding, breathing and excretion"* evolves in growing sophistication of tolerated doubt. The very sophisticated systems of hypothesis of science *"though hardly recognizable in their origins nevertheless retain the receptive qualities denoted by* ♀*"* (LE, 94). To grow, to think and to learn are at base an evolving experiencing of penetration into the unknown: *"Tolerance of doubt and tolerance of a sense of infinity are the essential connective of* ♂^{n} *if K is to be possible"* (LE, 94)

The sexual nature or Oedipal component of ♀ ♂ is implicit in the usage of the genetic symbol. Anyway, the term "sexual" may impart a sensuous and concretized sense that is alien to the theory (AI, 106). The unification of Freud and Klein in this theory of Bion performs a function in psycho-analysis that is analogous to that the physicists would like to see in a still non-existent theory in their own field—one that would integrate the quantum and relativity theories. Perhaps Bion obtained it because he was not looking for it as the physicists are—clinical facts and experience led naturally to it. The bisexual nature of the human mind is made clear:

> *I* [Idea] develops a capacity for any one of its aspects to assume indifferently the function ♂ or ♀ to any other one of its aspects ♀ or ♂. We must now consider *I* in its ♀♂ operation, an operation usually spoken of in ordinary conversation as thinking. From the point of view of meaning thinking depends on the successful introjection of the good breast that is originally responsible for the performance of α-function. On this introjection depends the ability

of any part of *I* to be ♂ to the other part's ♀ . . . briefly, explanation may be seen as related to the attitude of one part of the mind to another, and correlation as a comparison of content expressed by one aspect of *I* to content expressed by another aspect of I. [EP, 31–2]

That is, the breast may be the container of the baby but the baby is also the container of the breast. In terms of functions, there is no mother-in-abstractio, or a mother-in-itself. The entity "mother" exists because there is a baby that propitiates an environment for "motherness" (Winnicott is the other author who realizes this). Ditto, for a penis and a vagina, for masculinity and femininity as existent in any person irrespective of the biological or sensuous-concrete sex. It can be said that in the same way a PS⇔D exists, a ♀♂ has in its interior a functioning that is an ever-changing ⇔. It can be subsumed as "expulsion⇔ingestion" (EP, 42). Some of its realizations can also be stated by models other than the digestive system. *"Of these the most suggestive are (1) the respiratory system, with which is linked the olfactory system; (2) the auditory system with which is linked transformations such as music⇔noise, and (3) the visual system"* (EP, 95).

How can one state that ♀♂ is an "element of psycho-analysis"? The answer is important clinically. It must be duly weighed in the analytic session. Some apparently familiar statements display an unfamiliarity that is the clue to their emotional significance. *"Judgement of the importance or significance of the emotional event during which such verbalizations appear to be apposite to the emotional experience depends on the recognition that container and contained, ♀♂, is one of the elements of psycho-analysis. We may then judge whether the element ♀♂ is central or merely present as a component of a system of elements that impart meaning to each other by their conjunction.*

Considering now whether it is necessary to abstract the idea of a container and contained as an element of psycho-analysis I am met with a doubt. Container and contained implies a static condition and this impli-cation is one that must be foreign to our elements; there must be more of the character imparted by the words 'to contain or to be contained'. 'Container and contained' has a meaning suggesting the latent influence of another element in a system of elements" (EP, 7).

In *Attention and Interpretation* Bion furnishes a précis of his theories on thinking, container–contained in terms of their emotional origins:

> In the primitive phase, which Freud regards as dominated by the pleasure principle and from which he excludes the operation of memory, this last being dependent on the prior development of a capacity for thought, the prototype of memory appears to reside in one of the aspects of projective identification. This mechanism, employed to fulfil the duties of thought until thought takes over, appears as an interchange between mouth and breast and then between introjected mouth and introjected breast. This I regard as reaction between container ♀ and contained ♂. ♀ seems to be the element which is nearest in this phase to the memory . . .
>
> ♂ evacuates unpleasure in order to get rid of it, to have it transformed into something that is, or feels, pleasurable, for the pleasure of evacuation, for the pleasure of being contained. ♀ takes in the evacuations for the same motives. The nature of the relationship needs investigation. ♀, which may evacuate or retain, is the prototype of a forgetful or retentive memory, Pleasure may be retained if possession is the dominant concern; grievance if a store of ammunition is the main concern. Evacuation may be forcible as if to convert the evacuated object into a missile; introjection likewise as fulfilment of greed. [AI, 29]

Further expansion

The theory ♀ ♂ was expanded in 1970 and 1975. Bion suggested new possibilities for the nature of the link between ♀ and ♂. Hitherto it was described as "commensal". Now it is seen within a realm that admits more possibilities, thanks to insights into (−K). The new possibilities are called parasitic and symbiotic.

The whole issue is centred on the possibilities of the container being destroyed by the contained or vice-versa. There are many consequences to the group. Bion resorts again to the concept of "mystic", as an evolution of his observations that mystics have contact with truth in *Transformations*. Truth is seen as a potentially explosive container.

It seems that Bion relies, as ever, on his clinical experience, but his personal experience of having been subjected to co-option by the establishment is added. His words seemed prophetic: the establishment was unyielding and after his exclusion it decayed. The soil of England, which was able to contain "mystics" of the calibre of Freud and Klein, expelled local mystics such as Alan Turing, Oscar Wilde and Bion—to its own impoverishment.

Even a married couple can be uncreative if "*the sexual relationship ♀♂ plays such a part that there is **no room** for any of the other activities in which the married couple might engage*" (AI, 107—the same motto was to be expanded in *A Memoir of the Future*). The dynamic sexual intercourse represented by ♀ ♂ is the actual analytic session when the unknown is considered and doubt tolerated: "*The clue lies in the observation of the fluctuations which make the analyst at one moment ♀ and the analysand ♂, and at the next reverse the roles*" (AI, 108).

The evolving, transient, elusive nature of life itself is the next step in the evolution of the ♀ ♂ concept, as observable and "liveable" in the analytic session. In order to elicit it Bion resorts to a discrimination of "memory" and "remembering"; it also serves to display in here the flexible and dynamic use of the theory:

> ♀ or ♂ may represent memory. The container ♀ is filled with "memories" derived from sensuous experience . . . The ♂ memory is saturated accordingly. The analyst who comes to a session with an active memory is therefore in no position to make "observations" of unknown mental phenomena because these are not sensuously apprehended. There is something that has often been called "remembering" and that is essential to psycho-analytic work; this must be sharply distinguished from what I have been calling memory. I want to make a distinction between (1) remembering a dream or having a memory of a dream and (2) the experience of the dream that seems to cohere as if it were a whole, at one moment absent, at the next present. This experience, which I consider to be essential to evolution of the emotional reality of the session, is often called a memory, but it is to be distinguished from the experience of remembering. [AI, 107]

The theory of container and contained has some offshoots in groups and in some senses of inclusion and exclusion of the members of a group, as well as the possibility of some of the members of a group that glimpses reality as it is (the "mystics"). More considerations of the theory of the container/contained in regard to its usefulness in the practice of analysis can be found in the entry, "Real Analysis/Correct Analysis/Correct Interpretation".

The nature of that which links container with contained

The final development of the theory focused on the nature or quality of the link between container and contained. The first one was adumbrated in 1962, "commensal": *"By commensal I mean ♂ and ♀ are dependent on each other for mutual benefit and without harm to either. In terms of a model the mother derives benefit and achieves mental growth from experience: the infant likewise abstracts benefit and achieves growth"* (LE, 91). Eight years later, the definition was presented in a more developed form: *"By 'commensal' I mean a relationship in which two objects share a third to the advantage of all three"* (AI, 95).

The hasty reader or the concretized reader may feel a discrepancy. It is more apparent than real; the first definition already includes the third, albeit an immaterial one: it is called "mental growth"; it also has a materialness, it is called, "milk". The later definition is more true to the biological definition as well as more psycho-analytically explicit.

To the commensal Bion now adds, from clinical observation, two links: "symbiotic" and "parasitic". *"By 'symbiotic' I understand a relationship in which one depends on another to mutual advantage. By 'parasitic' I mean to represent a relationship in which one depends on another to produce a third, which is destructive to all three"* (AI, 95).

In *A Memoir of the Future* Bion would develop the concept further. Book I deals extensively with many disrupted and non-disrupted containers; at the end of the book, the characters of the book (Myself, Bion, Man, etc.) are put into his earlier theoretical terms of container and contained:

> MYSELF Terms like "mistress" and "maid", "husband" and "wife", are all "sensuously" meaningful and in the domain of sensuous relationships A + B can be meaningful in a macroscopic way. Even relationships which can be mathematically expressed, as the "pure" mathematician says they are in pure mathematics, become sensuous.
>
> BION Is that not saying that the mere fact of being able to formulate the relationship A+B makes it a macroscopic relationship? But *does* it? Is it more true to say that we are so used to formulate statements

only when they are macroscopic that we instantaneously assume that what **is** formulated must, by the fact of formulation, be macroscopic?

MYSELF The converse is thought to be true: that if we cannot formulate it, "it" must be ultra- or infra-sensuous; that concepts that are "empty" and intuitions that are "blind" must lack completion and that the "completion" which is not "complete", or is "unfulfilled", nevertheless exists. ♀ has ♂, and ♂ has ♀. In short, ♀ # [apart from] ♂ cannot be stable. It is the function of a discipline, any discipline, to fill or complete; it is the "job" of the link or synapse to join; it may be apart from a substitute used as a "link", but no substitute can do what the link does. Addiction in place of "marriage O" or "divorce O" fails; sooner or later any substitute for the real thing is bound to fail through instability. [AMF, I, 196]

That is, the emphasis is more and more in the "negative" as representing instability; "apart from", the realm of minus.

The container/contained relationship is exemplified, as in 1970 (in *Attention and Interpretation*), through some of its manifestations in the history of scientific ideas:

BION . . . If the "universe of discourse" does not facilitate the solution of 3 minus 5, then real numbers are no good, but must be enlarged by "negative numbers". If the mathematical "field of play" is not suitable for the manipulation of "negative numbers" it has to be extended to provide conditions for "games" with negative numbers. If the world of conscious thought is not suitable for playing "Oedipus Rex" the "universe of discourse" must be enlarged to include such plays. If serious psycho-analytic discussion cannot take place in the domain Freud found adequate, it must be enlarged. In fact, Freud enlarged it when he found that he could not believe what his experiences with patients seemed to suggest—that they had been assaulted sexually. He had to entertain the idea that events which had never taken place could have serious consequences. [AMF, 1, 176]

And finally he proposes a novel symbol for the container/contained that perhaps illustrates more aptly the sequence of the evolving life itself. The reader who followed the attempt to depict the evolution of the concept will see it in a most compacted form now, encompassing the genesis of thought in the movement of Ps to D and backwards: the realization of cruelty and the menace to life that life itself represents and the ensuing possibility of the inception of processes of thought. The novel symbol depicts Oedipus. It also includes a good deal of humour.

> MAN . . . God threw these presumptuous objects ♀♂ out of Eden. The Omnipotent opposes the extensions of the human ability to have intercourse. Babel opposed the extensions of power to the realm of mind. So extensions of plus-K are certain to reveal obstacles if extended to minus-K. The immortality achieved through reproduction by cell division leads to the mortality achieved by nuclear fission.
>
> BION What else?
>
> MAN I am not going to do your thinking for you. Sooner or later you will have to pay the price of deciding to think ±; whether, in Freud's formulation, to interpose "thinking" between impulse and action; or to interpose the two as a substitute for action; or interpose it between the two as a prelude to action.
>
> BION Oh, all right—let's get on with this enthralling and spectacular spectacle.
>
> (The darkness deepens. The skull-crushing and sucking object is overwhelmed by depression at the failing supply of nutriment from the dead ♀♂ and the failure to restore it to life. He formulates in stone an *arti*-factual representation, easily seen by Plato to be a lying representation of, a substitute for, pro-creation, a substitute for creation. The lying substitution is transformed into a prelude to action This whirling, swirling chaos to infinite and formless darkness becomes luminous and Leonardo da Vinci robs the hair, the brooding waste of waters, of its formless chaos.
>
> BION Disgusting! Mawkish! [AMF, I, 160–1]

Content of the patient's communications: This entry is wholly dedicated to commenting on that which may be seen as frequent distortion of Bion's texts. Some argue that Bion was not interested in the content of dreams and other verbalizations stemming from the patient. The same readers argue that he was not interested in the patient's life history and in the content of interpretations given.

The argument hardly sustains itself if one pays attention to texts that clearly refer to the matter in some parts of his work. Namely, those where he is dealing with a theory of observation in psycho-analysis, as different from theories of psycho-analysis. When he recommended a halt in the erection of hundreds of improbable theories of psycho-analysis, and emphasized a need to illuminate *"the psyche it betrays"* (AMF, I, 112), he was not deprecating existing theories that proved to be useful, such as Oedipus, which may or may not refer to contents.

> The content of the communication, so important in analysis, will be touched on only incidentally in discussion of transformations; it will depend on O as deduced from the material in the light of the psycho-analyst's theoretical pre-conceptions. Thus, if the content is oedipal material I do not concern myself with this but with the transformation it has undergone, the stage of growth it reveals, and the use to which its communication is being put. The exclusion of content is artificial, to simplify exposition, and cannot be made in practice. [T, 35]

The text is clear in stressing that the shift in emphasis is to purposes of exposition of just a theory—the theory of transformations. The wealth of clinical cases in his books displays an analyst keen on a number of theories that are clearly stated.

Controversy: Many entries in this dictionary display Bion's efforts to contribute to the study of the human being's struggle to make approximations towards reality ("inner" and "outer") as it is.

The attempts to apprehend reality soon made clear that different views and conclusions emerged. Like fingerprints, they varied as much as there were individuals. One's view of reality could differ from another one's to such an extent that it seemed that the two beings could not be talking about the same thing. In philosophy, this became known as the divergences between "subjectivists" (also called, "idealists" and "solipsists") and "realists". The use of the senses, defended by Aristotle and a long lineage after him, was criticized by Hume, Kant and also a long lineage after them.

In Bion's work, concepts such as common sense, constant conjunction, selected fact, invariances, the numinous realm of "O", scientific and artistic modes of apprehension of reality, also emerged as contrapuntal challenges to the subjectivist or idealistic tendency to privilege that may also be labelled as the "fingerprint view".

The "fingerprintians" tend to forget that the reality-O-"finger" is one and the same for any human being; the "fingerprintians" tend to forget that transformations and individuality are ensconced intrinsically in each fingerprint; but the transcendent reality, the quality of to-be-a-fingerprint, is quite independent from the infinite transformations of its outward appearance. The "realists" rely too much on outward appearances, identically to their seeming opponents. These controversies linger on and they are typical of theoreticians—science itself develops quite undisturbed by the musings of people who have no practical experiences. The fact that both realists and idealists rely on outward appearances, and that one defends the mind's creative and imaginative superiority over facts (recent tendencies, called post-modernist, argue that there is no such a thing as facts) and the other one defends the superiority of external reality as it is apprehensible by the sense apparatus over anything else, displays some paradoxes. Many try to resolve these paradoxes by partisanship. The latter is a main manifestation of controversy.

Controversy and judgmental values

Bion's work allows us to state that a psychic factor of controversy is the election of patterns. The pattern seems to be natural, but it is not. It is man-made. It depends on phantasies of superiority. Bion examines the origin of judgmental values in the human mind; he relates it to non-thinking. The issue can be seen as the triumph of paranoia, an abhorrence of reality as it is to the extent that it includes frustration of desire.

As early as 1961, he would illuminate this profound psychological issue:

> If intolerance of frustration is not so great as to activate the mechanisms of evasion and yet is too great to bear dominance of the reality principle, the personality develops omnipotence as a substitute for the mating of the pre-conception, or conception, with the negative realization. This involves the assumption of omniscience as a substitute for learning from experience by aid of thoughts and thinking. There is therefore no psychic activity to discriminate

between true and false. Omniscience substitutes for the discrimination between true and false a dictatorial affirmation that one thing is morally right and the other wrong. The assumption of omniscience that denies reality ensures that the morality thus engendered is a function of psychosis ... There is thus potentially a conflict between assertion of truth and assertion of moral ascendancy. The extremism of the one infects the other. [ST, 114]

In other words, when one loses sight of what true and false are all about, the lack of this kind of discrimination creates an unbearable vacuum. The vacuum itself is abhorred by the personality that puts fulfilment of desire above all else. This posture fuels a vicious circle. More hate of reality ensues. Truth seems to be exceedingly unattainable. Therefore one tries to resort to judgmental values in order to fill the vacuum.

The achievement of *correlation*, which would enable the psyche to tolerate the fact that paradoxes admit no resolution but forbearance, is hampered or precluded. The forbearance is of the very paradox, which excludes omniscience and demands tolerance towards the unknown that would remain as such, or the unconscious, id, "O".

Patients show* that the resolution of a problem appears to present less difficulty if it can be regarded as belonging to a moral domain; causation, responsibility and therefore a controlling force (as opposed to helplessness) provide a framework within which omnipotence reigns. In certain circumstances, to be considered later, the scene is thus set for conflict (reflected in controversies such as those on Science and Religion). This situation is portrayed in the Eden and Babel myths. The significance for the individual lies in its part in obstructing the PS ⇔ D interaction. [T, 64–65]

[* Bion's Footnote: And not only patients. The group is dominated by morality—I include of course the negative sense that shows as rebellion against morality—and this contributed to the atmosphere of hostility to individual thought on which Freud remarked.]

In 1969, Bion would write on controversy:

Much psycho-analytic "controversy" is not controversy at all. If listened to for any prolonged period, say a year, but preferably two or three, a pattern begins to emerge, so much so that I can write a chairman's address suitable, with the alteration of a phrase or two, for practically any paper by anyone at any time. Thus:

"Ladies and Gentleman, we have been listening to a very interesting and stimulating paper. I have had the great advantage of being able to read it in advance, and though I cannot say I agree with everything Dr X says" (chiefly because I haven't the faintest idea what he thinks he is talking about, and I am damned sure he hasn't either), "I found his presentation extremely—er—stimulating. There are many points that I would like to discuss with him if we had time" (thank God we haven't) "but I know there are many here who are anxious to speak" (in particular our resident ex-officio permanent bores whom no one has succeeded in silencing yet) "so I must not take up too much of our time. There is, however, just one point on which I would like to hear Dr X's views if he can spare the time." (At this point I prepare to give one of the favourite bees which reside in my own bonnet its periodical airing. It does not matter in the least how irrelevant it may be, or how unlikely Dr X is to have any views whatever on the subject, or how improbable that I would want to hear them if he had—the time has come and out it goes.) "It has often occurred to me" (and only the poor devils in my Society know how often that is) that . . . etc . . . etc. [C, 303]

This good-humoured record of reality was supposedly written in Los Angeles with no intention of seeing it published at the time it was laid down on paper. Twenty-three years later seemed to be a less delicate time to have it published, at least in the view of Francesca Bion. It embodies illumination about the fact that controversy itself demands to be viewed from a judgement-free vertex. At about the same time of that writing he would write the same thing in other terms, perhaps more palatable to the audience then. *"Controversy is the growing point from which development springs . . ."* (AI, 55).

There is a paradox to be coped with, to the extent that controversy seems to be a natural and necessary condition. But the paradox lingers on; it is necessary but not sufficient. The continuation of the phrase makes it clear:

. . . but it must be a genuine confrontation and not an impotent beating of the air by opponents whose differences of view never meet. What follows is a contribution to bringing different psycho-analytic views together in agreement or disagreement.

Hearing psycho-analytic controversy I have felt that the same configuration was being described and that the apparent differences were more often accidental than intrinsic; different points of view are believed to be significant of membership of a group, not of a scientific experience. Yet everyone knows that what is important is not the supposed use of a particular theory but whether the theory has been understood properly and whether the application has been sound.

It may be objected that to establish this would involve consideration of every individual analyst and of the circumstances of every individual interpretation. [AI, 55]

Bion suggests a way out: "*Even so, many difficulties could be obviated by more precise definition of the point of view (vertex)*" (AI, 55).

Years earlier, in 1962, he suggested a way to precision. Parts of the controversies were seen as a lack of precision in quoting the great authors. Once he thought that it was important to simplify communication between analysts. He recommended that it was preferable simply to quote a specific page and line of a standardized edition of a book instead of quoting theories or resorting to their verbal formulations and labels (LE, 38).

PAUL (soliloquizing) Anyone would think psycho-analysts never quarrelled. When the Wars of Psycho-analysis start we shall see something—and no holds barred. Santayana feared the day when the scientific beasts and blackguards would get hold of the world. What made him speak of the English as "sweet boyish masters?" [AMF, II, 273]

Manipulations of symbols

Perhaps much of the controversy stems from losing sight of the psycho-analytic vertex and ethos. This leads to a disarrayed situation of "one psycho-analysis or many" as Robert Wallerstein once considered. This leads to that which is known in mathematics as formalism, which almost destroyed mathematics at the beginning of the 20th century:

SHERLOCK . . . You heard that fellow Bion? Nobody has ever heard of him or of psycho-analysis. He thinks it is real, but that his colleagues are engaged in an activity which is only a more or less ingenious manipulation of symbols . . . There is a failure to understand that any definition must deny a previous truth as well as carry an unsaturated component. [AMF, I, 92]

Invariances and controversy

When Bion devised the application of the theory of transformations and invariances to psycho-analysis, he observed that "invariances under literacy", that is, the fact that a reader is alphabetized, does not suffice. He quotes Freud's example, of being regarded as a writer of *romans-à-clef* (T, 3). The theory of transformations and invariants seems to offer a different way to deal with controversies.

Analysts could realize that much of the controversy stems from a difficulty in realizing that the vertex or point of view influences the possibility or impossibility of realizing which invariance, or underlying pattern, flows "behind" the overt manifestation of whatever it is. Therefore the controversy, scholastic controversy, would be seen as based on tackling differences under the vertex of superiority. That is, a vertex that dictates that one vertex (and its consequent invariance) is superior to another vertex (and its consequent invariance): "*Kleinian transformation, associated with certain Kleinian theories, would have different invariants from the invariants in a classical Freudian transformation*" (T, 5). This statement has a revealing footnote, which bears out the issue: "*In practice I should deplore the use of terms such as 'Kleinian transformation', or 'Freudian transformation'. They are used here only to simplify exposition.*"

There is a difficulty in realizing that a different vertex may fill a gap left by another vertex. A point of view that admits mutual co-operation would replace the point of view of mutual destruction. There are some vertexes that reunite different vertexes. For example, the vertex of hallucinosis allows one to realize that transference and projective identification cover different ranges of hallucination. That is, projection of a desired state to repeat patterns of infancy in one case and projective identification of unwanted states into other people in the other. This would show that no real controversy exists at all: "*Since the invariants would be different so the meaning conveyed would be different even if the material transformed (the analytical experience or realization) could be conceived of as being the same in both instances"* (T, 5–6).

The invariances can be conceived of as "configurations". Loss of perception of the underlying configuration causes feelings of controversy; this can be seen as the loss of the scientific outlook, which construes general statements that encompass individual cases: *"The mathematical problem resembles a psycho-analytic problem in that it is necessary that the solution should have a wide degree of applicability and acceptance and so avoid the need to apply different arguments to different cases when the different cases appear to have essentially the same configuration. Any analyst will recognize the confusion that is caused, or at best the sense of dissatisfaction that prevails, when a discussion by members makes it quite clear that the configuration of the case is apprehended by all, but the arguments formulated in its elucidation vary from member to member and from case to case. It is essential that such a state of affairs should be made unnecessary if progress is to take place"* (T, 83).

And also: *"Most analysts have had the experience of feeling that the description given of characteristics of one particular entity might very well fit with the description of some quite different clinical entity"* (EP, 2).

Controversy and ad hoc theorizing

The texts quoted above contain perhaps the only point where Bion profits from Popper. This concerns his warnings about ad hoc theorizing: *"The search must be for formulations that represent the essential similarity of the configurations, recognized by all who deal with them, and thus to make unnecessary the **ad hoc** nature of so many psycho-analytical theories"* (T, 84). The similarity of configuration is the underlying invariance.

The abandonment, dismissal or pure lack of the grasping of existing theories seems to contribute to controversy:

> In practice, it is undesirable to discard established theories because they seem to be inadequate to particular contingencies; such a procedure would exacerbate a tendency to the facile elaboration of ad hoc theories at times when it were better to adhere to established discipline. It is therefore advisable to preserve a conservative attitude to widely-accepted theories, even when it has became clear that some adjustment needs to be made. [T, 4]

But how is one not to discard an already available theory when one cannot grasp it right from the beginning? *"The erudite can see that a description is by Freud, or Melanie Klein, but remain blind to the thing described"* (AMF, I, 5).

This can be seen in the dismissal of Oedipus, the sexuality of children and metapsychology by the psycho-analytic environment of the post-sixties era. Perhaps due to the fact that many are unable to experience it in their own analysis, many among the members of the movement created a controversy about Freud's work. André Green, who was much respected by Bion, stated that in some parts of the world many institutes of "psycho-analysis" forbade the teaching of Freud's work. This was not Bion's attitude, even though he actively made some adjustments to Freud's theories of the two principles of mental functioning and of dreams: *"The advantage of using the Oedipus myth to represent the row C category version is economy and avoidance of a whole series of ad hoc models and theories for different problems that have the same configurations"* (T, 96). In the above quoted text on erudition, the paragraph continues: *"Freud said infants were sexual; this was denied or reburied. This fate could have befallen the whole of psycho-analysis had there been no one to confer, as Horace said of Homer, immortality"* (AMF, I, 5).

The issue of dismissal of the most basic discoveries of Freud seems to warrant the question: are there deep-seated roots of controversy?

I am the discoverer of and inventor of homo alalu. I and my fellow homines with our opposable thumbs learned how to give birth and life by opposing penis to penis, vulva to vulva, till one of us began to swell up and up till the whole earth and sky was filled with the swelling and the roaring. It was decided that the monster should be destroyed. But some were lying and deceitful and resolved by their lying and deceit to continue their evil practices in secret and contribute their knowledge of pleasurable feelings to each other by rubbing. Some resolved to find this secret by learning from the secretive ones to do likewise, and others resolved likewise to deceive and lie so they could learn who and what they were that did those things so they could kill those who practised and taught these practices, and so confusion grew and it became impossible to tell good from evil. Some learned to talk, but again the same thing happened, for the language was used by some to perfect the arts of lying and deception and others to increase pleasure, but they could not agree which was which nor which was the sign by which what thing should be known. The monstrous swelling and roaring grew till the world was almost about to come to an end, but then it ceased. There came peace and quiet and the man was seen to be holding a deformed "thing". And he lied and said it came from inside him. And some said this was so and some said it could not be so and some sought to destroy the evil thing and some said, "Let us wait and then we shall be able to tell whether it is as they who say it is evil are right, or whether they who say it feels nice are right?" But no one could say because sometimes even those who said it was good admitted it was an evil brat, but they were not constant and the decision became so late that the brat, if it were evil enough, could slay those who came to kill it and so again confusion grew until even the confusion of tongues, even the counsel, was darkened until it covered the earth. And fear made men worship what they did not know and some said—Let us worship it in ignorance and fear—and some said—Let us worship it in daylight when we do not fear—and some said—Let us make ourselves afraid or we shall not fear—and some worshipped the sun and some the moon. Some likewise worshipped fear itself and some happiness and joy and light. And again they could not agree. And some worshipped what they made and some worshipped their cleverness, saying—We are the highest and best of all animals because we are tool-making animals—and some worshipped that part of themselves which they thought enabled them to make tools, the tools that made tools, but again they could not agree what that part was or how it should be treated. [AMF, I, 41–2]

Perhaps to keep controversy fit and ongoing—rather than using it as a starting point or jumping board—one must apply the rules of hallucinosis at work:

I do not believe that what separates scientists is their difference in theory, I have not always felt "separated" from someone who differs from me in the theories he holds; that does not seem to me to afford a standard of measurement by which the gap can be measured. Conversely, I have felt very far separated from some who, apparently, hold the same theories. Therefore, if the "gap" is to be "measured" it will have to be in some domain other than that of theory. The differences in theory are symptoms of differences in vertex and not a measure of the differences. [AI, 86]

Suggested cross-references: Transformations in hallucinosis, Vertex.

Correct analysis/correct interpretation: Refer to the entry Real Psycho-Analysis.

Correlation, relation, relationship: Correlation, the basic linking possibility of the mind, seems to be made between objects, persons, and persons and objects. Goethe called it "elective affinities". They seem to compose the stuff of that which we do not know what it is, but which we call life.

If the primitive particles of ammonia are in fact the birth of life on Earth, they represent a possibility of combination and correlation between that which we nowadays call nitrogen and hydrogen. The correlation—NH_3—seems to embody one (1)—(N); one (1)—(H), which composes two entities, (2)—N and H which in its turn makes for the third (3), (NH_3)—which is none of the former and is both. In psycho-analysis, Oedipus.

Correlation embodies an unresolved paradox: the mystery of life. It is manifested by music and mathematics, and by links (q.v.). It seems to allow a commonsensical view of reality as it is and of the **sense of truth** (q.v.).

At first Bion dealt with correlation through his investigation into the issue of communication in its most profound origin, that of the communication between baby and mother, or better, the infant and the breast. He elicited the existence of a primitive form of projective identification that is outside the realm of pathology and normalcy, namely, projective identification as a means of communication between the baby and its mother. He called it "realistic projective identification".

> In its origin communication is effected by realistic projective identification. The primitive infant procedure undergoes various vicissitudes including as we have seen debasement through hypertrophy of omnipotent phantasy. It may develop, if the relationship with the breast is good, into a capacity for toleration by the self of its own psychic qualities and so pave the way for alpha-function and normal thought. But it does also develop as a part of the social capacity of the individual. This development, of great importance in group dynamics, has received virtually no attention; its absence

would make even scientific communication impossible. Yet its presence may arouse feelings of persecution in the receptors of the communication. The need to diminish feelings of persecution contributes to the drive to abstraction in the formulation of scientific communications. The function of the elements of communication, words and signs, is to convey either by single substantives, or in verbal groupings, that certain phenomena are constantly conjoined in the pattern of their relatedness.

An important function of communication is to achieve correlation. While communication is still a private function, conceptions, thoughts and their verbalization are necessary to facilitate the conjunction of one set of sense-data with another. If the conjoined data harmonize a sense of truth is experienced and it is desirable that this sense should be given expression in a statement analogous to a truth-functional-statement. The failure to bring about this conjunction of sense-data, and therefore of a commonsense view induces a mental state of debility in the patient as starvation of truth was somehow analogous to alimentary starvation of truth. The truth of a statement does not imply that there is a realization approximating to the true statement.

We may now consider further the relationship of rudimentary consciousness to psychic quality. The emotions fulfil a similar function for the psyche to that of the senses in relation to objects in space and time. That is to say the counterpart of commonsense view in private knowledge is the common emotional view: a sense of truth is experienced if the view of an object which is hated can be conjoined to a view of the same object when it is loved and the conjunction confirms that the object experienced by different emotions is the same object. A correlation is established. [ST, 118–19]

This text matters to psycho-analysts, to philosophers and to mankind. It embodies an integration between Plato, Kant, Hegel, Freud and Klein. The text brings a comment that capacity for toleration of the self is that which in future works Bion would name as "atonement" (q.v.), to be one who one really is. This demands the inception of the depressive position. It seems that a Hitler-like personality, or an innate prevalence of death instincts, or violent life instincts, means that the beholder of such a tendency cannot tolerate its own self. Awareness of this paves the way for suicide or homicide. Oedipus-like blindness determined the impossibility of achieving correlation. Auschwitz's motto (*Arbeit machts frei*) subsumes the resolution of the dilemma through lies and denial.

The reader may ask, what is a "*truth-functional-statement*"? Perhaps its name was first given by Freud: "insight". The concept of sense of truth implies a total absence of judgmental values, implying emotional maturity, tolerance of paradoxes, diminishing omniscience and omnipotence, taming of envy and greed, forbearance and an enlightened humanity that perhaps marked the birth of psycho-analysis itself with Freud. It perhaps marked the inception of art, science, and humanity of man to man—hundreds and thousands of years earlier, together with its counterpart, man's inhumanity to man.

Correlation would be re-emphasized in *Transformations*: "*The theory of transformations is intended to illuminate a chain of phenomena in which the understanding of one link, or aspect of it, helps in the understanding of others*" (T, 34).

Suggested cross-references: Alpha-Function, Atonement, Controversy, Links, O, Sense of Truth, Truth.

📖 Sir Isaiah Berlin's The Sense of Reality.

Counter-transference: This term is included in this dictionary solely because of the misunderstanding that encircles its usage in many quarters around the world. Many readers try to enlist Bion's work (and in some writings, the person "Bion" himself, despite the fact that he has not been alive since 1979) as a supporter of the "counter-transference" movement. This is an undeniably influential movement, sometimes the basis of a kind of "pax romana" among parties who earlier waged true wars. For example, the self-called "annafreudians" and "kleinians/neo-kleinians", who, after the death of Anna Freud stopped quarrelling and reunited around some ideas. One of them is the idea of counter-transference. It was transformed into a common ground of belief. This movement can be seen as a trend, a fashion or perhaps as a bandwagon in the psycho-analytic movement. Many non-psycho-analytic schools, such as the so-called Jungians, also endorse it. It is outside the scope of this dictionary to study its real nature. It touches delicate political issues, alien to the realm of psycho-analysis. It is mentioned only to state in the clearest way possible that Bion never was part of this movement, as we shall soon see using his own writing.

The analyst's state of mind during the session

Bion seems to have been, after Freud and Ferenczi, the author who left the most remarkable contribution to the scrutiny of the **analyst's state of mind during the session**. His motivation was to improve the scientific status of psycho-analytic practice. This is also in the wake of Freud and Ferenczi; his attempts are contemporary with those of the Menninger brothers, who tackled the issue of trying to assess a theory of technique, and Theodor Reik.

The attempt is to improve the analyst's conditions to achieve at least some acquaintance with that which Freud called "personal factor" or "personal equation" (Freud, 1926, 1928). If this is possible at all, the analyst would be enabled to perceive his influences in the phenomena observed—namely, the patient's state of mind. This is as an ultimately unattainable goal. Nevertheless it may be feasible as a purposive attempt. The conditions worsen when primary narcissism and primary envy prevail.

The introduction of the analyst's analysis was a bold attempt to tackle the issue and have workable results, furnishing minimal conditions to the psycho-analytic endeavour. It is similar to the knowledge of the behaviour of certain particles in the realm of post-Planck and post-Einstein physics. One knows something about them and measures the interference that occurs when unknown particles are exposed to them.

Freud was somewhat ahead of the physicists in realizing the interference of the observer on the fact observed. That interference is also known as counter-transference. That is, the analyst's mistaking his patients with relevant figures from his (the analyst's) past. It can be dealt with, up to a point, exclusively in the analyst's own analysis. Findings about counter-transference belong to that analysis, from the unexpected and the unknown.

Counter-transference was defined by Freud. It differs from the conscious attempt to discipline a scrutiny of the analyst's mind as Bion presented it in his books *Elements of Psycho-analysis, Transformations* and *Attention and Interpretation*. The discipline that Bion proposes in those books includes:

(i)   some tools, such as the Grid (q.v.);
(ii) recommendations for attaining a posture, such as a discipline on memory, desire and understanding;

(iii) descriptions of consequences of this posture, such as:
- to be able to "dream the session",
- to train the intuition analytically,
- to discern the presence of transformations in hallucinosis during the session as a prelude for discriminating the dream from hallucination
- to perform acts of "faith" (q.v.)
- to get a "Language of achievement" (q.v.), which must necessarily be colloquial, in the sense of a colloquialism custom tailored to the listener, the patient,
- an ability to be seen or be called "mad".

All of this, though partially conscious, ought to reach, at least, the unconscious level. This is akin to the musician's exercises of scales and the sportsman or woman's off-competition exercises. There is a continuous movement between the analyst's unconscious and conscious, described as the functioning of the "contact barrier" (q.v.) (in *Learning from Experience*). It must include an ability to allow a free movement between PS and D and vice versa as well as tolerance for exercising an interaction between container and contained.

These processes of learning from experience and continuous exercising of the analytically trained intuition allow the development of the self-scrutiny of the analyst's state of mind. None of this has to do with counter-transference, which is, in a certain sense, a more general and complex issue. The counter-transference refers to the analyst's personality as a whole. It influences the analyst's state of mind during the session as it influences it in any instant of his life. But it is not the object of Bion's study. We shall soon see that counter-transference should be dealt with during the analyst's analysis.

The misunderstanding seems to be linked to the fact that for a few years Bion worked closely with some followers of Paula Heimann. He never explicitly espoused the "counter-transference bandwagon", as the author proposes to call this formidable movement of denial of the analyst's unconscious. Shades of it can be seen in the first version of Bion's paper on the language of the schizophrenic (then named, "Language and the schizophrenic"), published as chapter 9 of the book, New Directions *in Psycho-analysis*. In re-publishing the paper, twelve years later, whole sections of it that dealt with counter-transference in the typically heimannian/ hackerian way were omitted and modified (especially those of pages 224 and 225). The modifications appear in the newer and definitive version of the same paper, as published twelve years later in *Second Thoughts*. They leave no doubt about his abandonment of what seems to have been an initial interest in this fashion. Even in 1953 he had reserves about it: *"I would not have it thought that I advocate this use of counter-transference as a final solution; rather it is an expedient to which we must resort until something better presents itself"* (*New Directions in Psycho-analysis*, Tavistock Publications, 1955, p. 225). It is explicit in his later writings that for him the *"something better"* is still the analyst's analysis.

Lest any doubts be left, perhaps Bion's own words can be used to dissolve them. A useful text starts from the attempt to get near the numinous realm, or as Bion called it, "O":

I . . . postulate that O in any analytic situation is available for transformation by analyst and analysand equally.

I shall ignore disturbance produced by the analyst's personality or aspects of it. The existence of such disturbance is well known and its recognition is the basis for analytic acceptance of the need for analysts to be analysed and the many studies of counter-transference. While other scientific disciplines recognize the personal equation, or the factor of personal error, no science other than psycho-analysis has insisted on such a profound and prolonged investigation of it nature and ramifications. I ignore it therefore so as to keep an already over-complicated problem down to its simplest terms. I shall assume an ideal analyst and that Taα and Taβ are not disturbed by turbulence—though turbulence and its sources are part of O [T, 48]

A distinction must be made between the genesis of thought in the patient's life history and the genesis of expressions of thought in a given contingency. The emergence of the column 2 dimension may be observed in the contingency of the analysis as a step in the evolution of the statement and from it the analyst can judge that the conditions for interpretation have arrived; but it does not mean that an interpretation can be made; for the analyst's thought also must reach maturation. When he can see the column 2 element in his thoughts the conditions for interpretation are complete: an interpretation should be made. In terms of analytic theory it is approximately correct, but only approximately, to say that the conditions for the interpretation have arrived when the patient's statements provide evidence that resistance is operating; the conditions are complete when the analyst feels aware of resistance in himself—not counter-transference which must be dealt with by analysis of the analyst, but resistance to the reaction he anticipates from the analysand if he gives the interpretation. Note the similarity of the analyst's resistance to the response he anticipates from the patient to his interpretation and the patient's resistance to the analyst's interpretation [T, 168]

Freud, Bion and counter-transference

Counter-transference is a technical term, but as often happens with the technical term gets worn away and turns into a kind of worn out coin which has lost its value. We should keep these things in good working conditions. The theory about a counter-transference is that it is the transference relationship which the analyst has to the patient without knowing he has it. You will hear analysts say, "I don't like that patient, but I can make use of my counter-transference. He cannot use his counter-transference". He may be able to make use of the fact that he dislikes the patient, but that is not counter-transference. There is only one thing to do with counter-transference and that is to have it analyzed. One cannot make use of one's counter-transference in the consulting room; it is a contradiction in terms. To use the term in that way means that one would have to invent a new term to do the work which used to be done by the word "counter-transference". It is one's *unconscious* feelings about the patient, and since it is unconscious there is nothing we can do about it. If the counter-transference is operating in the analytic session the analysand is unlucky—and so is the analyst. The time to have dealt with it was in the past, in the analyst's own analysis. We can only hope that it does not use us too much and that we have had enough analysis to keep the number of unconscious operations to a minimum. [BLII, 87–8]

This does not mean that Bion was against anyone who wanted to study counter-transference. Up to the end of his life he tried to make clear his opinion on how to deal with it. This opinion is coherent with his overall attitude, which differentiated "to talk about" from "to be" or "to experience":

ROLAND You seem to suggest that as a psycho-analyst you are compacted of the best of both sexes

P.A. Would it were true. I hope that that desire does not obscure my inheritance of weaknesses. I have noticed a prejudice in favour of my patients and a related desire to share their excellences.

ROBIN Counter-transference?

P.A. Do not forget that "counter-transference" is by definition unconscious; it follows that I do not know the nature, in reality, of my counter-transference. I know theoretically, but that is only knowing *about* counter-transference—that is not knowing the "thing itself".

ROBIN Presumably, knowing "about" counter-transference is helpful. Isn't it inevitable that one learns much of which one has no direct experience? I learn about a trip to the moon, but shall certainly not experience it. It must have some value unless we are to believe that the process of the education is unrealistic [AMF, III, 515]

Freud thought it was—he included education among the three impossible professions.

Counter-transference, L and H

If the path towards an interpretation includes, linked to human frailty, aspects of L and H, the *"analyst is assumed to allow for or exclude L or H from his link with the patient, and Ta α and Ta β are assumed for purposes of this discourse to be free from distortion by L, H (i.e. by counter-transference.) Tp α and Tp β, on the contrary, are assumed always to be subject to distortion and the nature of that distortion in so far as it is an object of illumination through psycho-analytic interpretation, is the O of the transformation that the analyst effects in his progress from observation to interpretation"* (T, 49).

To be acquainted with the necessity of .Tp α, Tp β, L, and H, see the respective entries.

Suggested cross-references: Analytical view, Real Psychoanalysis, Scientific method.

Cure: In his first papers from the fifties Bion resorted to the traditional medical model of cure. In due course he left it aside, not unlike seasoned surgeons and the vast majority of clinicians, who also leave it aside. Medicine takes care of people; cure is a rare exception. The model of cure is replaced by those of "growth" (1962) and "becoming" (1965); from 1975 onwards another model is introduced: usefulness to life.

Bion's dismissal of the model of cure is a result of his scientific outlook. It demands respect for truth and real facts. Bion realized the hallucinatory nature of ideas of cure. It is an idealized goal that indicates a predominance of the pleasure principle. It may turn that which could be an analysis into colluded parasitic associations. These associations may be described as of mutual admiration; often they are indistinguishable from wishful thinking, panglossian reassurances and exercising of suggestion. To cure is an expression of hate of analysis in so far as it extinguishes investigation into the unconscious.

🕒 1950–57 The studies published in *Second Thoughts* rely heavily on models of cure, even though they contain the seeds of doubt.

1959–61 These doubts are allowed to flourish in his previously unpublished paper that surfaced in 1992, in *Cogitations*.

1963–66 The issues of truth, growth, mental functioning are brought to the fore.

1967 In "Commentary" to *Second Thoughts* Bion dwells on the inadequacies of the model of cure. In this text and in the short paper "Notes on memory and desire" cure is linked to desire.

1970 The ideas of cure are examined intra-sessionally.

> By definition and by the tradition of all scientific discipline, the psycho-analytical movement is committed to the truth as the central aim. If the patient constantly formulates −L and −K statements, he and the analyst are, in theory at least, in conflict. In practice, however, the situation does not present itself so simply. The patient, especially if intelligent and sophisticated, offers every inducement to bring the analyst to interpretations that leave the defence intact and, ultimately, to acceptance of the lie as a working principle of superior efficacy. In the last resort he will make consistent progress towards a "cure" which will be flattering to the analyst and patient alike ... Some forms of lying appear to be closely related to experiencing desire [AI, 99–100]

The idea of growth in emotional terms, identical to that of Freud, as a replacement to the ideas of cure, is offered:

"Since the experience of learning from which the patient is thus debarred is that of the parental relationship, the importance for the patient's development and for a successful outcome of analysis, depending on resolution of the Oedipus complex, are gravely prejudiced" (EP, 94); *"The psycho-analytic conception of cure should include the idea of a transformation whereby an element is saturated and thereby made ready for further saturation. Yet a distinction must be made between this dimension of 'cure' or 'growth' and 'greed'"* (T, 153).

Later on (1965) he would add the vertex of knowledge and truth. In commenting on the value of interpretations: *"Their value therapeutically is greater if they are conducive to transformations in O; less if conducive to transformations in K"* (T, 27).

In fact this was an idea that he was pursuing much earlier, having proposed a criterion of mental health:

> The man who is mentally healthy is able to gain strength and consolation and the material through which he can achieve mental development through his contact with reality, no matter whether that reality is painful or not ... The reciprocal view is that no man can become mentally healthy save by a process of constant search for fact and a determination to eschew any elements, however seductive or pleasurable that interpose themselves between himself and his environment as it really is. [C, 192]

One may conceive of mental disturbance as an incapacity to face truth; a continuous habit of lying brings decay: *"If analysis has been successful in restoring the personality of the patient he will approximate to being the person he was when his development became compromised"* (T, 143).

This leads us to his mention of treatment by psycho-analysis and the limiting factors presented by innate characteristics: *"Does it matter if intolerance of frustration, or any other dynamic characteristic is primary or secondary? The distinction indicates the limitation of any treatment effecting changes in the personality to secondary factors for primary factors will not be altered"* (LE, 29).

These conceptions must be duly weighed with everyone's tolerance of pain and frustration, which composes a paradox of the relationship of man with truth:

> By contrast it may be said that man owes his health, and his capacity for continuous health, to his ability to shield himself during his

growth as an individual by repeating in his personal life the history of the race's capacity for self-deception against truth that his mind is not fitted to receive without disaster. [C, 192]

Oedipus seemed to face this dilemma and was awarded with blindness; a woman who lost her 15-year-old boy fainted. "O" carries with it a potentially explosive load of truth to some people. The idea expressed circa 1960 would be developed in 1965, but with no deviation in the experience of the nourishing effect of truth:

My theory would seem to imply a gap between phenomena and the thing-in-itself and all that I have said is not incompatible with Plato, Kant, Berkeley, Freud and Klein, to name a few, who show the extent to which they believe the curtain of illusion separates us from reality. Some consciously believe the curtain of illusion to be a protection against truth which is essential to the survival of humanity; the remainder of us believe it unconsciously but no less tenaciously for that. Even those who consider such a view mistaken and truth essential consider that the gap cannot be bridged because the nature of the human being precludes knowledge of anything beyond phenomena save conjecture. From this conviction of the inaccessibility of absolute reality the mystics must be exempted. Their inability to express themselves through the medium of ordinary language, art or music is related to the fact that all such methods of communication are transformations and transformations deal with phenomena and are dealt with by being known, loved or hated. [T, 147]

This means that the capacity to grow implies intuiting O; the reality of personality. To intuit it is far from rational knowledge but it is near to living it, to living life as it is: "... *it is not knowledge of reality that is at stake, nor yet the human equipment for knowing. The belief that reality is or could be known is mistaken because reality is not something which lends itself to being known. It is impossible ... to sing potatoes: they may be grown, or pulled, or eaten, but not sung. Reality has to be 'been': there should be a transitive verb 'to be' expressly for use with the term 'reality'.*

When, as psycho-analysts, we are concerned with the reality of the personality there is more at stake than an exhortation to 'know thyself, accept thyself, be thyself', because implicit in the psycho-analytic procedure is the idea that this exhortation cannot be put into practice without the psycho-analytic experience. The point at issue is how to pass from 'knowing' 'phenomena' to 'being' that which is, 'real'" (T, 148).

Or, "*O, representing the unknowable ultimate reality can be represented by any formulation of a transformation—such as "unknowable ultimate reality' which I have just formulated. It may therefore seem unnecessary to multiply representations of it; indeed from the psychoanalytic vertex that is true. But I wish to make it clear that my reason for saying that O is unknowable is not that I consider human capacity unequal to the task but because K, L or H are inappropriate to O. They are adequate to transformations of O but not to O"* (T, 140).

Bion gives due consideration to the possible relationship between pain and cure: "*Pain cannot be regarded as a reliable index of pathological processes partly because of its relationship with development (recognized in the commonly used phrase "growing pains") and partly because intensity of suffering is not always proportionate to the severity of the disturbance ... Implicit in the discussion of reversible perspective as a means of preserving a defence against pain is the concept of growth. Growth is a phenomenon that appears to present peculiar difficulties to perception either by the growing object or the object that stimulates it, for its relationship with precedent phenomena is obscure and separated in time ... Difficulty in observing it contributes to the anxiety to establish "results", e.g. of analysis*" (EP, 62).

Bion's later view

ROBIN Doesn't your working day consist in discussing the qualities and defects of others?

P.A. I try to demonstrate the qualities of the individual. Whether they are assets or liabilities he can then decide for himself.

ROLAND I thought you were supposed to cure them.

ROBIN So did I.

P.A. "Cure" is a word which, like "illness" or "disease", is borrowed from physicians and surgeons to account for our activities in a comprehensible manner. [AMF, III, 541]

Suggested cross-references: Analytic view, Becoming, Correct analysis, Development, Mathematizing psycho-analysis, Truth.

Curiosity: Bion regards curiosity under two vertexes that imply two different meanings.

1) A first sense of curiosity is akin to that described by Freud and Klein. It is regarded as a manifestation of the development of the epistemophilic instinct. Infantile curiosity towards the sexual organs transforms itself into a curiosity about one's own mind. It may, in the next step, undergo a process of sublimation, and proceeds to a curiosity towards the external world, as a scientific or artistic curiosity. This kind of curiosity is linked to life instincts; it has a function in preventing senility. It is a specific manifestation of the K link (EP, 46, footnote)

2) A second sense corresponds either to a regression to or to a fixation of infantile sexual curiosity. It manifests itself as an arrogant, stupid curiosity that emerges when one feels that resorting to projective identification is hampered or impeded. In the clinic, this curiosity is displayed through an exaggerated interest in the analyst's private life. The patient behaves as if the most important person in the room is the analyst. The papers, "On arrogance" and "Attacks on linking" introduce the issue.

Suggested cross-references: Arrogance, Reversion of perspective.

D

D: A quasi-mathematical, shorthand symbol for the depressive position, first proposed in *Elements of Psycho-Analysis*, p.4. See entry PS⇔D.

depressive position Bion uses this term in exactly the same sense that Melanie Klein created it (see "Notes on some schizoid mechanisms", and *Envy and Gratitude*).

Misunderstandings: Depressive position and thinking processes—a whole tendency was created in a gross over-simplification of the term and especially in some readings of Bion's correlations of the depressive position and thought processes. Some authors attributed to Bion the idea that thinking occurs in the depressive position, and the paranoid–schizoid position is characterized by the lack of proper thinking. Trying to trace the origins of such a misunderstanding, it seems that it harks back to the days when psychoanalysis was tainted by ideas of pathology and cure. That is, the simplification and banalization happened when one equated the paranoid–schizoid position to pathology and the depressive position to cure. Please see the entry, PS⇔D, where his contribution to

rescue Melanie Klein's ethos of the concept includes a living movement, to and from. An ethos apparently lost after Klein's death, in
some published works about her writing. As early as 1955 (see the
final part of item 41 in *Second Thoughts*), when Bion still thought in
terms of pathologies of the mental apparatus, there is a statement
about the development of thinking processes in the depressive position. He gives a very extensive review of his ideas on pathology and
cure in the 1967 Commentary to this item. The text, consequently,
starts from the fact that Bion's idea was that thinking already
existed in the paranoid–schizoid position.

Both the apprehension of reality—and therefore thinking—and
all ego-functions, albeit embryonic, already exist there, as is clear in
Melanie Klein's suggestion of early phases of the Oedipus complex.
In Metatheory, when examining the paranoid and the delinquent
ways of dealing and not dealing with reality, Bion states that some
persons are able to perceive truth just to avoid stumbling into it by
accident—these people couple an ability to apprehend truth and
reality with no respect for love and life. Such a paranoid use
displays that highly sophisticated thinking does exist in someone
functioning under the paranoid–schizoid position. It will suffice to
intelligent people to find a suitable social locus to keep this way of
life seeming "normal", in a successful use of the neurotic part of the
personality by the psychotic part of the personality (q.v.). No
depression, in the sense of an insight into the damage done to the
object that is felt as good, is needed here; in fact it is abhorred, carefully avoided and circumvented.°

Suggested cross-references: P, PS⟺D.

Desire: Please refer to the entry, **Discipline on Memory, Desire and
Understanding**

Development: Together with "usefulness", growth (or development), it composes the double criteria to gauge if analysis is
happening.

Development and usefulness to life replaced the criteria of cure
(q.v.). The latter are based on ideas of unrestricted and stable
achievement of paradisiacal states whose description is clothed by
psycho-analytic wording—such as the prevalence of conscious over
unconscious, the achievement of the depressive position at the

expense of a demonized paranoid–schizoid position, the achievement of pleasure over anything else, the acquisition of "empathic"
self-objects or whatever theory of cure it may be. For example:

> The name given an object . . . is similar to a theory in that both
> imply that certain qualities are constantly conjoined; therefore, it
> cannot be properly described as true or false in its relationship to
> O; these terms express judgements on the health-giving effect of the
> theory to which they are applied, upon the personality entertaining
> the theory. The differentiation to be made to the name, or theory, is
> between "useful" and "not useful". . . [T, 53, 54]

Development is seen as the development of thinking (q.v.) and
emotional development according to Freud and Klein's observations: (i) the inception of the principle of reality, which translates
into tolerance of frustration and pain; (ii) the integration of the
Oedipal situation into the framework of the interplay between the
paranoid–schizoid and depressive positions. That is, the development of the mental apparatus in Bion's work is an integration of
Freud and Klein's discoveries.

> In psycho-analytic methodology the criterion cannot be whether a
> particular usage is right or wrong, meaningful or verifiable, but
> whether it does, or does not, promote development.

> I do not suggest that promotion of development provides a crite-
> rion without reservation; psycho-analytic theory and practice, in
> cases where thought shows serious disturbance . . . [LE, Intro-
> duction, end of item 7 and beginning of 8]

The papers and books written between 1942 and 1963 deal,
without exception, with issues of social and emotional growth, in
terms of mental and thought processes. They also deal with the
hindrances to it. They take for granted the reader's acquaintance
with Freud and Klein's theories of emotional development. Bion
focuses on the realm of the development of thinking and knowledge.

A whole new instrument, the Grid (q.v.), can be regarded as a
tool potentially useful to analysts and to psycho-analysis, in order
to enhance the latter's scientific value. It can gauge the development or non-development of thinking. The establishment of

categories is designed to measure *"degrees of growth"*. This development is seen as an increased ability to apprehend reality as it is; it seems to be possible to assess the truth-value of verbal statements through the use of this tool. The categories of this tool are specifically construed to assess development of thinking, either genetically speaking or in terms of its functions: *". . . it is useful for psycho-analysis to be able to signify degrees of growth and to represent these by stages with their proper sign. Hitherto I have spoken of 'growth' and 'increased sophistication' . . ."* (T, 43).

There is an endeavour: to choose useful theories in order to advance knowledge. The importance of this criterion is more outstanding even than the criterion of truth when applied to theories. A theory may be false but it may have a useful function in the development of science. The references to this are so numerous in Bion's work that to quote them extensively would overburden the reader.

In brief: hallucination is useful for the growth of cognitive processes or apprehension of reality. It provides a contrapuntal frame of reference, namely, that of error. Bion develops his earlier views of the phantasy of projective identification as a means of communication along these lines. They are now valued again in a non-pathological way and as an epistemological tool: *"The growth of insight depends, at its inception, on undisturbed functioning of projective identification"* (T, 36).

In the terms created by Shakespeare, "By indirections, find directions out" (*Hamlet* II, 1, 64).

> In practice it is undesirable to discard established theories because they seem to be inadequate to particular contingencies; such a procedure would exacerbate a tendency to the facile elaboration of ad hoc theories at times when it would be better to adhere to established discipline . . . For my present purposes it is helpful to regard psycho-analytical theories as belonging to the category of groups of transformations, a technique analogous to that of a painter, by which the facts of an analytic experience (the realization) are transformed into an interpretation (the representation)" (T, 4); ". . . we must be prepared to find the model of the painter misleading though still useful. [T, 36]

What does promote growth? In discussing the intolerance of frustration, intolerance of the no-breast and hypothesizing that the obtrusion of mathematical thinking in the form of the point as reflecting the tolerance of the no-thing, Bion writes:

> Why, then, to revert to the point and line, do these visual images lead in one case to the efflorescence of mathematics and in the other to mental sterility? And is it certain that "mental sterility" is a correct assessment? The question implies the validity of a theory of causation which I consider misleading and liable to give rise to constructions that are basically false; if it is fallacious we may discard it for one as fallacious—which may be true of the formulation, by Heisenberg [Heisenberg, W. Physics and Philosophy], of the problem of multiple causation. Both views have proved of value in the development of science, but developments of physics by the Copenhagen school appear to have made the theory irrelevant. If so, the logical step would be to bother no longer with causation or its counterpart—results. In psycho-analysis it is difficult to avoid feeling that a gap is left by its disappearance and that the gap should be filled. Over a wide range of our problems no difficulty is caused by regarding the theory of causation as fallacious but useful. When it comes to problems presented by disturbances in thought the difficulty cannot be met in this way ... The proposed chain of causation can then be seen as a *rationalization* of the sense of persecution. Furthermore, if the patient is capable of seeing that his proposed chain of causation is nonsensical he may use it to deny the persecution and thus evade any explanation that would reveal the depression he dreads. [T, 56–7]

When sincerely describing Klein's discordance with him in a particularly seminal example of his theory of pre-conceptions (q.v.) he emphasizes its "usefulness" rather than "truth": "*Melanie Klein objected in conversation with me to the idea that the infant had an inborn pre-conception of the breast, but though it may be difficult to produce evidence for the existence of a realization that approximates to this theory, the theory itself seems to me to be useful as a contribution to a vertex I want to establish*" (T, 138).

When describing the possible utility of the theory of transformations and the transformations in hallucinosis:

"*Transformations may be scientific, aesthetic, religious, mystical, psycho-analytical. They may be described as psychotic and neurotic also, but though all these classifications have a value it does not appear to me that the value that they have is psycho-analytically adequate I have chosen to write, though briefly, of transformation in hallucinosis because the description may serve to explain why I consider existing methods of observation, notation, attention and curiosity are inadequate, why a theory of transformations may aid in making these methods more nearly adequate* . . ." (T, 140). Obviously the words "aid", "to serve" convey meanings that are interchangeable with "useful".

Bion uses the exaggeration involved in science in order to get a better focus on a specific issue being researched; in connection, he develops the concept of hyperbole (q.v.). *"Just as exaggeration is helpful in clarifying a problem so it can be felt to exaggerate in order to gain the attention necessary to have a problem clarified"* (T, 141).

A sociologically oriented scholar may see the influence of Protestant ethics (in Max Weber's sense) as well as that of the so-called utilitarian philosophers who were contemporaneous to Freud.

📖 Chapters 6 and 7 of *Transformations*.

Direct evidence: Bion considers analytic practice as an empirical activity that furnishes direct evidence to the observer. This evidence is the unfolding emotional experiences taking place in the evolving session. *"The analyst's main concern must be with the material of which he has direct evidence, namely, the emotional experience of the analytic sessions themselves"* (T, 7).

Disaster: This word is used throughout Bion's work to depict at least five precisely defined emotional situations: (i) impairment in the acquisition of a sense of reality; (ii) splitting; (iii) an incapacity to dream, (iv) an excessive avoidance of pain; (v) Oedipus (both as a pre-conception and as a mental configuration).

Pain and Oedipus (iv and v) are seen as "elements of psychoanalysis", that is, they are basic and fundamental to the personality and to the analytical work. The remaining situations (i-iii) relate to basic functions of the mind. All of them relate to pain and attempts to avoid it. There is a technical issue involved. There is the possibility of the analyst bringing disaster to analysis if pain and manoeuvres to avoid it leads to an increased and unnecessary pain.

Disaster and the sense of reality

Disaster is also linked to failure to use the emotional experience to get a sense of reality: *"Failure to eat, drink, or breathe properly has disastrous consequences for life itself. Failure to use the emotional experience produces a comparable disaster in the development of the personality; I include among those disasters degrees of psychic deterioration that could be described as death of the personality"* (LE, 42).

Disaster and splitting

> Suppose the patient to be, or to have been, capable of normality: the conglomerate of fragments of personality which serves the patient for a personality can only be regarded as evidence of a disaster. The discussion of such a case is difficult because we are concerned not with the ordinary structures of the human personality for which terms such as ego, id, super-ego have been made available by Freud, but with the shattered fragments of these which have now been reassembled but not re-articulated. [C,74–5]

If one considers that splitting of thought is the single real effect of projective identification, its classification as a disaster is no exaggeration.

Disaster and a lack of capacity to dream

The three situations above are linked to this one: splitting and attacks on the perceptual apparatus damage the capacity to dream. Some patients of Bion—and this can be observed as a daily occurrence in analytical practice—objected to being exposed to sense impressions and consequently to "the thing his sense impression conveys to him. *The deprivation of sense impression must then lead to an inability to dream and a need to hallucinate sense impressions as a substitute for the dream"*. These patients hallucinate dreams and do not dream properly—its hallmark is a scarcity or lack of associations.

> A hallucination of a dream can no more yield associations than a hallucinated breast can yield milk.

> The failure to dream is felt as such a grave disaster that the patient continues to hallucinate during the day, to hallucinate a dream, or

so to manipulate facts that he is able to feel he is having a dream—which is the daylight counterpart of the night-time hallucination of a dream. But it is also the attempt to suck a dream out of an experience of reality or actuality. And in this respect the dream that yields no associations and the reality that yields no dreams are alike; they are similar to hallucinatory gratification. [C, 112]

Disaster and Pain

Pain cannot be absent from the personality. An analysis must be painful, not because there is necessarily any value in pain, but because an analysis in which pain is not observed and discussed cannot be regarded as dealing with one of the central reasons for the patient's presence. The importance of pain can be dismissed as a secondary quality, something that is to disappear when conflicts are resolved; indeed most patients would take this view. Furthermore it can be supported by the fact that successful analysis does lead to diminution of suffering: nevertheless it obscures the need, more obvious in some cases than in others, for the analytic experience to increase the patient's *capacity* for suffering even though patient and analyst may hope to decrease pain itself. The analogy with physical medicine is exact; to destroy a capacity for physical pain would be a disaster in any situation other than one in which an even greater disaster—namely death itself—is certain. [EP, 61–2]

The technical hint in dealing with pain relies on the concept of reversible perspective (q.v.). It is seminal in clinical practice. Reversible perspective is a special use of projective identification. The patient strives to render a dynamic situation static.

The work of the analyst is to restore dynamic to a static situation and so make development possible . . . the patient manoeuvres so that the analyst's interpretations are agreed; they thus become the outward sign of a static situation . . .

In reversible perspective acceptance by the analyst of the possibility of a capacity for pain can help avoidance of errors that might lead to disaster. If the problem is not dealt with the patient's capacity to maintain a static situation may give way to an experience of pain so intense that a psychotic breakdown is the result [EP, 60 and 62]

Disaster and Oedipus

Bion clinically observes a situation that can be described as the destruction of the Oedipal pre-conception (q.v.). It constitutes "*a disaster to the ego*" (EP, 93). Its clinical relevance is that such an observation enables the analyst to deal with a specific kind of material spoken in the session as debris, even though it may seem a whole, if taken at face value or sensuously apprehensible appearance.

> Analysts need . . . to consider that the Oedipal material may possibly be evidence for primitive apparatus of pre-conception and therefore possessing a significance additional to its significance in classical theory. I am postulating a precursor of the Oedipal situation not in the sense that such a term may have in Melanie Klein's discussion of *Early Phases of the Oedipus Complex*, but as something that belongs to the ego as part of its apparatus for contact with reality. In short I postulate an α-element version of a private Oedipus myth which is the means, the pre-conception, by virtue of which the infant is able to establish contact with the parents as they exist in the world of reality. The mating of this α-element Oedipal pre-conception with the realization of the actual parents gives rise to the conception of parents.

> If through envy, greed, sadism or other cause, the infant cannot tolerate the parental relationship and attacks it destructively, according to Melanie Klein the attacking personality is itself fragmented through the violence of the splitting attacks. Restating this theory in terms of the Oedipal pre-conception: the emotional load carried by the private α-element Oedipal pre-conception is such that the Oedipal pre-conception is itself destroyed. As a result the infant loses the apparatus essential for gaining a conception of the parental relationship and consequently for resolution of Oedipal problems: it does not fail to solve those problems—it never reaches them.

> The significance of this for practice is that scraps of what appear to be Oedipal material must be treated with reserve. If the evidence is related to a disaster to the ego, the destruction of the pre-conception and consequently the ability to pre-conceive, interpretations based on the supposition that fragmented Oedipal material is evidence of a destroyed object will be only partially successful. The investigation must be directed to distinguishing amongst the

elements of Oedipal material those that are fragments of Oedipal pre-conception from those that are fragments of the fragmented Oedipal situation. Since the experience of learning from which the patient is thus debarred is that of the parental relationship, the importance for the patient's development and for a successful outcome of analysis, depending on resolution of the Oedipus complex, are gravely prejudiced. [EP, 92–4]

This displays Bion's origin in the work of Freud in its most remarkable form. It is "*additional*", that is, it is not a replacement. It refers to the fulcrum of Freud's observations: Oedipus.

The observation was made possible by a lack of rigidity and ossification in the act of observing and interpreting. The results obtained when the professional practises a non pre-patterned observation seems to recommend the avoidance of scholastic interpretations. In this case, the prevalent scholasticism was "based" on object-relations theory. Bion suggests that Freud's theory, provided that it is employed in a more integrated way with Klein's theory, is more encompassing than Klein's theory if the latter is taken mechanistically or in an exclusive way.

To employ the theory of splitting in the clinic is expressed by the way that one looks for minute fragments. This is, so to say, "pure Klein". Looking for Oedipal material in unexpected places, or places where it may be unobservable is, so to say, "pure Freud"—to the extent that psycho-analytical material is not given to the senses. Its outward appearances are misleading. Again and again, he pushes both Freud and Klein's theory to their ultimate consequences—or at least, further than was imagined possible before him.

A final example of disaster was given in quasi-artistic terms. The situation depicts a woman unable to realize a parental couple:

Alice was not listening. Her attention had become wayward; since the outbreak of war she had noticed a deterioration . . . she could not sustain her train of thought . . . She knew this hall; with an effort she could visualize what had been its appearance when she dined there. Its drab, unfurnished condition established it as if a photographic slide had replaced the scene she knew . . . It was easier to believe that the inhabitants of the island had been wiped out and replaced . . . The village had been familiar since childhood. She had never known herself as anything but one of the gentry.

Now she stood naked, incongruous, alien, without a point of reference that made sense. True, there was defeat, but this was on a scale of defeat so disastrous that it would be necessary to suppose that something analogous to the Norman Conquest had taken place. [AMF, I, 27]

Misuses and misconceptions: (i) Disaster is often confused with the over-simplistic, positivistic "cause–effect" sense. The commonplace is the idea of trauma; (ii) Disaster is often confused with catastrophic change (q.v.).

The use of the word "cause" in the quotation (EP, 92–4) must be taken carefully both in the phrase and in the light of Bion's subsequent views of causes, as clearly stated in *Transformations and A Memoir of the Future*. In the text mentioned, the word corresponds to one or more causes of *"intolerance of the parental relationship"*, rather than a direct cause of the disaster.

The same applies to the term "result", that is clearly preceded by an "a". It is not a generalization. It is the observation of a specific situation. This is a novel formulation. It was implicit in Klein's work, but it seems that Bion was first to make it explicit and to operate it, namely, that some people never reach Oedipus.

The idea of trauma is a commonplace. It has a misleading penumbra of associations linked to its common social usage. Freud discovered psycho-analysis using three pillars: the abandonment of the idea of trauma, the interpretation of dreams and Oedipus. He realized that what matters to the analyst is not a hypothesized, believed or even real trauma during infancy. What matters is the patient's **use** of the facts of his life. This may be observed as a "past presented": how the material emerges in the here and now of the session. It emerges as actual events in the session: "scraps", debris. There is a need to detect the fragmented Oedipus, or even the non-existent, negative Oedipus in the debris spoken in the session. This debris assumes many forms. It can be logically stated in histories whose outward appearance is misleading.

Suggested cross-references: Analytic view, Catastrophic Change, Causes, Cure.

Discipline in memory, desire and understanding: The necessity for discipline in tackling the psycho-analytical task was recommended by Freud, who used some specific terms and analogies. As an example of a term, one may quote "abstinence". As examples of analogies, these of the archaeologist and of the surgeon. They are used in order to depict the analyst's work.

The interpretation of dreams demands a sophisticated mental discipline. The same applies to refraining from giving counselling, support. The same discipline is needed to perform a careful detection of hallucinated love based on transference.

Bion tries to rescue Freud's recommendations from oblivion and at the same time turns them into **technical tools**. He expands Freud's recommendations when he discovers that the discipline can rescue the freshness of the analytical experience. Ultimately, Bion disinters the "here-and-now" referred to by Freud.

His observation is that if the analyst recalls some specific kind of data he cannot exercise the free floating attention, freedom, intuition. This narrows his scope. Memory may be seen as a pre-emptive strike against the unknown. Bion would observe the hallucinated nature of memories; devoid of the truthful observation of hitherto unknown facts that unfold during the session, what is left to the analyst is to base him(her)self on hallucinated memories.

His stress on discipline in desire stems from the observation that subservience to the principle of pleasure precludes observing the patient as he or she is. Discipline in understanding is linked to the other two. It precludes the analyst's observations, respect and concern for the analysand's views and theories and explanations. Matters in analysis demand intuition and apprehension rather than understanding.

The three are products of denial of the unknown, anxiety and haste. The damages they make in the observation and apprehension of reality are vividly expressed in the "mistakes" and foolishness of the fictitious characters, Alice, Roland, Robin, and Tom in the opening chapters of *A Memoir of the Future*. The issue is expanded in the now classical paper, "Notes on memory and desire" and also in the "Commentary" of *Second Thoughts*, both from 1967.

Misuses and misconceptions Discipline about memory would be a "tabula rasa" idea. But Bion wrote that *"A bad memory is not enough: what is ordinarily called forgetting is as bad as remembering. It is necessary to inhibit dwelling on memories and desires"* (AI, 41).

Dispositions: Kant's formulation of the basic pre-conceptions of the human mind influenced Bion in at least two ways. An unfinished work was about a kind of disposition to be an analyst, and the tolls that are necessary to exercise psycho-analysis, which is both practical and scientific.

He does not define exactly what disposition is, in a philosophical or theoretical sense, but draws attention to the practical problems involved—both clinical and for scientific relevance. In other words, to what extent the terms employed by analysts have counterparts in reality, as expressing truth and relationships of the kind "I know X". One may see that Bion sets some premises and gives them empirical "flesh".

Dispositions" can be seen as a transient appreciation, rather than a diagnosis:

> A man may be disposed to envy, or to violence of emotion, or to regard truth and life highly, or to be intolerant of frustration . . . I shall call this state of mind at the time he is so disposed, his "disposition" . . . does this mean something in the psyche? Are there such things as dispositions? At once a problem is, what does one mean by "thing". He is disposed to be envious; he has an envious disposition; his disposition is to be envious. All these sentences mean something. It does not seem unreasonable to claim that there is such a thing as an envious disposition. Very well: then there are envious dispositions . . . loving dispositions—to take instances from the premises I have chosen. [C, 262]

Bion's attempt defines something, though this definition serves only as a mean, rather than an end-in-itself, it will allow the recognition of the necessity of a reliable form of scientific communication between analysts. It should not be treated as a new concept, but as an analogy, a conveyance:

> Since I want to say that there *are* such things, that is to say, things in actuality, in reality, which are represented by the word, "disposition", it is essential always to use the word in such a way that the reader will be correct in assuming that I mean what I meant on the previous occasion, that there is in reality something that is represented by the word, "disposition". [C, 262]

This point "*is inherent in psycho-analytic work and confronts the analyst at every turn*". It differs from the same problem that had already confronted the philosopher, at least until the advent of so-called post-modernism and its Kuhnian variety of epistemology. Both deny both mind and truth. Those tendencies see the former as not meriting being mixed with philosophy, lest it to be seen as a "psychologization" (since the difficulties Hume had in proving his point) of it, a downgrading. The latter is seen as non-existent or, at least, not a philosopher's problem. There seems to be confusion between the impossibility of accessing the ultimate truth, with fleeting but truthful intuitive approximations towards aspects of the noumena. The analyst cannot refrain from the issue: he is "*concerned with the practice of psycho-analysis, that is, he has to apply his theories in an empirical setting*".

This is the same when reiterating the scientific nature of psycho-analysis: "*this might amount to no more than the difficulties confronting the scientist who has to express his theories in terms of empirically verifiable data before subjecting them to experimental test*" (C, 263).

Suggested cross reference: Scientific Method.

Distance: Please refer to the entry, "hyperbole".

Disturbed personality: Bion at first employed the psychiatric view that divides normalcy from pathology. If one considers the whole of his work, from the beginning one spots the casting of doubts here and there. This occurred from his days as a tank commander. After his discharge from the army he voiced doubts about some psychiatric labels as applied to some of his fellows-in-arms who refused to carry on fighting. In the Trilogy *A Memoir of the Future* he states that some people were certified as insane but looked for him in amiable and kind terms many years after the war. He rated highly a member of his crew who tried to emulate him. Bion had won decorations for bravery, something he thinks he lacked. The man who tried to emulate him died in the attempt. In the "Commentary", *War Memoirs*, Bion made it plainly clear that he regarded this man as one who was endowed with a capacity for love that he lacked.

In the fifties disturbances of personality were seen by him as disturbances of thought. The fact that he tried to focus on different forms of development of the Oedipus complex, and his observation that in some cases the complex could not even form itself, seems to be an early way to give more attention to the fallacy involved in dividing pathology and normalcy.

As comprehension superseded judgement, the observation of specific, individual modes of functioning gradually replaced the idea of pathology. Eliciting the existence of psychotic and non-psychotic personalities (1956) indicates the development of a psycho-analytical view that echoes Freud's absence of judgmental values. Freud treated sexual development and sexual choices with no hint of judgement. Also, he saw symptoms as the last bastions of health—albeit unsuccessful.

Bion came to consider that a disturbed personality is a personality with lessened capacity to tolerate frustration. This view has nothing to do with "pathology". It means an allegiance to the principle of pleasure/displeasure and a denial of the principle of reality. In Bion's own terms, it means to function under the aegis of desire. There was a prevalence of death instincts. All of this depicts a mode of functioning rather than an illness.

The intolerance of frustration, or intolerance of the no-breast leads to disturbances of thought. Is "disturbance" the same as "illness"? If one throws a stone in still water and this initiates a disturbance, are the concentrically waves created "pathological"?

From there, Bion decidedly tackles the issue of truth. It is seen as forming the fundamental psycho-analytical ethos. This posture is identical to Freud's. Lack of it has a destructive effect on the development of the personality. Bion coins some aphorisms, in the wake of the French and British authors of the Enlightenment as well as Freud's style: "Truth is the food of mind"; and ": Mind hates truth".

He came to state that reality and truth are criteria for mental health. For example, in 1960, he warns about the inconvenient mixture of "knowledge" with "reality and truth", in a commentary about the fallacious positivistic view of science. He observed that some people who he then considered as disturbed tended to deal with the animate through means that were adequate to the inanimate. It is the same posture of the positivist "scientist":

> The scientist's mistrust of human intellectual effort tends to make
> him look longingly at the machine that can so often be made to

appear the ideal recording instrument ... how are we to find the truth ... if facts can be recorded only by an object incapable of ... anything we regard as thought on the one hand, and on the other if thought is possible only by an object incapable of recording facts?

The difficulty may not be real in any significant way, but seems so because the method of formulation, in terms of knowledge, truth, and reality, leads to fallacious exaggeration of some elements of the problem, to the exclusion of others. Progress is less impeded if we consider "know" to refer to a relationship, and reality and truth to refer to qualities of mental phenomena necessary to sustain mental health. [C, 146]

He defines mental health in terms of pain and truth: "*The man who is mentally healthy is able to gain strength and consolation and the material through which he can achieve mental development through his contact with reality, no matter whether that reality is painful or not*" (C, 192). The lack of judgmental values is seen when health—as different from mental health—may include hallucination and self-deception. This happens due to the fact that hallucination and self-deception are socially important. The group derives its sensations of well-being from hallucination (T, 5):

As a psycho-analyst I include the man's own personality as a part, and a very important part, of his environment. By contrast it may be said that man owes his health, and his capacity for continued health, to his ability to shield himself during his growth as an individual by repeating in his personal life the history of the race's capacity for self-deception against truth that his mind is not fitted to receive without disaster. Like the earth, he carries with him an atmosphere, albeit a mental one, which shields him from the mental counterpart of the cosmic and other rays at present supposed to be rendered innocuous to men, thanks to the physical atmosphere. [C, 192]

In other words, psycho-analytical understanding of the symptoms as adumbrated by Freud and Klein, led to a more precise insight into the paradoxical nature of illness, as a last resort for attempts at health. This translates into the compassion that marks the analytic attitude. Lack of compassion and love may be seen through one of its manifestations, which is more subtle than sheer delinquency. It consists in a blind pursuit of truth with disregard to oneself. Any practising analyst knows that to some people who are really intolerant of frustration the price of truth may be suicide or homicide.

Bion states this as early as 1960, in a paper in which he lists 14 points concerning compassion and truth. This paper is seen by the author as a seminal one. It seems to orient the whole of Bion's contributions to psycho-analysis.

Oedipus can be seen as the paradigm of a disturbed personality, victim of hubris, and in this sense the gluing or freezing in the paranoid–schizoid position, with no possibility for going back or forth to the depressive position, would be pathognomonic of disturbance. Points 8, 9, 10 and 12 illustrate the issue:

8. A man may lack capacity for love.
9. Similarly he may feel he lacks a capacity for truth, either to hear it, or to seek it, or to find it, or to communicate it, or to desire it.
10. He may in fact lack such a capacity.
12. Primary lack is inborn and cannot be remedied; yet some of the consequences may be modified analytically.
14. Applying (8) and (10) to the Oedipus myth, the death of the Sphinx is a consequence of such lack, as the question posed was not intended to elicit truth, and consideration for itself could not exist to erect a barrier against self-destruction. Tiresias may be said to lack compassion less than regard for truth. Oedipus lacked compassion for himself more than he lacked regard for truth [C, 125–26]

This means that truth and reality are to be taken in, to be lived rather than enforced. Compassion may be innate.

Disturbed personality is also applied to those who resort too much to hallucinosis:

The more the problem relates to the patient's inborn character the more difficult it is for him to modify his adherence to transformation in hallucinosis as *the* superior approach. If his solution were determined by a false belief that no real solution exists it would be easier for him to admit his mistake than it is when his solution is dictated by an inborn need to be "top". This would be unimportant were it not for the belief that certain disorders, notably schizophrenia, are physical and originate in pathological physical states. Their nature would be easier to grasp if seen to originate in a *normal* physical state and to spring from the very health and virility of the patient's endowment of ambition, intolerance of frustration, envy, aggression and his belief that there is, or ought to be, or will be (even if it has to be created by himself) an ideal object that exists to fulfil itself. The impression such patients give of suffering from a character disorder derives from the sense that their well-being and vitality spring from the same characteristics which give trouble. The sense that loss of the bad parts of his personality is inseparable from the loss of that part in which all his mental health resides, contributes to the acuity of the patient's fears. This acute fear is inseparable from any attempt to resolve the crux. Is the patient going to repeat the former error by becoming confirmed in his adherence to transformation in hallucinosis or will he turn to transformation in psycho-analysis? [T, 144]

The allegiance to hallucinosis is a special form of intolerance to frustration. The fabrication of an all-fulfilling object is directly linked to the addiction to lie. Lying is also seen as a manifestation of the disturbed personality: *"The disposition to lie may be regarded as a symptom of a severely disordered personality"* (AI, Introduction, page 2).

Suggested cross-references: Analytic view, Transformations in hallucinosis.

Dread, nameless dread: Please refer to the entries, Fear and (−K).

Dream: One of Bion's main expansions of Freud is the investigation of dream processes and dream work. The bulk of these explorations are in papers written in 1959, published in *Cogitations* (1992). Their synthesis and compaction are in *Learning from Experience*. In 1975, Bion would make his definitive contribution to the theme, with vols. I and II of *A Memoir of the Future*. They include dream-like verbal formulations and an attempt to depict verbally some of Bion's dreams and nightmares.

The main expansion is concerned with an observation that rescues a fact that was briefly mentioned by Freud in *The Interpretation of Dreams* (SE, VI, p. 491–3; 494n; 510; 534–5; 667). Namely, that dream work also exists during the day, not only during the night. This fact was already apparent when Freud observed the importance of the facts of the day in construing dreams. If there is a waking unconscious thinking and there is a daily activity called hallucination, why should day dreaming not exist? Free associations, children's play, are expressions of such an activity. The term "day dreaming" is usually understood as restricted to fantasising or reverie that is taken lightly. But Freud already puts it in more serious terms: those of phantasies and dreaming proper.

Bion explores the functions of dreams. In commenting on Freud's observation that *"people . . . overlook . . . the dependence of dreams upon waking life"* (Freud, 1900, SE, 4, p. 19) he states: *"My belief is that the dependence of waking life on dreams has been overlooked and is even more important. Waking life = ego activity . . . the dream symbolization and dream-work is what makes memory possible"* (C, 47).

Another expansion, still focused on the functions of dreams, is an original integration of Freud and Klein. A new function of dreams is observed: *"it is in the dream that the Positions are negotiated"* (C, 37); *"Certainly with the psychotic personality there is a failure to dream, which seems to be parallel with an inability to achieve fully the depressive position"* (C, 111).

These views do not depart from Freud, but improve him—especially as regards the functions of the dream. They are dealt with in more detail in other entries of this dictionary.

His final approach to dreams both in theory and practice can be illustrated with the help of some excerpts from *A Memoir of the Future*:

Theory

> P.A. "Talking about" dreams does not cause dreams. They exist—and some of us think, with Freud, that they are worthy of consideration and debate. The night, the dream, is a "roughness" between the smooth polished consciousness of daylight; in that "roughness" an idea might lodge. Even in the flat polished surface there can be a delusion, or an hallucination, or some other flaw in which an idea might lodge and flourish before it can be stamped out and "cured" . . .
>
> THEA I can't see why the truth is supposed to emerge in dreams.
>
> P.A. "In vino veritas" does not mean that the drunken man or the dreamer is speaking the truth. The drunkard, like the dreamer, is

less likely to be an efficient liar; he is unlikely to smooth the "rough place". But his inefficiency can be turned to good account.

ROBIN Dreamers and poets are credited with exceptional powers.

P.A. There is an ambiguity here because the dreamer is not distinguished from the sage or poet. The dreamer is like the drunkard—often in a state of decreased conscious efficiency. To be efficient the human has to be conscious, or, as we say, "has to have all his wits about him". We are concerned not with what the individual *means* to say so much as with what he does *not* intend to say, but does in fact say.

ROLAND This depends on your interpretation of *what* he says—not what he **says**.

P.A. I am concerned with what he says and what it is about. My interpretation is my attempt to formulate *what* he says so that he can compare it with his other ideas. [AMF, II, 267–8]

. . . We psycho-analysts think you do not know what a dream is; the dream itself is a pictorial representation, verbally expressed, of what happened. What actually happened when you "dreamed" we do not know. All of us are intolerant of the unknown and strive instantaneously to feel it is explicable, familiar. [AMF, II, 382]

Practice

The first volume of *A Memoir of the Future* is called *The Dream*. It is, as is a good deal of the last part of volume II, written in a kind of dream-like way. There are some parts of it that represent perhaps the nearest one is able to put into written form something akin to the real dream experience. It may be classed as a novel attempt at a "language of achievement" (q.v.). The reader may conclude for himself what kind of evocations or other impressions or feelings he or she has when reading the following quotation.

CAPTAIN BION I stared at the speck of mud trembling on the straw. I stared through the front flap at the clods of earth spouting up all round us. I stared at the dirty, strained face of my driver Allen—my strained face as I sat by me; at the boomerang that Allen sent me from Australia. I got out and hovered about six feet above us. I knew "they" would . . . and saw trees as woods walking. How "they" walked—walk! walk! they went like arfs arfing. Arf arf together, arfings the stuff for me, if it's not a Rolls Royce, which I'd pick out for choice. Then a nice little Ford bright and gay, and when they came to that ford, styx I say. Valiant for S'truth passed over and all the strumpets sounded for him on the uvver side. Cooh! What happened then? 'E talked a lot more about Jesus and dog and man and then 'e sez, all sudden like, Throw away the uvver crutch! Coo! Wot 'appened then? 'E fell on 'is arse. And 'is Arse wuz angry and said, Get off my arse! You've done nothing but throw shit at me all yore life and now you expects England to be my booty! Boo-ootiful soup; in a shell-hole in Flanders Fields. Legs and guts ... must 'ave bin twenty men in there—Germ'um and frogslegs and all starts! We didn't 'alf arf I can tell you. Let bruvverly luv continue. No one asked 'im to fall-in! No one arsed 'im to come out either—come fourth, we said and E came 5th and 'e didn't ½ stink. Full stop! 'e said. The parson 'e did kum, 'e did qwat. 'E talked of Kingdom Come. King dumb come. [AMF, I, 53–4]

One reader became impressed by the quality of this kind of universal dream to the point that he contacted Francesca Bion to share his impressions with her, two years after Dr Bion's death. Mrs. Bion said that this was a recurrent nightmare of Bion's for more than fifty years. The depiction of page 115 (AMF) displays the same quality.

Misuses and misunderstandings: Some readings of Bion's work, split from the whole context, favour an opposition between content and form of the patient's speaking and the analyst's inter-pretations (see for example, EP, 44–7). Does this reflect Bion's view as it is written in his books and papers? This reading was coupled with a particular reading of Bion's approach that illuminates func-tions of the mind and functions of the patient's verbalization in the here and now of the session. These readings state that Bion would oppose his view of dreams to that of Freud.

It may be that this kind of apprehension misunderstands both Freud and Bion's work. It reduces Freud's work to a pre-patterned symbol-decoding that characterized the bulk of papers published after Freud's death in establishment-backed "official" journals. In doing so they rejected Freud's warnings about this danger. The misunderstanding underrates Freud's theory and practice about dreaming processes and denies the non-hostile, non-rivalrous quality of Bion's extension of it.

The following quotation may dispel any doubts cast by readers prone to transforming different authors into characters in a kind of "who-is-who" fight for hallucinated supremacy in science:

> I turn now to a clinical experience in which analyst and analysand appear to be speaking the same language, to have many points of agreement and yet to remain without any tie other than that of the mechanical fact of continued attendance at analytic sessions. Progress of the analysis reveals a divergence which I shall sum up as follows:

> The analyst is, and thinks he is, in a consulting room conducting an analysis. The patient regards the same fact, his attendance in analysis, as an experience affording him the raw material to give substance to a day dream. The day dream, thus invested with reality, is that he the patient being extremely intuitive, is able without any analysis, to see just where his difficulties lie and to astonish and delight the analyst by his brilliance and friendliness. The patient reports, and the analyst believes, that he, the patient, has had a dream. The patient reports, but does NOT believe, that he has had a dream. The dream, an experience of great emotional intensity, is felt by the patient to be a straightforward recital of facts of a horrifying experience. He expects that the analyst, by treating it as a dream requiring interpretation, will give substance to his day dream that it was only a dream. In short, the patient is mobilizing his resources, and these include the facts of the analysis, to keep at bay his conviction that the dream not only was but is the reality and the reality, as the analyst understands it, is something to be appreciated only for those elements that are suited to refutation of the "dream".

> This account is not of a new theory of dreams, but is a description of a state, seen in an extremely disturbed patient, but probably of fairly common recurrence. [EP, 49–50]

When both are capable of waking from this kind of dream, sometimes the result may be felt as catastrophic:

> The patient who has no regard for truth, for himself, or for his analyst achieves a kind of freedom arising from the fact that so

much destructive activity is open to him for so long. He can behave in a way that destroys his respect for himself and his analyst, provided he always retains enough contact with reality to feel that there is some respect to destroy; and this he can always assume if his analyst continues to see him. If his analyst does not continue, then he has destroyed the analysis. But destruction of the analysis is to be avoided, for it entails loss of freedom—at least till a new object is found—thus introducing a need for moderation that is apparent at other points in the closed system that the patient strives to produce. An obvious instance of this is the need to avoid successful suicide or murder. [C, 249]

Recommended cross-references: Alpha-function, Dream the session, Dream-work-α, Beta-Screen, Contact-barrier.

Dream-like memory: A term first introduced in 1970. It clarified Bion's earlier warning about memory as a deleterious factor in the analytic session.

It is defined through a paraphrase of a verse of Shakespeare about dreams and life. Bion states that *"Dream-like memory is the memory of psychic reality and is the stuff of analysis. That which is related to a background of sensuous experiences is not suitable to the phenomena of mental life which are shapeless, untouchable, invisible, odourless, tasteless. These psychically real (in the sense of belonging to psychic reality) elements are what the analyst has to work with"* (AI, 70).

Dream-like memory partakes with free associations in the unknown nature of dreams—the stuff of the unconscious. With them the analyst may "dream the session" and the patient reaches a state that allows the analytic work to be done. Namely, his mind issues further free associations.

Suggested cross-references: Discipline in Memory and Desire, Dream, Dream-work-α, Memory, Real psycho-analysis.

"Dream", the patient's material: This entry has a motto. It resorts to a paraphrase of Freud and Bion: "There are more continuities between night-dreaming and day-dreaming than the formidable caesura provided by the state of being awake would make us believe".

To deal with the facts of the session and the patient's discourse in the here and now in the same way that Freud dealt with dreams.

It is a posture that perhaps is at the forefront of psycho-analysis. It is a scientific study of the relationship of conscious with unconscious. It is one among many attempts to investigate the unconscious. This is one of the extensions that Bion had made from Freud's theory; namely, their simultaneity rather than succession in time.

With hindsight, the formulation "to dream the session" can be regarded as the first step towards the theory of transformations in hallucinosis. The former and the latter may be regarded as a tool that enables analysts to:

(i)   apprehend the non-real nature of the emotional climates created during an analytical session;
(ii) profit more from the creative possibilities propitiated by free associations and dreaming;
(iii) apprehend the quality of resistances that the words uttered during a session have, as hiding truth and at the same time pointing to it.

> I have pointed out that it is essential to mental efficiency to be able to "dream" a current emotional experience, whether it is taking place while the person is awake, or while asleep. By this I mean that the facts, as they are represented by the person's sense impressions, have to be converted into elements such as the visual images commonly met with in dreams as they are ordinarily reported. Such an idea will not seem strange if the reader considers what happens in reverie—the word itself, chosen to name the experience, is significant of the widespread nature of the experience. Certain conditions are necessary for this work of conversion to be carried out . . . The analyst needs to have these conditions in his work, for smooth working of α-function is essential. He must be able to dream the analysis as it is taking place, but of course he must not go to sleep. Freud has described the condition as one of "free-floating attention" . . . [C, 216]

Bion's extensions of Freud's theory of dreams made explicit something that was implicit in Freud's theory. One of these extensions is the suggestion of a technical need, namely, "to dream the patient's material". This suggestion may be viewed as an integration of Freud's *The Interpretation of Dreams* and "Constructions in analysis". In this sense, the "dreaming of the patient's material" would be an equivalent of the analyst's work of metapsychologization of the session itself.

Bion observed that interpretations couched in Freud's terms—turning the unconscious, conscious—as well as interpretations couched in Klein's terms of projective identification, had some limitations, concerning the *"illuminations received from interpretations"* (LE, 21). These limitations were circumvented when it "occurred to him" that his patient was doing what he (Bion) had *"earlier described as 'dreaming' the immediate events in the analysis"*; or in terms of the theory of alpha-function, *"translating sense impressions into alpha-function"* (all quotations LE, 21).

*This idea seemed to illuminate sometimes but became dynamic only when I related it to **defective** alpha-function, that is to say, when it occurred to me that I was witnessing an inability to dream through lack of alpha-elements and therefore an inability to sleep or wake, to be either conscious or unconscious".*

The analyst is pressed to be the patient's conscious. For obvious reasons he is a conscious that is incapable *"of the functions of consciousness"*. Conversely, the patient is *"an unconscious incapable of the functions of **unconsciousness**"*. The clinical situation is rather typical: the patient can *"pour out a stream of material intended to destroy the analyst's psycho-analytic potency"*, or *"is concerned to withhold rather than to impart information"*.

The analyst finds himself overwhelmed by a *"plethora of interpretations that would occur to anyone with any common sense"*. He is invited to talk in non-psycho-analytical, socially-accepted phrases. The interpretations tend to be reassuring, either positively (laudatory) or negatively (accusatory). The patient makes heavy usage of that which Bion calls the "beta-screen" (q.v.), which *"has a quality enabling it to evoke the kind of response the patient desires, or, alternatively, a response from the analyst which is heavily charged with countertransference"* (LE, 21–24).

More and more the patient creates an environment whose main feature is a specific kind of acting-out: he tries to evoke *"interpretations which are less related to his need for psycho-analytic interpretation than to his need to produce an emotional involvement"* (LE, 25). The patient displays his inability to understand his own state of mind.

He tries by all means to fill the session with the analyst's state of mind. This contributes to the reversal of alpha-function and to the creation of bizarre objects (q.v.). One of them is that which could be analysis but is not; it is transformed into counselling, criticism, reassurance or the like.

The contact-barrier, in contrast to the beta-screen (q.v.), *"may be expected to manifest itself clinically—if indeed it is manifest at all—as something that resembles dreams. As we have seen the contact barrier permits a relationship and preservation of belief in it as an event in actuality, subject to the laws of nature, without having that view submerged by emotions and phantasies originating endo-psychically.*

> Reciprocally it preserves emotions with endo-psychic origin from being overwhelmed by the realistic view. The contact-barrier is therefore responsible for the preservation of the distinction between conscious and unconscious and for its inception. The unconscious is thus preserved. [LE, 26–7]

One may remember that the so-called psychotics one finds interned in hospitals display straightaway in their contact a kind of skinless or "overt" unconscious all the time. They seem to be relentlessly devoid of resistances. Applying Bion's contributions to that observation, in these patients the unconscious is absolute and cannot be made conscious. The person is an unconscious-in-itself. The person is unable to dream.

This state is felt as unbearable; it calls for denial, splitting and projection into someone else. The capacity to dream, so to speak, as well as the capacity to think, is projected into the analyst. The analyst is at once called to dream for his patient as well as being forced not to be able to dream, thus alleviating the patient of the pain involved in dreaming and therefore in having access to the unconscious activities of his or her mind.

These conclusions are presented as such in Bion's four basic books, published in 1962, 1963, 1965 and 1970. Thanks to Francesca Bion's efforts, in *Cogitations* we have at our disposal the preparatory studies that considerably expand Bion's paths to a novel formulation. It stems from his clinical experience, which is also depicted in much more detail in *Cogitations* than in the four basic books.

The contribution is to make explicit something that was included in Freud's work but could not be used unless the professional could see the issue by himself. It corresponds to Freud's quotation of Goethe in "Constructions in analysis", a "call to the witches". It enlarges Freud's observations on dreams in proposing that the dream processes—that function during the day, as Freud stated in *The Interpretation of Dreams*—should be used by the analyst as they unfold in the session. In short, the analyst must "dream the patient's material" in order to catch a glimpse of the unconscious processes at work—in the here and now and during the emotional experiences lived in the session.

Klein seems to have been the first to put into practice the day-dreaming capacity of the human being when she intuited the possibility of play technique. The child both hallucinates and dreams when it plays. To differentiate this on the spot enhances Klein's contributions.

In bringing together Freud's observations on dreams, the development of thought processes and functions of the ego (always according to Freud) with Klein's positions, Bion unified the two theories. This happened in 1959, based on pure empirical data, that is, clinical experience. This unification can be seen in his own words. He was dealing with a patient who had "*an ability to see what everyone sees when subjected to the same stimulus*"; a patient who resorts to projective identification almost all the time; "*an ability to believe in survival after death . . .*" In other words, this kind of patient has no conception of death at all. This is an omnipotent feature of anyone's personality. The functions of the ego are both impaired and exaggerated when paranoid–schizoid phenomena prevail.

Omnipotence also surfaces when the patient displays "*an ability to hallucinate or manipulate facts so as to produce material for a delusion that there exists an inexhaustible fund of love in the group for himself*". Interpretations are feared for they mean "*that elucidation of illusory, delusory, or hallucinatory mechanisms for making the patient feel loved, lest such elucidation should show him that such love as he wishes to feel that he receives does not in fact exist . . . In so far as the patient is successful in evading the attacks on his narcissism, he experiences a hallucinatory gratification of his craving for love. This, like all hallucinatory gratification, leaves the patient unsatisfied. He therefore greedily resorts to a strengthening of his capacity for hallucination, but there is naturally no corresponding increase in satisfaction*" (C, 29–30). All of this led to "*an inability to dream and hatred of common sense*" (C, 31).

Bion observed that he had to keep circulating freely in areas that seemed incommunicable to the patient, namely, the areas of the ego and of the id, in the actual session. The patients also have to circulate freely through them. This ability became visible, as occurred in psycho-analysis, in patients who seemed unable to do this. A theoretical detour seems to be necessary; it reproduces Bion's own path. He makes a choice, stating that Freud's final theory of guilt "*is a more fruitful theory*" than Klein's theory of guilt. Freud's theory states denial of guilt linked to the Oedipal situation; Klein puts it as the effect of a "*loved injured object*" which "*may very swiftly change into a persecutor*" (Klein, 1952, p. 285).

In a certain sense, Freud pushes the issue back towards the ego; Klein returns it towards the id. The id was where Freud started from (even though he did not call it "id" then), when he talked about repression as a result of deflected cathexis. But he had modified the theory in *Inhibitions, Symptoms and Anxiety*, in terms of the Oedipus complex in which the death instincts function. This includes the areas of the ego and the super-ego, which are partially unconscious. To study the dynamics of object relations as Klein did, even though it includes the whole mental apparatus, is tilted towards examining the object cathexis, which is instinctual (area of the id); the ego and super-ego are not under close scrutiny when this focus is prevalent.

The idea of a cruel, murderous super-ego, a "*mass of super-egos— the bizarre objects*" is seminal in illuminating the inability to dream. It led Bion to deal with the matter tolerating the paradox of a conscious and an unconscious functioning simultaneously. He leans neither towards the id nor the ego; the obtrusion of the super-ego is more clearly perceived.

There is no hostile criticism in Bion's evaluation of Klein's theory, as well as that of Freud. Its effect is that both theories emerge stronger and expanded. He continues integrating and unifying them, as we shall see soon.

The dream is not regarded as a boxed, compartmentalized unconscious activity. It is dealt with as belonging to both realms, id and ego. Freud did this with the concepts of manifest and latent contents, but Bion seems to push the issue further in the actual moment of the session. It is not only a case of dreams that are reported as having occurred hours or days earlier. It is rather a dream being dreamt during the session—or an inability to do this.

The suspicion that the actual events of the session are being turned into a dream came back to me today with X when at one point I suspected that my interpretation was being made into a dream . . . I suspect that Freud's displacement etc. is relevant; he took up only the negative attitude, dreams as "concealing" something, not the way in which the *necessary* dream is *constructed* (C, 33). . . . I shall assume that the patient's fear of the murderous super-ego prevents his approaching the Positions [paranoid–schizoid and depressive positions]. This in turn means that be is unable to dream, for it is in dream that the Positions are negotiated. He therefore postpones this experience till the analytic session in which he hopes he will have support, or perhaps, feeling he has support, dares to have the dream he cannot have without the consciousness of support.

He has to dream—the important thing here is not the content of the dream, but his having to "dream" . . . the essential difference between the resistance as something peculiar to the neurotic and relegation to the unconscious, and psychotic destruction of the means for understanding which is associated with an apparently full consciousness of what is ordinarily the furniture of the unconscious. "I do not understand", or "do not know why", or "do not know how", etc. may be taken either as a *positive* statement of *inability* to dream, or a defiant assertion of a capacity for *not* dreaming. [C, 37]

The link between dreaming and Klein's observations about the Positions is made with the aid of a formulation borrowed from the philosophy of mathematics, that of the selected fact. It matters because projective identification and other manifestations of the paranoid–schizoid position as well as depressive phenomena are ubiquitous in analysis: *"the interplay between paranoid–schizoid and depressive positions is made possible by a selected fact which is known as the 'harmonizing or unifying fact' spatially, and the 'cause' temporally . . ."* (C, 44). The selected fact must be, so to say, intuited and "dreamt".

The importance of these is that much that passes for "normal" during the session may in fact be pure hallucination. Indeed, a few years later these observations would lead to the theory of transformations in hallucinosis (q.v.). This makes the difference between real analysis (q.v.) and a colluded or hallucinated practice.

In other words, the dream-work we know is only a small aspect of dreaming proper—dreaming proper being a continuous process

belonging to the *waking* life and in action all through the waking
hours, but not usually observable then except with the psychotic
patient ... At any rate the hypothesis that in an analytic session I
can see the patient dream has proved to be very valuable especially
with its counterpart of seeing the contrasting activity of hallucination. [C, 38]

The basis that seems to have given Bion a hint of the kinship and
differences between dreams and hallucinations—something that
occupied a great deal of Freud's work—may be seen in statements
such as this: "*Freud says the state of sleep represents a turning away from
the world and 'thus provides a necessary condition for the development of
a psychosis'. Is this why X talks of losing consciousness?*" (C, 43). Bion
was coming from a lengthy and profound experience with
psychotics and was able to see the value of observing the function
of seemingly minor verbalizations.

Thus Bion comes to his proposal that is a recommendation
concerning the analyst's state of mind that, if present, propitiates
analysis; if absent, precludes it: "*Anxiety in the analyst is a sign that
the analyst is refusing to 'dream' the patient's material: not (dream) =
resist = not (introject)*" (C, 43).

The extension of Freud's theory of dreams and of the unconscious as epistemologically previous to the conscious are extended:
"*It may be worth considering, when a patient is resisting, whether the
resistance bears characteristics relating it to phenomena Freud described
as 'dream-work'. But **Freud** meant by dream-work that unconscious material, which would otherwise be perfectly comprehensible, was transformed
into a dream, and that the dream-work needed to be undone to make the
now incomprehensible dream comprehensible* [New Introductory
Lectures, 1933a, SE 22, p. 25]. *I mean that the conscious material has to
be subjected to dream-work to render it fit for storing, selection and suitable for transformation from paranoid—schizoid position ... **Freud** says
Aristotle states that a dream is the way the mind works in sleep: I say it
is the way it works when awake* [New Introductory Lectures, 1933a, SE
22, p. 26–7]" (C, 43).

Therefore the day-dreaming activity, already adumbrated by
Freud, is now put to practical use. The simultaneous functioning of
conscious and unconscious is established—rather than a time-
succession between them. Those issues would be developed more

in *Learning from Experience*. The appreciation of the unconscious is heightened. It is as if Bion were "out-freuding" Freud; perhaps he was stretching Freud's observations in a sense that he pushes its limits further than was thought possible. Let us see a quotation that vouches for these statements. Bion reminds us of Freud again and again, in order to further the issue:

Freud says,

It is easy to see how the remarkable preference shown by the memory in dreams for indifferent, and consequently unnoticed, elements in waking experiences is bound to lead people to overlook in general the dependence of dreams upon waking life and all events to make it difficult in any particular instance to prove that dependence. [The Interpretation of Dreams, 1900a, SE 4, p. 19]

My belief is that the dependence of waking life on dreams has been overlooked and is even more important. Waking life = ego activity, and in particular the play of logical thought on the synthesis of elements, i.e. particles of the paranoid–schizoid position . . . the dream symbolization and dream-work is what makes memory possible. [C, 47]

One may feel that Bion subverts Freud. But one may also see that what he does is to find the other side that complements that which Freud illuminated; an implicit situation is made explicit, in terms of antithetical pairs.

From unconscious to conscious or unconscious ⇔ conscious?

Bion states that there is a need to make something unconscious as a condition for enabling this something to be conscious at all. In other words, nothing can be conscious without a sojourn in the unconscious. It is a change from sticking exclusively to the formula, "turning the unconscious, conscious" (or "where the id was, ego shall be"). This expansion of Freud would appear a few years later in *Learning from Experience* in the guise of the theory of the "contact-barrier" (q.v.). Bion quotes two examples: the learning of walking and the learning of the word "Daddy".

The unconscious appears at full bore in its quality or nature of being an "unknown". This quality, made apparent by the German name-*unbewußt*—was gradually lost by the psycho-analytical environment. This quality obtrudes in the proposal of thoughts without a thinker and the search for a selected fact. Later it would emerge in the concept of invariances—underlying immaterial facts that call for research into the unknown to be discovered. The psycho-analytical movement persistently falls back into a posture that takes the patient's words at their face value, dealing just with the manifest content; no underlying facts are detected.

In doing this, our practice undergoes a psychologization in the academic tradition of psychology. Perhaps the inability to dream the session, to deal with thoughts without a thinker that float in the air, the allegiance to the conscious words uttered, accounts much more for the present day so-called "crisis" than has been considered.

The attempt to display that nothing can be conscious without having been unconscious would remain alive to the end of Bion's life. The last attempt was the Trilogy, *A Memoir of the Future*. It contains a dream-like verbalization that may help the reader to find the way back to conscious **for himself (please refer to the entries Analytic View, Atonement, Real Analysis).**

There are some conditions for dreaming the patient's material: (i) The exercising of personal freedom with no resorting to a priori and ad hoc theorizing; (ii) analytically trained intuition, meaning, experience of personal analysis as profound as possible, reaching the analyst's psychotic personality coupled with experience with the patient's psychotic personality. (i) and (ii) bring with them sensations of impending madness or actual madness.

> One way of dealing with the problem of scientific evidence for dream theories would be to restrict the search for data to experience shared by analyst and patient, or at which analyst and patient are both present. Such occasions might be all those on which the patient said he had had a dream, or all those on which there appear to be events taking place, e.g. the patient sits up and looks around in a dazed way; the analyst, identifying himself with the patient, feels that the experience the patient is having would be more understandable if the patient were asleep and dreaming.

> "More understandable." Why? Because it is more appropriate to the facts as the analyst sees them. But this means that if the analyst were feeling what the patient seems to be feeling, than he, the analyst, would be disposed to say, "I must have been dreaming".

Just then I found I had been asleep; just before I woke I seemed to be saying to F that I was feeling I was going mad because I could not sort out the feeling I was having in the dream about having a dream and who I was. The dream seemed to be that I was trying to solve the problem I am in fact trying to solve, but with the addition of the fear of going mad—a sort of mental disintegration. [C, 51[

The same issue was put very explicitly in *A Memoir of the Future*. This links up with what was said earlier in this entry about projective identification and the demand that the patient makes on the analyst, that he must dream in place of the patient.

The non-psychotic, and the non-psychotic part of the personality, is afraid of making something conscious—the typical neurotic fear in psycho-analysis—because making it conscious is feared as the same as "bringing it out into the open"; this in turn is felt to be the same as evacuating it and making it conscious in such a way that it can never be made unconscious again, and therefore unavailable ever again for unconscious waking thinking. And this in turn is felt to be indistinguishable from being psychotic. This is one of the reasons for the neurotic fear that successful analysis will make him mad. [C, 71]

The patient's necessity to dream during the session and its paradoxical companion, namely, the fear of dreaming, displayed by patients, led Bion to two discoveries:

1. That the analyst should also have a capacity to dream the session.
2. That the actuality of hallucinosis is more frequent than formal appearances led us to suppose (please refer to the entry, "Transformations in hallucinosis").

Since it is essential that the creative worker should keep his α-function unimpaired, it is clear that the analyst must be able to dream the session. But if he is to do this without sleeping, he must have plenty of sleep. [C, 120]

To dream is at once to apprehend reality through a non-real *real* experience. It is non-real because it is *only* a dream; and it is *real* because to dream, as an act, is real, even though its manifest content is not.

Having two sets of feelings about the same facts is felt as madness and disliked accordingly. This is one reason why it is felt necessary to have an analyst; another reason is the wish for me to be available to be regarded as mad and used to being regarded as mad. There is a fear that you might be called an analysand, or reciprocally, that you may be accused of insanity. Should I then be tough and resilient enough to be regarded and treated as insane while being sane? If so, it is not surprising that psycho-analysts are, almost as a function of being analysts, supposed to qualify for being insane and called such. It is part of the price they have to pay for being psycho-analysts. [AMF, I, 113]

Recommended cross-reference: Dream.
Suggested cross-references: Alpha-function, Dream-work-α, Beta-Screen, Contact-barrier.

Dream-work-α: This concept of dream work-α is relevant to the student of the work of Bion in terms of a history of ideas. In the opinion of the author it must be put into its historical perspective. It is not possible to define it without introducing a gross distortion. Its definition varied in time and in the end it was discarded.

It furnishes an example of learning from experience and error, and also of the outcome of a non-rivalrous, but critical approach to the works of the great masters. By "critical", here, is meant, in the sense of not being submitted to authoritarianism or idealization.

The concept of dream-work-α arose from Bion's scrutiny of the mysterious nature of that which we accustomed ourselves to call "dreams". During the last century thousands of artisans (practising analysts) around the world repeated Freud's observations. This repetition is valuable to the extent that it furnishes an example that fulfils Popper's criterion of reproducibility: it scientifically confirms, at least in part, Freud's work, but it cannot be seen as furthering it. Perhaps no other author in the history of the psycho-analytic movement tried to further Freud's observations on dreams as did Bion.

The study of the history of this concept offers an opportunity to see:

(i) Bion's use of Freud's observations under a non-idealized, non-authoritarian and non-rivalrous way.

(ii) His gradual replacement of philosophy with philosophy of mathematics.

(iii) How his anchoring in clinical work helped him to correct and improve his views; consequent to this, the evolution of the concept offers an opportunity to see a scientist at work. In other terms, Bion avoided flights of imagination, hasty and unwarranted formation of ad hoc theories. Knowing too well that his proposals *"may seem to introduce a dangerous doctrine opening the way for the analyst who theorizes unhampered by the facts of practice", Bion warned that "unfettered play of an analyst's phantasies has long been recognized; pedantic statement on the one hand and verbalization loaded with unobserved implications on the other mean that the potential for misunderstanding and erroneous deduction is so high as to vitiate the value of the work done with such defective tools"* (T, 39, 44). Even though Bion would make this warning six years after having proposed and discarded the concept of dream work-a, one may see that he not only claimed, but practised it.

℗ During the fifties and until 1960 Bion was critical of Freud's idea that consciousness had the qualities of a sense-organ. In chapter VII of *The Interpretation of Dreams*, Freud leaves to consciousness the role of a sense organ for apprehending psychic quality.

Bion's criticism paralleled his attempt to improve Freud's differentiation of hallucination and dream. At that time Bion attempted to create a new, all-encompassing theory that could account for mental states that have the nature of dreams. In this theory, dreams would be a partial aspect of mental activity. In the end Bion gives up the attempt; he finally adopts Freud's definition. From then on he displays a distinct preference for adopting established theories that may not be completely satisfactory but at the same time no better replacement is available.

It became clear to him that the confusion he was trying to resolve in theoretical terms was in fact a confusion made by his patients. Bion realized that these patients cannot dream and therefore they cannot be awake. He matches this observation with that of the use that the psychotic personality (q.v.) makes of the non-psychotic personality (q.v.). This indicates that there is no need to modify Freud's theory, but rather indicates the need to examine in more detail Freud's observations on cognitive development, in terms of perception and apprehension of sense data and their transformation into non-sensuous data. Bion starts from Freud's concept of dream-work. Theoretically, he states that the dream is where Klein's positions are negotiated. Practically, he hints that the analyst must "*'dream' the patient's material*" (C, 43).

In focusing on the patient's and the analyst's difficulties in dreaming, Bion rescues Freud's observation that dream-work exists during the whole day, even when the person is conscious, wide awake. The patient cannot dream and puts the dream-yet-to-be-dreamt into the analyst, via projective identification. The analyst is tempted to dream for the patient. He must not do this; he must "dream the session". More than rescuing Freud's observation, he expands the duties of the dreaming activity. As with night-dreaming, day-dreaming may be more near reality than worldly values and social conventions, that may be hallucinated.

The nature and function of resistance may be that of a negative: there's always another side that goes beyond appearances; this includes the formal, manifest content of the patient's discourse. In 1977 (*A Memoir of the Future*) Bion would put this in clearer terms: resistances simultaneously betray and disguise truth. This "another side" of whatever it is may corresponds to day-dreaming.

> It may be worth considering, when a patient is resisting, whether the resistance bears characteristics relating it to phenomena Freud described as "dream-work". But *Freud* meant by dream-work that unconscious material, which would otherwise be perfectly comprehensible, was transformed into a dream, and that the dream-work needed to be undone to make the now incomprehensible dream comprehensible. *I* mean that the conscious material had to be subjected to dream-work to render it fit for storing, selection, and suitable for transformation from paranoid–schizoid position to depressive position . . . *Freud* says Aristotle states that a dream is the way the mind works in sleep: *I* say it is the way it works when awake. [C, 43]

His research makes parts of Freud's work more explicit: "*Contact with reality is **not** dependent on dream-work; accessibility to the personality of the material derived from this contact **is** dependent on dream-work. The failure of dream-work and the consequent lack of availability of experience of external or internal psychic reality gives rise to the peculiar state of the psychotic who seems to have a contact with reality but is able to*

*make singularly little use of it either for learning by experience or for
immediate consumption.*

*In this respect the dream seems to play a part in the mental life of the
individual, which is analogous to the digestive processes in the alimentary
life of the individual. Why?"* (C, 45).

The dream is seen as an epistemological function of the mind: it
has, so to say, introjective properties. It introjects reality itself, external or internal. The analogy with the digestive system is hinted at.
It was to remain lurking until it was embodied into the theory of
α-function.

The first mention of alpha dates from 5 August 1959. It had to
do with dreams and the psychotic's inability to dream—which was
seen as an attack on α: *"The dream-elements in the psychotic dream are
really the discarded residue of α-elements that have survived mutilations
of α"* (C, 53). At first, α was a somewhat vague entity that operated
just on sense impressions. Despite its still somewhat vague nature,
it was duly defined: *"α is concerned with, and is identical with, unconscious waking thinking designed, as a part of the reality principle, to aid
in the task of real, as opposed to pathological, modification of frustration"*
(C, 54).

A clinical fact, namely, a striking inability that some patients had
to dream, led him to investigate the issue. Bion observed these
patient's attempts to compensate for this inability through dreaming during the session:

> I wish now to extend the term, "dream", to cover the kind of events
> that take place in an analysis of a schizophrenic—events that
> appear to me to merit the description, "dreams".

> One of the points I wish to discuss is related to the fact that the
> actual events of the session, as they are apparent to the analyst, are
> being "dreamed" by the patient *not* in the sense that he believes that
> the events observed by him are the same as the events observed by
> the analyst (except for the fact that he believes them to be a part of
> a dream, and the analyst believes them to be a part of reality) but
> in the sense that these same events that are being *perceived* by the
> analyst are being perceived by the patient and treated to a process
> of being dreamed by him. That is, these events are having some-
> thing done to them mentally, and that which is being done to them
> is what I call being dreamed . . . [C, 39]

In defining α Bion integrated the writings of Freud in 1911 to those of 1900. To put α as part of the unconscious as well as part of the reality principle is an expansion of Freud's contributions. It elicits the existence of the day-dreaming activity. The hypothesis here is that dreams are not only the royal road to the knowledge of the unconscious processes of the mind—but they are also a royal road to the knowledge of reality as it is; meaning, both the reality of the self and external reality. Summing up, dreams can be seen as a self-epistemological tool at the service of the epistemophilic instincts.

Reality itself is (i) amenable to be apprehended, albeit unwittingly and partially, by the senses; (ii) then it is dreamt, and therefore it is made unconscious in order to return later to consciousness.

Bion leaned heavily on Freud's observation of a choice, namely, the crossroads of modifying reality or evading it. α was first seen as the device that would make it possible to modify reality. In 1959 it was not seen as a function. It did not have the status of something that was not to be confused with dreaming activity proper.

α was a first attempt to solve something in Freud's work that puzzled Bion. How could it be that consciousness performs the function of a sense-organ for the apprehension of psychic quality? In the end Bion makes peace with the concept and accepts it. His critical attitude helped to improve Freud's theory. He realized that the acquisition of that which can be seen as a psychic quality itself depends on modification of frustration. He integrates Klein's observation of projective identification into Freud's theory: projective identification can be used as an evacuation that serves to evasion of frustration.

Simultaneously with the construction of an "α project" that could replace Freud's theory of consciousness and its attendant modes of apprehension of reality, Bion was increasingly extending Freud's theory of dreams. *"How does a dream evade frustration? By distortion of facts of reality . . . by dream-work on the perception of facts . . . Freud attributes to dream-work the function of concealing the facts of internal mental life only—the dream-thoughts only. I attribute to it the function of evading the frustration to which the dream-thoughts, and therefore the interpretation of dream-thoughts, would give rise if allowed to function properly—that is, as mechanisms associated with the legitimate tasks involved in real modification of frustration"* (C, 54).

α thus opened the road to a more precise study of waking unconscious thinking, during a time that the psycho-analytic movement made a sensible detour towards conscience and conscious ego. During that epoch the establishment began to despise or ignore the unknown, the id-*unbewußt*. A few days after trying to introduce his alternative, Bion asks: "*Does this [waking unconscious thinking] have the function I attribute to α or does α carry out the transformation of sense impressions which makes these storable in such a form that they are available for waking unconscious thinking?*" (C, 55).

At this moment he sharply denies to α the task of symbol formation. This is a first step towards separating α from dreams. Did his firm grasp of Klein and Segal's perceptions on this issue, coupled with his experience with excessively concretizing psychotics who could neither dream not wake, help him to reach this point?

This separation of α from dreams puts α as a *precursor* of dreams—later to be seen as the factory of raw material to be used in dreams. It was just the existence of *hostile* criticisms against Freud that seemed to furnish him with a hint. He quotes page 54 of *The Interpretation of Dreams*, SE 4, where Freud observes that there are people who use the "*need in a waking state to disparage the dream*"; Bion emphasizes an often overlooked statement of Freud, namely, **the dependence of waking life on dreams** (SE 4, p. 19; C, 47). Bion joins this with his idea that thinking, which Freud thought was originally unconscious, was in fact "*still unconscious*" (C, 54).

That is, Bion comes up with the idea of a "*dream-work-α*", which replaces, in a mere two days, the α theory. "*Most of the criticisms cited* [he is referring to Freud SE 4 p. 54] *are hostile and indicate the need in a waking state to disparage the dream. This is compatible with α-theory that there is a failure of 'digestion mentally'. It would explain partly why the 'facts' and their ideational counterpart had not been digested if the rational conscious attitude was so hostile to the ideational counterpart of the stimulus, wherever in reality it originated. For such hostility would be likely to inhibit dream-work-α, and in so far as the inhibition failed—for after all the patient has dreamed—the hostility now extends to the product of the dream-work*" (C, 56–7).

Four days later another invariance that permeates the whole of Bion's work obtrudes in the construction of the theory. Epistemologically, he used Bacon, Locke, Schlick, Prichard, Braithwaite, Bradley and part of Popper's contributions to science. Bion was looking for a generalizing theory that could spot Hume's constant conjunctions and/or Poincaré's selected facts. They could endow the theory of the "generalizing" or "unifying" powers.

In the path that would lead Bion to the theory of α-function we are now in an intermediate phase: "dream-work-α". We have already seen that from "alpha" to "dream-work-α" the modification was to separate "alpha" from "dreaming". The next step is duly described: *"Under the title dream-work-α I propose to bring together a number of mental activities all of which are familiar to practising psychoanalysts, although they may not have previously associated them together in this way"* (C, 62).

In other terms, this is a practical application of Poincaré's selected fact; Bion draws it from the philosophy of mathematics. His extension of Freud: *"The title, 'dream-work', has already a meaning of great value. I wish to extend some of the ideas already associated with it and to limit others"* (C, 62). His affiliation is clearly stated: Freud's *The Interpretation of Dreams*, "Formulations on the two principles of mental functioning", "Instincts and their vicissitudes" and the *New Introductory Lectures on Psycho-Analysis*; he unifies them with Klein's "Notes on some schizoid mechanisms". He attributes to the sign α the value of a notation *"for the sake of brevity"* (C, 63), to the more cumbersome term *"dream-work-α"*.

The theory has features that would be transmitted to its replacement, the theory of alpha-function. It was not regarded as a function. It contained no definition. It included too many intentions: to differentiate dreams from hallucinations, to include something still ill-defined that was neither dreaming proper nor waking thinking. In this sense, this term "functioned" exactly as that which Bion observed in psychotics—who can neither wake nor dream. If it is true that it is clinical work that nourishes the best psycho-analytic concepts, it is also true that the elevation of a clinical finding to the status of normal functioning entails some risks. Perhaps this was the case with this theory and perhaps it was superseded in part for this reason.

In this case, clinical observation paved the way to realizing that psychotic functioning is a deeper layer of that which we call normalcy. The posture had its finest hours in the elucidation of the psychotic personality and its final development in the theory of transformations in hallucinosis (q.v.). During the fifties Bion still had an allegiance to a view that believed that the scheme "pathology or health" could be applied to suffering. Bion's questioning this scheme as well as the idea of cure was far in the future. These views contributed to some of the inconsistencies one may find, as Bion found, in his theory about dream-work-α.

The theory tried to resolve the function of dreaming and to resolve Bion's doubts about Freud's theory of consciousness. It also tried to integrate Bion's view that some dreams were at the service of projective identification. In trying to resolve all those problems in a single frame, the theory of dream-work-α contained some contradictions. For example, it was important to illuminate the existence of day-dreaming; it also illuminated the problems consequent to the failure to dream. The key lay in restricting its goals and also in making clearer its origin in sense impressions. But this key was well ahead.

Let us look at these problems in some detail and the way Bion resolved them. The resolution was not theoretical. Clinical work furnished the clues. The observation that dream activity or mechanisms occurred during the day is present in the theory of dream-work-α: "Dream-work-α is continuous night and day" (C, 63). *Freud said this from the beginning, when he stated again and again the continuities between everyday occurrences and their "remains" in dreams. Despite Freud's remarks the layman's idea prevailed; namely, that of a separation of day-dreaming activity and night dreaming activity. It corresponded to the separation of conscious from unconscious. Even Freud at a certain point capitulates and separates them, for example, when he posited a succession in time: from unconscious to conscious.*

Bion says that dream-work-α "*. . . operates on the mental counterpart of events of external reality, or on what Bradley calls the ideational counterpart of external fact*" (C, 63). Here resides a difference between dream-work-α and α-function. Bion was trying to use Bradley's ideas on mental functioning. Bion seemed to think that the philosopher of science could help to solve a problem he saw in Freud's work. In saying that dream-work-α operates on *mental counterparts* rather than on *sense impressions* he was not using clinical work, but philosophy. He would change it later when defining α-function: it acts on sense impressions. This was a stumbling block: his proposed device, α, operated in the stuff that the mind is made of—*mental counterparts*—rather than in sense impressions, as he would state later. Let us say that α and dream-work-α were too broad, all-encompassing attempts; they tried to replace dreams; for dreams operate in the stuff of the mind.

Did his experience lead him to undervalue for a while the sense impressions? *"Various kinds of tic, including a stammer, reports of supposed dreams in which there is apparently no content but a powerful emotional experience, reports of dreams in which visual images are devoid of associations of emotion—these for the present appear to be as near as we are likely to get to an understanding of the mental material on which α works"* (C, 65).

Was Bion separating psychic from material reality? *"The ideational counterpart on which α operates appears to be consciousness associated with certain sense impressions, which Freud calls the consciousness attached to the sense organs . . . What this is I am not able to suggest"* (C, 63). There was an overriding factor in the constructive criticism of Freud's theory of consciousness. His objection about this specific part of Freud's work was the lack of clinical grounds that could confirm Freud's theory in practice: *"I have no clinical experience that I feel would be valuable to differentiate from other clinical experiences and label as a part of that which constitutes the consciousness attached to the sense organs"* (C, 63).

This is a consideration that shows Bion's scientific bent. It would be just this scientific *Weltanschauung* that furnished him with a clue to resolve those issues—in the end, to get on peaceful terms with Freud's theory of consciousness. It also marked, with the replacement of the theory of dream-work-α by the theory of α-function, his giving-up of a theory that had become overloaded by too many simultaneous goals.

In *Transformations* he recommended not abandoning a theory that could have some shortcomings; but he seemed to have been doing exactly this when he toyed with the theories of dream-work-α and α. One of the clues that led him to abandon his own all-encompassing theories rather than Freud's was his perception that different people can use the **same words** with different senses. Later he would see that even the same person can use the same word with different senses, according to the context. The observation of psychotic patients led him to realize that some people utter phrases and words *"devoid of undertones or overtones"*. One may say "table"; but it *"seems to be a **lack** of associations . . . as if, meaning nothing but 'table', it came near to meaning nothing at all"* (C, 63).

At this time, Bion was very near to discovering the existence of something he would a little while later name "β-elements". The description was ready. What was lacking was a concept. Both psycho-analytically and philosophically, it lacked the verbal counterpart of the numinous realm, the unconscious (*unbewußt*) realm. The following paragraph of the same text introduces the reader to this realm:

There are other experiences that appear to be those of emotion, fear, anxiety, dread, to which the patient seems unable to attach either a name or an image" (C, 63). In this text, Bion follows a route that is the same route that the patient followed in his suffering; Bion as a writer (and probably as an analyst) also suffered from this. The reader is invited to experiment with the taste of the "psychotic way". The psychotic way cannot differentiate conscious from unconscious, cannot realize their filtering unification (see the entry, "contact barrier") as an ever-flowing, back and forth situation. "*These experiences also appear to be untransformed by α. . . it is an undigested fact; it has not been 'dreamed', it has not been transformed by α*" (C, 63–4).

Another step is taken towards the theory of α-function: "*Is it possible to get nearer to describing what α does? It pays attention to the sense impressions*" (C, 64). α-function, in its turn, does *pay attention to the sense impressions*; moreover, it actively uses them. It transforms the sense impressions into elements that will be useful to store in the memory, to think, to dream etc.

In putting α as something that *pays attention to the sense impressions* and thereafter considering that feelings are internal sense impressions, Bion is able to put aside Bradley, Braithwaite and others. It is fair to say that in the same work that he courts those philosophers he also points out critically where psycho-analysis cannot be in agreement with them. Taking into account that those texts are in the book *Cogitations* and therefore they represent an intermediate stage in the development of theory, one may conjecture that he realized how near-sighted and unsuccessful is the attempt to replace psycho-analysis with philosophy. One would also think that this attempt enabled him to perfect his use of philosophy as an inspiring analogical tool rather than a replacement.

He would not resort to terms such as "ideational counterparts of events of external reality" any more. He would instead see that both dreaming as we know it and sense impressions as soon as they have entered into the psyche **are** those counterparts. They need to be construed by the person. They cannot be taken for granted as existing. The philosopher does not bother investigating how they are construed clinically and in real life.

Bion thought that the sense impression "must be ideogrammaticized". In proposing this, Bion values—as did Freud—the visual component. The ideogrammatization is also valued due to the fact that it confers "*durability*" on the sense impression. Bion is trying to see how an external or internal stimulus loses its material aspect; he is on the verge of enunciating the "de-sense-fying" function of the mind. It will be his mastery of Freud and Klein that allows him to further the research: "But now there enters a new feature depending on whether the pleasure–pain principle or the reality principle is dominant. If the reality principle is dominant, then the object of the ideogram will be to make the experience suitable for storage and recall; if the pleasure–pain principle is dominant, the tendency will be to have as the object of the ideogram its value as an excretable object" (C, 64). *The quest for ideograms would occupy Bion for the rest of his life as one can see in AMF, volume I, pages 85ff.*

All his experiences with psychotics as depicted in the clinical papers written from 1950–58 could not give him the unification of the theory: "*So far I have to confess that I cannot really do more than indicate the kind of material that is worked on by α*" (C, 65). During this time he observed many acted-out and other concrete manifestations and was able, as an analyst, to extract the communicative power they had. He worked on "mental material" that was delivered in the form of "material material". He, as an analyst, deconcretized the communication. And the patient? On which material did his α work? Had the patient any α to count with? Again, he still did not see that α worked exclusively on sensuous impressions.

Unable to go further, Bion examined "*the relationship of α to the mechanisms of projective identification and splitting . . . The immediate point is the adverse effect on the personality when the dream-work-α is associated with the pleasure principle and excessive projective identification . . . the true dream* **is** *felt as life-promoting, whereas the dream employed as a container for projective identification is felt to be an artefact, as deficient in life-promoting qualities as a hallucinated breast is felt to be deficient in food*" (C, 66–7).

Now the theory had a problem: dreams are both "introjectory" (through dream-work-α) and excretory (when used as a container for the unwanted, for projective identification). When a theory has to be too amended and fixed it becomes stretched. It loses its boundaries: Bion saw the need to posit two types of dreams. This would constitute no problem if he was working within the boundaries of the theory of dreams. Is not the attributing of too many functions and purposes to a theory a sign that it lacks a proper definition? In this case, the two functions are contradictory: one serves the reality principle and one serves the pleasure principle. When thinking in dreams, it is easy to reconcile them, for dreams may *express* both; but when it comes to thinking in *functions* of dream-work, this fact becomes contradictory.

One sees that when Bion attributed a closer kinship with dreams to α the theory became complicated and all-encompassing. When he returned to see it as an activity that is nearer the port of entry of stimuli, that is, sense impressions, it became less complicated. He tackles dreams again and makes a suggestion: let us return to the old definition of dreams, namely, that which occurs during the night. But let us see it as *"a symptom of mental indigestion"*.

Bion proposes that dreams—as they are commonly understood, reported dreams—are a symptom of *"a failure of dream-work-α"*. The key seemed to him, now, the difference between dreams and hallucination at the point of confusion of dreams and hallucination: the creation of visual imagery: *"The failure may of course be due to precisely such causes as the use of visual imagery in the service of projective identification which I have just been describing, but there are . . . also degrees of frequency with which the patient resorts to the use of dream imagery in the service of projective identification. Investigation of the dream as a symptom of a failure of dream-work-a means that we have to reconsider the series of hypotheses that I have grouped together under the heading of dream-work-α"* (C, 68).

He was dissatisfied with the theory and was trying to approach it through the psycho-analytical method that blends the positive, phenomenal, the sensuously apprehensible manifestations of whatever it is, with the negative (q.v.). That is, Bion was trying to test his still foggy hypothesis through observing the *lack* (negative, minus) of it. The first observation was linked to a murderous superego: *"One of the dangers of the failure to dream α in the session is that the patient then splits the murderous super-ego and evacuates it"* (C, 69). The failure to dream means to act out the dream in day-time hallucinations, usually of a murderous quality. His careful empirical attitude is well depicted during the time he tries to examine the possibilities of establishing a theory; his first considerations on truth that were to come to fruition in *Transformations* (C, 70) date from this time.

A new approach was made two weeks later. Again it was his experience with psychotics that helped him: *"The inability of the psychotic to 'digest' his experience mentally because of his lack of capacity for α contributes to the situation with which most observers are familiar, namely the easy accessibility to the **observer** of what should be the psychotic's unconscious. These elements remain detectable because the patient cannot make them unconscious. They are therefore also, as I have shown, not available to **him** because there has been no dream-work-α done to make them unconscious and therefore available to him. He is a man both unable to make these elements unconscious and unable to profit by experience, for profiting by experience means being able to make the material consciously perceived into material that can be mentally stored in such a way that it is susceptible of both concretization and abstraction"* (C, 71).

That which was called "abstraction", could be seen under the vertex of clinical experience as the possibility to "de-sense-fy" and de-concretize in order to think. Bion observed that psychotics did *not* do this; but he still could not see how to *do* this. Instead of being crushed by the psychotic's acting-out, Bion seemed to be able to maintain at least part of his mind free from the patient's projective identification. This may serve as an example to his contemporaries and following generations of analysts. Perhaps he was aided by his analysis with Melanie Klein to realize the phantastic nature of projective identification. He gradually became enabled to have a finer observational appreciation of the function of the psychotic's concretized bombardments that created specific emotional climates. They had emotional contents that could be decoded from the dreamless acted-out events.

The quotation serves as a hint of things to come. It displays the ancestor of his yet-to-be-written book's title. In it the phrase *"learning from experience"* would replace the phrase *"profit by experience"*. The model resorts again to the analogy with the digestive system; the reference to dreams is displaced by an observation of the interplay between conscious and unconscious. Dream-work-α now has a function as a kind of transporter in conscious-unconscious travelling—a function it would retain thereafter. This "travel" is analogous to digestion; the mention of "storing" as a function of dream-work-α is a step towards the formulation of α as a function itself. It further differentiates α from dreaming proper.

One month later, October 1959, Bion finally divorces α from dreams: he accepts Freud's use of the latter term: "*The term, 'dream', I shall always use for the phenomena described by Freud under that term*" (C, 95). He begins his career, so to speak, of furnishing new forms that seem both to rescue Freud's insights and to facilitate their apprehension: "*The dream is an emotional experience that is developmentally unsuccessful in that it is an attempt to fulfil the functions which are incompatible; it is in the domain of the reality principle and the pleasure principle, and represents an attempt to satisfy both. That is to say, it is an attempt to achieve frustration evasion and frustration modification and fails in both. In so far as it is an attempt at modification of frustration, it requires an interpretation; as an attempt at frustration evasion, it has failed to satisfy because the wish fulfilment in it leaves the personality aware that the wish has not been fulfilled in reality. The dream thus occupies a conspicuous role in treatment; it contains, and is itself a manifestation of, painful stresses.*"

These statements further his proposal of attributing a (mental) function to α. The dream is seen as a tool in the treatment. It is not seen as an event that could serve all psycho-analytical purposes and therefore can resolve anything—practically and theoretically. In adumbrating that the dream fails both as an attempt to achieve frustration evasion and frustration modification, Bion or any other researcher would be justified if they tried to look for another theoretical tool to take care of some phenomena. The issue is not just theoretical; perhaps the human mind, realizing the dream's failure, also "looked for" another practical tool. The researcher would be just trailing a path which analogically corresponds to the mind's path. To look for another tool means to leave the dream-theory as it is, with its capacities and limitations. There is no replacement. At the same time, a new theory—such as α—will have its own uses and right from the start will be unencumbered by "all-encompassing" tasks that had already been overstretching it:

But for this same reason its [the dream's] *importance is less central amongst the processes involved in the maintenance of smooth development; the crucial mechanisms are those associated with rendering the perceptions of experience fit for storage in the psyche, namely α, and for making these stored transformations of experience available again when the psyche needs them. The problem is, what are these crucial mechanisms?"* (C, 95). The phrase *"smooth development"* stresses that a process more basic and primitive than dreams may be at work; perhaps it propitiates conditions to dreaming activity itself. It is an exploration into the functions of the dynamic unconscious (unknown, *unbewußt*). It takes Freud's theory to its ultimate "Freudian" consequences.

In a certain sense, the dream, if regarded as "consciousness-bound" (starting from the unconscious and becoming conscious) will always be interpreted as something too compromised by consciousness. It cannot deal with some phenomena that Bion is forced to deal with, when dealing with patients who display their psychotic personality more clearly. The "unconscious-bound" sense is still a mystery—even to dreams. This is an issue that Freud emphasized. Dream-work seems to be the main device that turns the conscious into unconscious; but it also fails in doing this. Thanks to its failure one may interpret dreams. The phenomena Bion tries to deal with are, *"the crucial mechanisms are those associated with rendering the perceptions of experience fit for storage in the psyche"*. Such a mechanism must turn that which is conscious into unconscious. Such a mechanism is neither the dream nor dream-work. The former uses elements already stored in the psyche; the latter has a function in construing the storable elements but does not store them.

Freud dealt with this issue when he was confronted with the fact that mechanisms that send sensory perceptions to memory must be differentiated from those which send them to consciousness. This thread is left loose in Freud's work; this is exactly the issue that Bion is tackling now. (See Freud, "Regression", chapter VII of *The Interpretation of Dreams*, SE, 539–40. In 1920 Freud would separate the two mechanisms.)

Bion's way is an example of scientific research in the psycho-analytical field. It is similar to Planck's creation of his "constant of nature" and Einstein's creation of the constant "c": *"It may be that we can never know* [the crucial mechanisms], *that we can only postulate their existence in order to explain hypotheses that are capable of translation into empirically verifiable data, and that we shall have to work with these postulates without assuming that corresponding realities will at some time be discovered. I regard α as a postulate of this nature"* (C, 95).

These postulates helped Bion when he examined α in the light of its negative, that is, its destruction. *"One consequence is starvation of the psyche in its supply of reality. There is therefore nothing that can be opposed to phantasy . . . since its [α] destruction makes it impossible to store experience, retaining only 'undigested' facts, the patient feels he contains not visual images of things but things themselves . . . regarded by him in the same way as non-psychotics and the non-psychotic part of his personality regard 'thoughts' and 'ideas'. . ."* (C, 96–7).

The next phrase allows one to see the differentiation between the α processes and dreams, and the hallucinated character of the production of such images during the day: *"they are expected by him to behave as if they were visual images in his mind . . . the result I want to consider here is the patient's inability to dream . . . The starvation of the psyche of all elements needed for growth and development gives extreme urgency to the patient's inability to dream . . . this activity is extra-sessional . . . the fear is of nothing less than annihilation. Consequently the patient...needs to restrict these attempts to sessions . . . The combination of incapacity to dream with the urgency imposed by psychic starvation gives rise to . . . the hallucinated dream which affords no associations"* (C, 97–8).

An inability to dream is itself so serious that the patient is compelled to have a dream, a "queer dream" that is a counterpart, on the level of dream thinking, of the hallucinatory gratification experienced in waking life when true gratification is impossible . . . The failure to dream is felt as such a grave disaster that the patient continues to hallucinate during the day, to hallucinate a dream, or so to manipulate facts that he is able to feel he is having a dream—which is the daylight counterpart of the night-time hallucination of a dream . . . .in this respect the dream that yields no associations and the reality that yields no dreams are alike; they are similar to hallucinatory gratification. [C, 111–12]

Step by step Bion is approaching, through the empirical nourishment of clinical material, a process that is distinct from dreams but is seminal to their formation. In the parts quoted, the two clinical situations that led him to the observations were omitted, namely, the cruel and annihilating super-ego that menaces to emerge extra-sessionally, and the analyst's function in the session (please refer to the entry, "Analytic View").

In January 1960 a proto-α-element is hypothesized for the first time. It was not called element but "object". As ever, the empirically collected clinical data both bear and illuminate the formulation: a patient brings *"together two sets of objects"* (C, 113). One of them is a continuously fragmented object, *"similar to, if not identical with"* the bizarre objects (q.v.); they are amenable to juxtaposition but not combination; they are *"useless for dream thoughts, for storage as memory, or, as Freud said, for notation, and therefore no good for unconscious waking thinking"*. The other one is called α-object, which is endowed with *"suitability for dream-thoughts"* and can make the depressive position imminent.

Resorting to a hypothesis of the existence of α-objects completes the divorce of dream-work-α from dreams. The α-objects assume the function of raw material for the construction of dreams. With them α has comparatively less "dreaming" functions; it still has functions regarding the movement from PS to D. In due course those functions would also be left aside; the definition of α-function, α-elements and β-elements assumes a self-supporting character. Nevertheless, even if their previous functions were changed, they would remain linked both to the formation of dreams and to the interplay of the positions. They remain there as factors of the latter. Dreams, PS⇔D, α-function will, as we shall see soon, acquire (in the case of α-function) or recover (in the case of dreams and the positions) a status of their own. Their relationship became clearer when Bion got an inspiration from the mathematician. He examined the relationships of dreaming, PS⇔D and α-function in terms of factors and functions.

In February 1960, after having defined "α-elements", Bion defines β-elements for the first time: *"objects are felt to be alive and to possess character and personality presumably indistinguishable from the infant's own . . . the real and the alive are indistinguishable; if an object is real to the infant, then it is alive; if it is dead, it does not exist"*.

He hypothesized the model of such elements in order to discuss verbally objects that are in a pre-verbal state; moreover, they are not felt as alive because of being, so to speak, "extinguished" by the infant's rage: *"If the object is wished dead, it is dead. It therefore has become non-existent, and its characteristics are different from those of the real, live, existing object; the existing object is alive, real and benevolent"*. Bion proposes *"to call the real, alive objects α-elements; the dead, unreal objects I shall call β-elements"* (all quotations, C, 133).

One day later Bion made another improvement in the theory. It had to do with the functions of dreaming, day-dreaming activity and the flow of impressions and experiences from consciousness to unconsciousness and the obverse. *"The occasions when the patient expresses a number of feelings verbally—'I am anxious, I don't know why'. 'I am feeling a bit better, I don't know why.'—may be an expression of an experience such as I suggest takes place when he has a dream. That is to say, he has an emotional experience on which dream-work-α is done so that the emotional experience can be made available, stored for use in consciousness. Ordinarily α operates to enable a conscious emotional experience to be stored in unconsciousness"* (C, 135). The definition of α-function is already here, albeit still unnamed.

Bion was still tempted to continue using the concept of dream-work-α. What it is? It is not intended to be a replacement for dream or dream-work. It is an in-between process that converts experiences—loosely defined—into α-elements. They retain those emotional experiences that cannot be experienced during the day, when one is wide awake. They must be dreamt in order to be, so to say, accessible to the dreamer who could not access them when awake. The concept is important in the sense that it states that things are not flowing one-way from unconscious to conscious, but it is the other way round and back. It corresponds exactly to that which Freud described in his study of dreams (for example, item B, "Regression", of the chapter VII, *The Interpretation of Dreams*) as well as the neurophysiological path of the stimuli that impact our sensuous apparatus: *"I wonder if dreams, i.e. the actual emotional experiences, are not the emotional experiences I do not have, or cannot allow myself to have, during wakefulness. They then have to be retained, if I am to learn from the experience, by being converted through dream-work-α into α-elements, and then these α-elements are combined according to certain rules to make them approximate to what in daytime wakefulness would be narrative of the event in which I am participating and which I need to record"* (C, 149).

Besides the patient's state of mind, the analyst's state of mind is under constant scrutiny too. The theory of dream-work-α provided Bion with a seemingly useful tool for this endeavour that is part of almost the entirety of his contributions to psycho-analysis: *"Free-floating attention, regarded as necessary in analytic work, might be described as that state of mind in which the analyst allows himself the conditions in which dream-work-α can operate for the production of α-elements"* (C, 150).

A scheme

Emotional experience → dream-work-α → α-elements → rationalization and "narrativization" → dream.

Sensation of waking event in which personality is participating as in an unfolding narrative → dream-work-α → α-elements → dream-thoughts.

Dream-work-α is now seen as a factory for α-elements. It appears in the scheme as a "logical" component that is expressed explicitly through the words, "rationalization" and "narrativization". This logical component would be excised and dispensed with later in the theory of α-function. One may notice that it would be increasingly left aside in his later works, especially in the Trilogy.

The logical component makes this theory more palatable to those who are used to believing in rational thinking. It is a logical scheme that is concerned with logical constructs such as narratives. It reflects an attempt, albeit already critical, to endow psycho-analysis with a scientific status. Bion was highly critical of that which was considered science in his epoch—positivism. He made full use, and displayed a rare grasp of insights as diverse as Hume's and the Copenhagen School/Heisenberg's about the false objectiveness of this self-titled science. He writes this, for example, in a text, "Criticism of psycho-analysis also applied to other sciences" (C, 152), that was written just when he was trying to establish the dream-work-α theory (these criticisms would be more profound in *Transformations*, p. 4, and in many parts of the Trilogy).

His awareness of the limitations of logical thinking was nourished both by his analytical experience and his life experience. Nonetheless it was not wholly developed during the late fifties and early sixties. It seems that fear of mistaking non-rational with irrational was a fact to be reckoned with. The romantic influence in social movements such as Nazism and Stalinism were too fresh and vivid then. The scheme reproduced above was devised (1960) when

Bion was trying to sort out some issues linked to logic and its function in the mind. The attempt to insert logical thinking into a psycho-analytic theory was at the service of the wish that psychoanalysis could partake of the features of a deductive scientific system. The credibility of analysis, in the same way that occurred in Freud's epoch, was at stake and continues to be so.

Bion tried at that time to endow the theory of a logical form, which deals with day-time dream-like states. He tried, for example, to depict verbally an α-element stating that his verbal depiction was an image. He proposed to call the image an α-element. This happened, as I have tried to adumbrate, just when he was trying to contend with a serious question: "what should be the content of a psycho-analytic interpretation?" (C, 175). He was trying to determine the truth-value of the analyst's statements. He would pursue this path in his books *Learning from Experience*, *Elements of Psychoanalysis*, devising the Grid (q.v.); *Transformations* uses this tool. To determine the truth-value of a statement differs from positivism. It was developed more in *Attention and Interpretation*.

Let us examine his depiction of an α-element. In it, the scientific approach (after Prichard, Bradley and Braithwaite, three independent-minded epistemologists), the analyst's mind and the dreamwork in action are constantly conjoined. It is as if a "scientific function of the personality" is at work. It is at work in a patient who genuinely looks for analysis; it is at work in an analyst and in the intuitive scientist. Also visible are the processes of projective identification and hallucination, as opposed to dreaming:

> But I seem to have involved myself in some kind of contradiction. This is intended to be a scientific communication, and I have already expressed the view that as such it should be addressed to a hypothetical concept, the non-psychotic part of the personality which is endowed with certain unspecified immutable characteristics. I feel I am addressing it to an actual person—intelligent, friendly, engrossed in what I am writing and, to be frank, quite warmly appreciative of my effort. Analytic experience tells me this is really myself and that I shall be in for a rude awakening when I find out the real response. "A rude awakening": am I then asleep? By no means. But this figure, these characteristics with which I have endowed it and you, might very well exist in a dream.

I propose to call this image an α-element. (This does not refer to its function as part of a phantasy; it applies only to the visual image itself.) The hypothetical concept, the "non-psychotic part of the personality", I consider to be a version of the α-element which belongs to a level of increasing generalization in the hierarchy of hypotheses that form the theory to which both the α-element and the hypothetical concept belong. Conversely, the α-element approximates to a level of decreasing generalization, or increasing particularization, thus having a relationship with the hypothetical concept somewhat similar to that which exists between the level of empirically verifiable data and the hypotheses of the scientific deductive system related to it. [C, 178]

Thereafter Bion continues his attempt to reach a definition of dream-work-α. Let us try to summarize the context: he was at odds with the functions of dreams (seen, for example, in the failure of dreams both to modify and to evade frustration; quoted above, October 1959). He unearthed its presence during the day; he was still at odds with Freud's definition of consciousness. He had a firm grasp of Freud's definition of dream work, and agreed with it (that is, all the mental tricks such as condensations, transformations into the contrary, denial, displacement, etc. that make up the "manifest content"). And finally he was trying to endow the latent content— the analyst's interpretation—with validity.

Dealing with latent content, his next attempt was a suggestion to modify Freud's term dream-work "*to describe a related but different series of phenomena*". Why does he suggest the modification? "*To avoid confusion with the concepts already established in psycho-analytic usage . . . I propose for my purposes to modify Freud's term by calling it dream-work-α*" (C, 179).

Bion re-establishes forgotten neurological paths, identical to those used by Freud: from the sensuous apparatus to the psyche. He reverses the process called by Freud, "regression" (*The Interpretation of Dreams*, item B, chapter VII). Regression, after Freud, is the return, so to speak, of a thought that cannot be thought at all in a visual (or verbal) image in dreams. The reversion made by Bion corresponds to the neurological pathway of the apprehension of reality, which Bion names "observation": "*In the state of mind of relaxed attention necessary in making observations, the individual is able through his senses to establish contact with his environment*" (C, 179).

This contact also occurs in contexts more complicated than that of the dreaming during sleep. The example given by Bion is that of a conversation with a friend. He reminds us that when a person is talking with another person, the talk—a verbal formulation that provokes an acoustic stimulation—is invested with a creation of dream-like images. These images are formed when one is wide awake. In his example, the friend asks about the place where Bion proposes to spend his holidays. Bion visualizes *"the church of a small town not far from the village in which"* he proposes to stay.

The dream-like visualization has another important kinship with night-dreams: namely, the mnemic debris that composed it and was stored in experiential memory: *"The image of the church has been established on a previous occasion—I cannot now tell when. Its evocation in the situation I am describing would surprise no one, but what I now wish to add may be more controversial. I suggest that the experience of this particular conversation with my friend, and this particular moment of the conversation—not simply his words but the totality of that moment of experience—is being perceived sensorially by me and converted into an image of that particular village church."*

That is, an immaterial fact—an emotional experience, and the experience of thinking—is, as any stimulus, first harboured by the sensuous apparatus. It is the same way that Freud described the pathway of dream formation. Identically, the sensuous experience is transformed in the realm of other mental processes that Freud calls pre-conscious and unconscious. When—according to Freud— dream work functions, there is a return (regression) to a sensuous phenomenon. *"I do not know what else may be going on, though I am sure that much more takes place than I am aware of. But the transforma- tion of my sense impressions into this visual image is part of a process of mental assimilation. The impressions of the event are being re-shaped as a visual image of that particular church, and so are being made into a form suitable for storage in my mind"* (C, 180). In other words: mind func- tions in a dream-like way, if allowed to, in states of a paradoxical "relaxed attention".

The *re-shaping* and *storage* that Bion refers to constitutes the evolution of the concept. Bion looks for irreducible, elemental units—later called, "elements". As he refines the concepts of α and β he finally bridges the last gap that hitherto precluded him from reaching a theory of α-function. Namely, the equating of sense impressions—be they either external stimuli of the psychotic's tendency to sensuous-concretization—to β-elements, or things-in-themselves. In a certain sense he applies Freud's method, that is, the same that led him to replace the idea of concrete trauma by that of imagined phantasies as products of the mind. For β-elements are now seen as the psychotic's productions too:

> By contrast, the patient might have the same experience, the same sense impressions, and yet be unable to transform the experience so that he can store it mentally. But instead, the experience (and his sense impressions of it) remains a foreign body, it is felt as a "thing" lacking any of the quality we usually attribute to thought or its verbal expression. [C, 180]

The definitions are correspondingly improved: α-elements continue to be regarded as the products of dream-work-α; they are precursors of dreams; dream-work-α is seen as a fact different from dream-work; β-element is still seen as a dead object, but with important differences and amendments now; they transcend pathology and compose a function of the mind:

> To the first of these products, that of dream-work-α, I propose to give the name, "α-element"; to the second, the unassimilated sense impression, "β-element" It may be wondered why I should need to consider β-elements at all in an inquiry into scientific method if they are a characteristic of a disturbed personality. My reason is that while I have been led to observe β-elements through treating disturbed patients, their occurrence is by no means restricted to their use by disturbed individuals . . .

> If my contention is correct, the production of α-elements is of the first importance: on an adequate supply of these elements depends the capacity for what Freud calls "unconscious waking thinking", the ability to entertain and use dream-thoughts, the capacity for memory, and all the functions . . . that Freud tentatively suggests come into existence with the dominance of the reality principle ("Two principles of mental functioning" [1911, SE12]). [C, 181]

Then Bion reaches that which would be the final definition of the β-element. It embodies Freud's work on the two principles, neurology, and Klein's formulation of projective identification. The concept was developed as a continuously improved formulation blending observation and clinical data: *"The β-elements are characteristic of the personality during the dominance of the pleasure principle: on them depends the capacity for non-verbal communication, the individual's ability to believe in the possibility of ridding himself of unwanted emotions, and the communication of emotion within the group"* (C, 181).

This element started by being a dead object that was dead because the infant felt it is as dead as long as it was frustrating. It was unacceptable due to the fact that it was a source of pain. That is, it was "made dead". From there the β-element acquired a "deadness" due to the fact that it was concretized. It was now seen by Bion as partaking of the features of the thing-in-itself. Or, to put it better, its "concreteness" led to the situation that it is felt as the thing-in-itself. The "concreteness" seems to be necessary if the object is to be felt as fulfilling rather than frustrating. The person who has only β-elements to cope with would correspond to Kant's "naïve idealist".

Dreaming, the apprehension of sensuous stimuli, waking unconscious thinking, dream-work, and processes of knowledge are **expressions** of Aristotle's "urge to know". Bion shows that the individual's processes of knowledge can be put into sophisticated epistemological terms (those of Prichard, Braithwaite, Schlick and Carnap; Bion does not quote the last two):

The α-elements may be presumed to be mental and individual, subjective, to a high degree personal, particular, and unequivocally belonging to the domain of epistemology in a particular person. The example I have given of the visual image of the church is to a high degree particular, and must be regarded as belonging to the lowest level of empirically verifiable data. [C, 181]

To keep this quotation in mind may help avoid misunderstandings that actually occurred years later. Some descriptions of these misunderstandings may be found elsewhere in this dictionary (please refer to the entries, Alpha-function, alpha-element). For example, mistaking α-elements with thinking, or with symbols. One should keep their nature in mind, that of "raw material", suitable to be employed in dream-thoughts:

In the context in which I have cited it, it is not even a symbol, although once the individual has experienced such a visual image

there is nothing to prevent its appearance in other contexts fulfilling the functions usually associated with symbols. What I wish to
emphasize is that its character as an α-element is its suitability for
employment in dream-thought and unconscious waking thinking,
and not the way in which it may be employed. I may have more to
say about the characteristics of the α-element that makes it suitable
for use as a symbol or an ideogram, but for the present I emphasize
its character as an element—an irreducibly simple object. [C, 181]

The search for "elements of psycho-analysis" began in this
paper. "*Without α-elements it is not possible to know anything. Without
β-elements it is impossible to be ignorant of anything: they are essential
to the functioning of projective identification; any unwanted idea is
converted into a β-element, ejected from the personality, and then becomes
a fact of which the individual is unaware . . .*" (C, 182).

Even though Bion did not specifically quote Freud's definition
of the ultimate unknowability of the unconscious (*The Interpretation
of Dreams*, SE, VI) as well as the definition of proto-phantasies (in
Beyond the pleasure principle), these seem to be the origins of his
concept.

It may well be that this early learning, or first stage of any learning,
is effected by dream-work-α on the one hand, and the mechanism
of projective identification on the other. This supposes that the β-
elements can be employed when α-elements do not exist, and the
α-elements are a later stage of β-elements—that is to say that
dream-work-α operates on β-elements and not directly on sense
data. [C, 183]

The last statement differentiates the intermediate stage of the
theory from its latest, readied version. At this time β-elements were
not equated to the thing-in-itself. One may conjecture when Bion
perceived that β-elements shared the qualities of the Kantian category, the thing-in-itself. Following this, use of Kant also contributes
to Kant's theory. Bion came to regard β-elements as sense data
themselves. A final difference between the theory of dream-work-α
and α-function is that the latter *does* operate on sense data. One may
conclude that there remained some vague ideas about the nature of
elements that belonged to the realm of thinking and those that
didn't. Are those elements which serve to be discharged through

projective identification, elements that belong to the area of thinking? Bion realized that it was convenient to consider the existence of un-thought elements, and that the difficulty in thinking such elements was based on the paranoid–schizoid idea that they were the absolute truth. Thus armed, Bion could finally discard the term dream-work-α altogether. While conserving the definition of α-elements, there was the need to develop further the definition of β-elements, as un-thinkable things-in-themselves.

He was aware that the arrangement of the dream-work-α"*did not cover a mechanism in which the α-element is used to explore the emotional experience in which the person finds himself*" (C, 183). This would depend on a mental function, of considering inner stimuli such as feelings as sensuous experiences to be decoded by consciousness—exactly as Freud proposed—and of the consideration of un-thought but existent pre-conceptions. The reconciliation with Freud's original and fundamental definition of consciousness and the ultimate unknowability of the unconscious would oppose Bion to the psycho-analytic movement of his time. The latter was concretizing Freud's method into a kind of mechanistic, thoughtless decoding of previously known symbols, running against the very ethos of psycho-analysis.

In August 1960, more light was thrown on this. His resorting to a graphical recourse in order to try to enhance the communicative powers of that which he wished to communicate may be observed, namely, his sparing use of hyphenated terms that enlivened the verbal formulation. One may only hope that future followers and disciples will not ape this hyphenation. This abuse would turn something useful into a debased, common-place non-communicative device.

> It is advisable to revert to the patient's dream over and over again—elaboration 1, 2, 3 . . . n; but not simply as dreams to be interpreted and related to a stimulus. *They must be related to the dream-work that the stimulus has stimulated* . . . the methods of dream-work-α are not the same as those of dream-work which is related to interpretation of dreams, but are the *reciprocal* of dream-work and are related to the capacity to dream, i.e. to transform into dream, events that are grasped only on a rational, conscious level . . . the element of "resistance" in dream-work, as elucidated by Freud, is a compound of two elements: resistance, as described by

> Freud: and a felt need to convert the conscious rational experience into dream, rather than a felt need to convert the dream into conscious rational experience. The "felt need" is *very* important; if it is not given due significance and weight, the true dis-ease of the patient is being neglected, it is obscured by the analyst's insistence on interpretation of the dream. [C, 184]

Once Freud's contributions were differentiated from the distortions made in Freud's name, it seemed to be easier for Bion to devise the final form of α theory. In the view of the author, even resorting to Kant was simply a way to make Freud's usage of Kant explicit.

📖 The influences of Freud, Planck and Einstein still did not win widespread use outside psycho-analysis and physics if compared with the easier grasping of the positivist's ideas of causes, effects, and the adoption of deductive systems. Quite independently of popularity, deductive systems proved to be far less scientific than their creators wished them to be. Modern scientists and epistemologists know that deductive systems cannot go beyond their own assumptions, falling into a circularity that hampers real scientific development—provided that scientific development is regarded as research into the unknown. Bion would abandon this attempt from 1965 onwards (please refer to the entry, "Common Sense"). There are a number of good primers for the interested layman: Max Planck's *Scientific Biography*; Jules-Henri Poincaré's *Science and Method*; Werner Heisenberg's *Physics and Philosophy*; Bertrand Russell's *ABC of Relativity*, Roger Penrose's *The Emperor's New Mind*. For a work dedicated to the analyst, this author's *A Apreensão da Realidade Psiquica* (The apprehension of psychic reality).

Suggested cross-references: Alpha-function, Dream, Dream the session, Mind.

E

Elements of psycho-analysis: Bion looked for elements, something that could qualify to be seen as fundamental and basic, *"irreducible"*, to psychic reality. In order to do this he resorted to mathematical analogies. This kind of analogy had already proved itself when Bion applied the theory of functions to the study of thinking.

The "elements" are scientific abstractions, rather than concrete entities. If they are so regarded, Bion's proposal would be indistinguishable from that of the alchemists. Bion read Euclid's Elements; this is the sense of such a term in his work (C, 111).

> I propose to seek a mode of abstraction that ensures that the theoretical statement retains the minimum of particularization . . . The elements I seek are to be such that relatively few are required to express, by changes in combination, nearly all the theories essential to the working psycho-analyst . . . The combination in which certain elements are held* is essential to the meaning** to be conveyed by those elements . . . The task is to abstract*** such elements by releasing them from the combination in which they are held and from the particularity that adheres to them from the realization which they were originally designed to represent. [EP,2]

[Footnotes:

*Compared with the tendency to produce *ad hoc* theories to meet a situation when an existing theory, stated with sufficient generality, would have done. Compare Proclus, quoted by Sir T. I. Heath, on Euclid's Elements—Heath, T. I. *The Thirteen Books of Euclid's Elements*, Chap. 9, CUP 1956).

** A consequence of PS⇔D. See Chap. 18.

*** A consequence of PS⇔D. See Chap. 18 [see also the entries Container/Contained, PS⇔D]

This is a psycho-analytic task in a compacted form: it is valid during a session as well in the building of real analytic theories—in order to get "*the realization which they were originally designed to represent*".

To state that the elements are not concrete entities but rather abstractions does not mean that they are inventions, fictional, or unreal. They maintain the mathematical nature of an immaterial, dynamic function; they "have a functioning":

> The elements are functions of the personality . . . In so far as each **is** a function the term "function" has a meaning similar to that which it is associated in mathematics . . . In so far as each function *has* a function the term "function" is used as the name for a set of actions, physical or mental, governed by or directed to a purpose. Whenever I use the term "function" I use it to denote something which is and has a function. [EP, 9]

Mathematics being a primitive manifestation of mind itself, to state that the elements are, and have a function, or are real immaterial fact, is the same as to state that they share the basic qualities of mental phenomena. They are abstractions in the mind; nevertheless, in a paradox that demands tolerance, in a certain sense they are observable, or there are realizations that correspond to them: "*The sign representing an abstraction must therefore represent a function that is unknowable although its primary and secondary qualities (in the Kantian sense) are. As I propose to consider the elements as observable phenomena it must be assumed that I am talking about primary and secondary qualities of elements and not the abstractions or signs by which I represent them*" (EP, 9).

Being phenomena, the elements are observable; Bion describes some of their characteristics. The elements, their quasi-mathematical notation and their realizations are encompassed in Table 1.

Table 1   The elements and their realizations

Name of the element	Quasi-mathematical notation	Realizations
1 A dynamic relationship between container and contained		1. A baby and a mother who may communicate with each other through projective identification 2. a creative person 3. penis, breast and vagina 4. the apparatus for thinking (EP, 31)
2 Selected fact	PS⇔D	a free movement between paranoid–schizoid and depressive position, insight, sense of truth
3 Links	L, H, K	love, hate and processes of knowledge
4 Reason and Idea	R and I	R, reason, is a function that serves passions, leading to the latter's domination in the realm of reality ; I corresponds to α-element; R and I are related in the extent that I is an interpolation between impulse and action (EP, 4); it is the negative of acting-out; the Grid
5 Pain		reversion of perspective, negation of pain, disagreement between analyst and analysand only appear when the analysand is less able to hallucinate; attempts to deny movement and to transform dynamic into static (EP, 54, 60, 61)

How can we observe these phenomena? There is an old tradition that recommends the use of common sense (q.v.). Its definition appears in many parts of Bion's work; two or more senses must be used:

I shall consider an object to be sensible to psycho-analytic scrutiny if, and only if, it fulfils conditions analogous to the conditions that are fulfilled when a physical object's presence is confirmed by the evidence of two or more senses. [EP, 10; the complete version is in C, 9ff.]

The psycho-analytic investigation of psychic and material reality achieves a formulation through psycho-analytical interpretations. It demands some regard to the "dimensions" that characterize psycho-analytic space-time. Bion describes three of those "dimensions" and their extensions:

1.   A dimension in the realm of senses.
2.   A dimension in the realm of myth.
3.   A dimension in the realm of passion.

Reason and passion are discussed in regard to the elements:

When thoughts have to be used under the exigencies of reality, be it psychic reality or external reality, the primitive mechanisms have to be endowed with capacities for precision demanded by the need for survival. We have therefore to consider the part played by the life and death instincts as well as reason, which in its embryonic form under the dominance of the pleasure principle is designed to serve as the slave of the passions, has forced it to assume a function resembling that of a master of the passions and the parent of logic. For the search, for satisfaction of incompatible desires, would lead to frustration. Successful surmounting of the problem of frustration involves being reasonable and a phrase such as the "dictates of reason" may enshrine the expression of primitive emotional reaction to a function intended to satisfy not frustrate. The axioms of logic therefore have their roots in the experience of a reason that fails in its primary function to satisfy the passions just as the existence of a powerful reason may reflect a capacity in that function to resist the assaults of its frustrated and outraged masters. These matters will have to be considered in so far as dominance of the reality principle stimulates the development of thought and thinking, reason, and awareness of psychic and environmental reality. [EP, 35–6]

Elements of psycho-analysis are unsaturated elements in search of saturation; once saturation is achieved, or meaning, the saturated element must become an unsaturated one—in search of new saturation. Those elements were represented by Bion in *Learning from Experience* by the sign (ξ). It represents an unsaturated element that determines the value of a constant (which he called ψ as soon as it is identified. Therefore elements of psycho-analysis are closely related to that which Bion earlier named psycho-analytic objects (q.v.). Psycho-analytic objects are *"derived from"* the psycho-analytic elements (EP, 11). Being derived from elements, elements are a part of those objects. *". . . If they are elements, despite any appearance to the contrary, it is necessary to know of what psycho-analytic object they are part"* (EP, 104). As a practical example one may quote one of his studies on transference, where both the concepts of object and element seem to be useful clinically:

> The elements of the transference are to be found in that aspect of the patient's behaviour that betrays his awareness of the presence of an object that is not himself. No aspect of his behaviour can be disregarded; its relevance to the central fact must be assessed. His greeting, or neglect of it, references to the couch, or furniture, or weather, all must be seen in that aspect of them that relates to the presence of an object not himself; the evidence must be regarded afresh each session and nothing taken for granted for the order in which aspects of the patient's mind present themselves for observation are not decided by the length of time for which the analysis has endured. For example, the patient may regard the analyst as a person to be treated as if he were a thing; or as a thing towards which his attitude is animistic. If ψ(ξ) represents the analyst's state of mind vis-à-vis the analysand it is the unsaturated element (ξ) that is the important one in every session. [EP, 69]

The elements of psycho-analysis are an intrinsic part of Bion's epistemological tool, the Grid. The Grid can gauge the truth-value of statements made by the participants of the analytical act. It also gauges the function and the genetic (or ontogenetic) state of development of some thoughts, ideas, objects and elements. The formulation of the elements of psycho-analysis is important in the sense that those elements are capable of growth, even though their "elementary" quality lingers on. They are amenable to be "saturated" with meaning, and in this sense they can be screened and "seen" through the aid of the Grid (q.v.). It is not a simple coincidence that Bion developed both theories, the Grid and the elements, in the same book. The Grid tracks the development or decay of an element and furnishes its state at a given point of time.

> The elements of psycho-analysis are ideas and feelings as repre-sented by their setting in a single grid category. [EP, 103]

Elements of psycho-analysis and the analyst's personal analysis

> Search for the elements of psycho-analysis is restricted to that aspect of them that it is the business of the psycho-analyst to discern. They cannot be represented , either by abstract signs, such as I have suggested, or by mythological narratives evoking visual imagery, in such a way that anyone other than a trained and prac-tising psycho-analyst could recognize the realization approximat-ing to the representation. [EP, 67]

& Bion describes some of the "elements'" intrinsic features. The author once proposed some labels or generalizing names for those features; they were not given by Bion but they may be help-ful, for they depict the features he described:

1. **Transcendence**: The elements need to be able to maintain *"the realization which they were originally designed to represent"* (EP, 3 and 4).
2. **Valence or a capacity to relate**: *"they must be capable of articula-tion with other similar elements"* (EP, 3). This depends on *"tropism"* (C, 34; T, 109), of *"elective affinities"*.
3. **A sense of truth**: the elements are thoughts without a thinker rather than products of an imaginative mind. They are not the product of desire either: *"when so articulated they should form a scientific deductive system capable of representing a realization suppose one existed"* (EP, 3).
4. **Paradox**: an element of psycho-analysis needs to be able to contain a basic paradox, the supreme creativity of a couple; in this sense an element is pregnant.

The "dimensions" of a psycho-analytic interpretation are simi-lar to the "phase space" described by Hamilton (Sandler, 1997, pp. 44, 51); they are not philosophical, pedagogic, psychological or theological postulates.

Emotional experience: The inclusion of the term "emotional experience" in the work of Bion is directly linked to the issues of apprehension of reality. It is a verbal form that makes more explicit that which Freud and Klein observed about the breast as a (is it **the**?) fundamental experience of all human beings.

Perhaps the first time that Bion publishes anything about it is when he develops his theory on thinking, about the fact that a real breast is offered—the realization of a breast: a particular experience, in the purest empirical sense of the word. Namely, that the entity breast was not just another figment of the baby's imagination; that a real breast does exist as a matter of fact. This experience gets its emotional quality if and when it matches with the baby's preconception of the breast. It may be said that when **the** breast turns into **a** breast the prototype of all emotional experiences occurs: "... *I shall suppose that an infant has an inborn pre-conception that a breast that satisfies its own incomplete nature exists. The realization of the breast provides an emotional experience*" (LE, 69).

Three years later, he would reaffirm the same and would name some of its representations in the adult world: "*The infant's experience of the breast as the source of emotional experiences (later represented by terms such as love, understanding, meaning) means that disturbances in relationship with the breast involve disturbance over a wide range of adult relationship*" (T, 81).

That is, emotional experience is not an event that occurs exclusively independent of the internal milieu. It has a seminal link with external reality too; it provides the stuff that this link is made of. The term "experience" indicates that. One may notice that Bion chooses a phrase—borrowed from Freud and Klein (who used it extensively)—that denotes something that is not just an emotion. The latter is a term that expresses a dynamic, moving influx, like object cathexes, which are linked to instinctual sources. The added term, experience, denotes the link with something more, which may be either external or internal.

His efforts towards a theory of thinking are the root of that which he names "emotional experiences". He goes along lines that differ from those of academic psychology: thinking at its inception depends on an emotional experience. In this Bion profits from Freud and Klein: this emotional experience is the contact with the breast. This experience is constituted with its simultaneous negative companion: the loss of this same breast, or the "no-breast". This is a way to see the issue as dependent on emotional experiences from its inception. *"We must assume that the good breast and the bad breast are emotional experiences"* (LE, 35). Bion states that this is an assumption. In scientific terms, it constitutes a hypothesis, to be verified.

The term has some problems; one must catch its gist experientially. Anyone who tries to "understand" its definition is at a loss: "it" must be experienced. One should try to intuit and apprehend, through experience, its counterpart in reality. In that it shares the animate—experiential—qualities that are a hallmark of all definitions linked to the sciences. One may "define" a crocodile or the cooking of an egg, but this differs from experiencing an actual crocodile or trying to boil an egg.

It is an experience that demands to be described in its entirety. For example: Oedipus is not a feeling—even though it is accompanied by a myriad of often contradictory feelings. Oedipus is not an emotion—even though basic human emotions are involved in its origin. Oedipus is an emotional experience that demands to be described in its entirety according to each person's individual structuring of it. This structuring is transitory; it can be glimpsed transitorily during an analytic session. Many have accustomed themselves to some repetitive patterns, which become lifeless. This way of life seems to correspond to that which Freud called transference and Riviere called defensive organizations.

Emotional experiences present overt features that are usually misleading. To quote the example of Oedipus again: it can be seen as an extreme attraction between parents and their progeny. This attraction may present itself as mutually repulsive overt behaviour. In order to realize the emotional experience it is necessary to look for the underlying experience. It underlies the overt, manifest appearances. As is customary in Bion's work, his interest in emotional experiences was aroused by his clinical experience with psychotics. In 1959, he wrote:

"The contact with a psychotic patient is an emotional experience, presenting some precise features that differentiate it from the experience of contact of a more usual kind: the analyst does not meet a personality, but a hastily organized improvisation of a personality, or perhaps of a mood. It is an improvisation of fragments; if the impression is predominantly of friendliness, there will nevertheless be easily discernible fragments of

hostility embedded in the conglomerate that has been assembled to do service, for the occasion, as a personality. If the impression is predominantly of depression, the mosaic of fragments will reveal incongruous bits of a smile without context other than a kind of contiguity with surrounding fragments: tears without depth, jocosity without friendliness, bits of hate—all these and many more fragmentary emotions or ideas jostle each other to present a labile façade" (C, 74). That is, Bion describes the emotional experience—which in any given case demands to be described—and he does not use a concept.

The theory of alpha function deals with the inception of emotionality itself. How do sensuous impressions, which are the port of entry of any stimulus, come to be a psychic experience, or match possible pre-existent phenomena belonging to the psychic realm? Bion's theory of thinking posits that no emotion can even exist without a not-me, or external stimulus; this is in agreement with Freud's formulations of psychic cathexes directed to objects as well as purposes and goals of instincts. It is also in agreement with the observations about autistic states. Bion furthers this early object-relations formulation with the Kantian hypothesis of pre-conceptions. The sense of reality is what matters when Bion talks about an emotional experience, rather than "emotional experience" *per se*, as if it were a concrete entity or a concept-in-itself.

> A central part is played by alpha-function in transforming an emotional experience into alpha-elements because a sense of reality matters to the individual in the way that food, drink, air and excretion of waste products matter. Failure to eat, drink or breathe properly has disastrous consequences for life itself. Failure to use the emotional experience produces a comparable disaster in the development of personality; I include amongst those disasters degrees of psychotic deterioration that could be described as death of the personality . . . An emotional experience cannot be conceived of in isolation from a relationship. [LE, 42]

What is the relationship here? The study of Bion's work, especially of his book *Learning from Experience* (the quotation from *Cogitations* is one of the many preparatory papers to *Learning from Experience*) considers that objects, animate and inanimate, are *"in relationship with each other"*. It is easy to see this through many examples: we are born when a male and a female relate; matter and energy relate with each other and from these relationships the universe we live in emerged: common sense is a conjunction of at least two senses; mathematics and music are made of relationships.

Emotional experiences: they require the physical presence

There is a paradox here: an emotional experience is immaterial but to occur it does not dispense with the materiality of the persons involved. One cannot have analysis through the telephone or internet in the same way that one cannot have a sexual relationship or a meal through telephone or internet.

> The psycho-analyst who undertakes a schizophrenic analysis undergoes an experience for which he must improvise and adapt the mental apparatus he requires. He has one great advantage in his relationship with his analysand which he lacks in his relationship with his colleagues and others outside the experience—the analysand has the experience available to his intuition if he will permit the psycho-analyst to draw his attention to it. Those excluded from the psycho-analysis cannot gain from the psycho-analyst's formulations because they are formulations dependent on the presence of the experience being formulated. They are thus in the position analogous to one whose mathematical ability has not reached a point where it can deal with the problem of objects when the objects are not there. [ST, 146]

With the perception that psychosis is an ever-present feature, this remark serves any analysis.

Misuses and misunderstandings: There seems to be a tendency to reify the concept. This seems to occur in at least three forms: (i) "I work **in** the emotional experience"; (ii) "I work **with** the emotional experience". (iii) a system of notation.

(i)   To work "in the emotional experience" seems to embody the idea that emotional experiences are "things" that would exist and be available to some people. As a matter of consequence they would not be available to other people. Another vertex may consider that emotional experiences may always exist, as the air that surrounds us and is amenable to being breathed—

in variable individual degrees. Under this vertex, both analysts and any individual being in any context would be working "in emotional experiences". What is at stake is not to work in or out of something that is not even a thing, but it is the ability to apprehend it (them) and thereafter be able to endow them with a verbal form.

(ii) To work "with the emotional experience" may also be reifying to the extent that it assumes that an emotional experience is something that can be touched, grabbed, etc.

(iii) To deal with a system of notation as if it were a thing-in-itself is also to reify such a system. Bion states in an unmistakable way that the denomination "emotional experience" is just a notational system—notation being one of the functions of ego (SE, 10); (LE, 42). To deal with it as if it were a concrete thing itself means missing the fact that it is just an aid for getting a *"sense of reality"* (LE, 42).

One should say that all great authors' great books and papers—as those of Freud, Klein, Winnicott and Bion—provide opportunities for undergoing intensive and extensive emotional experiences. Like young medical students in their first reading of medical books, many report that they see themselves in these authors' texts. Among Bion's works, the remarkably powerful evocative property of his later works may account for their lack of popularity (*A Memoir of the Future* and its companions, *War Memoirs and The Long Week-End*).

📖 *Second Thoughts* , p. 119: sense of truth.

&; There seems to remain scarce awareness of the necessity to discriminate emotional experiences from affects, emotions, and feelings—both in written works and in the way professionals regard them. Freud and Klein differentiated them, up to a point. The German language allows more precision to do it. Bion thought that it was not possible, for the time being—1965—to differentiate them. But thanks to his work, perhaps today we are in a better position to do this. The author proposed such a classification in a paper presented at S.B.P.S.P., 1998.

Suggested cross-references: Links, Mathematization of psychoanalysis, Models, Sense of Truth.

Emotional turbulence or psychological turbulence: Emotional turbulence is a phenomenon of life; it occurs when human beings meet each other. It involves "O", ultimate truth: it is the real contact or apprehension of reality. The concept tries to depict fears and resistances to turbulence associated with "becoming". Emotional or psychological disturbance—fear of emotional turbulence—means resistance to transformations in O. By it Bion means a state of mind with a painful quality.

The concept of emotional turbulence and/or psychological turbulence was formulated with the aid of two expressions. It mixed a quasi-jargon ("psychological") with a physical fact ("turbulence"). These terms were already part of common language when the concept first appeared. Even though this specific conjunction of terms is an uncommon one, it keeps a pervasive penumbra of associations with the common language—it is made from two well-known words. Therefore it may be, to some ears, evocative of those associations. This may be misleading.

Bion used the terms "psychological turbulence", "emotional turbulence" and "turbulence". They are used in three ways, even though they retain the same basic sense: change and resistance to change. This appears at three important moments of his work; 1965, 1975 and 1977. In 1977 he introduces the term "emotional turbulence". He illustrates the turbulent emotions in other parts of his work, mainly in *A Memoir of the Future*.

🕭 The term is first introduced through an analogy, and later defined in *Transformations*. It is used as an aid to define the concept of "Transformation" (q.v.). Turbulence is the inverse of tranquillity. It is defined through a fact studied by physicists: the reflection of the image of a tree in the water of a lake (T, 47). The atmospheric conditions can change "*from calm to turbulence*" and this would "*influence the transformation*" in a reflection of the image of the trees.

The model is applied to the analyst's state of mind. If it is turbulent it hampers or even precludes the analytical view (q.v.). Bion considers the processes through which the analyst effects his interpretations; to use his parlance in *Transformations*, they are the processes of transformations, Ta α These processes lead to a final product, the interpretation or construction, Ta β. "*I shall assume an ideal analyst and that Ta α and Ta β are not disturbed by turbulence—though turbulence and its sources are part of O*" (T, 48).

Another factor is introduced: even though examining the analyst's need to be analysed in this part of the book, turbulence is part of O. The issue is not a rule, "one must avoid turbulence". He would return to the point emphasizing that the attempt to avoid turbulence is an obstacle to making interpretations. At this time, he creates the concepts of circular argument (q.v.) and hyperbole (q.v.). He focuses the case of interpretations made *"mainly because it is available as a column 2 statement intended to prevent 'turbulence' in the analyst"* (T, 167). All the other mentions of turbulence and attempts to avoid it are discussed under the heading "proto-resistance".

Emotional turbulence and catastrophic change

Bion encircles a state in which a status quo that is felt as pleasurable or simply static is so maintained and forced to remain undisturbed. But the move into the unknown obtrudes. It is akin to catastrophic change (q.v.) but differs from it in the fact that it installs itself *after* the change was effected. An inner truth that is feared is elicited with catastrophic change, as for example, the psychotic nature of seemingly psychosomatic phenomena such as those depicted in the first pages of *Transformations*. Emotional turbulence is a phenomenon involving "O", ultimate truth, in another way: it is the real contact or apprehension of reality. Emotional turbulence tries to depict fears and resistances to turbulence associated with "becoming". Emotional or psychological disturbance thus means resistance to transformations in O; catastrophic change means leaning towards transformations in hallucinosis. In some cases the intolerance of states of emotional turbulence can lead to a catastrophe.

The term is also used and duly defined with the aid of a real episode in the history of science. Science is seen as a way to apprehend reality as it is. Bion transformed the episode into a parable, much akin to that of the "tomb-robbers" he describes in "Caesura". It seems that the tomb-robbers were more successful than Sir Isaac Newton—who in his forays into knowledge experienced a psychotic breakdown.

The episode was used a number of times and in different ways in Bion's work (please refer to the entry Container/Contained). This time, Bion focuses on a human event linked to Newton's theory of fluxions, which today is named differential calculus:

Bishop Berkeley's sarcastic reaction against it. The following convention enables the reader to read the text:

K = a link that people maintain with persons and things, named, "knowledge"; in this link one knows someone or something.

T = transformation.

T Newton = transformations made by Newton.

T Newton β = the final product of the transformation made by Newton.

H_3 refers to a category of the Grid (q.v.), namely, the notation of algebraic calculus.

Col. 1 refers to column 1 of the Grid, definitory hypotheses and things-in-themselves.

Col. 2 refers to column 2 of the Grid, statements known to be false.

Thus the quasi-mathematical notation, "T Newton β H_3" means a final algebraic calculus as transformed by Sir Isaac Newton. Correspondingly, "T Newton β col. 2" means "a final lie expressed by Newton's transformation", or "a final resistance expressed by Newton's transformation". And "T Berkeley β col. 2" means "a final lie expressed by Berkeley's transformations".

F_3 means notation of a concept. Please keep these definitions firmly in mind when reading what follows.

One must keep in mind the polemic as it was historically recorded: Newton was able to develop a mathematical device, named fluxions, which could be discarded as soon as a given result (finite lines proportional to the device, fluxions) was found. The discarding was compared, as an analogy, to the scaffolding of a building, which is also disposable in the same way that it is indispensable to the erection of a building. This device functioned as increments: evanescent increments. Today it is known as differential calculus.

Bishop Berkeley became upset and called those evanescent increments "ghosts of departed quantities" in a hostile, defiant way. Bion considers that the differential calculus as formulated by Newton was a "transformation in K", or an advance that developed mathematical knowledge. *"The transformation in K is effected by discarding the 'scaffolding' of fluxions, 'the ghosts of departed quantities'. The discarding of the scaffolding may be regarded as a step to achieve finite*

*lines 'proportional to them', a category H$_3$ formulation; or, the 'finite lines
... proportional to them' may be regarded as an F$_3$ formulation used as a
column 2 formulation to prevent emergence of the 'ghosts of departed
quantities' and the psychological turbulence that such an emergence would
precipitate"* (T, 157).

At the time that Newton was developing differential calculus
and involved himself in this polemic with Berkeley he underwent
a nervous breakdown; his office went up in flames and he never
fully recovered. He was not able to resume his activities as a physicist again. *"Berkeley's formulation may be regarded as an F$_3$ contribution. The polemical tone gives it a column 2 category, denying, though he
acknowledges the truth of Newton's result, the validity of the method: the
ironic tone denies the reality of 'the ghosts of departed quantities'. . ."*

T Newton β H$_3$ furthers mathematic inquiry; T Newton β col. 2
denies the "ghosts". T Berkeley β col. 2 denies, by irony, "ghosts",
and, by polemic, the scientific approach. In both instances the
column 2 dimension is directed against psychological turbulence;
why? for fear of the turbulence and its associated "becoming". Put
in other terms, transformations in K are feared when they threaten
the emergence of transformations in O. [T, 158]

My term "psychological turbulence", needs elucidation. By it I
mean a state of mind the painful quality of which may be expressed
in terms borrowed from St John of the Cross. I quote: [The Ascent
of Mount Carmel]

"The first (night of the soul) has to do with the point from which
the soul goes forth, for it has gradually to deprive itself of desire for
all the worldly things which it possessed, by denying them to itself;
the which denial and deprivation are, as it were, night to all the
senses of man. The second reason has to do with the mean, or the
road along which the soul must travel to this union—that is, faith,
which is likewise as dark as night to the understanding. The third
has to do with the point to which it travels—namely, God. Who,
equally, is dark night to the soul in his life."

I use these formulations to express, in exaggerated form, the pain
which is involved in achieving the state of naïvety inseparable from
binding or definition (col.1). Any naming of a constant conjunction
involves admission of the negative dimension and is opposed by

the fear of ignorance. Therefore at the outset there is a tendency to precocious advance, that is, to a formulation which is a col. 2 formulation to deny ignorance—the dark night of the senses. The relevance of this to psychological phenomena springs from the fact that they are not amenable to apprehension by the senses; this tends to precipitate transformation into such objects as *are* and so contributes to Transformation in hypochodriasis . . .

Similarly the intuitive approach is obstructed because the "faith" involved is associated with absence of inquiry, or "dark night" to K. [T, 158–9]

In 1975, Bion furnishes other analogies. An example is the famous Leonardo da Vinci sketches of human hair. The onlooker sees living, turbulent waters. The journey from sensuous to non-sensuous through a sensuously apprehensible artistic transformation (please refer to the entry "container/contained" to see the quotation).

In 1976 he would introduce the term "emotional turbulence"—which is also the title of a short paper. At this moment the term acquires a descriptive value. It depicts the emotions that pervade two human beings whose ways cross: when two personalities meet there is a period of anxious turbulence and many emotions are aroused. The difference between **knowing** and **being** is implicit: sexual situations can emerge, as well as situations of survival, for hostility and aggression can obtrude. The sexual situation appears through its negative, that is, it is latent. In his papers ("Emotional turbulence" and "On a quotation from Freud", CSOW) there is a scrutiny of the then fashionable concept of "borderline" together with a fuller exploration of the period of latency, where the latent is emotional turbulence itself.

Usefulness The concept would have nothing to do with the vehicle Bion uses to convey it, a part of the history of science, in a concrete way, except in one important sense: that each individual repeats in his private history the history of science and its vicissitudes. Moreover, it marks the clinical utility of the concept in analysis. It is a kind of epistemological practice, a way to know: *"Resistance to an interpretation is resistance against change from K to O. Change from K to O is a special case of Transformation; it is of particular concern to the analyst in his function of aiding maturation of the person-*

alities of his patients"(T, 158). It marks the difference between "talking about analysis" and "being analysed", suffering the experience of analysis. It marks the difference between patients who learn many things about themselves but do not get in touch with themselves. It marks the difference between an intellectualized practice and a real analysis.

Suggested cross-references: Catastrophic change, Negative, Proto-resistance.

Enforced splitting: An extensive separation of material from psychic reality.

Bion used this term once. It is in *Learning from Experience*, chapter V. *"If the emotion is strong enough it inhibits the infant's impulse to obtain sustenance.*

> Love in infant or mother or both increases rather than decreases the obstruction partly because love is inseparable from envy of the object so loved ... The part played by love may escape notice because envy, rivalry and hate obscure it, although hate would not exist if love were not present. Violence of emotion compels reinforcement of the obstruction because violence is not distinguished from destructiveness and subsequent guilt and depression. Fear of death through starvation of essentials compels resumption of sucking. A split between material and psychical satisfaction develop. [LE, 10]

Enforced splitting is a step further from the observation that there are people who deal with the animate with methods that could succeed with the inanimate. Since the forties Bion had been observing it in patients with severe disturbance of the thought processes.

The excessive concretization and lack of getting in touch with psychic reality are linked to this enforced splitting. It precludes symbol formation and contributes to a special mode of mental (dis)functioning, namely, symbolic equations. Symbolic equation is a term created by Melanie Klein and popularized by Hanna Segal.

The enforced splitting differs from the splitting *"carried out to prevent depression"* as well as *"from splitting impelled by sadistic impulses"*. It is aroused by a violent fear of hate, envy and fear itself which are violently maintained and are born from violence. Those feelings are so feared that steps are taken to *"destroy awareness of all feelings"*, even though the price to be paid is *"taking life itself"*. This constitutes the stuff that enforced splitting is made of. In enforced splitting, the person has contact with some external manifestations of reality—such as the need to survive—but little regard for truth (q.v.)

> If a sense of reality, too great to be swamped by emotions, forces the infant to resume feeding, intolerance of envy and hate in a situation which stimulates love leads to a splitting . . . in that its object and effect is to enable the infant to obtain what later in life would be called material comforts without acknowledging the existence of a live object on which these benefits depend . . . The need for love, understanding and mental development is now deflected, since it cannot be satisfied, into the search for material comforts. Since the desires for material comforts are reinforced the craving for love remains unsatisfied and turns into overweening and misdirected greed . . . the patient greedily pursues every form of material comfort; he is at once insatiable and implacable in his pursuit of satisfaction.
>
> . . . the patient appears to be incapable of gratitude or concern for himself or others. This state involves destruction of his concern for truth . . . his pursuit of a cure takes the form of a search for a lost object and ends in increased dependence on material comfort; quantity must be the governing consideration, not quality. [LE, 10–11]

Such a patient invariably regards the interpretations as bad but he *"must have more and more of them"* (LE, 11). This seems to be the basis of consumerism, and seeking bureaucratic and political posts.
Suggested cross-reference: Truth.

Envy: The term is used in the same way as Klein. A kind of "bread and butter" conception in Bion's work, it means that violent love together with intolerance of frustration have odious effects. In *A Memoir of the Future* one finds some comments on envy and its link with cruelty. The latter is aimed both against oneself and exterior bound. *"Envy lay waiting, single-celled, to become malignant"* (AMF, 1, 10). Therefore, its objectless nature, having annihilated the object, is stressed. The envious invasion and disrespect that characterizes indifference as well as inhumanity appears in a quasi-medical "examination": *"Rosemary, exasperated by an unusually painful scrape between her fingers-they were usually too expert to inflict pain unless with*

intent . . . the medical examination was minute and thorough. The wishes
of the two girls were of no consequence" (AMF, 1, 28).

Establishment:

> BION At Oxford, when I wrote the account, we were not so critical.
> I don't think it was because it was against orders, but because it was
> less awful to think all was well than to believe our bigger enemy
> was what you later called . . .
>
> MYSELF . . . the Establishment. Certain gross words would have
> been—still are—more appropriate. [WM, 205–6]

> Plato seemed to think that the Socratic Greeks might at least under-
> stand the parable of the cave. But between then and now many
> hundreds of people have tried, oh "ever so hard", to understand
> what it means. And some people, like Jesus, have continued the
> naïve idea. "If you can't understand the parable, what am I to tell
> you?" he complained when his disciples were not stupid enough to
> be simple. All that they could do was to decide that Jesus was God
> and shut him up under a tombstone of heavy, cold, religious adora-
> tion. [AMF, I, 47]

Bion, following Freud, introduced this term in psycho-analysis,
borrowing from sociology. While Bion introduced the term, Freud
dealt with the issue itself. In *Totem and Taboo* he studied some institutions, such as the Church and the Military. The institutional issues
are relevant both to psycho-analysis itself and to the psycho-
analytic movement.

Bion studies some features of the establishment—or interests of
the herd—as issues that affect the individual. They can be
subsumed under at least three headings: vogue, co-option, and the
extinction of the individual. As analytic experience unfolded, Bion
observed an introjected establishment. These have more psycho-
analytical relevance to the extent they can be dealt with—in
contrast with macro-social situations—in the analytical setting.
This "introjected establishment" was observed in his analysis of
psychotics. It has as its orbit the subservience to the pleasure/
displeasure principle: *"superabundance of primary narcissism"*, which
demands endless love from the group; fear of the unknown, or the
analyst's narcissism, his clinging to his own established codes, and

the imbalance of narcissism and social-ism. Ultimately, that which is always at stake is the survival of the herd versus the survival of the individual.

The vogue seems to instil habits of mind, established forms of thinking and non-thinking that repeat themselves; people become addicted to them. Marx, in observing religion, called it the people's opium. The vogue has paradoxical effects: it can empower a real scientific or artistic eruption; but it also can extinguish scientific and epistemophilic curiosity. The vogue, once at the service of creation, can also put the person who is under the aegis of memory, desire and understanding into a repetitive, non-creative state.

Among the powerfully destructive vogues, there is one that stands out in Bion's contributions. He follows Kant and Freud in explicit (EP, 35, AI, 103, C, 189) critiques of the Cartesian vogue in western "thinking". This vogue manifests itself in at least five powerfully-established ideas:

(i)   The idea of cause in the scientific movement.
(ii)   The idea that the thinker creates thoughts.
(iii) The idea that conscious logical thinking is all that exists.
(iv)   The idea of a separation between matter and mind.
(v)   The idea that time and space are separated.

In *Attention and Interpretation* Bion develops the idea that the establishment tends to co-opt and to kill the geniuses and mystics, as Bion calls them. Those are the people who are able to glimpse "O", the numinous real. One of his examples is the history of Christ's thinking. In *A Memoir of the Future* Christ is seen as being buried under a cold stone of adoration. It debased that which Christ tried to convey into a dead legacy. Bion quotes many revolts against this, especially the movement of Port Royal. He was greatly impressed by Jansenism. Bion also has a mature grasp that revolts against the establishment producing new establishments that imitate that which they criticized. This is brought home in his view of John Milton's commitment to Cromwell's policies.

> . . . apparently primary narcissism [Freud, "Instincts and their vicissitudes", 1915c, SE 14] is related to the fact that common sense is a function of the patient's relationship to his group, and in his

relationship with the group the individual's welfare is secondary to the survival of the group. Darwin's theory of the survival of the fittest needs to be replaced by a theory of the survival of the fittest to survive in a group—as far as the survival of the individual is concerned. That is, he must be possessed with a high degree of common sense: (1) an ability to see what everyone else sees when subjected to the same stimulus, (2) an ability to believe in survival of the dead after death in a sort of Heaven or Valhalla or what-not, (3) an ability to hallucinate or manipulate facts so as to produce material for a delusion that there exists an inexhaustible fund of love in the group for himself. If for some reason the patient lacks these, or some similar series of capacities for attaining subordination to the group . . . which is known to be indifferent to his fate as an *individual*—by destroying his common sense or sense of group pressures on himself as an individual, as the only method by which he can preserve his narcissism. [C, 29–30]

FORTY YEARS You are too personal, Twenty-five. You've learnt that from P.A. He is always being personal.

FIFTY YEARS Not personal—specific.

P.A. I have great respect for the individual. Do you think that is wrong?

FIFTY YEARS No, but it is not in keeping with the growth of the Herd. I can see P.A. will be in serious trouble if the Herd develops faster than he does.

P.A. If the development of the Herd is incompatible with that of the individual, either the individual will perish, or the Herd will be destroyed by the individual who is not allowed to fulfil himself. [AMF, III, 461]

The establishment also tries to extinguish the individual in other ways. They seem to have been elicited through Bion's use of his own life experiences. Early in his life he had been separated from his parents due to an establishment-backed initiative that seemed not to be subjected to second thoughts. After his experiences as a tank-officer in WWI he saw the establishment's deeds as identical with criminal attitudes of the various countries' governing bodies (WM, 205–6). The establishment's interest ran against the individual's needs.

Clinical sources and implications

This has serious implications for the analyst's task—beyond socio-logical considerations. In the group of two, analyst/patient, "*the psychotic defence against interpretation . . . which constitutes, or is felt to constitute, an attack on the patient's narcissism. In practice this means evading the elucidation of illusory, delusory, or hallucinatory mechanisms for making the patient feel loved, lest such elucidation should show him that such love as he wishes to feel that he receives does not in fact exist. This in turn means that the analyst has to convey by various means that he loves the patient, and that in this respect he is a representative of the common sense of the patient's social group, which loves the patient more that it loves itself. This latter belief can, of course, be supported by the patient by his believing that analysis itself is an expression of such group love for him. Or, in early infant terms, that the breast is a gift to him from the family group.*"

The problem is the same emphasized by Freud since *The Interpretation of Dreams*. One resorts to hallucination as a source of "well-being": "*In so far as the patient is successful in evading the attacks on his narcissism, he experiences a hallucinatory gratification of his craving for love. This, like all hallucinatory gratification, leaves the patient unsatisfied. He therefore greedily resorts to a strengthening of his capacity for hallucination, but there is naturally no corresponding increase in satisfaction*" (C, 30).

This feeling that hallucination can furnish solace also has socio-logical implications; many people hallucinating simultaneously produces a huge shared hallucination. Both in *Experience in Groups and Transformations*, one gets a sense that all groups are halluci-nated; in a certain sense, it seems that one of the features that composes the "introjected establishment" is an allegiance to lies, in the form of hypocrisy:

> The assumption underlying loyalty to the K link is that the person-ality of analyst and analysand can survive the loss of its protective coat of lies, subterfuge, evasion and hallucination and may even be fortified and enriched by the loss. It is an assumption strongly disputed by the psychotic and *a fortiori* by the group, which relies on psychotic mechanisms for its coherence and sense of well-being. [T, 129]

Finally, concerning the analyst's state of mind, the establishment can be regarded as the established ideas, theories, theories on a specific patient, codes, cultural habits and anything that disguises itself as a reason to say, "*Thus far and no further*" (AMF, II, 236–7, 242, 265).

> ROBIN The whole of psycho-analytic theory seems to be vitiated—as shown by the structured nature of the system itself—by favouring only those phenomena which appear to conform to classical logic, the sort of logic with which we are already familiar.

> PAUL Timidity is a fact of our nature. We cling to anything which gives us the chance of saying "Thus far and no further". Any discovery is followed by a closure. The remainder of our thoughts and endeavours is devoted to consolidating the system to prevent the intrusion of yet another thought. Even any roughness of our system that might facilitate the lodgement of the germ of another idea is smoothed and polished. [AMF, II, 265]

The analyst who feels established by his memory, desire and judgmental values cannot do research and cannot help his (her) patient to further research into the unknown.

⊕ This term, even though it can be traced from Bion's adolescent experiences at war, is an evolution of the term, "public view".

Among some of his last thoughts on the issue one may quote:

> EDMUND I don't doubt it, but I want to go on with my astronomical hobbies.

> P.A. There is nothing to stop you provided you are not so terrified by your imagination or your scientific activity that you cannot think at all.

> ROBIN The government might become so terrified that they stopped you. But perhaps they are too ignorant to be terrified; that also would act as a cloak to protect the tender shoots of scientific speculation till they become "theories".

> ROLAND If they become strongly established theories they become too strong for the tender shoots of social speculation. Panic can be a powerful solvent of discipline.

> ALICE No government would dare to stop astronomers doing astronomical research.

P.A. If I were the government and wanted to stop astronomical research I am sure I could do it in a subtle enough way to escape criticism. I could say there was not enough paper to spare for the printing of astronomical articles. I could attack the availability of materials which were essential for the manufacture of certain instruments. I could discourage grants for the education of potentially gifted astronomy students.

ROLAND Which goes to show that it would be inadvisable to let you into government posts of power!

ALICE I think it would help if an astronomer stood for Parliament.

ROBIN But the principle stands—it is dangerous to allow men of such mischievous power authority which they can use to prevent mental development.

P.A. Suppose astronomers could convince the majority of human beings that the sun showed signs of imminent catastrophe; that at any moment we would be enveloped in whirlpools of immense temperatures. Would you allow that to be broadcast when nothing could be done? [AMF, III, 284–5]

Suggested cross-references: Common sense, Herd, Public view.

F

Factors and functions: The concept of factors and functions belongs both to the philosophy of mathematics and to geometry (which can be seen as one of the "practical" applications of mathematics). Bion borrowed this concept as an aid to the development of the theory of thinking and its offshoot, the theory of learning from experience. In chronological terms it is the second time that Bion borrowed from philosophy of mathematics. The first time was Frege's theory of numbers, which was used in "A theory of thinking" (q.v.). Bion wants the reader to be reminded of the philosophical, mathematical and current usage of these concepts.

One may state that almost the entirety of Bion's contributions to psycho-analysis has its roots in Freud's "Formulations on the two principles of mental functioning". The concept of function uses it in so obvious a way that it probably passes unnoticed. Something functions when it is seen *vis-à-vis* other something else.

Those who are reminded of elementary school or college mathematics and physics will recognize here a description of the Euclidean system of co-ordinates. The linear function may be the simplest example of it. It is represented by an equation with two variables (x and y) which function under some rule, one vis-à-vis the other. For example, one x equals two "ys". The ethos of the mathematical function has some features that are ever-present in any human endeavour, to the extent that mathematics is one of the oldest human attempts to create a formulation that presents or represents some counterparts in reality. Namely, the binding capacity to formulate relationships.

One may be reminded of factoring, odd numbers, the lowest common denominator, the highest common divider. I suppose that Bion was able to perceive and rescue the fact that Freud investigated the functioning of the mental apparatus. The term "functioning" usually brings associations with machinery. But this is part of the history; there is an abstraction linked to it, the concept itself. Freud observed two **factors**, which he named "principles". Bion emphasizes Freud's perception of the existence of mental **functions**, especially the function of attention (LE, 5). In fact Freud established for the first time the "functions of the ego" as well as the functions of human sexuality.

The theory of functions in Bion's work, even though some of the inspiration for its formulation is drawn from mathematics, has nothing to do with mathematics *per se*. It is pure Freud in its roots. Any applied science studies functions; this is true for biology, physics, medicine and engineering. Lest the reader think that this statement is a creation of the author, Bion's own statement will suffice to dispel such a misgiving: *"The term 'function', used in the sense of a function of the personality, has not the meaning it possesses for the mathematician or the mathematical logician though it has features partaking of the meaning of both"* (LE, 89).

The concept of function underlies other basic contributions by Bion, namely, the concept of relationships or links. The relations between objects and beings as well as beings and other beings would mark a seminal step taken by him (see the headings Links, H, L, K, Commensal, Parasitic, Symbiotic). The concept of factors comes together with the concept of function, and both subsume the concept of constant conjunction (which is used exactly as Hume proposed using it). The factors are subordinate to the function.

The theory of functions is intended to furnish more precision and rigorousness to psycho-analysis as compared with that which can be furnished by the use of colloquial formulations. This concept would emphasize the complexity of mental functioning and would be a kind of preview of another concept, that of binocular vision. Binocular vision (q.v.) and Links would be developed in the same book, *Learning from Experience*. There was no place for "absolutes" of any kind in the work of Bion right from its start: one studies *relationships*.

He defines function and factors in an intertwined way: *"To call an action by the name of the person of whom it is thought to be typical, to talk, for example, of a Spoonerism as if it were a function of the personality of an individual called Spooner, is quite usual in conversation. I take advantage of this usage to derive a theory of functions that will stand up to more rigorous use than that for which the conversational phrase is employed. I shall suppose that there are factors in the personality that combine to produce stable entities which I call functions of the personality"* (LE, 1).

He furthers the definitions: *"'Function' is the name for the mental activity proper to a number of factors operating in consort. 'Factor' is the name for a mental activity operating in consort with other mental activities to constitute a function. Factors are deducible from observation of the functions of which they, in consort with each other, are a part"* (LE, 2). It follows that factors are subordinate to functions, even though an element or trait can be a function under a given vertex and a factor under another. Functions appertain to the realm of phenomena and are observable; factors appertain to the realm of noumena and are not observable: "Factors are deduced not directly but by observation of functions" (LE, 2).

Flexibility is demanded when using these concepts; they are not ultimate realities and they must not be reified: *"They can be theories or the realities the theories represent. They may appear to be commonplaces of ordinary insight; they are not because the word used to name the factor is employed scientifically and therefore more rigorously that is usual in conversational English"* (LE, 2).

Suggested cross-reference: Mathematizing psycho-analysis.

Facts:

P.A. Being aware of facts has, I am sure, had an effect on me analogous to that of food on my physique. [AMF, II, 330]

This entry will offer further evidence for the statements made in the entries Analytic view, Opinion (of the analyst), Scientific method. They are included in this dictionary as an effort to help to dispel any doubts on the necessity of not attributing to Bion non-scientific views about the analyst's work. By non-scientific views, idealistic (also called, solipsistic or subjectivist) views as well as a blind relativism that denies the very existence of truth and reality themselves is meant.

Observation and facts

In inviting the reader to use an observational theory to improve the scientific value of psycho-analysis, Bion tries to assess the stuff that the patient's verbal formulations are made of.

One must remember the conventions of Bion's proposed notational system before reading the following quotation:

(i) T (patient) stands for the transformations made by a patient around and with an original emotional and physical experience, or invariance.

(ii) The two other symbols, T (patient)α, and T (patient)β stand for the processes of those who would like to have more details about these quasi-mathematical terms, see entries in this dictionary, Transformations, symbols: T, T α, and T β.

Bion tries to assess what the words convey, beyond the manifest, outward appearance of discourse and/or acting out during the session. He is concerned with the *"nature (or, in other words, meaning)"* of a series of phenomena. Namely, *"the material provided by the analytic session"* which *"is significant for its being the patient's view (representation) of certain facts which are the origin (O) of his reaction"*.

> In practice this means that I shall regard only those aspects of the patient's behaviour which are significant as representing his view of O; I shall understand what he says or does as if it were an artist's painting. In the session the facts of his behaviour are like the facts of a painting and from them I must find the nature of his representation . . . From the analytic treatment as a whole I hope to discover from the invariants in this material what O is, what he *does* to transform O . . . As I am concerned with the *nature* (or, in other words, meaning) of these phenomena, my problem is to determine the rela-

tionship between three unknowns: T (patient), T (patient) α, and T (patient) β. Only in the last of these have I any *facts* on which to work. [T, 15]

Seventeen years later he used a literary-philosophical form to express his view, which dispensed with the quasi-mathematical terms: *"P.A. I find it useful to make a distinction between meaning and fact. 'Facts' are the name we give to any collection of constantly conjoined experiences which we feel temporarily have a meaning;* **then** *we consider we have discovered a 'fact'"* (AMF, II, 236). In other words, facts that are available to the analyst's observation are the final products—or manifest content—of the analysand's transformations of his experiences, sensuous and psychic.

An increasingly larger number of Bion's readers—following a trend in the psycho-analytical movement—do not have a medical or other kind of scientific experience of contact with facts and observation. Some of them have been adopting a partisan attitude favouring structuralist and post-modern views, meaning, relativistic idealism. These readers conclude that Bion was under the sway of a positivistic idea of the existence of a neutral observer when he uses the term "observation". The same is true when Bion's texts display his concern for truth and life, when uttering the word "facts". A *verboten* word in our post-modern and Kuhnistic days. The following quotations may help those who are used to the critical debate to entertain second thoughts about this idea.

The same issue was already presented in some of the diatribes that Aristotle had with his master Plato—diatribes that would be better resolved only when an older Aristotle, now at flight trying to save his life, matured emotionally, from personal suffering.

One of the Aristotle versus Plato arguments had to do with the word representing "point" as used by the former, which meant "puncture"—therefore too tied to sensuously apprehensible factual reality. Aristotle, who defended non-physical metaphysics, in practice returned to the concreteness of it, when he tried to deny feelings.

Bion reminds us that Plato was attacked by Aristotle when the former defined the point by an emotional experience, a negative aspect, in the sense of the non-existence of whatever it be in order to attain existence: that a point was "the beginning of a line". Whereas Plato seemed inadequately "feelingful" to Aristotle,

Aristotle seemed to favour a "feelingless" view that also calls for critical scrutiny. This is Kant's "criticism". Nietzsche and Freud were inspired by the "critical posture".

> Now the associations of a statement include feelings: indeed many of the associations of a verbal statement represent feelings . . . [Aristotle's objection] suggests that the importance of a definition is to mark a constant conjunction without the evocation of feelings; but something seems real only when there are feelings about it. The negative quality of a definition, then, relates to the need to exclude existing emotions as well as ideas. [T, 77]

Some facts are seemingly basic and simple, such as a point. It is one of the earliest mathematical objects made available to us. Being a mathematical object it can be used as a reality that does not depend on the concrete object to be dealt with. This simple fact has as *"the realization which will approximate to it"*. . . *"an emotional experience"* (T, 77). Perhaps it may be argued that the point needed some millennia to have finally been experienced. Nevertheless it remains mathematically basic and simple.

In an imaginary dialogue between the place where instincts spring from, "Soma", and the psychic reality, "Psyche", one finds a reference to a lack of intuition. In his earlier forms of expression, written in the books before 1975, Bion resorted to Kant's aphorism, "concepts without intuitions are empty, intuitions without concepts are blind". Now he resorts to an event that could had killed him when in action at war:

> SOMA . . . If you had any respect for my "feelings" and did what I feel you, you wouldn't be in this mess.

> PSYCHE I am in this mess because I was squeezed into it. Who is responsible—your feelings or your ideas? All that has me is yours—amniotic fluid, light, smell, taste, noise, I'm wrapped up in it. Look out! I am getting absorbed! [AMF, III, 434]

Facts and feelings

Respect towards the existence of real facts can be accompanied by, and is no denial of doubting, the human ability to perceive them.

Also, they may be accompanied by doubts about the human ability to communicate them beyond the realm of feelings:

ROSEMARY ... Scientific bunkum. What do *you* know about the waves emitted by my feet when I chose to make them twinkle, twinkle on the hard, hard slum pavements of my street? I have seen the natural, unspoiled louts and blackguards of my slum follow my heels, threads of invisible steel hooking their eyes and dragging them helpless at my feet till I chose to release them. Love! You don't know what is it—none of you.

P.A. Your beliefs are expressions of great confidence in your powers; how you come to such "beliefs" and what evidence has convinced you they are "facts" I don't know ...

ROSEMARY I feel it; I know it. [AMF, II, 400]

The analyst's feelings may be scrutinized in order to determine if they have counterparts in reality:

P.A. People frequently assume that I am devoid either of culture or of technical equipment—or both.

ROLAND You sound hardly used.

P.A. No; it is part of the analyst's profession to be familiar with the real world, whereas laymen think they can afford to be deaf and blind to these unpleasing components of real life.

ROLAND What solution do you suggest? Psycho-analysis seems to be available only for the wealthy, and even so only to confirm those analysands and their analysts in the belief that the world of riches is the best of all possible worlds.

P.A. I think this is the best of all possible worlds because I know of no other world that is possible. That is not the same as thinking, like Pangloss, that there is no way in which we could strive to improve it. We consider the attempt to improve humans both worth while and urgent. [AMF, III, 528]

P.A. .... It is assumed that the character or personality corresponds to the physical boundaries which we can see and touch, but that does not seem a wise assumption—if there is in reality such an entity as a mind or character. For example, if one of us went out of the room and spoke we would recognize that it was ...

ROBIN Oh surely! We should only recognize the sound and interpret that to be evidence of an individual, not a "character".

P.A. Perhaps. But I think that we would soon learn to distinguish between a recording, however faithful, and the real thing . . . I do not believe that a mother, being requested to act the part of a mother to her child while a record of her voice was being played, would not betray her deception. I suspect that the baby would react to that sense of falseness in the mother.

ROLAND But this is pure conjecture! Is there no scientific proof?

P.A. It is conjecture; but I am not sure that it is "pure" conjecture any more than I consider "pure" truth to be available to mere human beings like ourselves. Psycho-analysts have to be cautious about their claims of scientific truth. The nearest that the psycho-analytic couple comes to a "fact" is when one or the other has a feeling. Communicating that fact to some other person is a task which has baffled scientists, saints, poets and philosophers as long as the race has existed. [AMF, III, 536]

P.A. It appears—to us—to be the case. But is what appears to "us" to be regarded as identical with fact? Priest and others seem to think we psycho-analysts claim to know. I regard any thing I know as transitive theory—a theory "on the way" to knowledge, but not *knowledge*. It is merely a "resting place", a "pause" where I can be temporarily free to be aware of my condition, however precarious that condition is. [AMF, III, 462]

The search for facts always stumbles on belief—or paramnesias to fill the void of ignorance:

ALICE I thought you were a scientist.

ROSEMARY I thought scientists spoke the truth and believed in facts.

P.A. I wouldn't waste my capacity for belief on facts—I only believe when there is no fact available.

ROBIN You mean that when there is nothing factual you fall back on beliefs—like the Christian religion and such rubbish. No wonder psycho-analysis is such a tissue of lies.

P.A. No, I don't mean that. I mean I am careful to choose what I know and what I believe and, to the best of my capacity, not to mix them up. Because I do not take to be true what humans tell me are the facts, it does not mean that I fall back on "believing" a lot of twaddle as if I had to keep my mind full at all costs. Or the reverse—empty—like a kind of mental anorexia nervosa.

ROLAND I always thought anorexia nervosa was supposed to be mental.

P.A. Not by me. It is reputed to be a fact like all these masses of psycho-analytic theories which are not facts at all though their representations, like the pages in a book, are facts. They fill a space as paramnesias fill an amnesia. [AMF, II, 294–5]

Therefore, facts are unfolding events; to know them is a transient act before the very fact to be known is also amenable to decay or development. The prevalence of habits extinguishes curiosity and leads to precocious senility. The feeling of the "already known" or perhaps the dangerous syndrome of the "I do know" leads to disaster. This is a menace to the very perception of the existence of facts—that perception decays and can die. Facts cannot be created individually. In contrast, hallucination, hallucinosis and delusion—or lies—can be known, filed, memorized and above all can be created by individual minds with no regard to living or inanimate objects of the "not-me" kind.

This kind of disaster was depicted with the aid of the imaginary characters Alice and Roland, in the first chapters of *A Memoir of the Future*. Bion resorts to some kinds of facts that are the stuff whence psycho-analysis springs—hate, love, envy, warfare—to enhance further our perception of what a fact is all about, in sharp contrast with imagination (q.v.).

The following quotations can be seen as summarizing his final views of real facts, as they unfolded to him. The various characters represent how old he was when confronted with the facts as well as his reflections. The factual—objective or object-dependent truth—is no more important than the truthful recollection:

P.A. Right—let's start. I remember now how I felt when I was Twenty-one. We had just been ordered up the Line; I was terrified. I did not like the prospect at all. The orders were that we must not allow the enemy any rest, but carry on the pursuit now he had been beaten and a great gap torn in his lines by our victory on August

8th. Unfortunately I had been decorated for gallantry, Twenty-one knew I was terrified and hadn't the courage do get the doc. to invalid me out. I knew I had not the courage for "heroic" deeds. Besides, I had 'flu; my runner was given a bottle of phyz. to dose me with. No one knew what I was suffering from so it was called p.u.o.—pyrexia of unknown origin. I hoped my death would be painless and sudden. The infantryman by my side had a hole in his belly. We looked at him coldly. "He's a gonner—why waste time looking at him? Come on—zero hour." I scrambled out of the trench and started walking forward. I inhibited—as I learned to call it later—any whisper of fact to burst through my p.u.o. A grey-haired man with his legs worn around his neck like a scarf wanted me to "help" him. It was annoying to be expected to disentangle his neckwear. Besides, I was busy. "*No*—stretcher bearers coming." I knew they weren't; only regimental stretcher bearers help. Why did I tell him that? I had been taught—disciplined—so that in just such a crisis I would not have an unfamiliar, unthought-out problem to solve in inadequate conditions for its solution. As a doctor I now understand; as an influenza-sodden tank officer, "S.B.'s coming!" I lied. "Kamerad kaput!", yelled the little Boche as he ran towards me, his bottom wiggling furiously as he tried not to fall. I could tell the hideously disarticulated old Tommy to go to Hell—"S.B.'s coming!"—but I allowed the horrible little Boche to drag me to his cubby hole. No discipline—I knew he would murder me. I entered; in the dark another Boche with his legs wrapped round his neck for scarfwear. "Kaput?" He dragged me to touch—"Kaput?" I did. "Yes, kaput." He burst into tears. I told myself, "Now—damn fool—get *out*." Only then I snapped out—out of the hole, out into the air, out into the sense to carry my Smith & Wesson where I had been taught to carry it.

Priest You would not have felt any better if you had been a parson. I remember our pink-faced, jolly, card-playing padre and how scornful you were—you and that red-faced, non conformist private—because he would not come up and bury the dead. Poor Smith! He was so rigorous mortis that we could not force his arms into our grave; we were in a hurry too.

P.A. He preferred bridge with the colonel in H.Q. mess.

ROLAND Oh, don't be so hypocritical—so would you if you had been able to play bridge and hadn't been commanding a tank.

P.A. True—I was not scared—I was nothing. I thought I would be court-martialled. I was surprised that I told such an articulate, coherent story that I couldn't detect a chink of falsehood in it—and my men were so grateful and so full of admiration. I was amazed that I could not believe a word of it. All lies and so completely factual that even now—

ROLAND Well, what happened?

P.A. I caught up with my leading tank. I knew the long-range naval guns must get us. "Get out!" I told them, "and walk behind till it gets hit". I set the controls at full speed and got out myself. It raced—for those days—ahead so we could hardly stumble up with it. And then—*then!*—the full horror came on me. Fool! What had I done? A I scrambled and tripped in my drunken influenza to catch up with the tank, in the shadow of which I had ordered my crew to remain sheltered, my ice-cold reality revealed a *fact*: The tank, in perfect order, with guns, ammunition and its 175 horse-power engines, was delivered into the hands of the enemy. Alone, I alone, had done this thing! My pyrexia left to rejoin its unknown origin.

PRIEST How did you get in—by beating your hands on the cold steel doors?

P.A. I was in; I did get in. A high-velocity shell struck; without thought I shot out of the hatch as the flames of petrol swathed the steel carcass. Are you hurt, sir? No—fell on my arse. Are you all right, sir? Of course! Why? Home—quick!

PRIEST Do you really remember this? It sounds most unlikely—but I cannot claim to attach so much importance to what you scientists call facts.

ROLAND Both Robin and I regard facts as facts. If I did not remember to sow corn and harvest "facts", the crew you "saved" would not have anything to eat. Not would the rooks be blown cawing across the evening sky.

ROBIN I remember P.A. and his doctor friend as boys driving Curley to Munden when she did not want to be separated from her calf. Poor unintelligent animal! No one had told her about "Separation Anxiety", but she knew all about the way *not* to Munden.

P.A. My twelve-year-old hadn't heard of "separation anxiety" either, but "remembered" not to be separated from my intelligently disciplined 175 horse-power acquired
{conscious
conscience}

Even now I have to risk being heard by some damned psychiatric neologism-shooter.

ROBIN You speak with bitterness that I more usually hear conjoined with evacuation of hatred. In fact, if you hated psychoanalysis I would not be surprised to hear what I heard you say. As it is, I am almost shocked.

ROLAND If you were twelve years old I would not be surprised to hear that Curley had not arrived at Munden. I am shocked that as a psycho-analyst you are angry that your "meaning" has not driven into what you think is the right verbal pen.

P.A. I know, and have reason to fear that the "pen" into which it has entered will imprison both me and my meaning—inescapably. You think this is all talk and that talk is nothing. I know—thought I cannot prove—it is *not*. [AMF, III, 474–7]

Suggested cross-references: Real psycho-analysis, Sex.

Faith, act of faith: Faith is a term borrowed from Lurianic/Christian cabbala. Bion uses it to describe a "*scientific state of mind*" (AI, 32). It was devised to use at the decisive moment of interpretation.

It refers to a sense of experiencing the existence of reality and truth. Even though truth is not wholly reachable, comprehensible or amenable to being uttered or owned, its existence can be intuited and used. The experiencing of an evolving truth or reality as it is, is a transient one—but unmistakable. It is not the mystical posture it may seem, but an acknowledgement that trained intuition can be developed and put into practice. It expresses a faith that truth exists.

The intuition is exercised during the experience of deprivation (St John of the Cross' "three dark nights of the soul"), of the nothing. This deprivation includes, first, a discipline in memory, desire and understanding: "*The 'act of faith' depends on disciplined denial of memory and desire. A bad memory is not enough: what is ordinarily called forgetting is as bad as remembering. It is necessary to inhibit dwelling on memories and desires*" (AI, 41).

The term was introduced further to differentiate "to know about" and "to be" (or "being") whatever it is. It deals with attempts at apprehending reality as it is. It was devised (in an implicit way) in *Transformations*, where an appeal to the mystic tradition was made for the first time. It was depicted in *Attention and Interpretation* and it was expressed vividly in *A Memoir of the Future*. More specifically, faith tries to depict the state of mind that is "welcome" when one tries to discipline oneself from memory, understanding and desire. Still more specifically, "faith" allows one to travel from K (processes of knowledge) to O (origin, ultimate truth), or K⇨O. All those definitions of faith are in *Attention and Interpretation*, pages 31ff.

Its intuitive nature is akin to that which must be practised by the infant who, equipped with a pre-conception of a breast, looks for a real breast to match it. The real matching is possible when the baby tolerates the "no-breast" part of the experience.

> It must "evolve" before it can be apprehended and it is apprehended when it is a thought just as the artist's O is apprehensible when it has been transformed into a work of art.

> But, the act of faith is not a statement . . . has no association with memory or desire or sensation. It has a relationship to thought analogous to the relationship of a priori knowledge to knowledge . . . It does by itself not lead to knowledge "about" something, but knowledge "about" something may be the outcome of a defence against the consequences of an "act of faith". A thought has as its realization a no-thing. An "act of faith" has as its background something that is unconscious and unknown because it has not happened. [AI, 35]

It is "pure Freud" and "Pure Kant", where psychic reality is concerned (*"the analyst whose aim is O"*, AI, 29), material reality, or manifest content and latent content, or noumena and phenomena.

> A term that would express approximately what I need to express is "faith"—faith that there is an ultimate reality and truth—the unknown, unknowable, "formless infinite". This must be believed of every object of which the personality can be aware: the evolution of ultimate reality (signified by O) has issued in objects of which the individual can be aware. The objects of awareness are aspects of the "evolved" O and are such that the sensuously derived mental functions are adequate to apprehend them. For them faith is not required. For O it is. An The analyst is not concerned with such sensuously apprehended objects or with knowledge of such objects. Memories and desires are worthless but inevitable features that he

encounters in himself as he works. He **is** concerned with these objects in his analysand because he is concerned with the working of the analysand's mind. His analysand will express his awareness of O in people and things by formulations representing the inter-section of evolutions of O with the evolution of his awareness . . .

There can be no rules about the nature of the emotional experience that will show that the emotional experience is ripe for interpreta-tion . . . I can only suggest rules for the analyst that will help him to achieve the frame of mind in which he is receptive to O . . . then he may feel impelled to deal with the intersection of the evolution of O with the domain of objects of sense or of formulations based on the senses. Whether he does so or not cannot depend on **rules** for O . . . but only on his ability to be at one with O.

My last sentence represents an "act" of what I have called "faith". It is in my view a scientific statement because for me "faith" is a scientific state of mind. [AI, 31–2]

This experience can be felt as fearful: *"by eschewing memories, desires, and the operations of memory he can approach the domain of hallu-cinosis and of the 'acts of faith' by which alone he can become at one with his patient's hallucinations and so effect transformations O⇒K"* (AI, 36).

It allows for catastrophic change and atonement.

Misuses and misconceptions: Adding to the solipsistic/rela-tivistic trend, superficial readings see Bion as a religious writer. He is not: *"An 'act of faith' is peculiar to scientific procedure and must be distinguished from the religious meaning with which it is invested in conversational usage"* (AI, 34–5).

The term is simply an attempt to express just *"approximately"* and convey Bion's observations on a state of mind that is conducive to scientific (that is, truthful) interpretations and insights in the analytic setting and is not to be taken as a concept.

To quote Bion's writing again, which may—hopefully—pre-clude preconceived interpretations of his work: *"A term that would express approximately what I need to express is 'faith'—faith that there is an ultimate reality and truth—the unknown, unknowable, 'formless infi-nite' . . . But the act of faith is not a statement"*. It is not a learnable statement to be bettered in the session, it is not a theoretical or tech-nical statement either; it *"approximately"* depicts a posture.

Suggested cross-references: Analytical view, Atonement, Catas-trophic change, Hallucinosis, K, O, Transformations in K and O.

Fame:

> P.A. There is no such thing as a "well-known analyst"; an analyst is one who at one stage of fashion is famous, at another infamous; the barrier between "famous" and "infamous" is as slight as the verbal "in". It is unimportant—except to the psycho-analyst who cannot afford to be unaware that it is a "built-in" part of his profession. [AMF, III, 520]

There are a sizable number of references like this, that put fame and its attendants such as Gloria into human terms; Bion tries to display its basic fallaciousness, following Milton, who saw it is as a seed that does not grow in mortal soil. (One may refer to AMF I, 55, 91–2, 158; II, 396, among others.) His final comment about the delusional state of importance and fame that is endowed with an unsurpassed clarity is in *Cogitations*, 377.

Fear: Fear is one of the manifestations of abhorrence to pain. The links between fear and cowardice and paranoid states, in terms of saving one's own skin first, a kind of "self-love" which is fused with "self-hate" in an absolute state, are well known since Freud.

Too much love for oneself produces self-protection at the cost of one's ethical values. Fear is ingrained in the human condition. The links between masculinity, femininity and fear, or "sub-thalamic fear", are a final attempt by Bion towards a theory of psycho-analysis. It is just adumbrated in many parts of *A Memoir of the Future*. One of the most synthesizing passages may be the following quotation. It is based on a background of sensuous realizations: the invasion of a country by an army (represented by the character "Man"), a former maid who transforms herself into a mistress of her former mistress, "Rosemary" and "Alice" respectively, but the underlying invariance—a sado-masochistic relationship—remains unalterable; and a psycho-analyst named "Bion":

> BION According to Rosemary, Alice is able to have a masochistic relationship with her former maid.
>
> MAN This is a psycho-analytic formulation.
>
> BION I agree. I do sometimes express my views in terms which can themselves be characterized; in this instance my formulation is

called theoretical. But let me tell you something in more conversational terms about a man I knew in the army. He was highly educated at a well-known public school and, as far as I could see, had the opportunity common to people of the privileged classes of taking up an occupation of responsibility and power. He did not do so. He failed his chance of being trained as an officer, became an officer's servant and stayed in that position till the end of the war, by which time I had no means of knowing his further career.

ALICE Are you suggesting my career is comparable?

BION The thought occurs to you; if you are willing, and others likewise, this could be debated. If so, it is not an obstacle to the discussion that my case was a man and Alice is a woman; that kind of behaviour is not restricted to one sex. Yet is can be described, both in the man and now Alice, as "sexual". This is a classification familiar to me; in psycho-analysis the relationship between Rosemary and Alice could be discovered or demonstrated or classified as sexual. Suppose we consider Rosemary and Alice as welcoming, for their individual reasons, the country's downfall; their nation or culture undergoes a change which makes it possible to each individual to pursue a life which they would not otherwise have been free to do. I can see that the defeat makes that freedom possible. The desire to achieve such freedom, if shared amongst a sufficient number of people, could contribute to a defeat.

MAN What would be described as a defeat brought about by the decadence of the society or group; although I have known a society to be decadent *and* victorious. Reciprocally, the victory is regarded as a sign or symptom or "result".

ROSEMARY Men seem to attach great importance to conflict, rivalry, victory. Even in private affairs I couldn't make a man think that there was any importance in what I thought or felt about him. He talked and acted as if the only matter of consequence was whether he was successful. I suppose he thought I would then be bound to fall in love with a man of such capacity and brilliance. To the end he never entertained the possibility that I loved *him* and couldn't care less about his successes.

BION Is that true? I would be surprised if you did not find, if you are honest with yourself, that you cared a lot about his success.

ROSEMARY He had some distinction; it was the most boring part about him. Why, even in sexual love he was convinced he had to be potent. He couldn't believe that I might love him and therefore be capable of helping him to be potent.

BION I am sure there are many men who have no doubt of the woman's ability to make fools of them. In technical terms, there are plenty of men who are sure the woman can "castrate" them. All states exist, from primitive fears of the female genital—as expressed in visual prototypes of a vagina dentata—to fears that the woman would rejoice in triumphing by humiliating the man.

MAN There is certainly a profound belief in the pleasure of triumphing over and humiliating a rival. That state of mind is common enough and it is feared by man or woman. It, and the fear of it, can be generated by the experiences of the child.

BION Its efficiency depends on belief. But there can be innumerable reasons for fear, including fear of the pleasures of cruelty.

MAN You are again talking of "reasons"—"one reason", "innumerable" reasons. Don't you think *Belief* is the action-generator analogous to "numbers generators'? Man, like animals, is capable of fear. You can have "reasons" for being afraid; you can fear death and believe you will die. Belief is the action-generator; what generates belief?

BION If that state has been part of you, you must be familiar with the constantly conjoined elements. We can suppose that the constant conjunction has a "great deal to do with it"—or is "constantly conjoined with"—the fact that we are still alive. I would go further; I have owed and shall owe my continued existence to my capacity to fear "an impending disaster." The question is not "where is one to draw the line?" but where has the line been drawn? Between conscious and unconscious? By the phrenes? The thalamus? [AMF, I, 173–175]

Fear and dread, a primitive intuitive reality of the human mind, seems to be, together with passionate love, the nearest "O" formulation that Bion made. It corresponds to Klein's "anxiety of annihilation", and is usually extruded:

In a civilized world it is more comfortable to believe in its civilized qualities, to obscure the cruel laughter . . . which might evoke, through memory and desire, the configuration evocative of dread. It seems clear that the attempt is inherent to ward off, or to ward off awareness of, something which is dread and terror, and behind that the object that is nameless. There are many formulations of dread, unformulated and ineffable—what I denote O. [AMF, 1, 77]

Feelings: Feelings are seen as sensuous stimuli coming from the self (LE).

(Please refer to the entries, Alpha-function, Emotional Experience, Facts, Sex, Ultra-sensuous.)

Frustration, tolerance of: It would not be an exaggeration to state that all of Bion's contributions to psycho-analysis have a fulcrum, namely, the issue of tolerance and lack of tolerance of frustration. Subservience to desire, allegiance to memory and understanding, are some of its manifestations. It seems that this capacity or lack of it is genetically determined or in any case, innate. It manifests itself through regard for truth and a capacity for compassion.

Endogenous or primary narcissism and envy is the most profound formulation hitherto achieved that illuminates the existence and quantity of a basic endowment: a capacity to tolerate frustration and not to tolerate it. A violent feeling of love enhances the latter.

One phantasizes that the world (originally the breast) must be that which it desires one to be, and phantasizes that it cannot be that which it is in reality. Intolerance to frustration indicates a prevalence of the principle of pleasure/displeasure. It implies intolerance to pain. The person feels the pain but it cannot be said that he suffers it (AI, 9); the person is always trying to evade it. This action further worsens his or her predicament. The issue is not limited by the imposition of desire, for it may well be that a necessity is at stake; again, due to the prevalence of innate paranoid and narcissistic traits the person phantasizes that all his or her needs must be satisfied.

The disorders of thinking that Bion studied in his first contributions to psycho-analysis and the ensuing exploration into the realm of hallucination and hallucinosis—intolerance of the no-breasts— can be said to stem from Freud and Klein's basic contributions to psycho-analysis.

Historically speaking one may rely on the autobiographical 6-volume series composed of the Trilogy *A Memoir of the Future*

(1975–78), the two volumes of *The Long Week-End* (published posthumously during the eighties) and *War Memoirs*(ditto, in the late nineties) to see the origin of his contribution and the help he probably obtained from his own analysis.

One may say, from Bion's opinions about himself, that two of his life experiences, namely, (i) his un-thought out and impulsive enlisting with the hosts of young English men to fight WWI; (ii) his abandoning of his first wife and first daughter, again to serve his countrymen; gave a mix of a stimulating social environment and self-indulgence to his own desire. These experiences provided him with authority to use, in a straightforward way, with no parallel in the history of the psycho-analytic movement, Freud's observations about the two principles of mental functioning.

The purely psycho-analytical approach is obtained when one writes, as Bion did, a work that is not dazzled by external causes. Within certain limits (for example, the existence or absence of physical harm, or outrageous social conditions linked to differences of social classes, distribution of wealth that imposes famine on children or warfare directed against unarmed civilians, to quote a few examples) the issue is not exactly the quantity of pain, but the capacity to endure it.

G

godhead: A term used interchangeably with truth.

grid: The Grid is a device intended for a conscious, **extra-analytic session,** critical scanning of psycho-analytic material (T, 128) as well as an unconscious **intra-analytical** scanning. The conscious use of the Grid **is not** appropriate for *"the actual contact with the patient"* (please refer to the entry **Idea** for the unconscious use of the Grid).

It may be used as a prelude as well as an aftermath: it trains the analyst's assessment of the analytic work done and it also may help future work. It *"provides practice, analogous to the musician's scales and exercises, to sharpen and develop intuition"* (EP, 73). This intuition is seminal and necessary because of the immaterial nature of psycho-analysis: *"What psycho-analytic thinking requires is a method of notation and rules for its employment that will enable work to be done in the **absence** of the object, to facilitate further work in the **presence** of the object"* (T, 44)

This assessment is made in terms of the success, or lack of it, in approximating, albeit partially and transiently, to the patient's truth as well as the truth of what occurs in a session. In other words: to what extent and under what parameters were the insights gained, intrapsychically and in the relationship of analyst and analysand, truthful? The raw material to be examined are the analyst's and the patient's **verbal statements**. *"The two axes should thus together indicate a category implying a comprehensive range of information about the statement"*. The reader who accepts Bion's invitation may become interested in examining the scientific basis of his own practice.

The Grid is an attempt to simplify the communication between analysts as well as a personal communication of an analyst with himself (LE, 38). Its formulation dates from circa 1960 (C, 195); it integrates, in a hitherto unavailable form, Freud's "Two principles of mental functioning" with Klein's "Interplay of positions" (Freud, 1910, 1920; Klein, 1940, 1946, 1947). It was first published in*Elements of Psycho-Analysis* and was subjected to extensive explanations in *Transformations* (pp. 39–47, 167–169) through clinical use having as its hallmark a mobile, dynamic non-patterned form (pp. 50, 66, 74–75, 88, 94, 96–100; 126). To read those selected parts of *Transformations* seems to me essential for using the Grid. Bion tried to improve the tool in 1967 and 1971 (published in 1992, pp. 325, 357); fourteen years later two of its "categories" (line C and column 2) were considerably developed (Bion, 1977b; 1977d, pp. 57 and 92). The Grid is a commonsensical tool to the extent that it uses commonality of senses—each axis provides one sense. Bion looked for a psycho-analytical method to discriminate elemental *"facts as they are"* (Bacon, 1620, 1625; Johnson, often quoted by Bion; for example, *Cogitations*, pp. 6, 13, 114; circa 1959; also 1970, 1975). One may ascribe some category of the Grid to a given analyst or patient's statement, couple it with his previous experience with the patient, or a free association; from the communion—common sense—of those two different senses, one may gauge the truth-value of a given statement. The two axes of the Grid *"may appear arbitrary"* but they *". . .stem from the analytic situation itself"* (EP, p. 91). They take into account the use the analysand *"makes of the analytic situation"* through scrutinizing the patient's most evident activity in analysis: thinking and lack of it. The two axes measure **uses** and **functions** (horizontal axis) of statements *vis-à-vis* the **ontogenetic value** (vertical axis) of statements, which reflects growth (EP, pp. 63, 92). The statements, being verbal statements, are a function of thinking processes. The realness of a clinical occurrence is stated in clearly explicit terms: the various Grid categories.

The Grid contains dynamically linked **categories** formed by the **intersection of two axes** in a representation of Euclid's bi-dimension (fig. 1). Those categories represent constant conjunctions. *A statement may fall simultaneously in different categories and one category may fall into another* (T, 116). This can change kaleidoscopically at the next "decisive moment". Each axis expresses basic psycho-analytic theoretical-practical, intra-session activities and may be regarded as a synthetic **epistemological tool** that illuminates the underlying rationale of the psycho-analytic endeavour.

i. The horizontal axis determines the columns that are, for purposes of notation, numbered from 1 to 6. It depicts the functions of the ego according to Freud (Freud, 1910): notation, attention, enquiry and action. To them, Bion added two Kantian categories akin and more primitive to the ego-functions adumbrated by Freud. I surmise that those two categories were implicit in Freud's work but they were not yet named:

(1) Column 1 is a primitive equivalent of intuitive pre-conceptions, which Bion names *definitory hypothesis*, probably linked to instinctual endowment.

(2) Column 2 is a non-saturated category full of the unknown, named "ψ". It corresponds to *false* statements *known as such*" by analyst and analysand. If its begetter is the analyst, it indicates his need for further analysis. The statements appertaining to this category are not amenable to be understood, but rather to be perceived and used as pointers. A telling example of statements appertaining to column 2 are explanations and rationalizations. They are full of feelings, sound and fury but, being devoid of emotional experiences that only exist in a relationship (LE, 42), they mean nothing (after *Macbeth*, V, v, 19). The emotions that are amenable to being represented by it are no-emotions at all, for "their fundamental function is denial of another emotion" (AI, 20).

During the development of the Grid, Bion stressed the phantastic nature of projective identification, already stated by Melanie Klein herself (Klein, 1946, p. 298) as well as its relationship with hallucination (Bion, 1977b, p. 11). Successful projective identification depends on collusion, the stuff of column 2. Bion proposes to typify lies in order to differentiate them sharply from false state-ments: "*the false statement being related more to the inadequacy of the human being, analyst or analysand alike, who cannot feel confident in his ability to be aware of the 'truth' and the liar who has to be certain of his knowledge of the truth in order to be sure that he will not blunder into it by accident*" (Bion, 1977b, p. 11). He synthesizes: "*it is simplest to consider column 2 as relating to elements known to the analysand to be false, but enshrining statements valuable against the inception of any development in his personality involving catastrophic change*". The Grid helps us to deal with lies under a scientific vertex, rather than a moral one: a scientific endeavour, the apprehension of reality, is at stake.

A central role in column 2 events is performed by "*reversion of perspective*", a fact dependent on the presence of projective identifi-cation in a session of analysis. Reversion of perspective is one of the tools to see beyond the material, overt, acted-out appearances (EP, pp. 54, 60; 1975, p. 11–37). An example of reversed perspective at work is the scrutiny of emotions of hate and love during an analy-sis, under the vertex of tolerance of paradoxes (Sandler, 1997b). It is expressed by the analyst's realization that "*if the hate that a patient is experiencing is a precursor of love, its virtue as an element resides in its quality as a precursor of love and not in its being hate*" (EP, p. 74). This includes the appearances of manifest discourse, talk. Resistance, in Freud's sense, expresses itself even in discrete words uttered by our patients, which are counterparts during the actual session of the manifest discourse as it is traditionally regarded in dreams. Therefore the words, phrases, facts, events, reported by the patients might well be dreams being dreamed during the actual session. But they may be hallucinations and delusions too: it is a matter of discrimination. If they constitute dreams, resistance and manifest content simultaneously point to the truth and equally disguise this very same truth. We psycho-analysts are ever at the risk of aping a dog that looks at his master's pointing hand instead of paying attention to the object the hand points to (AMF, 2, 267). It is a matter of intuiting the existence of the moon's dark side, of intuiting the obverse of whatever it is that remains hidden, lurking—but **is** there. This allows us to formulate statements that avoid descriptions of "*particular clinical entities*" being subjected to fit "*some quite different clinical entities*": "*Correct interpretation therefore will depend on the* *analyst's being able, by virtue of the grid, to observe that two statements verbally identical are psycho-analytically different"* (EP, 103).

ii. The vertical axis (rows) of the Grid is construed according to the Euclidean system of coordinates. It is to be **constantly conjoined** with the horizontal axis of functions and is used to reach a common sense between two senses (the two axes). The falsity of a statement as well as its truth is a *"function of its relationship to the other element in the scheme"* (Bion, 1977b, p. 9). *"A possible approach may therefore be provided by considering the nature of the match between the stage (or row) and the use matching row and column in terms of the appropriateness of one to the other, but this only shelves the problem by postponing it to a later stage in the discussion, for it necessitates criteria by which to judge appropriateness"* (T, 44).

This axis has lettered categories, A to H. It furnishes an (onto)genetic view of the development of the thinking apparatus, a spectrum that ranges from primitive sense stimuli to the most sophisticated expression of human thought hitherto known. At that time, Bion, influenced by neo-positivism, ascribed this status to scientific deductive systems and algebraic thought. The "A" line shelters that which is felt as things-in-themselves: psychotic feelings of attainment and ownership of absolute truth, which Bion named "β-elements". The "H" line corresponds to **algebraic calculus**. In between A and H we have:

Line "B", "α-elements", that is, "de-sense-fyed" β-elements that have undergone a "digestion" by "alpha-function" (Bion, 1962a, b). They are building blocks that can be used to think and to dream work; to build dream thoughts; also to store in the form of memories.

Line "C", that comprises **dreams, myths, dream thoughts**, to which I would add metaphors. It corresponds simultaneously to Plato's Ideal forms **and** to Aristotle's "nous": the mind thinking about itself and presenting the real universe, human nature and, above all, itself to itself. This is a remarkable category; myths are powerful enough to convey macro, universal truths and they are also valid at the micro, individual level, as part *"of the primitive apparatus of the individual's armoury of learning"*. Bion considers the myth as a *"fact-finding tool"* and states explicitly: *"I wish to restore its place in our methods so that it can play the* *vitalizing part there that it has played in history (and in Freud's discovery of psycho-analysis)"* (EP, 66). Bion scrutinizes the Oedipus Myth (EP) and the myth of Babel (Bion, c. 1960, published in 1992, C, 226). This Grid category would be noticeably expanded in 1977 to the point of meriting a Grid of its own.

Line "D" lodges Kantian **pre-conceptions**, which correspond to Freud's protophantasies (Freud, 1920). *"Since self-knowledge is an aim of psycho-analytic procedure the equipment for attaining knowledge, the function and apparatus of pre-conception, must be correspondingly important"* (EP, p. 91). They are, probably, phylogenetic introjections, and thus inborn. For example, the pre-conception of a breast.

Line "E" lodges **conceptions**. This evolution of thought processes was first adumbrated in "A theory of thinking" (ST, 110). It is the product of the frustrating (or partially satisfactory) mating of pre-conceptions with a realization. If the thought is bound to further development, line E leads to

Line "F", **concepts**, which are conducive to

Line "G", **scientific deductive systems**. In order better to apprehend the *ethos* of the C line onwards, one should firmly grasp the conception of psychic reality as a different form of existence of material reality (Freud, 1900) and must not be "too concrete" as Hanna Segal says (Segal, 1979, p. 62; Sandler, 1997b). This leads to *line "H"*.

I suggest that one must bear in mind that both sides of the Grid are open-ended. They allow the construction of negative Grids, Tri, Four and n-dimension Grids, for example.

& Bion's second thoughts about the Grid included an expansion into a grating (BNYSP, 91) as well as the eliciting of some of its shortcomings (both in *Elements of Psychoanalysis* comments and in *Taming Wild Thoughts*). The author of this dictionary proposed an expansion that included three- and four-dimension views of the Grid (1987, 1999), already included implicitly in Bion's original formulation.

Suggested cross-references: Idea, Intuition.

group: Please refer to the entries, Basic Assumptions, Establishment, Two-body psychology.

growth: Bion mentions growth in all of his books, from *Learning from Experience, Elements of Psychoanalysis, Transformations, Attention and Interpretation* and *A Memoir of the Future*. "*'Growth' here refers to the growth of a mental formulation*" (T, 42, fn1).

There is an approach to a scientific psycho-analysis; this is explicitly mentioned in the titles of and throughout the texts. This approach is made to the transformation between conscious thinking and unconscious dream activity and vice-versa as a condition for growth and development. At first, growth was seen as a reflection of the overcoming of the primitive stages of non-thinking due to the prevalence of the desirous drives and natural helplessness of the baby.

The link between purely concrete feeding and emotional experiences ranges from symbol formation to the realization of Oedipus. The first symbol is the immaterial inner counterpart of the breast, the no-breast. Therefore the pattern of growth is given by the extent to which the baby tolerates the frustration provoked by the no-breast.

Perhaps the earliest mention of Growth can be found in *Learning from Experience*. In defining the psycho-analytical object, Bion extends the concept to include "*phenomena related to growth*" (LE, 70)—"*like the extensions of all biological concepts . . . Growth may be regarded as positive or negative. I shall represent it by ($\pm Y$). The plus and minus signs are employed to give sense or direction to the element they precede in a manner analogous to their mode of employment in coordinate geometry . . . Whether (Y) is preceded by plus or minus sign will be determined only by contact with a realization*" (LE, 70).

Y may be plus or minus when seen, for example, against the background of the "*resolution of the conflicting aims of narcissism and social-ism. If the trend is social (+Y) abstraction will be related to the isolation of primary qualities. If the trend is narcissistic (-Y) abstraction will be replaced by activity appropriate to $-K$ . . .*" (LE, 70).

Bion had many suggestions stemming from clinical work that thinking can be viewed according to degrees of sophistication. He represented the varying degrees, representing growth, by their reflections when one scans the Grid (q.v.) (EP, 86). Categories run from A to H and from 1 to 6, as well as from a constantly conjoined scrutiny of both axes, from A1 to H6. This kind of development meant a development of thought processes. Growth was thereafter seen as related to an increased capacity to face the unknown, to abandon cravings for explanations and understanding of perception of one's destructiveness, in Klein's sense of a transition between the paranoid–schizoid and depressive positions. Growth would include, from the time that Bion wrote *Transformations*, a respectful awe towards the existence of truth, "O"; he introduces the term "atonement" to the relationship between the human being and "O":

> The psycho-analyst accepts the reality of reverence and awe, the possibility of a disturbance in the individual which makes atonement and therefore, an expression of reverence and awe impossible. The central postulate is that atonement with ultimate reality, or O, as I have called it to avoid involvement with as existing association, is essential to harmonious mental growth. It follows that interpretation involves elucidation of evidence touching atonement, and not evidence only of the continuing operation of immature relationship with a father ... Disturbance in capacity for atonement is associated with megalomaniac attitudes. [ST, 145]

Growth is equated in psycho-analysis with an evolved capacity to love, hate and know; to know that we shelter aggressive feelings without being overwhelmed by satisfying them or by denying them. In other words, it means emotional growth.

Growth is linked to diminishing the allegiance to hallucinosis; it means casting doubts on the ideology of the superiority of hallucination over reality, on the ideology that receiving is superior to giving, in renouncing the search or election of a superior idea, being, image, issue (see Transformation in Hallucinosis). Growth depends on realizing that life is not restricted to its material nature.

> The psycho-analytic conception of cure should include the idea of a transformation whereby an element is saturated and thereby made ready for further saturation. Yet a distinction must be made between this dimension of "cure" or "growth" and "greed." [T, 153]

> Dream-like memory is the memory of psychic reality and the stuff of analysis. That which is related to a background of sensuous experience is not suitable to the phenomena of mental life which are shapeless, untouchable, invisible, odourless, tasteless. These

psychically real (in the sense of belonging to psychic reality) elements are what the analyst has to work with. . . .the sacrifice of memory and desire is conducive to the growth of dream-like "memory" which is a part of the experience of psycho-analytical reality. The transformation of the emotional experience into mental growth of analyst and analysand contributes to the difficulty of both to "remember" what took place; in so far as the experience contributes to growth it ceases to be recognizable; if it does not become assimilated it adds to those elements that are remembered and forgotten. Desire obstructs the transformation from knowing and understanding to being, K → O. [AI, 71]

This is a step from "knowledge" (K), to talk about something and understand it, to O, to be at one with reality as it is, an ever-evolving situation. This seems to be difficult: "*The systematic separation into two objects, good and bad, conscious and unconscious, pain and pleasure, ugly and beautiful, had provided a framework which seems to have facilitated the development of knowledge, but the element of growth appears to have escaped formulation especially since it resembles maturation*" (AMF, I, 77).

Growth, + or −, remains inaccessible to thought, if unmistakable to feeling. Conceptual thought and passionate feeling are impossible to relate within the confines of existent universes of discourse [AMF, I, 138]

Is to grow to tolerate paradoxes, the prototype of those paradoxes being the internal object that demands to be perceived in its loved and hated aspects as the one and only object? All texts of Bion seem to indicate this, to the extent that he usually displays at least two faces of the situation; in some cases, more. Growth is also seen as a growth of meaning, accretions of meaning, in thinking processes and in the relationship of container and contained, resulting in growth of container and contained. This is extremely important in a single session of analysis, to the extent that an authoritarian, supportive, idealized professional can work as an analyst. He and the patient will evolve and grow into the unknown through "*tolerated doubt*" (LE, 92) to the extent they allow each other to hear, to associate freely and to "inseminate" each other.

Bion uses models to depict this growth of contained and container (which he denotes by ♀♂) and of the evolving cycles of pre-conceptions in their march to conceptions: that of reticulum, from Elliott Jaques and Tarski's questionnaire with blanks to be filled in, and that of a medium in which *"lie suspended the contents"* protruding, or sprouting from a *"basis which is unknown"*. This model has as its counterparts in reality a baby who sucks, a baby in the uterus, a penis and a vagina, and the model for learning from experience and the accretions of it.

He proposed the signs $♀^n$ and $♂^n$ to the growing ♀♂. The possibility to learn *"depends on the capacity for $♀^n$ to remain integrated and yet lose rigidity"* (LE, 93).Ideally, the evolving learning tends to increased sophistication and tends to infinity (LE, 94). In the growth of knowledge, it is inseparable from the decay, destruction of it, or "minus K". Growth, being related to the stuff of unconscious, is feared: *"Mental evolution or growth is catastrophic and timeless"* (AI, 107–8).

Growth is intrinsically related to pain—commonsensical and medical wisdom observes *"growing pains"* (EP, 63). In discussing the reversible perspective (q.v.), that is, the attempt to turn a dynamic situation into a static one (EP, 60), Bion states that the reversion of perspective, through the excessive use of projective identification, is *"evidence of pain"*. Any development has painful aspects; it can lead to catastrophic changes and abandonment of cherished habits. But to study growth, one refers to events separated in space and time in unbridgeable ways: *"Growth is a phenomenon that appears to present peculiar difficulties to perception either by the growing object or the object that stimulates it, for its relationship with precedent phenomena is obscure and separated in time"*. To help this situation myths are seen as providers of succinct statements *"of psycho-analytic theories which are relevant in aiding the analyst both to perceive growth and to achieve interpretations that illuminate aspects of the patient's problems that belong to growth"* (EP, 63). In myths, growth and pain are constantly conjoined in tolerable ways and may have been an attempt to work through both. Bion suggests at least three myths as primitive models for mental growth: that of the Tree of Knowledge, the Tower of and the city of Babel, and the Sphinx. Growth is also linked to the imbalance or even conflict between narcissism and social-ism as components of the Oedipal situation.

Misuses and misconceptions: A common misunderstanding of the concept of Growth in the work of Bion is mixing it up with a therapeutic/pathologic vertex, implying that growth happens from pathology to cure. The harmony to which Bion refers is a commonsensical harmony of the person with him(her)self, within him or herself. With this, with one he naturally and really is, one must be at one. For some people this state may imply murder—auto-murder or hetero-murder.

The explicit eliciting of the double arrow that represents the interplay quasi-mathematically, in the sense of a to and fro tandem-functioning of Klein's positions, the paper on "Memory and desire" (1967), the second thoughts on cure (ST, 1967), the chapter "Medicine as a model" in *Attention and Interpretation* and the many remarks on cure or yearnings for a better life included in *A Memoir of the Future* furnish many disavowals of such an understanding of growth. Many readers tend to replace some realizations or counterparts of growth in material reality for the growth that Bion refers to. *"It is interesting to consider the relationship that exists when the growth of a mental formulation appears to be matched by a realization of growth that approximates, or is 'parallel' to, the mental formulations"* (T, 42, fn 1).

Difficulty in observing growth *"contributes to the anxiety to establish 'results,' e.g. of analysis"* (EP, 63).

Difficulties in growing

Emotional development, in Bion's view, is impaired by desire, which feeds hallucination:

> Saint Augustine resorted to using the equipment of religion, which is available in many Religions, to express the separation of good from evil. The systematic separation into two objects, good and bad, conscious and unconscious, pain and pleasure, ugly and beautiful, has provided a framework which seems to have facilitated the development of knowledge, but the element of growth appears to have escaped formulation especially since it resembles maturation. [AMF, I, 77]

The concept of "psycho-analytical object" (q.v.) has intrinsic to it the idea of growth; it is discussed more fully in that entry.

Synonym: Development.

Suggested cross-references: Binocular View, Cure, Development, Grid, Psycho-analytical object, Reversion of perspective.

Guilt: Please refer to the entry, Science versus Religion.

H

H: The negative of hate is not love. It may be grasped by its manifestations: seduction is one of them. The hateful nature of the link is disguised; the gossiper, the manipulator, the politician, the overprotective parent. Also, the parents who exercise cruelty when letting their expectations about the children's behaviour prevail.

Recommended cross-references: Links, Minus.

H-link: Please refer to the entry, Links.

Hallucination: Bion uses the term exactly in the same sense that it is classically defined by psychiatry and academic psychology. Bion's contributions are part of a bygone, perhaps golden epoch of a mutually fruitful contribution between psycho-analysis and psychiatry. This epoch lasted from Eugen Bleuler to Silvano Arieti, having as its great contributors professionals of the stature of the brothers Menninger, Harry Stack Sullivan, Donald Winnicott, Herbert Rosenfeld, Henry Ey, André Green, Clifford Scott, among others. During the time of the writing of this dictionary this cross-pollination was brought to a halt. (It does not belong to the scope of this dictionary to conjecture or investigate if this halting is the first sign of extinction or what factors contributed to it.)

Hallucination defines perceptions that have no real object to stimulate a sensuous receptor; in other terms, it is objectless, false perception. The mind creates images or other sensuous manifestations from nothing, in a process akin to that one observes in dreams. Starting from this definition Bion broadens its scope and investigates its nature.

He notices that patients who cannot dream, or hallucinate dreams, resort, in waking life, to a special form of imaging (sometimes also other sensuous manifestations). These images seem to function as a means of communication of the unthought, undreamt—that which seems not to be tolerated intrapsychically.

Bion states that in his experience "*such observation of the hallucinatory process is essential and rewarding*". His reconsideration of the term does not modify it but augments its scope. It illuminates a function and the *nature* of hallucination, eliciting its "group" character, that is, a process involving two people rather than one, as if it were a neutral observer "observing" the other being's madness.

Function

Hallucinatory activity seemed to be "*an attempt to deal with the dangerous parts*" of the personality (ST, 71). In the wake of this and also as its leitmotiv, hallucination "*is an attempt at cure*". This is in line with Freud's observation about the paths to the formation of symptoms (*New Introductory Lectures*).

His first published analytic observation of hallucination makes full use of Klein's perceptions on the phantasy of projective and introjective identification: patients hallucinate to be able concretely to both eject and engulf feelings and ideas and even a whole person: "*It may have been that he was so manipulating the analysis and myself that I felt I was no longer an independent object, but was being treated by him as an hallucination*".

He observes a patient who felt that "*his eyes could suck something out of me*"; the eyes could also make an "*expulsion*" of that which he had sucked in, hallucinatorily (ST, 67). One may observe that Bion was able to exercise both practically and theoretically a basic psycho-analytic ability first exercised by Freud, namely, a dynamic view that allows a tolerance of paradoxes: in this case, the openness that allowed for the observation of an "in" and "out" phantasy, occurring simultaneously.

One of the practical applications can be regarded as a practice akin to preventive psychiatry: *"An awareness of the double meaning that verbs of sense have for the psychotic sometimes makes it possible to detect an hallucinatory process before it betrays itself by more familiar signs"* (ST, 67). The more familiar signs correspond to overt disturbance known in psychiatry as schizophrenia and malignant feelings of persecution. Bion's allegiance to Freud's view on the "curative" function of symptoms shows him to be a helper who aids the psychiatrist, avoiding a judgmental posture:

> Hallucinations and the fantasy of the senses as ejecting as well as receiving, point to the severity of the disorder from which the patient is suffering, but I must indicate a benign quality in the symptom which was certainly not present earlier. Splitting, evacuatory use of the senses, and hallucinations were all being employed in the service of an ambition to be cured, and may therefore be supposed to be creative activities. [ST, 68]

Nature

> Hallucination may be more profitably seen as a dimension of the analytic situation in which, together with the remaining "dimensions", these objects are sense-able (if we include analytic intuition or consciousness, taking a lead from Freud, as a sense-organ of psychic quality). [T, 115]

In 1965, Bion would insert the classical definition of hallucination into his expansion of Freud's framework of the functions of the ego—which include definition, notation, attention, memory. To these Bion added the pre-conception, the *"intuitive psycho-analytic background"* (T, 138).

He *"may now reconsider the term 'hallucination'. It must be distinguished from an illusion or delusion because both these terms are required to represent other phenomena, namely those that are associated with pre-conceptions that turn to conceptions because they mate with realizations that do not approximate to the pre-conceptions closely enough to saturate the pre-conception, but closely enough to give rise to a conception or misconception"* (T, 137).

Illusion is thus a misrepresentation stemming from a false perception with a factually real stimulus; it is a false perception from an existent object due to distortion by feelings. In his terms, it is a mating of a pre-conception with an external realization that leads to a mis-conception. Delusions are logical illogicalities. The deluded person builds with the aid of rationality stories stemming from false premises; this also leads to mis-conceptions.

A pre-conception must form a concept: *"The pre-conception requires saturation by a realization that is **not** an evacuation of the senses but has an existence independent of the personality"* (T, 137). This requirement is a kind of insurance against hallucination. In theoretical terms, Bion is using Melanie Klein and Freud's contributions. In this point, psychiatry is enriched by analysis—for the first time the *mechanism of formation* of hallucination is investigated. Hallucination, in its turn, *"arises from a pre-determination and requires satisfaction from (a) an evacuation from the personality and (b) from conviction that the element **is** its own evacuation"* (T, 137).

The "groupish" nature of hallucination, that is, its dependence on an interaction of at least two points of view, from the patient and from the analyst, introduces the awareness of the interference of the observer in the phenomenon observed, brought to light by Freud, Planck and Heisenberg. It also relates to Bion's affiliation to John Rickman, i.e. a "two-body psychology" (q.v.). This kind of tolerance of "two-ness" is a hallmark of Bion's contributions to psycho-analysis.

> Confusion occurs if due weight is not given to the fact that the total conjunction bound by the term hallucination is associated with two different points of view, or, as I prefer to call it, with two different vertices, one represented by the patient, the other by the analyst. [T, 137–8]

From the beginning Bion was able to use Freud's hint in "Constructions in analysis", namely, Freud's inspiration by Goethe, which seemed to enable him to compare the analyst's constructions with the delusions of the patients, *"delusions may be the equivalents of the constructions which we build up in the course of an analytic treatment—attempts at explanation and cure"* (ST, 82).

This hint helped him to refine the observation of the analyst's state of mind; and he did this through fuller profiting from the observation of hallucination. The refinement includes the differentiation of dreaming and hallucination. First, as those activities appear in the patient, and thereafter, as they appear in the analyst.

Both patient and analyst could—and should—"dream the session" (q.v.) as he saw from 1959 to 1965. From then on it became clear that the issue was not just a dream-like one. A fact that characterized Bion's own path in psycho-analysis also showed itself as a necessary path of any analysis. At least an analysis that considers the research into the unknown (meaning, *unbewußt*, unconscious) made with unknown limits (meaning, with a tendency to the infinite) as an integral part of the very act of analysing. A turning point was his final abandonment of the psychiatric criteria in pathology and cure. Psychiatry seems to be helpful to psycho-analysis with regard to diagnosis but not to conduct. Another seminal issue was his realization of the states of hallucinosis. That is, states apparently normal or socially acceptable, which coincide with the analyst's habits or codes of conduct. In those states the omnipotent phantasies of superiority occurring in the session may pass unnoticed— both to analyst and analysand. When an analytic couple can push the eliciting of the psychotic personality as far as possible, the patient realizes his capacity to hallucinate, and the analyst should accompany him(her). In 1967 he would put the issue thus:

> The proper state for intuiting psycho-analytical realizations . . ..can be compared with the states supposed to provide conditions for hallucinations. The hallucinated individual is apparently having sensuous experiences without any background of sensuous reality. The psycho-analyst must be able to intuit psychic reality which has no sensuous realization. The hallucinated individual transforms and interprets the background of reality, of which he is aware, in different terms from those employed by the psycho-analyst. I do not consider that the hallucinated patient is reporting a realization with a sensuous background; equally I do not consider an interpretation in psycho-analysis derives from facts accessible to sensuous apparatus. How then is one to explain the difference between an hallucination and an interpretation of an intuited psycho-analytical experience? The charge is sometimes loosely and lightly made that psycho-analysts psycho-analysing patients who are psychotic are themselves psychotic. I would seek a formulation to represent the difference between the intuition (in my sense of the term) of a realization, which has no sensible component, and a hallucination

of a realization which is similarly devoid of a *sensible* realization. The psycho-analyst has at least the opportunity which would allow him to contribute an answer; many supposedly sane and responsible people transform thoughts into actions which it would be charitable to call insane and are often, charitably, so called . . .

Ordinarily the sense organs have their own objects of sense . . . In the mental realm, the "sense organ of psychic quality", to borrow a phrase from Freud, has no such limitation. It can indifferently appreciate *all* the counterparts of *all* the senses. The mental counterparts of smell, sight, etc., can all, apparently be intuited by the same apparatus. The issue is of practical importance to the psycho-analyst whose analysand says, "I see what you mean" when he has a hallucination, say, of being sexually assaulted; what *he* means is that the *meaning* of what the psycho-analyst said appeared to him in a visual form and *not* that he understood an interpretation [ST, 163–4]

Or, still more synthetically, three years later:

Receptiveness achieved by denudation of memory and desire (which is essential to the operation of "acts of faith') is essential to the operation of psycho-analysis and other scientific proceedings. It is essential for experiencing hallucination or the state of hallucinosis.

This state I do not regard as an exaggeration of a pathological or even natural condition: I consider it rather to be a state always present, but overlaid by other phenomena, which screen it. If these other elements can be moderated or suspended hallucinosis becomes demonstrable . . . Elements of hallucinosis of which it is possible to be sensible are the grosser manifestations and are of secondary importance; to appreciate hallucination the analyst must participate in the state of hallucinosis. [AI, 36]

Misuses and misconceptions: A prevailing idea in some quarters is that hallucination for Bion differs from hallucination in psychiatry. It seems that those readers could not realize that Bion illuminates two different uses, that of the psychiatrist and that of the analyst, of the same phenomenon. For example, when trying to show that "the analytic situation requires greater width and depth than can be provided by a model from Euclidean space", he stresses that there is an extensive usage of unfamiliar and unfamiliarly vague undefined (for the analyst) expressions. Those are the beta-elements at work; "Such a patient can talk of a 'penis black with rage' or an 'eye green with envy' as being visible in a painting. These objects may not be visible to the analyst: he may think the patient is hallucinating them. But such an idea, perhaps sound to the view of a psychiatrist, is not penetrating enough for his work as an analyst" (T, 115).

He would state this again: "I explain that existing descriptions of hallucinations are not good enough for practising psychoanalysts" (ST, 160). Only closed minds would read it as if it disparages existing views. To amend, to improve, differ from to eliminate. Bion states that the existing analytic—not only psychiatric—explanations of hallucination are not enough—including his own. Again, not enough does not mean, "psychiatry is wrong".

Another serious misconception is a kind of praise of folly. There are readers who think that the analyst must hallucinate in the session; they mistake the idea of the analyst's participation in the state of hallucinosis (see above, in the quotation of AI, 30) with the analyst's hallucinations. The latter must be dealt with in the analyst's analysis; the latter means a state of sympathy, concern for life, discernment on projective identification, forbearance to the patient's envy and greed and omnipotence and realization of hyperbole (q.v.). To participate in hallucinosis is a step towards the realization of the patient's hallucination and a discrimination of the participants of the couple.

Lest any doubts remain, one may see the last clear definition of hallucination:

> Verbal, musical, artistic modes of communication all meet with realizations that they appear to represent only very approximately. Hallucination may be regarded, wrongly, as a representation and therefore as unsuited to some activities. As verbal, musical, and artistic transformations have compensating values arising from their being *transformations of O*, it is natural to consider the like possibility with hallucinosis. But hallucinations are *not* representations: they are things-in-themselves born of intolerance of frustration and desire. Their defects are due not to their failure to represent but to their failure to *be*. [AI, 18]

⊕ Echoing Freud's view about his own work with dreams, Bion's views on hallucination did not change throughout his life.

Anyway, he strongly hoped that readers could find functions other than those of hallucinated evacuation (ST, 160). The revision in *Second Thoughts* is used to re-affirm the need to *"'intuit' hallucinations"* and to respect the evolving nature of the analytical experience. The clinical study that he made is used to re-confirm this living nature of the analytical experience: *"The psycho-analyst must not allow himself to be deflected from the vertex from which the emotional events, when they have evolved, become 'intuitable'. The study of hallucination is at its beginning, not its end"* (ST, 161). The expansion in *Transformations* and the enlivened depiction of hallucinated characters (for example Alice, who hallucinated a marriage) in *A Memoir of the Future* shows some of the possibilities.

📖 As this entry does not include detailed clinical experiences (empirical data) that support the theory, it would be useful to consult them, even taking into account the difficulties in putting a psycho-analytical experience down on paper (ST, 65–81; C, 15; 23, 82, 83, 88. 89). In the opinion of the author, a firm grasp of the definitions of hallucination in psychiatry is mandatory.

Hallucinosis:

> This state I do not regard as an exaggeration of a pathological or even natural condition: I consider it rather to be a state always present, but overlaid by other phenomena, which screen it. If these other elements can be moderated or suspended hallucinosis becomes demonstrable. [AI, 36]

Bion's use of the psychiatric concept of hallucinosis does not modify it but expands its scope. Seen under the vertex of mental functioning, it is one of the forms that transformations assume. As occurs since Freud's perceptions about symptoms as the last bastions of health and the universality of neuroses, it is not restricted to the realm of pathology. Analysis provides a condition to observe it in so-called normal people. In psychiatry, hallucinosis is the presence of hallucinations in an otherwise conserved personality.

The first time that Bion mentions hallucinosis is when he comments on the manifestations of the intolerance of the no-breast and its subsequent procedures after provocations to substitute the *"thing for the no-thing, and the thing itself as an instrument to take the place of representations when representations are a necessity as they are in the realm of thinking. Thus actual murder is to be sought instead of the thought represented by the word 'murder', an actual breast or penis rather than the thought represented by those words, and so on until quite complex actions and real objects are elaborated as part of acting-out. Such procedures do not produce the results ordinarily achieved by thought, but contribute to states approximating to stupor, fear of stupor, hallucinosis, fear of hallucinosis, megalomania and fear of megalomania"* (T, 82).

One may perceive that the elaborate acting-out in outer reality is accepted as normal by the encircling milieu. This association gives the appearance of an otherwise conserved personality the exact meaning of the psychiatric category of hallucinosis—the presence of hallucination in a generally conserved personality.

Experiencing a state of hallucinosis is possible and necessary when the analyst or any scientist has as their aim, "O" (AI, 29, 36). When one denudes oneself of memory and desire, one attains a state of *"receptiveness"* (AI, 34). In experiencing this state, one is able to perform an *"act of faith"*. *"It is essential for experiencing hallucination or the state of hallucinosis"* (AI, 36). Bion does not regard this state *"as an exaggeration of a pathological or even natural condition"*. He rather considers it *"to be a state always present, but overlaid by other phenomena, which screen it. If these other elements can be moderated or suspended hallucinosis becomes demonstrable; its full depth and richness are accessible only to 'acts of faith'. Elements of hallucinosis of which it is possible to be sensible are the grosser manifestations and are of secondary importance; to appreciate hallucination the analyst must participate in the state of hallucinosis ... By eschewing memories, desires, and the operations of memory he can approach the domain of hallucinosis and of the 'acts of faith' by which alone he can become at one with his patient's hallucinations and so effect transformations O⇒K"* (AI, 36).

Misuses and misconceptions: Many readers mistake the very clear statement of Bion as praising folly, arguing that an analyst must hallucinate. "Must participate", "at-one" means a sympathetic observation, rather than an acting-out. One must not do something that happens by itself.

Suggested cross-references: Faith, Transformations in hallucinosis.

Hate: Please refer to the entry, Links.

Herd:Please refer to the entry, Establishment.

📖 *Instincts of the Herd in War and Peace*, by Wilfred R. Trotter. This is one of the most basic foundations of Bion's thought, together with Freud, Klein and the philosophers of the Classical era and of the Enlightenment.

Hyperbole: The term defines a fact that does not constitute a theory of psycho-analysis, but as with the vast majority of Bion's contributions, it is a theory of psycho-analytic observation. It is based on Klein's theory of projective identification:

> ... I shall regard the Kleinian theory of Projective Identification as a psycho-analytic formulation ... based on a background of realizations encountered in analytic practice and in every-day life: these realizations I shall call "hyperbole". "Hyperbole" is a term belonging to the system of Theories of Observation in contrast to the theory of Projective Identification, which I regard as a term belonging to the system of Psycho-analytical Theory ... The domains of Theories of Observation and Theories of Psycho-analysis overlap but the problem is simplified if a distinction is made and can be preserved ... "Hyperbole" is the term I give, in theories of observation, to the realizations that correspond to the theory of projective identification. [T, 160]

The observational concept of hyperbole uses a visual image drawn from algebraic geometry in order to try to depict a violent over-exaggeration of feelings. It aims to force the container to tolerate those very feelings that appear exaggerated. The exaggeration tries to ensure attention. The container may react in many ways. Sometimes the result is reverie (q.v.); sometimes it reacts with more evacuation.

⊕ The term was suggested in 1965. The clinical situation it refers to was the object of Bion's studies in earlier times. It constitutes one of the many examples in the work of Bion (repeating that which happened with Freud and Klein's work) of the purely empirical approach to psycho-analysis, drawn from clinical experience. A fact that was already existent but remained unobserved, has been gradually intuited, perceived and only after considerable work, gained the status of something that could be named. It is the scientific posture in contrast to the religious posture, which usually names the unknown before knowing even small parts of it. It is a posture that avoids transforming psycho-analysis into a vast paramnesia to fill the void of our ignorance, as he would state in 1976, 77 and 79 (in the short papers, "Evidence" and "Emotional turbulence" as well as in *A Memoir of the Future*). One can see that its still un-named counterpart in reality is that which Bion described as the *"fate of the expelled fragments"* of personality after the phantasized expelling that was described by Melanie Klein. In 1956 he described a "fate" characterized by fragments which *"consist of a real external object which is encapsulated in a piece of personality that has engulfed it"* (ST, 39). This referred to the "final" status of the particles, as bizarre objects; from there on he proceeded to describe the "trajectory" and the features of the deployment. To describe this he follows Freud's suggestions about symptoms being the last bastions of health: *"Hallucinations and the fantasy of the senses as ejecting as well as receiving, point to the severity of the disorder from which the patient is suffering, but I must indicate a benign quality in the symptom . . . Splitting, evacuatory use of the senses, and hallucinations were all being employed in the service of an ambition to be cured, and may therefore be supposed to be creative activities"* (ST, 68).

In 1957 he came to realize that the objects were thrown in hallucination to distant places in space and time (ST, 75). In 1958 he focuses his attention on the patient's strivings *"to force"* parts of his personality into the analyst *"with increased desperation and violence"* when the patient *"felt"*—the word is here seminal, it is just a feeling—that the analyst *"refused to accept parts of his personality"* (all quotations ST, 103–4). What does this mean? It means that Bion was keeping track of both the patient's movements and the analyst's reactions and the extent they could influence the patient's communications. The catch 22 situation was that *"in the patient's belief . . . the analyst strives, by understanding the patient, to drive him insane"* (ST, 107). This paradox that typifies psychosis, when primary envy and primary narcissism are a fact, would mark the rest of his investigations, which would lead him to the formulations of transformations in hallucinosis and hyperbole. He was able to see that a *"constant conjunction of increasing force of emotion with increasing force of evacuation"* was continuously evolving in a kind of self-feeding process of envy and greed, akin to an atomic chain reaction (he had already used the image before, in 1956). The phrase was used in 1960 and was to be repeated in 1965, when finally he was able to use a term derived from geometry that depicted this ever-swelling process (C, 249; T, 142). The term hyperbole finally binds this constant conjunction.

Its definition and use is wholly contained in the book *Transformations*. Remarkably, it is defined in more than one place. In this author's view, the clearest definition appears late in the book, in the last chapter:

> The term "hyperbole" has a history which fits it for compact representation of a number of clinical statements which (i) occur frequently, (ii) are easily recognizable as instances of hyperbole and (iii) are almost certainly symptomatic of a constant conjunction which has significance for the personality being analysed and for the main body of psycho-analytic theories of idealization, splitting, projective identification, rivalry and envy ... it has a wide spectrum, is flexible and lends itself easily for use by the analyst as a "selected fact" to aid in displaying coherence which, without it, may not be apparent. "Hyperbole" can be regarded as representing hyperbole, and hyperbole is projection conjoined with rivalry, ambition, vigour which can amount to violence and hence to "distance" to which an object is projected. [T, 162]

The term **distance** is defined by Bion not just in the sense of Euclidean tri-dimensional space but also in the sense of differential calculus. In 1965 he was fully able to integrate his view that the mathematician's problems shared the quality of the psychotic's problems; space and time are not units that can be recognized in the unconscious, but are rather conscious unreal constructions of the rational mind—a discovery made almost simultaneously by Freud in psycho-analysis and by Einstein in physics. In terms of psychic reality, this distance admits no measurement; it is "*a non-existent quantity*" constantly conjoined with a hallucination; "*it could be where quantity was or where it will be but not where it is*, it represents an unsaturated element, an evanescent increment" (all quotations from T, 162).

Its realization is more feasible through the depiction of clinical experiences; Bion furnishes it with a series of four statements made by a patient:

1. I have always believed you are a very good analyst.

2. I knew a woman in Peru, when I was a child, who had second sight.

3. It seems to me psycho-analysts would do better if they believed in God: God *can* cure.

4. There ought not be so much pain and suffering in the world. What can a mere human being do?

The interpretation of these statements would depend on circumstances which I cannot report here; the suggestions I make must be seen as related to exposition and not clinical experience.

Comment:

1. (a) The goodness of the analyst stops short, as it were, in my person. I am "it".

(b) The goodness of the analyst is incarnate in me. I am the embodiment of analytic goodness.

(c) The goodness of the analyst is incorporated in me. Either I have obtained possession of the goodness of the analyst by "taking it into" myself or some force has "put it into" me.

Which of these statements represents the facts most closely depends on the judgment the analyst forms in the emotional experience itself.

2. (a) The goodness of the analyst has been projected a long way in time and place. This is hyperbole; there is something in the experience with the analysand that makes this term suitable for binding the particular conjunction, and none other . . . the early meaning of hyperbole as a "throwing beyond" someone else, signifying rivalry.

(b). The goodness of the analyst has been thrown "into" the woman, or Peru, or the past. [T, 160–161]

There is a justification, now in scientific terms, to use the expression hyperbole:

It is a commonplace that any attempt at scientific inquiry involves distortion through the exaggeration of certain elements in order to display their significance. This characteristic is present in L and H as much as in K. In order to link its phenomenological counterpart in analytic practice, with the penumbra of associations that I regard as significant. I shall call this characteristic hyperbole. I mean the term to convey an impression of exaggeration, of rivalry and, by retention of its original significance, throwing and out-distancing. The appearance of hyperbole in any form must be regarded as significant of a transformation in which rivalry, envy and evacuation are operating. There is a profound difference between "being" O and rivalry with O. The latter is characterized by envy, hate, love, megalomania and the state known by analysts as acting out, which must be sharply differentiated from acting; which is characteristic of "being" O.

Just as exaggeration is helpful in clarifying a problem, so it can be felt to be important to exaggerate in order to gain the attention necessary to have a problem clarified. Now the "clarification" of a primitive emotion depends on its being contained by a container which will detoxicate it. In order to enlist the aid of the container the emotion must be exaggerated. The "container" may be a "good breast", internal or external, which is able to detoxicate the emotion. Or the container may not be able to tolerate the emotion and the contained emotion may not to be able to tolerate neglect. The result is hyperbole. That is to say, the emotion that cannot tolerate neglect grows in intensity, is exaggerated to ensure attention and the container reacts by more, and still more, violent evacuation. By using the term "hyperbole" I mean to bind the constant conjunction of increasing force of emotion with increasing force of evacuation. It is immaterial to hyperbole what the emotion is; but on the emotion will depend whether the hyperbolic expression is idealizing or denigrating. [T, 141–2]

The term was used to help the formulation of transformations in "O"; in the wake of Freud, one cannot know what sanity is without realizing what insanity is. To the reader who still is not acquainted with Bion's concepts of K, O and transformations in O, the contents of the following quotation ought to be fully grasped if read conjointly with the entry "O":

It is possible through phenomena to be reminded of the "form". It is possible through "incarnation" to be united with a part, the incarnate part, of the Godhead. It is possible through hyperbole for the individual to deal with the real individual . . .

The "cause" O may be felt to be present or absent, single or multiple, independent of the personality or hallucinated. O, in its "caused" dimension, as in all others, may be located in the Platonic Form, of which people and things are "reminders"; in a deity, of which people and things are "incarnations"; in hyperbole, of which people and things are containers. [T, 148 and 152]

Recommended cross-references: O, Saturation, Transformations in Hallucinosis.

Suggested cross-reference: Mathematization of psychoanalysis.

I

Idea: One of the names assigned to the Grid (q.v.) at the decisive moment that it is being used consciously after or before a session; or unconsciously as a result of the analyst's free floating attention during a session (EP, 28). This may be the only intra-session "use" of the Grid, which cannot be characterized exactly as such due to its unconscious nature. This use partakes of the qualities of the dream. Bion denoted it through the use of the sign *I*.

> The grid and the concept of transformations are altered by the situation they are devised to examine in proportion as they are brought to bear on it. They retain their character so long as they are employed *away* from the tense situation; after a session in which they have been employed, though so transformed by Taαand by the tension of the session that the analyst may not be able to see that grid and transformation are in use, they resume the characteristics they possess extra-analytically. This is disquieting, but no one who tries to use the grid or transformation concepts in a session would doubt that it is true. Unless transformed so that the instrument (O = the grid) has become Taβ it loses power to illuminate during the session, but regains it afterwards.

No one can understand the grid or transformations without experience of their use as part of psycho-analytic practice . . .

Although home work is not done in an atmosphere of emotional tension, grid and transformation theory are applied to the recollection of such situations. The analyst's intuition, which it is the object of these reviews to exercise and develop, is operating in contact with the tense situation. It is important to distinguish between the grid (as it appears in my scheme) operating in tranquillity on recollections, and the grid as part of the analyst's intuitive contact with the emotional situation itself. [75–76]

With *I* Bion tries to represent either the whole Grid or one of its components distinguished by the coordinates of the Grid's horizontal and vertical axes. *I* also applies to the patient and this living functioning is called by Bion the very *"apparatus for thinking"*.

In introducing *I* Bion introduces a novelty in his early model for the apparatus of thinking. He couples the model of the human digestive apparatus that was adumbrated in *Learning from Experience* with the reproductive apparatus that is involved in the model of container and contained. The full cycle of integration between the two models would be closed in 1970, in his book *Attention and Interpretation*.

For now he states that this apparatus for thinking deals with *"primitive categories of* **I** *. . .* **I** *develops a capacity for any one of its aspects to assume indifferently the function* ♀ *or* ♂ *to any other one of its aspects* ♀ *or* ♂*. We must now consider I in its* ♀ ♂ *operation, an operation usually spoken of in ordinary conversation as thinking"* (EP, 31). This encompasses bi-sexuality (after Freud, 1905) and primitive sexuality (after Klein, that is, the relationship between the breast and the infant: *"From the point of view of meaning thinking depends on the successful introjection of the good breast that is originally responsible for the performance of α-function. On this introjection depends the ability of any part of* **I** *to be* ♂ *to the other part's* ♀*"* (EP, 32).

& The author proposed a more explicit integration of the two models to the apparatus of thinking in 1997, published in 2000 (Sandler, 2000). This integration is an attempt at illuminating the operation of both the analyst and the patient's feminine and masculine aspects at the moment that the analyst must perform a receptive, containing function when he or she intuitively exercises his

capacity for free floating attention as well as the patient's need to be masculine when he or she expresses his or her free associations prodigally.

Suggested cross references: Container/Contained, Grid, Intuition.

Imagination: This entry intends to make clear the uses of the verbal term, "imagination", in the work of Bion. Its etymological meaning corresponds to the human being's ability "to make images". The colloquial use had suffered a stretching of its semantic field. It seems to have been influenced by the idealistic/relativistic/solipsistic or subjectivist trend in philosophy. It came to express and to defend the creative powers of the individual mind.

The fact that psycho-analysis deals with immaterial facts seemed to have created a fertile soil for an early adoption of a kind of "praise of folly", in the wake of idealism, subjectivism and solipsism. The vicissitudes of the idealist seem to be forgotten or ignored by most of the psycho-analytic movement. This occurred despite the warnings of Freud in, for example, "The question of a *Weltanschauung*". Many other authors such as Ferenczi, Menninger and Reik contributed to the perception of this trend. Nevertheless there was praise for imagination.

Bion's thrust into the unknown and into the imaginative powers of the human being seemed to entice the idealism-prone professional; the same occurred with the work of Melanie Klein and Donald Winnicott. Those original authors did not defend a "creativity" exclusively based on an individual mind. Quite to the contrary, it is easily demonstrable that creativity for them meant an encounter with the person with his or her own unconscious self. In Freud's terms, the meeting of unconscious and conscious, the meeting between ego and id. The "two-ness" is a condition of life, both in material and psychic reality. In Bion's work, as in that of Freud, there is always the presence of antithetical pairs and their outcome, the synthesis. The theory of object relations is a model that depicts the inception of an alternative to autism.

In Bion's work, one may quote many passages that vouch for his allegiance to the scientific, rather than to the idealistic vertex:

A theory of transformations must be composed of elements and constitute a system capable of the greatest number of uses (represented by the horizontal axis of the grid) if it is to extend the analyst's capacity for working on a problem with or without the material components of the problem present.

This may seem to introduce a dangerous doctrine opening the way for the analyst who theorizes unhampered by the facts of practice, but the theory of transformations is inapplicable to any situation in which observation is not an essential. Observation is to be made and recorded in a form suitable for working *with* but is inimical to wayward and undisciplined fabrications . . . In short, the theory is to aid observation and recording in terms suitable for scientific manipulation without the presence of the objects. [T, 39–40]

That is, many defend the idea that imagination should exist independent of facts. Or that which one calls "facts" are just constructions of the mind. The interference of the observer in the object observed is mistaken for the non-existence of the object observed—a distrust of truth and reality in the end run. For sure the mind is able to do that which the idealist thinks is the one and only way; it imagines while detached from reality in states of autism, delusions and hallucinations.

Very early on Bion was able not to fall into this trap that confounded and still confounds sizable parts of the philosophical movement. The philosopher is spared from facts, practical issues; he tries to denounce both the "psychologization" and the "essentialism". But the more he does this, the more exposed he is to the risk of falling into those very psychologizations and essentialisms that he dreads. In denying the existence of ultimate realities—instead of perceiving their unknowability—he defines and knows the "ultimatest" reality of them all: that of the non-existence of whatever may be outside the creative powers of the individual unrestrained mind. The issue is perhaps deep-rooted: it may lie in the denial of the supremely creative pair, the parental couple, as Melanie Klein tried to show.

Reality always provides stimuli that are felt as offences to a man or woman's narcissism. Bion tried to avoid this millennia-old philosophical conundrum (realism versus idealism), a false issue, in observing the issue psycho-analytically. When examining a case where a patient seems to challenge common sense, he resorts to the philosophy of science. His patient sees blood everywhere, and he tries to integrate the philosopher's contributions with the psycho-analytical vertex. The reading of the case is important and can be found in the second chapter of *Cogitations*, on Scientific Method. Just the parts that are relevant to the discussion of imagination will be quoted. Bion asks, "*Where is the patient's common sense? What has happened to it?*" (C, 17) (see the entry, Common Sense, in this dictionary).

In discussing this, in searching for an inner truth in the psychotic's production that seems to be too painful for the psychotic mind to bear, he brings to the fore the fact that positivism or classical logic, the self-called "realism" can be at the service of the wildest idealism:

I have accepted as scientifically sound the idea that common sense may be, and should be, accepted as the arbiter that decides what are the facts in external reality to which these mental activities relate. The philosopher of science has always been brought to a standstill at this point, caught between the logic of the idealist philosopher on the one hand, and the feeling of unreality to which an acceptance of such logic would expose him on the other. There is essentially no difference between the reactions of Braithwaite and Doctor Johnson to the demands of the idealist. . .

I know the patient's hatred of reality is strongly coloured by the feeling that a sense of reality carries with it a stimulation of the socially polarized aspect of his emotional drives, and that this stimulation is felt to menace the ego-centric aspect of his emotional drives and therefore his narcissism, thus increasing his fear of annihilation. I know, therefore, that a belief that his common sense has been lost, destroyed or alienated is quite compatible with and illuminant of his previously expressed hatred of reality or the mental apparatus that might link him with it. . .

Before Hume's insistence that there is nothing in a scientific hypothesis but a generalization and that any added element does not belong to the scientific generalization properly speaking, but is only the psychological factor in the observer which he recognized as a tendency in the human mind for certain ideas to be associated together, philosophers of science were not prepared to admit either that this something extra to the generalization did not exist, or that its existence lay in the personality of the human being. It was supposed that this something was analogous to the logic of the human mind. My view diverges from the view that the scientific hypothesis or law includes more than a generalization and that that something is a function of external reality. It approximates to the views of those epistemologists—Kant, Whewell, Mill, Peirce, Poincaré, Russell and Popper—who tend to the beliefs compatible with the idea that scientific knowledge is the result of the growth of common-sense knowledge. My agreements—and disagreements—with these epistemologists are a direct consequence of a psycho-analytic investigation of the phenomena known to all of them under various synonyms for scientific common sense. It is my view that the impasse in which the scientists and philosophers of science find themselves is not capable of further adumbration, let alone resolution, without the employment of psycho-analytic research, and more precisely research into the phenomena collectively called common sense ... In fact I do not consider that the elaboration of a deductive system from facts declared by common sense to be so can be separated from the earlier phenomenon which is a precondition for the elaboration of a deductive system, namely the inspiration ...

Analysis and synthesis are both involved in understanding. If the act is carried our lovingly it leads to understanding; if carried out violently, i.e. violently with hate, then it leads to splitting and cruel juxtaposition or fusion. [C, 15, 19, 21, 22]

In other words, because of his psycho-analytical formation and experience with psychosis, Bion was not prone to accept the over-simplistic positivistic approach. But he also was not—also due to this contact with real facts provided by clinical work—prone to accept the easy way out of the problems created by the positivists, namely, nihilistic idealism.

Bion was able to see that the scientific hypothesis or law could not be more than a mental formulation, in the wake of Hume's perceptions of constant conjunctions. What often passes unobserved is that the scientific hypothesis is not reality itself, even though it purports to depict some realities and pretends to have a counterpart in reality. This fact, that the law is a mental formulation, does not deny that a reality exists. That reality remains stubbornly outside the reach of human schemes—as Kant called them, or models—as Freud and Bion called them. This means that the models cannot acquire a reality of their own as if they could replace the reality they purport to describe. There are people who believe that id or super-ego exist in factual concrete reality; Freud was not among them.

Years later Bion would state the flights of imagination disguised as science in a dialogical form:

P.A. . . . I do not see why an infinitely small biological particle being whirled round the galactic centre on a speck of dirt—called by us the Earth—should, in the course of an ephemeral life that does not last even a thousand revolutions round a sun, imagine that the Universe of Galaxies conforms to its limitations.

PAUL The laws of nature are only the laws of scientific thought.

ROBIN It is readily assumed, filled with meaning, that these colossal forces "obey" these laws as we obey social conventions. [AMF, II, 229–30]

It was not for nothing that Bion brought to the psycho-analysts' awareness a then-forgotten aphorism of Kant, "*concepts without intuition are empty; intuition without concepts are blind*". Again, the use of intuition seemed to be fertile soil for hasty idealistic interpretations of Bion's work. This intuition is seminal and necessary due to the immaterial nature of psycho-analysis, but to dissociate intuition from the scientific approach is alien to Bion's work:

What psycho-analytic thinking requires is a method of notation and rules for its employment that will enable work to be done in the *absence* of the object, to facilitate further work in the *presence* of the object. The barrier to this that is presented by unfettered play of an analyst's phantasies has long been recognized; pedantic statement on the one hand and verbalization loaded with unobserved implications on the other mean that the potential for misunderstanding and erroneous deduction is so high as to vitiate the value of the work done with such defective tools. [T, 44]

The quotations included in the entries, "Atonement, "The Minus Realm" and "Mathematizing psycho-analysis" further illuminate the issue.

Imagination also strikes unobserved in socially shared conventions—hallucinosis. The following text can perhaps represent the ultimate views of Bion concerning facts and imagination as well as the qualities of the language to convey truth:

ROLAND Don't be a bloody cunt. Do you want me to tell you the dream or not?

P.A. Do go on—

ALICE Well, really! Are you supposed to listen to language like this? It is not even sexual—as P.A. would agree.

ROLAND All right Xanthippe, darling. Socrates' complaint is comprehensible if we are not allowed to discuss naturally and spontaneously

ALICE I have no objection at all, but surely it is not necessary to talk like that. Yes, I know—you are going to say "like what?", but I shan't repeat such . . . such . . . language, though you are trying to make me use the words. You know very well what I mean, but I have to think of Rosemary. I am sure she agrees.

ROSEMARY Oh yes, Ma'am, I do. My mum was very particular how she brought me up. When I asked her what she and her gentleman were doing—I had come into the room innocently because Patricia our dog was barking so loud—Trixie we used to call him because it sounded less girlish if you see what I mean—him being a dog and not a bitch if you excuse the expression, Ma'am.

ROBIN Oh God-all-fucking-mighty—do get on will you.

ALICE There you go again—is it necessary to be blasphemous to make yourself clear?

P.A. He is speaking rhapsodically—not with social or scientific precision.

ROLAND Robin will agree with me that he is being no more blasphemous than I am when I say "bloody cunt"; bloody is only a quick way of saying "by Our Lady"—which is sacred. Go on, Rosemary, for Christ's sake.

ROBIN Oh Cripes!

ROLAND "Schoolboy" for Christ. Anyhow, *please* get on.

ALICE Now he has become sufficiently civilized to say "please", go on Rosemary.

ROSEMARY Oh, yes, Ma'am—my mum was always most particular and wore a crucifix all the time because she told me I should never forget Our Lord, especially when the gentlemen came to see us. That was how I found out that she *only* had high-class gentlemen like lords to see her though my friend Faith—she was called that out of Faith, Hope and Charity—

ALICE I won't ask you two what you are thinking because I can see it in your faces.

ROBIN There must be something wrong with the small muscles of our faces Roland.

ROLAND "Myasthenia gravis", no doubt. But Rosemary's story is so exciting that I can hardly wait to hear.

ALICE Then why don't you two fucking bastards shut up and let her get on? Can't you control your face muscles? See—I can talk that stuff as you can.

ROLAND I am sure P.A. knew you always could.

ALICE Go on, Rosemary—don't take any notice of the ugly faces they make.

ROSEMARY That's what my mum always used to say me. "Rosemary", she says "don't you take any notice of what people say. You may as well be killed for a Lion as a Cockroach"—now what was I saying?—forgotten—oh yes, Faith and me used to have many a laugh about the gentleman my mum knew and we used to watch and laugh till one day Trixie flew at the gentleman because he thought he was being cruel to my mum. I was frightened because my mum was so pale and she told me that if it hadn't been for Trixie the gentleman would have beaten her to death with a leather stick he had.

ROLAND P.A. would call it "pure phantasy".

P.A. Not only phantasy, but phantasy certainly.

ROBIN Do you mean you don't believe it happened?

P.A. I mean that I do not doubt it was a real phantasy and a real fact—in so far as I am capable of knowing what a fact is and of respecting the factualness of a fact however "realized". Phantasies sometimes burst through into articulated words when the individual is "off guard" as when he is asleep; they break out also when the individual is conscious and fully awake. Sometimes they break "in" to articulate speech, conventionally acceptable art or music, and sometimes into conventionally acceptable "behaviour"—in this instance unacceptable muscular action. Sometimes the "acceptable conversation" has to stretch, alter, to accommodate the thing that "breaks through"; sometimes the "conventionally acceptable" crushes the "outbreaking impulse". Usually it is a compromise between the two. Just now Alice allowed her ears and lips to be degraded by "bloody cunt" and "fucking bastard"; the rest of us have had to allow ourselves to be limited by being polite and saying "please".

ROSEMARY —the gentleman had to run away.

ALICE He was lucky. Or was he?

P.A. This language, which clearly we all know though we have forgotten it, are forgetting it, and hope in future to forget it, makes an unrecognized—an unrecognized archaic and still vital—contribution to our intercourse. [AMF, III, 483–5]

Suggested cross references: Analytic View, Atonement, Facts.

Ineffable: The word means an event that cannot be confined to the limits of any verbal formulation known to man.

It is a word used by Bion to talk about the numinous realm, or, in his quasi-mathematical notation, "O". In bringing the realm of the noumena to psycho-analytic considerations, the wording traditionally used to deal with it was used too, as a matter of consequence.

The word may seem new to analysts—even alien to the analytic movement. It is not true if one remembers Freud's firm Kantian basis, as expressed, for example, in his statement that the unconscious is the true psychic reality. There he compares its ultimate unknowability—and hence its ineffable character—with that of material reality, which remains ultimately unknowable to our sense organs. Freud writes this in Chapter VII of *The Interpretation of Dreams* (p. 690).

Model making in science—constructs that purport to depict some parts of their counterparts in reality—is always a limited and flawed task. Even to them, ultimately, the word "ineffable" applies. In Plato's terms, that which appertains to the Demiurge's work is, in its perennial reformation, an attempt to utter the ineffable.

Misuses and misunderstandings: Ineffable means just that: some fact that cannot be put into words. Emotional experiences are ineffable; that which is intuitable and "experienciable" is ineffable. It does not link with esotericism or mysticism, even though the mystics were among the first, after Plato, to recognize the existence of that which is not amenable to be put into words or any religious, artistic or scientific formulations.

Infra-sensuous: Please refer to the entry, Ultra-sensuous.

Interpretation: *"Nothing is to be gained from telling the patient what he already knows . . ."* (T, 167).

Bion deals with interpretations throughout all his work under a specific vertex. He focuses on the bias that turns them into formulations that, given a specific vertex, turn them away from truth.

He tried to furnish some epistemological tools to gauge the truth-value of interpretations. In other words, the ability to issue an interpretation that can help a person to "become **O**" (c.f.)—that transiently glimpses the numinous, unconscious realm. Interpretations try to represent "O".

He advanced comparatively few new theories in psychoanalysis. He suggested epistemological devices to improve the validity of interpretations in a given context. He stressed that the fact or "O" (c.f.) must be available to the analyst and to the analysand equally. The analytic context provides a unique opportunity for that availability. This seems obvious enough at least in science, where it is a—perhaps *the*—basic principle. How could a scientist study a phenomenon that is not available to him?

The quest is something that surpasses the necessity for an availability that is just measured by its concrete, sensuously apprehensible component. Both analyst and analysand *must* be physically present. This is a necessary condition that functions like a harbour. But it is not enough. Following suit, the analyst deals also with nonconcrete facts that belong to psychic reality. The immaterialness of the facts we deal with seemed to facilitate that which Bion calls the analyst's *"unhampered"* fantasizing activity. It seemed necessary to him to warn analysts that they had better steer away from facts they do not witness.

Bion did not fall into the trap of proposing a "definitive", superior theory that could originate interpretations which would solve once and for all the quest for "O". Instead, he devised an observational theory independent of specific theories:

> For my present purpose it is helpful to regard psycho-analytical theories as belonging to the group of transformations, a technique analogous to that of a painter, by which the facts of an analytic experience (the realization) are transformed into an interpretation (the representation). Any interpretation belongs to the class of statements embodying invariants under one particular psycho-analytic theory; thus an interpretation could be comprehensible because of its embodiment of "invariants under the theory of the Oedipus situation". [T, 4]

> What the psycho-analytic thinking requires is a method of notation and rules for its employment that will enable work to be done in the *absence* of the object to facilitate further work in the *presence* of the object. The barrier to this that is presented by the unfettered play of the analyst's phantasies has long been recognized: pedantic statement on the one hand and verbalization loaded with unobserved implications on the other mean that the potential for misunderstanding and erroneous deduction is so high as to vitiate the value of the work done with such defective tools . . . [T, 44]

The bulk of the psycho-analytic literature in periodicals for at least two decades preceding Bion's contributions instantaneously became endangered; his warnings were warded off by the psychoanalytic establishment. The next three decades witnessed a growth of the publication of those unfettered relativistic, idealistic and subjectivist approaches. They are today called hermeneutic, postmodern and textualist interpretations; even those that cannot be seen as such, do enshrine the analyst's individual imagination or opinion, fuelled by desire. In fact, many analysts do think that they can interpret their patient's parents, relatives, partners without having ever seen them: "*In psycho-analysis, any O not common to analyst and analysand alike, and not available therefore for transformation by both, may be ignored as irrelevant to psycho-analysis. Any O not common to both is incapable of psycho-analytic investigation; any appearance to the contrary depends on a failure to understand the nature of psycho analytic interpretation*" (T, 48–9).

Therefore, the concept of analytic interpretation in Bion's work is the same concept of interpretation that Freud used in his last phase. It carries with it the sense of a "construction". The constructions in analysis endeavour to make approximations to underlying truths that are not given directly to the senses. Those truths—the truth about oneself—are dependent on insight, which calls for intuition and a capacity to dream (Freud quotes Goethe, in his quest for the "witches' help"). Bion also profited fully from the possibilities opened up by Klein, with regard to observation of the here-and-now "total transference situation" and the interplay between paranoid–schizoid position and depressive position. Many patients attempt to control or narrow the analytic scope through heavy resorting to projective identification as a preferred way of relating with the analyst. The finer discrimination of projective identification, that is, the unconscious phantasy that one can be rid of painful feelings or other stimuli, comprised his approach to the work of interpretation.

In that which can be seen with hindsight as his earlier phase, Bion scrutinized carefully the non-verbal clues to an interpretation. This can be seen in the so-called clinical studies on schizophrenia. Many among the patients' acted-out manifestations such as stares, silences and others were used to good account in order to improve the understanding of what was going on (see Analytic View) with the patient and in the session.

During 1959–64, he actively sought the scientific basis for interpretations, examining Plato, Locke, Hume, as well as the neo-positivist approaches to science, such as Braithwaite, Popper and others. He also leaned on Descartes and other mathematicians such as Pascal and Poincaré, having made an analogy with the insight obtained by the mathematician and by the analyst. This can be seen in the use he makes of the concept of selected fact (q.v.), making a novel integrative approach between this concept from Poincaré (a fact that gives coherence to elements hitherto dispersed or seen as dispersed) with Klein's concept of the paranoid–schizoid position, with regard to the fragmentation of the self. Therefore interpretation is an act of thought and depends on the personal capacity for integration.

The next step was an examination of the interference of feelings and emotions in interpretation. This is expanded in *Learning from*

Experience. Bion was able to see that the patient can feel his feelings; later (in *Attention and Interpretation*, p. 9) he would see that they can feel them but cannot suffer them. During 1959–64 he was trying to see why one cannot learn from experience. He observes that the mind has functions; but there are people who cannot respect those functions.

With respect to interpretation: "*In practice the theory of the functions and the theory of alpha-function make possible interpretations showing precisely how the patient feels that he has feelings, but cannot learn from them; sensations, some of which are extremely faint, but cannot learn from them either . . . Sense impressions can be seen to have some meaning but the patient feels incapable of knowing what the meaning is.*

Interpretations derived from these theories appear to effect changes in the patient's capacity for thinking and therefore of understanding" (LE, 18).

Bion considers that with patients with severe disturbances of thought, transference interpretation, in Freud's original sense as well as interpretations based on anal eroticism, theories of splitting, projective identification and false self, had only a slight effect—if any. He observed that the situation was not one where he was called to be a depository of parts of the personality of the patient; but rather he was being used as a repository of *mental functions*, including "being" (in hallucination) the patient's consciousness (LE, 20–1).

Therefore, one may say that Bion proposes interpretations that include interpretation of the living experience of functions of the mind at the moment they happen in the analysis. It is an extension of Klein's observation of projective identification. It ensues that if an analysis goes far or deep enough, one is allowed to display one's psychotic personality (q.v.). That personality demands a novel approach to the interpretive activity in analysis that is of seminal importance to any subject in analysis. It is especially important if the patient is one who wishes or needs to be an analyst.

This second phase, which can be seen as the "late Bion", implies an amendment—rather than a replacement—of his analogies between the analyst and the mathematician through the analogy of the analyst and the painter (and the artist in general as a matter of consequence). The analytic interpretation is now seen as being part of the group of transformations, in the same sense that a painter transforms into imagery that which he sees.

The patient states one or more sentences or construes situations. Something underlies it—the invariances. They can be intuited or detected through the help of a scrutiny of the patient's moves from definitory hypothesis and sensations of grasping ultimate reality to more sophisticated and developed modes of thinking, which includes the functions of the ego (attention, notation, memory) and a range that reaches algebraic calculus (see **Grid**).

Bion considers that an interpretation is a particular form of transformation. With the aid of the theory of transformations he dwells on some aspects of the interpretation. He does this in particular forms made apparent with patients with disturbances of thought who are intolerant of frustration, of the no-breast, and deny to the analyst the very foundations of his interpretations when couched in transference as well as in projective identification, which is *"placed in a vertex that will be inoperable"*.

How can we interpret when the parts of the patient's personality occupy *"the place of"* the analyst to *"deny that vertex to the analyst"*? (T, 135). How can we interpret when there is a fundamental difference of levels of the statements of patient and analyst, namely, *"for the medium of the analysand's transformation lies in the sphere of action, that of the analyst in the sphere of thought and its verbal representations"* (T, 136)?

The theory of transformations offers an alternative to approaching those patients, to the extent that it elicits that the nature of transformations in this kind of patient is neither that of transference nor of projective identification, but of hallucinosis (T, 137). Moreover, an interpretation should help the patient and the analyst to expand Freud's tool, namely, "turn the unconscious, conscious" into a tool that helps to illuminate *how* this turning is done.

> If I am right in suggesting that phenomena are known but reality is "become", the interpretation must do more than increase knowledge. It can be argued that this is not a matter for the analyst and that he can only increase knowledge; that the further steps required to bridge the gap must come from the analysand; or from a particular part of the analysand, namely his "godhead", which must consent to incarnation in the person of the analysand. [T, 148]

In Freud's terms, insight is the patient's task and the analyst is a kind of midwife. Bion expressed it many times, and some parts of his work are indeed very clear about this: *"Since psycho-analysts do not aim to run the patient's life but enable him to run it according to his lights and therefore to know what his lights are, Taβ either in the form of interpretation or scientific paper should represent the psycho-analyst's verbal representation of an emotional experience"* (T, 37).

Ten years later, that which can be seen as a kind of theory would be expressed in experiential and novel forms. If *Transformations* can be regarded as the theory, *A Memoir of the Future* is a kind of practical lesson:

MYSELF Perhaps I can illustrate by an example from something you *do* know. Imagine a piece of sculpture which is easier to comprehend if the structure is intended to act as a trap for light. The meaning is revealed by the pattern formed by the light thus trapped—not by the structure, the carved work itself. I suggest that if I could learn how to talk to you in such a way that my words "trapped" the meaning which they neither do nor could express, I could communicate to you in a way that is not at present possible.

BION Like the "rests" in a musical composition?

MYSELF A musician would certainly not deny the importance of those parts of a composition in which no notes were sounding, but more has to be done than can be achieved in existent art and its well-established procedure of silences, pauses, blank spaces, rests. The "art" of conversation, as carried on as part of the conversational intercourse of psycho-analysis, requires and demands an extension in the realm of non-conversation . . .

The "thing-in-itself", impregnated with opacity, itself becomes opaque: the O, of which "memory" and "desire" is the verbal counterpart, is opaque. I suggest this quality of opacity inheres in many O's and their verbal counterparts, and the phenomena which it is usually supposed to express. If, by experiment, we discovered the verbal forms, we could also discover the thoughts to which the observation applied specifically. Thus we achieve a situation in which these could be used deliberately to obscure specific thoughts.

BION Is there anything new in this? You must often have heard, as I have, people say they don't know what you are talking about and that you are being deliberately obscure.

MYSELF They are flattering me. I am suggesting an aim, an ambition, which, if I could achieve, would enable me to be deliberately and precisely obscure: in which I could use certain words which could activate precisely and instantaneously, in the mind of the listener, a thought or train of thought that came between him and the thoughts and ideas already accessible and available to him. [AMF, I, 189–191]

Resistance to interpretations

The issues subsumed by the term, resistance, were expanded by the formulation of the Grid's category column 2: falsities or statements known to be false. They also include manifestations of the paranoid–schizoid position. Therefore they are marked by the presence of fear. Ultimately, fear of truth itself. Column 2 events are indispensable for reaching an interpretation: "*Epistemologically a statement may be regarded as evolved when any dimension can have a grid category assigned to it. For purposes of interpretation the statement is insufficiently evolved until its column 2 dimension is apparent. When the column 2 dimension has evolved, the statement can be said to be ripe for interpretation; its development as material for interpretation has reached maturity*" (T, 167).

The analyst must cope with the paradox that truth is attainable when its "lie" face is allowed to evolve. Freud said the same when he resorted to Goethe's already-mentioned invocation to the witches, in "*Constructions in Analysis*". He compared the analyst's constructions to the patient's delusions.

ROSEMARY You are not sorry; nor am I bored. But—

ROBIN But what? Or is that a secret between you and Alice?

P.A. If it is, I might suggest a psycho-analytic interpretation., But this is not a psycho-analytic occasion and therefore the minimum conditions for a verbal, audible interpretation don't exist.

ROBIN Something sexual, I bet.

P.A. A sexual situation affords the conditions for a sexual interpretation, an analytical situation affords an opportunity for a psycho-analytic interpretation.

ALICE What *is* a psycho-analytic interpretation?

P.A. It must be perspicacious and perspicuous. That is—

ROLAND These long words!

P.A. —an expression of a scientifically accurate insight which is phrased in a language comprehensible by the listener. It must be believed to be true by the analyst, and his formulation should be in terms that would penetrate the barriers of the listener's incomprehension.

ALICE Oh, I know—that would get through my thick feminine skull.

ROSEMARY Well, I *don't* know!

P.A. You both give an example of the difficulty I am talking about. Alice, hostile, "thinks" I am an obtuse male; Rosemary "remembers" my learnedness. Both—feelings, and ideas remembered— produce an obscurity. [AMF, III, 459]

From this obscurity, clarity eventuates—in a paradoxical cycle determined by the tandem movement between PS and D and vice versa.

Misuses and misunderstandings: As usual they stem from oversimplified, canonical readings. Some think that Bion outdated Freud just in respect of interpretations. The conundrum rages in some parts of the world concerning a pseudo-war "in the name of Bion" or "Freud" that opposes form versus content of interpretations, stating that Bion despised the content. Is it a reflex of little learning (see, for example, **Oedipus**)? But perhaps it is useful to remember that Bion in fact emphasized more than anyone else since Freud and Klein, the function of the patient's actions and statements in the here and now of the session. Sometimes and with a certain class of patients, to overlook the function is a sure way to error. Bion's amendment is not a substitution for interpretations of content. The content calls to be elicited, perceived and dealt with as its function unfolds in the here and now. The difference with those cases is that the work does not end here. To intuit the meaning of the content is a prelude to the eliciting of the function. The issue is not "content versus function", but to take the context into detailed and careful account. For example, one finds content of rivalry in a session. The content is just a part; there is a *"distorting effect produced by the approach to a configuration through one if its parts. Rivalry is an important element but its significance depends on the particular constant conjunction or configuration of which it is part. 'Rivalry' signifies a constant conjunction but the constant conjunction it signifies is not the* *relevant one in this context. It is common to find some feature, such as the cruelty of the super-ego, and to suppose that one has discovered the key to a baffling situation only to find that the same feature occurs in other situations which bear no marked resemblance to the situation to which one hoped the key has been discovered. In my experience this difficulty arises because the* **key** *has been detected in the elements of a second, third or subsequent cycle of psycho-analytic (that is, analyst's) transformations when it should be sought in the nature of the transformations effected by the analysand. What matters in the present context is not rivalry so much as rivalry under transformations in hallucinosis"* (T, 136–7).

If the reader denies, splits off and forgets the expression *"in the present context"* he is prone to generalize the recommendation unduly. If the reader entertains phantasies of superiority and loses a sense of truth he or she will transform a recommendation into a judgmental, authoritarian rule of a "Gospel according to St. Wilfred", made by the reader.

The same applies to readings of the limitations of interpretations couched in transference and projective identification.

Suggested cross references: Analytic view, Correct Interpretation, Grid, Hallucination, Interpretation, content, Transformations in Hallucinosis.

Interpretation, content: In some places in the world there is a very specific reading of Bion's work that tries to impinge an idea, namely, that there could be a dispute between interpretations of content of communication and other interpretations.

There are people who argue that the content of communication as well as the content of dreams and the content of interpretations is of no interest to a "Bionian analysis". They would be quite correct, if a "Bionian" analysis could ever exist outside the realm of hallucinated idolization and distortions of Bion's writings. This argument is endorsed by some followers as well as detractors. The latter often complain about an alleged scarcity of clinical descriptions in Bion's written work.

There is at least one phrase in his work that can illuminate the question and perhaps the origin of the distorted reading. (In fact, any reading that tries to replace the original text is a distortion, for it means that the reader impinges his own meanings instead of looking for those of the author, as John Ruskin once realized.) The phrase is: *'The content of the communication, so important in analysis, will be touched on only incidentally in the discussion of transformations; it will depend on O as deduced from the material in the light of the psycho-analyst's theoretical pre-conceptions. Thus, if the content is oedipal material, I do not concern myself with this but with the transformation it has undergone, the stage of growth it reveals, and the use to which its communication is being put. This exclusion of content is artificial, to simplify exposition, and cannot be made in practice"* (T, 35).

Thus, an artifice he used when he was introducing and therefore trying to communicate a theory of observation in psycho-analysis, the theory of transformation (q.v) was distorted as if it were an intra-session posture.

Suggested cross-reference: Interpretation.

Intuition: *"The analyst conducting a session must decide instinctively the nature of the communication that the patient is making"* (T, 34).

Kant's definition of intuition (*Anschauung*) has precision and wide acceptance: it means the contact with reality without brokerage of rational thinking. Taking into account the Kantian ethos of Freud's discoveries (which were made explicit by Freud himself) and more than this, the quotations that Bion makes from Kant about intuition, perhaps it is not unwise to adopt this definition.

Intuition is a word that Bion brought back to the analytic vocabulary. It happened after decades of the psycho-analytic movement's distrust and abhorrence of it. The attitude is explainable because of at least two factors:

(i) Difficulties in the translation of the word, as used by Freud, from German to other languages.

(ii) The existence of an obnoxious misuse of the term in Germany during Freud's formative years. This misuse debased it, allowing it to turn into a banal vulgarization of a very precise definition by Kant. The followers of Schelling's version of an esoteric *Naturphilosophie* (in itself a far cry from a discipline of the same name created by Goethe) as well as the criminal development of pagan religions such as Nazism, were responsible for this debasing of the term, one of the many offshoots of too little learning that characterized the excesses of Romanticism. Freud wanted to keep psycho-analysis safe from those tendencies. Some other authors, notably Ferenczi, did not shun stating that they relied on their intuition to deal with patients and even to make discoveries in the field of psycho-analysis.

Other fields of research also suffered from this during Freud's time, especially when he discovered the possibility of analysing dreams. This is brought home to one who is informed about Max Planck and Albert Einstein's tribulations with Ernest Mach. The latter explicitly condemned a science that relied on intuition. Mach came to the point of founding an entire movement against it, which became known as "neo-positivism", whose development, incidentally, developed in surprising ways, judging by the work of its three principal authors, Wittgenstein (who abandoned it), Schlick (who died too early to review all his initial positions but had time to begin it) and Carnap.

☾ The first time (as far as this author's research goes) that Bion uses the term "intuition" is in his paper "Differentiation of the psychotic from the non-psychotic personality" [Francesca Bion notes: see ST, 135—used in "The Imaginary Twin"]. It has to do with the minute splitting the person does on his ego, trying to expel those parts that could make them "aware of the reality he hates" (ST, 47). This act damages his perception and self-perception: *All those features of the personality which should one day provide the foundation for intuitive understudying of himself and others are jeopardized at the outset*" (ST, 47).

Intuition is something we use when we must make explorations into the unknown; the unconscious, in other words. Again, the apprehension of the semantic field of the word in German helps the analyst here: *unbewußt* means not-known (from *wissen*, knowledge). This is possible through consciousness, or as Bion illuminated, through a two-way selective flowing from conscious to unconscious and back through the contact-barrier (q.v.).

The analyst must tell the patient that which he does not know (Freud): "*The emotion to which attention is drawn should be obvious to the analyst, but unobserved by the patient; an emotion that is obvious to the patient is usually **painfully** obvious and avoidance of unnecessary pain must be one aim in the exercise of analytic intuition. Since the analyst's capacity for intuition should enable him to demonstrate an* *emotion before it has become **painfully** obvious it would help if our search for the elements of emotions was directed to making intuitive deductions easier"* (EP, 74).

. . . the analyst must have a view of the psycho-analytic theory of the Oedipus situation. His understanding of that theory can be regarded as a transformation of that theory and in that case all his interpretations, verbalized or not, of what is going on in a session may be seen as transformations of an O that is bi-polar. One pole of O is trained intuitive capacity transformed to effect its juxtaposition with what is going on in the analysis and the other is in the facts of the analytic experience that must be transformed to show what approximation the realization has to the analyst's preconceptions—the preconception here being identical with Taβ as the end-product of Taα . . .

Freud stated as one of the criteria by which a psycho-analyst was to be judged was the degree of understanding allegiance he paid to the theory of the Oedipus complex. He thus showed the importance he attached to this theory and time has done nothing to suggest that he erred by over-estimation; evidence of the Oedipus complex is never absent though it can be unobserved.

Melanie Klein, in her paper on 'Early Phases of the Oedipus Complex', made observations of Oedipal elements where their presence was previously undetected" (T, 49–50).

Analytically trained intuition makes it possible to say the patient is talking about the primal scene and from the development of associations to add shades of meaning to fill out understanding of what is taking place" (T, 18). Intuition being the exercising of the mind's ability to apprehend reality with no interference of logical thinking, this analytically trained intuition alone makes possible the allegiance that Freud told us was needed to entitle a person to call himself an analyst, that is, allegiance to the Oedipal configurations. It is not a puzzle or something to be understood—for any human being is born of a Mother and a Father and experiences it. The experience is unconscious and is forgotten. But it must be intuited and seen through the analyst's own analysis. In Bion's words, learnt from experience.

The Grid was devised to help the analyst train his intuition:

Although home work is not done in an atmosphere of emotional tension, grid and transformation theory are applied to the recollection of such situations. The analyst's intuition, which it is the object of these reviews to exercise and develop, is operating in contact with the tense situation. It is important to distinguish between the grid (as it appears in my scheme) operating in tranquillity on recollections, and the grid as part of the analyst's intuitive contact with the emotional situation itself. [T, 75–6]

If the psycho-analytical situation is accurately intuited—I prefer this term to "observed" or "heard" or "seen" as it does not carry the penumbra of sensuous association—the psycho-analyst finds that ordinary conversational English is surprisingly adequate for the formulation of his interpretation. [ST, 134]

Intuitive psycho-analysis depends on the analyst's relationship with the breast:

The rules governing points and lines which have been elaborated by geometers may be reconsidered by reference back to the emotional phenomena that were replaced by 'the place (or space) where the mental phenomena were'. Such a procedure would establish an abstract deductive system based on a geometric foundation with intuitive psycho-analytic theory as its concrete realization. The statements (i) the resumption by the psyche of an emotional experience that has been detoxicated by a sojourn in the good breast (Melanie Klein) and (ii) the transformation of the emotional experience into a geometrical formulation and the use of this geometrical formulation as the counterpart of a concrete realization for a geometrically based, rigorously formulated, deductive system (possibly algebraic), may now be regarded as the (i) intuitive psycho-analytic and (ii) axiomatic deductive representations of the same process. [T, 121–122]

In terms of communication, Bion was not satisfied, as the continuation of the phrase makes clear. The replacement of this quasi-mathematical notation by a quasi-artistic notation as attempted in *A Memoir of the Future* would confirm his dissatisfaction:

Both statements are verbal representations of a realization and neither of them is satisfactory; nor is much improvement likely by mastery of the medium of verbal expression. The intuitive statement lends itself to the representation of genetic stages: the axiomatic formulation lends itself to the representation of a use. [T, 122]

Mathematics, science as known hitherto, can provide no model.
[AMF, I, 61]

Concreteness coupled with "enforced splitting" (*Learning from Experience*, chapters V–VI) are real obstacles to exercising intuitive psycho-analysis or real psycho-analysis in the absence of the object. The problem echoes the baby's problem when it must introject an object that is deprived of its concrete aspect. There is a basic weakness in the verbal formulations of elements suitable to represent genetic stages of thinking (see entry "Grid"). The basic weakness partakes of the nature of the basic weakness of a beta-element, that is, a thing-in-itself. But things-in-themselves have no capacity for saturation as they are already saturated. The nature of those elements is material and there is no "No", no negative that allows newness to enter the scene.

The element that represents genetic stages appears to have or to require a capacity for saturation, for becoming pregnant. I have phrased my last sentence in terms that illustrate the difficulty that arises when a term that in some contexts gains by its metaphorical quality (a 'pregnant statement') loses communicative quality if it is employed in a context where its metaphorical quality ceases to be metaphorical because its context has approximated it to a α-element—it is, relative to its context, saturated" (T, 122). Therefore intuitive psycho-analysis is an impossible task for those professionals who deal with the verbalization of patients at their face value. This is especially significant in "reconstructions" (by the so-called analyst) and "recollections" of the past (by the patient) as well as in the creation of an impossibility for dealing with free associations and with dreams. The interpretation of dreams turns out to be an a priori or ad hoc manipulation of signs and theories. The metaphorical value of the theory is lost too and the theory is taken as a thing-in-itself. No theory seems to be spared from this.

What are the obstacles to exercising intuition? There are at least two: (i) the prevalence of desire, memory and understanding; (ii) the idea that transformations in K can replace O—rather than being a step towards O.

The formalist tradition in psycho-analysis dictates an a priori application of pre–Learned theories. It provoked a multiplication of verbal formulations and theories that preclude the intuition of the invariants, pointers to O, amidst the material; the same multiplication precludes the description of the same basic configurations. Fear of the unknown is at the basis of all of that and was depicted years later:

> SHERLOCK The simple part of it has been dealt with by Watson. You heard that fellow Bion? Nobody has ever heard of him or of Psycho-analysis. He thinks it is real, but that his colleagues are engaged in an activity which is only a more or less ingenious manipulation of symbols. There is something in what he says. There is a failure to understand that any definition must deny a precious truth as well as carry an unsaturated component. [AMF, I, 92]

All attempts to keep a theory free of this, to arrive at fresh formulations of that which Freud discovered, were doomed to meet the same fate. The self-titled "-ians" of all brands did this with their preferred great author's work:

> P.A. We are all scandalized by bigotry. We are none of us bigot-generators; that is, we none of us admit to being the spring from whom bigotry flows. As a result we do not recognize those of our offspring of whose characters we disapprove. Indeed, Melanie Klein discovered that primitive, infantile omnipotence was characterized by fantasies of splitting off undesired features and then evacuating them.
>
> ROLAND I am sure you don't mean that children *think* like that?
>
> P.A. It would be inaccurate and misleading to say so. That is why Melanie Klein called them "omnipotent phantasies". But although I found her verbalization illuminating, with the passage of time and further investigation which her discoveries made possible, her formulations were debased and became inadequate. These primitive elements of thought are difficult to represent by any verbal formulation, because we have to rely on language which was elaborated later for other purposes. When I tried to employ meaningless terms—alpha and beta were typical—I found that "concepts without intuition which are empty and intuitions without concepts which are blind" rapidly became "black holes into which turbulence had seeped and empty concepts flooded with riotous meaning". [AMF, II, 228–9]

In 1965, Bion would insert the classical definition of hallucination into his framework proposed after Freud, to form the "*intuitive psycho-analytic background"* (T, 138). Hallucination is seen *"as a dimension of the analytic situation in which, together with the remaining 'dimensions', these objects are sense-able (if we include analytic intuition or consciousness, taking a lead from Freud, as a sense-organ of psychic quality)"* (T, 115) . . . *"The psycho-analyst must not allow himself to be deflected from the vertex from which the emotional events, when they have evolved, become "intuitable". The study of hallucination is at its beginning, not its end"* (ST, 161).

> The rules governing points and lines which have been elaborated by geometers may be reconsidered by reference back to the emotional phenomena that were replaced by "the place (or space) where the mental phenomena were". Such a procedure would establish an abstract deductive system based on a geometric foundation with intuitive psycho-analytic theory as its concrete realization. [T, 121]

The "intuitive psycho-analytic" representation of a basic emotional experience—infantile helplessness—is expressed by the following statement: "the resumption by the psyche of an emotional experience that has been detoxicated by a sojourn in the good breast (Melanie Klein)" (T, 122). The "intuitive statement lends itself to the representation of genetic stages". In Bion's text there is an expansion of axiomatic formulations (transformations of emotional experiences into points, the place where a breast was and other more sophisticated formulations) that lead themselves to representations of uses.

Intuition and geometry

> . . . as part of an intuitive psycho-analytic theory, that the patient has an experience, such as an infant might have when the breast is withdrawn, of facing emotions that are unknown, unrecognized as belonging to himself, and confused with an object which he but recently possessed. Further descriptions only add to the multiplicity of which I already complain as the reader will see if he consults any analytic descriptions of infantile behaviour. The relationship of these representations with the realizations approximating to them may be compared with the axiomatic geometric deductive space that I wish to introduce as a step towards formulations that are

precise, communicable without distortion, and more nearly adequate to cover all situations that are basically the same. I suggest
the following comparisons: (i) "Unknown", in the model afforded
by the intuitive psycho-analytical theory, with "unknown", in the
mathematical sense in which I wish to use 'geometric space'. (ii)
"Variable", as applied to the sense of instability and insecurity in
the model of infantile anxiety, with "variable", as I wish to apply it
to geometric space ... The relationship of geometric space to the
psycho-analytic intuitive theory that I propose as *its* realization; the
further relationship of the psycho-analytical intuitive theory to the
clinical experience which I consider is *its* realization; together these
represent a progression such as that in the transformation of an
experience into a poem—emotion recollected in tranquillity. The
geometric transformation may be regarded as a representation,
"detoxicated" (that is, with the painful emotion made bearable) of
the same realization as that represented (but with the painful
emotion expressed), by the intuitive psycho-analytical theory. This
implies that any individual capable of making the transformation
from O, when O is a psychic reality, to $\{Ta\}\beta$ is capable of doing
for himself something analogous to projective identification into
the good breast, he being identified with himself and the breast.
[T, 124–5]

In other words, if one does not realize what a breast and a
mother is—in cases of primary narcissism and envy—one perhaps
cannot be an analyst, or an artist, or scientist.

In discussing bizarre responses to interpretations that would be
quite correct in connection with hallucination and hallucinosis,
Bion states: "... *the psycho-analytical game may develop the analyst's
intuition (as a musician's exercises facilitate his capacity to perform an
actual musical creation though not themselves being more than scales and
other manual exercises) in preparation for the work required of it in analysis*" (T, 130) ... "*that state of mind in which ideas may be supposed to
assume the force of sensations through the confusion of thought with the
objects of thought, and the excess of passion animating the creations of
imagination (I use Shelley's formulation of his poetic intuition to provide
the background realization for the statement 'hallucinosis'*" (T, 133–4).

What is needed to form a background to exercise the intuitive
psycho-analytic approach? Those functions that Freud saw as
belonging to the ego, or the consciousness as a sense organ for the

apprehension of psychic qualities: "*The intuitive psycho-analytic back-ground is that which I have 'bound' by terms such as preconception, defi-nition, notation, attention*" (T,138).

One of the metaphors that Bion resorted to was that of St John of The Cross. Intuition can be exerted when one allows oneself to experience the "Dark night of the soul". This corresponds to Freud's abstinence from worldly values, which include knowledge: "*. . . the intuitive approach is obstructed because the 'faith' involved is associated with the absence of inquiry, or 'dark night' to K*" (T, 159).

On Gist—and feminine intuition

The following formulations, made approximately three years before Bion's death, perhaps subsume his latest postures, including in a clinical situation:

ROBIN I should be interested to know what P.A. thinks of mater-nal intuition. Do you think that paternally gifted psycho-analysts would be capable of such fine discrimination? (AMF, III, 515).

P.A. Sometimes I think they do, but not often. Nevertheless psycho-analysis enables the psycho-analyst to learn something and even to pass it on. There are occasions when a resistance is surmounted with astounding speed; a number of facts display their relationship for the first time. It is almost a revelation.

PRIEST You use a term which is part of our technical equipment.

P.A. I thought you would notice that. I would that we could make clear both the verbal fact you mention and the psychic reality which corresponds. The concentration of meaning would require the concision which can be achieved in music or painting. Would my analysand undergo the work necessary to understand if I could achieve such precision? Audiences rarely listen to music or look at pictures; still less do they think it worth while listening to what an analyst says.

PRIEST These difficulties have been familiar to the religious for many centuries. Music, painting, poetry, vestments gorgeous and austere—all have been used as auxiliaries.

P.A. I have found that the auxiliary can easily be transferred by the receptor from the periphery to the centre. Messages intended to convey profound truth—the Iliad, the Aeneid, Paradise Lost, The Divine Comedy—have all in turn become famous as gorgeous settings for the precious "stone" which is outshone by its attendant splendour. Krishna warned Arjuna that he might not be able to survive the revelation of the godhead which he, Krishna, was prepared to vouchsafe. Dante has only rarely found a reader able to discern the vision to which he points in Canto XXXI of the Paradiso. Milton's mind was overshadowed by a doubt whether he could pass beyond the "evil days" on which he had fallen; it was indeed his tragedy.

PRIEST The most profound expression of despair known to us was, "Why has thou forsaken me?"

P.A. This discovery is one which all are afraid to make. A theory that the human animal is not going to call on God to do for him what he must do for himself in loneliness and despair cannot be formulated; any formulation is a substitute for that which cannot be substituted.

ROLAND Do you suggest that *that* psycho-analytic interpretation is the explanation of Christ's reported call on the Cross?

P.A. You show that I have failed to make it clear that I attach the utmost importance, in the practice of analysis, to the presence of analyst and analysand at the same time and in the same place in conditions in which the consciously discernible facts are available to both people. These are the *minimum* conditions, not the maximum. Only then does psycho-analysis become an activity open to the two participants. You suggest that I am making a statement about events reported to have taken place almost two thousand years ago; if you believe that to be the gist of my remarks, what might you not say about my opinions when I am not present to defend them?

ROBIN I don't see why you are angry. Roland's mistake seems to me to be natural and understandable. I had not observed that he was misrepresenting you.

P.A. As I see the situation I would be lacking in proper feeling if I were not angry.

ROLAND That's your opinion.

P.A. That is what I said. Whose else should it be? Yours? Well, why not? I hope I am not doing anything to obstruct your freedom.

ROLAND Your answer is hostile and I can detect, even though you may not, impatience, sarcasm and irony in it too.

P.A. I shall not deny or confirm your observations; I think you want me to be so impressed by the facts that you observe, that I would not dare to make an interpretation at all.

ROSEMARY Like your interpretation of Man's holster.

P.A. I still think it would be wiser to interpret it as containing a gun than to accept his offer to interpret it as containing chocolate.

ROBIN & ROLAND So do we.

P.A. We have many facts available; if we interpret each one in isolation, the facts and the interpretations do not amount to much; taken together, the "gist" can be interpreted. The Mathematical sum cannot be mathematically expressed, yet the "gist" can be.

ROLAND What is your definition of "gist"?

P.A. I have none, because a definition would add to an already overwhelming vocabulary of formulations that seem to be precise where no precision exists. If you listened to my talking you could probably feel that the 'gist' of what I meant when I used the word "gist" was a constant conjunction of your impressions. Your interpretation of my communications might be something you could formulate.

ROLAND Can you give me an example of something—an interpretation say—which expresses the "gist" of an idea?

P.A. I was called to see a patient who was suspected of being "schizophrenic". As I approached his bed I was aware of a flurry of movement. When I reached his bed he had hidden himself beneath a blanket so that only one eye was visible. With this eye he observed me intently. He maintained silence for weeks—it may have been a month or more.

ROLAND Yes, but can't you give me the "gist" of your definition? I don't want to be rude, but our time here is very limited.

P.A. That is why I said "intently". Sometimes, as in this instance, the gist of an experience may take a long time to grasp. An eye seen in isolation conveys nothing; seen for some weeks as I saw it, "intently" is a fair summary of what I saw—the "gist" of the experience. Psycho-analysis may convey the "gist" of what two people are doing if both are satisfied that the name "psycho-analysis" conveys enough meaning for immediate needs. But what I want to communicate to you would require other conditions and time which you will not spare.

ROLAND Go ahead then. What about your dotty patient?

ROBIN Have we time to discuss dotty patients?

ROSEMARY Yes, I'm interested.

ROLAND These aren't the days for pursuing interests.

ROSEMARY Not for you perhaps. When I was the servant here I never had time for anything that might have interested me. You can think yourself lucky that I allow you and the rest to participate when I am following my interest. Go on P.A. Alice—you may stay in case I want you; it may do you good.

P.A. One day, after I had given many interpretations apparently without effect, the man suddenly said, "I want help". [AMF, II, 333–5]

Smelling danger

ROBIN Surely you do not seriously mean that an analytic session is comparable with going into action?

P.A. Comparable, yes. Imminent death is not expected, although there is that possibility. That does not weigh the anxiety—fear in a low key. One shrinks from giving the unwelcome interpretation.

ROBIN Is it not just fear that the patient is going to be angry at being criticized?

P.A. I don't think so; the patient may be angry at a critical comment, perhaps even murderously angry, but I do not think that possibility consciously deters.

ROBIN Is it some unconscious fear—the counter-transference of which you spoke?

P. A. It is, though one is not "conscious" of it—to obviate that is one reason why we think analysts must themselves be analysed—there is an inherent fear of giving an interpretation. If a psycho-analyst is doing proper analysis then he is engaged on an activity that is indistinguishable from that of an animal that investigates what it is afraid of—it smells danger. An analyst is not doing his job if he investigates something because it is pleasurable or profitable. Patients do not come because they anticipate some agreeable imminent event; they come because they are ill at ease. The analyst must share the danger and has, therefore, to share the 'smell' of the danger. If the hair at the back of your neck becomes erect, your primitive, archaic senses indicate the presence of the danger. It is our job to be curious about that danger. . .—not cowardly, not irresponsible. [AMF, III, 517]

Suggested cross-references: Analytic view, Atonement, Interpretation, Transformations in K and O, Transformations in Hallucinosis.

Intuitive psycho-analysis, trained psycho-analytic intuition: These terms refer to the analyst's intuition of the multifarious possible outward presentations of the underlying Oedipus situation. It cannot be dealt with under the criteria of positivism. Later the term was used to describe the situation of intuiting the presence of hallucination. Trained intuition depends on the personal analysis of the analyst and a capacity to grasp the numinous realm of the immaterial, non-sensuous psychic reality (the unconscious).

Suggested cross-references: Analytical View, Atonement, Intuition, O, Oedipus, Real psycho-analysis.

Invariance: A concept borrowed from the philosophy of mathematics, first established at the end of the nineteenth century by two mathematicians, James Joseph Sylvester and David Cayley, who lived in London and Baltimore. Sylvester died in 1897 and Cayley in 1895. The concept was first used in physics by Paul Dirac, in 1930; it was first used outside physics by Bion, in 1965. It was used for the first time in philosophy by Robert Nozik in 2001. For a more detailed account of those origins, please refer to the entry Transformations.

The concept is seminal to any scientific endeavour, for science has regard to truth. Invariances refer to some truthful quality that characterizes the innermost nature of whatever it is, independently of the position of the observer. Invariances refer to no less than the Platonic forms and the numinous realm unearthed by Kant.

Even though Bion does not use this term before 1965, as a built-in, necessary part of the concept of transformations as it was used by its original authors, one can spot it in the first chapter of *Learning from Experience*. There, the issue is taken right from the beginning, using a colloquial formulation: *"To call an action by the name of the person of whom it is thought to be typical, to talk, for example, of a Spoonerism as if it were a function of the personality of an individual called Spooner, is quite usual in conversation"* (LE, 1).

Even though in this place Bion uses the concept to develop a theory inspired by the mathematical concepts of factors and functions, it is easy to see that the "typicality" refers to an invariance that marks, in this example, that Mr. Spooner is Mr. Spooner and no one else due to the invariance "Spoonerism"—his hallmark. Invariances are hallmarks of whatever it is.

. . . **something** *has remained unaltered and on this* **something** *recognition depends. The elements that go to make up the unaltered aspect of the transformation I shall call invariants"* (T, 1). The concept of invariance is an evolution of the concept of "selected fact" (LE, 72; C), now free from the earlier borrowing of mathematical philosophy by Poincaré. It is more psycho-analytically encompassing too. It refers to a possibility of transient access, glimpses of a path to "O", the numeric field that generates events in psychic and material reality (material = sensuously apprehensible). Invariances can be intuited, detected and up to a point, named. They are the mental counterpart of a given reality that is *existent, intuitable and usable* (one may see the remark on the impossibility to *"sing potatoes"* [T, 148]) but ultimately unknowable. They can be partially known and conserve a fundamental feature of "O": its **transcendence** (to time, space, individualities).

The example on the first page of the book *Transformations* refers to a "poppy-ishness", **the quality of being a poppy**, ineffable but "intuitable" and existent. It pervades **without variations in its essence**; nevertheless, it paradoxically **varies in its form** (transforms). The forms are phenomenal expressions. In Bion's example: a field of poppies is concretely regarded; in contrast we may have an impressionistic painting of this field of poppies and a realistic painting of the same field. (Impressionism and Realism as schools of painting.) The choice of such a subject bears more that a passing resemblance to Monet's painting and the fields of the Somme, where Bion fought in the First World War.

The forms (images in the retina, a painting by an impressionist artist, a painting by a realist painter) do vary. Paradoxically, "binocularly", the "poppy-ishness" does not vary. The paradox that demands to be tolerated is that transformations and invariances vary *and* do not vary. To detect an invariance is a step towards the apprehension of a reality—that is that and no other thing (cf. **Transformations in "O"**). The invariances are a mark of recognition—of a school of painting, of a vertex in psycho-analysis, even of a particular psycho-analyst. *"Invariants make . . . representation comprehensible"'* (T, 5). One can apply different sets of theories to the same material; different invariants can convey different meanings but the material transformed *"can be conceived of as being the same in both instances"* (T, 5–6).

Bion would make it explicitly clear in *Attention and Interpretation*—as if he had observed that an idealistic use was debasing his concept.

> From the material discussed it should now be possible to detect a pattern that remains unaltered in apparently widely differing contexts. It would be useful to isolate and formulate the invariants of that pattern so that it could be communicated.

> Freud formulations do just that. Thinking, developed through psycho-analysis, has led to discoveries that were not made by Freud, but that reveal configurations resembling those discoveries he *did* make. [AI, 92]

Suggested cross-reference: Transformations.

J

Jargon:

> P.A. His Satanic Jargonieur took offence; on some pretence that psycho-analytic jargon was being eroded by eruptions of clarity. I was compelled to seek asylum in fiction. Disguised as fiction the truth occasionally slipped through. [AMF, II, 302–3]

Freud was awarded the Goethe Prize, perhaps the most coveted literary prize of the German-speaking world. This was for his contributions to the German language. Perhaps this language has a similarity to the Russian language and some of the dialects that stemmed from them, for example the Yiddish language. These languages have a remarkable plasticity, and the building of words for specific purposes does not necessarily share the nature of neologisms.

Unfortunately the rich wording that Freud was able to create in a rich language, in order to try to express that which is ultimately non-expressible, namely, mental life itself, suffered unexpected fates. It was transformed too early into jargon; too early it was used as an a priori pattern. That which was devised as a tool to be used in scientific research into the unknown was used to deny this same unknown. A few years before dying, Bion asked if the whole of psycho-analysis was a vast paramnesia destined to fill the void of our ignorance ("Evidence", 1976, "Emotional turbulence", 1977 and *A Memoir of the Future*, pub. 1979, written over a period of approximately five years). Jargon, like slang, gives to the beholder the hallucinated sensation that he "knows" something that he in fact does not know; it gives to the group a sense of coherence and beholding. The word, even if it means nothing or means many different things to different people, has those differences or nothingness duly overlooked. A sense of "clarity", indistinguishable from paranoid and religious states is obtained when the word is uttered. Is jargon a sign of the adolescence of any given field?

> ROBIN Good heavens! Can't one talk simple literate English?
>
> P.A. You should hear my psycho-analyst aspirants talking "simple literate" English.
>
> PAUL But you surprise me. Do you really think anyone expects psycho-analysts to talk "simple" English? I thought it was understood that it was a point of honour to talk incomprehensible jargon.
>
> P.A. It is a point of honour when we are playing the game of Who's Top of the Psycho-analytical League Tables, but that is when we are "talking about" psycho-analysis (AMF, II, 227–8).
>
> BION I was speaking conversationally.
>
> SHERLOCK Ah! In my kind of work you have to be precise.
>
> MYSELF So you have in ours. Unfortunately we have to talk conversational English and that is not a language intended to be used for the purposes for which we have to use it.
>
> SHERLOCK I, alas, have to use the language my author puts at *my* disposal.
>
> MYSELF You—meaning both of you—don't do badly. My characters are not fictional and they are very dissatisfied with such means of communication as I put at their disposal.
>
> SHERLOCK "Means of communication"! Do you mean English? If not—

MYSELF No, I don't. If it is English, that is *not* enough. I am aware that conversational English is inadequate; but you should hear what they say about anything else.

BION Jargon, for example.

SHERLOCK HOLMES Why not paint or draw or compose music, or—

BION —play the violin. Did you ever try your violin playing on your clients or criminals or courts of law? [AMF, I, 202]

Or its development, two years later:

ROBIN Well, I have a mind of course.

ROLAND That is what we are discussing.

ROBIN If we could speak the language of mathematics . . .

PAUL If we could speak the language of religion . . .

ALICE If we could learn to look at what artists paint . . .

ROLAND What is wrong with not talking at all and listening to the music?

EDMUND Once it would have been understood when we were exhorted to hear the music of the spheres.

ROBIN I wouldn't object if I could speak the "mathematics" of the spheres.

P.A. There may be something to be said for the language of the psycho-analyst.

ROLAND He hasn't got a language—only "jargon".

P.A. That is not so. I try to talk English because it is the best I know. But I do not know it well enough to speak it for the purpose of what I want to convey. I do not talk Jargonese any more than Paul talks Journalese . . . This is my lack and misfortune in so far as you want me to talk a language *you* can "understand" and I want you to meet me at least half way by talking a language *I* can understand. [AMF, II, 230–31]

Sometimes jargon may be useful provided it is a shorthand and the conversants are attuned to using it as a caricature. Then it can serve as a communication among professionals. Continuous usage can debase meaning; in the psycho-analytical field, the continuous appearance of Freud-substitutes who looked at the field under the vertex of rivalry complicated the situation extraordinarily.

Take the word "transference": many tried to debase it, to attribute new meanings to it, and many succeeded. The only result was to destroy its use for the purposes of scientific communication among peers.

> Terms like "excessive", "hundreds of times", "guilt", "always", have a meaning provided that the object discussed is present. It is not present in a discussion between psycho-analysts; when it is not present intercourse between psycho-analysts tend to jargon, that is to an arbitrary manipulation of psycho-analytical terms. Even when that does not happen it presents an appearance of happening. [ST, 148]

Jargon becomes an end-in-itself and seems to be an attractive lodging for self-feeding erudition. Many think that to build skilled talk about analysis can replace the practice of analysis: ". . . *the erudite can see that a description is by Freud, or Melanie Klein, but remain blind to the thing described*" (AMF, I, 5).

Perhaps if and when analysis develops out of its *"fumbling infancy"*, it will be free from jargon.

> SHERLOCK The simple part of it has been dealt with by Watson. You heard that fellow Bion? Nobody has ever heard of him or of Psycho-analysis. He thinks it is real, but that his colleagues are engaged in an activity which is only a more or less ingenious manipulation of symbols. There is something in what he says. There is a failure to understand that any definition must deny a previous truth as well as carry an unsaturated component (AMF, I, 92).

> PAUL . . . St John of the Cross even said that reading his own works could be a stumbling block if they were revered to the detriment of direct experience. Teachings, dogma, hymns, congregational worship, are supposed to be preludes to religion proper—not final ends in themselves.

> P.A. This sounds not unlike a difficulty we experience when psycho-analytic jargon—"father figures" and so forth—

> ROBIN: Touché!

P.A. —are substituted for looking into the patient's mind itself to intuit that to which the psycho-analyst is striving to point: like a dog that looks at its master's pointing hand rather than at the object the hand is trying to point out" (AMF, II, 267).

P.A. Mystery is real life; real life is the concern of real analysis. Jargon passes for psycho-analysis, as sound is substituted for music, verbal facility for literature and poetry, trompe l'oeil representations for painting (AMF, II, 307).

ROLAND Or Pythagoras, buried under his triangle—

P.A. Or Freud buried under his oedipal triangle, or Melanie Klein under a mass of evacuated identifications—

ALICE Or a mass of Kleinian Theories treated to "introjective projections" or even what I say interpreted, diagnosed, relegated to the lavatory bowl as psychotic distortions by virtue of the neologisms of psychiatry. Time that antiquates antiquity; the neo-news allowed to calcify in the realms of oblivion until the mental archaeologists scrape the arteries free of their horny integuments and display the dead jargons of the past to be admired, re-diagnosed, re-interpreted and re-interred.

P.A. James Joyce tried to break out of the mental ossifications in which his tender shoots of animation were enclosed by the Clongowesian wrappings of Roman Catholicized semitic Zeus.

PRIEST Zeus was a juvenile vulgarian anyway. Truth always has to break out of the wrappings of the latest Enthusiast who wants to bring his pet mummy to life. [AMF, III, 466–7]

To talk about analysis and to experience analysis

P.A. . . . I find that any rational explanation that is "reasonably" proffered has only ephemeral effect. Environmental factors leave virtually no lasting lesson in the recipient's mind—to trace.

ROBIN Then what does have lasting effect?

P.A. Anything which stimulates, mobilizes, creates feelings belonging to the love⇔ hate spectrum.

ROBIN I don't know what you mean—it sounds like jargon. I find it difficult to see what differentiates your statements from other jargonese statements.

P.A. You are right—and I don't know what to do about this difficulty when I am "talking about" psycho-analysis. If I were practising psycho-analysis with you I could try to demonstrate an emotional experience you were having and say, "What you are *now* feeling is what I call 'hate', or 'love', or some subdivision between the two." *Here* I can elaborate what you have called "jargon" by this rather long-winded story—'construction' as Freud might have called it—. [AMF, II, 361–2]

Suggested cross-references: Bionian, Kleinian.

Judgmental values:

> In psycho-analytic methodology the criterion cannot be whether a particular usage is right or wrong, meaningful or verifiable, but whether it does, or does not, promote development. [LE, Introduction, 3]

In *A Theory of Thinking* Bion offers a view of judgmental values. They are seen as originating at a point in time that is simultaneous with the inception of the processes of thinking; which obtrudes as learning from a specific experience, namely, that of the mating of pre-conceptions and realizations. From this mating a conception can ensue. It *"does not necessarily meet a realization that approximates sufficiently closely to satisfy"* (ST, 113).

Conceptions, thus, are that which stems from those primitive processes of thought. There is an amount of frustration involved; if it *"can be tolerated the mating of conception and realizations whether negative or positive initiates procedures necessary to learning by experience"* (ST, 113–4).

Some different developments may take place, when a negative realization takes place. There is always a parcel of negative realization. It is something that Bion would develop later. Tolerance of frustration may not be so great; therefore, it does not activate the mechanism of evasion. Nevertheless it can simultaneously be too great to bear dominance of the reality principle. In this case, *"the personality develops omnipotence as a substitute for the mating of the pre-conception, or conception, with the negative realization"* (ST, 114). It is now that judgement emerges, as a kind of last resort institution:

This involves the assumption of omniscience as a substitute for learning from experience by aid of thoughts and thinking. There is therefore no psychic activity to discriminate between true and false. Omniscience substitutes for the discrimination between true and false a dictatorial affirmation that one thing is morally right and the other wrong. The assumption of omniscience that denies reality ensures that the morality thus engendered is a function of psychosis. Discrimination between true and false is a function of the non-psychotic part of the personality and its factors. There is thus potentially a conflict between assertion of truth and assertion of moral ascendancy. [ST, 114]

It is necessary to discriminate ethics from morals; the former, in the same way as the super-ego, are linked to Kant's "categorical imperatives"; the latter is the phenomenon that Bion focuses on.

ALICE ... Perhaps we should discuss it with Priest when he returns. He's been away a long time but I understand he is coming back in time for our next meeting.

ROLAND Oh my ... good.

ALICE You don't sound pleased; what is the matter?

ROLAND I'm glad he is coming, but I don't want to be involved with God and the rest of that pious stuff.

ROBIN To do him credit he does not try converting us; to be fair to P.A. he doesn't try to convert us to psycho-analysis either. [AMF, III, 541]

The analytic posture may be sharply differentiated from pedagogy, justice and law, ministering and the like. Transference phenomena are an invitation to mistake analysis for those activities. Personal analysis of the analyst's narcissistic traits helps to make due differentiation. The analyst does not judge; he or she perceives, appreciates and describes. An analysis shows how it is rather than how it ought to be. Judgement is relevant to analysis when it is an issue in the session, originating from the personality of the analysand. The following quotations perhaps illustrate the issue, in terms of the analyst's posture:

Since psycho-analysts do not aim to run the patient's life but to enable him to run it according to his lights and therefore to know what his lights are, Taβ either in the form of interpretation or scientific paper should represent the psycho-analyst's verbal representation of an emotional experience. [T, 37]

ROBIN Doesn't your working day consist in discussing the qualities and defects of others?

P.A. I try to demonstrate the qualities of the individual. Whether they are assets or liabilities he can then decide for himself.

ROLAND I thought you were supposed to cure them.

ROBIN So did I.

P.A. "Cure" is a word which, like "illness" or "disease", is borrowed from physicians and surgeons to account for our activities in a comprehensible manner" (AMF, III, 541).

ROLAND Either you are being very modest or psycho-analysis is not much good.

P.A. Neither. Psycho-analysis is a fine instrument: psycho-analytic experience makes poor capacity for some things greater than yours.

ROLAND Thank you; you *are* complimentary.

P.A. I did not expect you to like my opinion, and your contempt is not lost on me. If I were prey to depression I would despair of your impenetrable complacency. It brings home to me how impossible it is for me to get the help of a critical attitude. It would help if I could rely on the purifying effect of austere criticism. I cannot. Fantastic admiration and complacent hostility, both are available in quantity and both are so much mental rubbish. I do *not* value either your praise or blame.

ROLAND Do you think I value yours?

P.A. I know you do not; in my opinion you cannot. It was the hundreds of cultured, educated, well-meaning "yous" which constituted a liability that England could no longer support but sank under the weight. (Rosemary enters unexpectedly and unnoticed. She sits and listens).

ROLAND I thought you people were supposed to be impartial.

P.A. In the practice of my job I am; even when I am not engaged in my profession I retain habits of impartiality. Whatever the contingent circumstances my natural impulse would incline me to justice rather than injustice. But that is not what *you* mean when you speak of impartiality—you mean partiality to your views. It is not natural to me to be partial to your views as far as I have reason to know them (AMF, II, 308–9).

P.A. You may not envy the kind of eminence which stimulates my envy, but you nevertheless have feelings of envy. The fact that I may not be able to define feelings, either yours, mine or those of others which are neither yours nor mine, does not mean that they do not, did not, or may not in the future exist. They may at some stage become so obtrusive that it is possible to attach a name to them.

ROBIN Although I have been aware of the pressure of what I can now call sexual or envious feelings, I would have been outraged had I been told that I was sexual or envious.

ROLAND What other people can verbalize about my feelings, especially if I can't, is particularly exasperating.

P.A. That is one component of the practice of psycho-analysis that is constant even if not constantly perceived. Guilty feelings are unwelcome and even in infants easily evoked. It is difficult to give an interpretation which is distinguished from a moral accusation.

ROLAND Surely this is a defect of psycho-analysis?

P.A. Certainly; but when I agree, you and others are therefore liable to assume that it is psycho-analysis only that suffers from that weakness, whereas I believe that this is a fundamental experience. It is this fundamental experience that underlies Plato's dialogue between Socrates and Phaedrus which is being revived here—a few hundred years later—in this discussion. [AMF, III, 480]

In *Attention and Interpretation*, the privilege of the individual under the analytical vertex (*"Psycho-analysts accept their field to be the individual"* (AI, 127) is compared with that of moral agencies of society-at-Large. *"Freud's scheme of id, ego, super-ego suggests one view of the organization of the personality, though there is nothing to suggest that the scheme represents a preference and not an observation"* (AI, 127).

ADOLF What the devil have you got all this armour plate for?

ALBERT Call me Albert. I've got it *for* the Devil. What the devil do you s'pose? I'm resting; it's my spore stage.

ADOLF But I got these teeth for spores. Your vegetative existence is an offence. It's provocative, blast you! It's a resistance! You put ideas into my head. I was all right before you stirred up the ten commandments. Since then I have not been able to sleep for the itch to commit adultery. It's all your fault.

ALBERT There you go! Now you are making *me* feel guilty. Why can't you keep your conscience to yourself? Now I am filled with the gnawing of conscience and re-conscience and remorse. World without end—Amen.

ADOLF Keep your religion to yourself! Now you make *me* want to attend mass. All right, serves you right if I *do* eat you!

ALBERT You have wak'd me too soon. I must slumber again.

ADOLF Do wake me—in a few thousand years' time.

ALBERT By that time I shall have reached your anus.

ADOLF The right place for anyone's remorse—keep right away from my mouth and teeth! Right up the other end of my alimentary canal.

ALBERT Don't blame me if you have digestive pains. You mustn't blame me if you devour me. My armour plate, my resistances, my spores are pretty tough. Are you sure your anus can take it? [AMF, 83–4]

Suggested cross-references: Analytical view, Establishment, Tool-making animal.

Jung: There is a discrete, critical reference to Carl Gustav Jung's work in the writings of Bion. He is said to have been present at Jung's lectures in London; later readers are prone to identify Jung's mysticism with Bion's use of the model of mystics.

PRIEST Has not Jung said this?

P.A. He said he agreed with Freud's description of the transference; he talked also of archetypes and a collective unconscious. I don't see why he should not call the Oedipus figure an archetype if he wants to, or say that an equivalent of the Oedipus figure exists in every human being. But I do not see any need to augment Freud's facts and theory; if I saw a better way of demonstration I would not hesitate to use it. The postulate of a collective unconscious seems to me to be unnecessary. I would not say that because two people see a mountain *that* is evidence of a "collective eye"; it is simpler to say both people have eyes that function in a similar manner. I would not use an expression which might risk an increase in ambiguity—which is bad enough at best. [AMF, II, 422]

K

K link; Knowledge–Link; *"knowing"* (LE, 50), or *"know"* (EP, 3). The latter expression conveys with added precision its transient, dynamic nature rather than a static, teleological knowledge— or *"piece of knowledge"* (LE, 47).

This link displays one of Bion's integrations of Freud and Klein's theories; namely, that of the two principles of mental functioning and that of projective identification.

Concern for knowledge is a fundamental feature of psychoanalysis. It is an attempt to know our inner lives beyond our material existence. Irrespective of the word used to label that which Freud called, "psychic reality" (mind, internal world, emotional life, personality or character, ego, id, etc), it is our task to know psychic reality as well to know what hampers this task. To know—and to deal with the unknown—is an activity that originated science.

This concern marked all of Bion's work. It is affiliated to the Freud-Aristotle lineage, whose invariance is the human being's "urge to know" (as expressed in metaphysics). Bion includes this urge in his study of the inception of cognitive and thinking processes. Bion does not dwell on the "philosophicalities" of that which Ernst Cassirer named "the problem of knowledge":

The problem with which philosophers of science have become associated has been given added significance by psycho-analysis and this for two main sets of reasons: x has the strength and is shown in detail to have the weakness of which he has always been suspected when he embarks on an investigation of y that is related to y's capacity for contact with reality. I do not propose to spend time on the philosophical problems involved as they can be found dealt with in Kant, Hume and their successors. [LE, 48]

The issue is dealt with using psycho-analytical tools in order to tackle psycho-analytic issues: *"I wish to emphasize that all that has been said about the problems of knowledge applies with particular force to psycho-analysis and that psycho-analysis applies with particular force to those problems"* (LE, 48); *"I am convinced of the strength of the scientific position of psycho-analytic practice"* (LE, 77). The scientific position is warranted by clinical observation.

Freud's contributions coupled with further clinical experience has shown Bion the **way** that emotions interfere with problems of knowledge—that of pain. Pain is an ever-present factor that obtrudes in analysis. Indeed, if the knowledge of a real breast is feasible to the extent one tolerates the no-breast, pain is an unavoidable accompanying fact of the experience. Also, if the schizophrenic's disturbances of thought are visible in anyone whose analysis is extended enough, pain emerges—ultimately, in facing and realizing truth, people fear feeling crazy. Therefore pain qualifies as a selected fact (q.v.) or invariance in the processes of knowing.

According to Kant, the five basic human senses and "pure reason" are not enough to ensure knowledge. Hume noticed that "constant conjunctions" are psychological constructions. They indicate more the reality of the onlooker's state of mind than real features of reality. In analytical terms, to get sensations of knowledge means that evasion of frustration is operating, rather than modifying it.

In Bion's example, x K y (x knows y) is a painful emotional experience, to the extent that it includes the no-knowledge. If it goes forward there emerge feelings of x getting a piece of knowledge of y. When one is successful in getting those feelings of knowledge, *"x K y no longer represents the painful emotional experience but the supposedly painless one"* (LE, 49).

In developing his theory of α-function (please refer to this specific entry as well as Dream-work-α, β-elements and Thinking) Bion would make his first verbal formulations on knowledge. This was made after serious consideration about the scientific method as it was seen in 1959–60: "*I reserve the term, 'knowledge', for the sum total of α-and β-elements. It is a term that therefore covers everything the individual knows and does not know*" (C, 182).

His main source was the clinical experience with patients with remarkable disturbances of thinking. This translates into the participant observation of a session's key emotional experiences. Those are conveyed through the relationship and non-relationship of the patient with the analyst.

Bion introduces his first detailed model about the K link in chapter sixteen of *Learning from Experience*. Please refer to the entry, "Link", to have a clearer idea of his model of links. The K link is discussed here to the extent that it is "*germane to learning from experience*" (LE, 45).

Science and mathematics study relationships between things. In our case, Bion studies the relationships of elements of a model: "*The choice of L or H or K is not determined by a need to represent fact but by the need to provide a key to the value of the other elements that are combined in the formalized statement. In psycho-analysis where a statement depends on other statements for its value the need for recognition of such a key statement is pressing*" (LE, 47).

L and H are relevant—or may be—to K, but if the purpose is K, "*neither is by itself conducive to K*" (L, 47). The "K purpose" is not an abstract love of knowledge but rather a need to know the patient. Bion represents this necessity as "*analyst K patient*". It is a formulation that denotes a relationship. The statement, "*analyst K patient*" is a statement that "*represents an emotional experience*". The emotional experience itself is given by the session. There is a suggestion in which "*if x K y then x does something to y. It represents a psycho-analytic relationship*" (LE, 47).

From knowledge to processes of knowing

K activity resorts to abstraction, in contrast to that reverse process of concretization by which words cease to be abstract signs but become things-in-themselves. Abstraction and formalization are essential in order to make an attempt to demonstrate a relationship.

> As I propose to use it, it does not convey a sense of finalit;, that is to say, a meaning that x is in possession of a piece of knowledge called y but rather that x is in the state of getting to know y and y is in a state of getting to be known by x. [LE, 47]

This includes the idea of a process that allows research into the unknown. Therefore it *"covers everything the individual knows and does not know"* (C, 182). In Bion's view a paradox did exist and was tolerated: knowing includes not knowing. Or, to experience truth includes to experience lying; or to experience reality, includes to experience hallucination.

> The question "How can x know anything?" expresses a feeling; it appears to be painful and to inhere in the emotional experience that I represent by x K y. An emotional experience that is felt to be painful may initiate an attempt either to evade or to modify the pain according to the capacity of the personality to tolerate frustration. Evasion or modification in accordance with the view expressed by Freud in his paper on Two Principles of Mental Functioning are intended to remove the pain. Modification is attempted by using the relationship x K y so that it will lead to a relationship in which x is possessed of a piece of knowledge called y—the meaning for x K y repudiated by me on p. 47. Evasion on the other hand is attempted by substitution of the meaning "x is possessed of piece of knowledge called y" so that x K y no longer represents the painful emotional experience but the supposedly painless one. [LE, 48–9]

Therefore, the K link runs a risk: a manoeuvre to get knowledge *"is intended not to affirm but to deny reality, not to represent an emotional experience but to mis-represent it to make it appear to be a fulfilment rather than a striving for fulfilment. The difference between the aim of the lie and the aim of truth can thus be expressed as a change of sense in x K y and to relate to intolerance of the pain associated with feelings of frustration . . . it is possible to increase understanding of the insane by considering his failure to substitute a misrepresentation of the facts for the representation that corresponds to, and therefore illuminates, reality. The motive is likely to be explained in Freud's statement that "hallucination was abandoned only in consequence of the absence of the expected gratifi-cation"* (LE, 49).

The K link was hitherto seen in the light of Freud's two princi-ples of mental functioning. The key here is the hallucination of fulfilment and its obverse, namely, the possibility of tolerating an urge that is doomed to dissatisfaction. To resort to misunderstand-ing and misrepresentation to ensure a continuous evasion is exam-ined under the entry, "minus K" (−K).

This theory of knowledge under the analytical vertex had undergone an amendment in the final chapters of *Learning from Experience*. It is constituted by the inception of one of the few theo-ries of psycho-analysis that Bion made, that of the container and contained (q.v.). This area is covered in its specific entry of this dictionary and the reader may refer to it. Of importance here is the continuous attention to intrapsychic functioning. The K model is used in conjunction with his earlier theory of thinking (q.v.)—that of pre-conceptions mating with realizations to give concepts. K, in terms of container and contained, is permeated by emotions; growth is the formulation that depicts the changes of container and contained which conjugates through emotions. This growth includes increments of knowledge/non-knowledge (or doubt) in a process of knowing. This process is called by Bion, "learning from experience". It is a process that has analogies with the digestive and the reproductive systems.

☺ K is associated with curiosity (T, 67) and its practical applica-tion meets with the Grid. Knowledge cannot be obtained through reason, which is the *"slave of the passions"* (T, 73); Bion suggests the use of intuition to experience *"transformations in O"* (q.v.).

The analytic aim evolves from K to O; please refer to the specific entries. Bion would resort more heavily to Hume concerning constant conjunctions and in considering reason as a slave of the passions. *"The process of binding is a part of the procedure by which something is 'won from the void and formless infinite'; it is K and must be distinguished from the process by which O is 'become'. The sense of inside and outside, internal and external objects, introjection and projec-tion, container and contained, are all associated with K"* (T, 151).

The living transient character of the processes of knowing was described at the end of his life: *"P.A. It appears—to us—to be the case. But is what appears to 'us' to be regarded as identical with fact? Priest and others seem to think that we psycho-analysts claim to know. I regard any thing I 'know" as transitive theory—a theory 'on the way' to knowledge, but not knowledge. It is merely a 'resting place', a 'pause' where I can be temporarily free to be aware of my condition, however precarious that condition is"* (AMF, III, 462).

K space

K seems to be the *"space in which what is normally regarded as classical analysis takes place and classical transference manifestations become "sense-able"* (T, 115).

Misuses and Misconceptions:

1. To see K as a piece of knowledge: Bion himself warned against this use.

2. To use K (and the theory of links altogether) as a proof of Bion's affiliation to an imagined "relationist" school within the psycho-analytic movement. When introducing the theory of container and contained, he writes: *"Reconsidering K in the light of previous discussion although K is essentially a function of two objects it can be considered as a function of one"* (LE, 90).

3. K and interpretation: there are readers who like to eschew L and H and state that the correct interpretation is made exclusively under K. This precludes the intuitive approach and the evaluation demanded by each case that was recommended by Bion (EP, 51). Also, it mistakes a recommendation clearly directed to the analysis of psychosis and psychotic phenomena with a general posture. The psychotic personality challenges K and can even display contempt for it; it favours emotional climates full of projective identification and reversion of perspective (q.v.). Therefore in those cases and moments it is necessary to attempt *"to establish a K link"* (T, 61). This applies to *"the emotional tone accompanying the interpretation"* (T, 60) and relates to the *"patient's apparent demand for exactitude both with regard to the verbal communication itself and the emotional accompaniment"* (T, 61). Even though Bion considers that to establish a K link is, *"after all the case with any interpretation"*, and therefore in trying to establish the K link *"there must be no emotion belonging to the H or L group"*, this refers to a specific moment of the act of interpreting, in which H and L can well be a prelude or an aftermath of the interpretation. Extra care must be taken with exacting patients, who, in

making no *"allowance for human frailty"* behave as if verbal communications, when received (many times they are not) are conveyors
of aspects of the analyst's L and K. *"In successful analysis the patient
brings to bear quite brilliant intuitive grasp of the possibilities that his
analyst's deficiencies offer his super-ego for demolition of the analyst"* (fn
T, 61).

&: This author has proposed integration between the two
models of Bion's theory of thinking (Sandler, 2001).

−**K**: A quasi-mathematical sign to denote the negative realm of
greedy misunderstanding that manifests itself through a specific,
purposive mode of knowledge. It is a function of envy. Envy and
violence of emotion are two factors of this kind of negative knowledge. Are there other factors in −K? This question awaits further
clinical research.

A model may be useful in order to grasp what minus K is all
about. A baby feels fear that it is dying. It splits off and projects such
feelings into a breast; envy and hate go together to the extent that
the breast remains undisturbed. Taking into account that *"envy
precludes a commensal relationship"* (LE, 96) the breast cannot be felt
as a moderator of the dreadful and annihilating feelings. It cannot
allow a re-introjection that could be growth-stimulating.

In this case it continues being a breast, but in fact it is a minus
breast or a breast in the minus K domain. It is felt as *"enviously to
remove the good and valuable element in the fear of dying and force the
worthless residue back into the infant"*. The violence of emotions (q.v.)
adds to the situation, in affecting the projective processes *"so that far
more than the fear of dying is projected"* (LE, 97). The process of denudation must be seen under the vertex of K (knowledge); therefore it
is a denudation of meaning. This denudation of meaning is *"therefore more serious . . . The seriousness is best conveyed by saying that the
will to live, that is necessary before there can be a fear of dying, is a part
of the goodness that the envious breast has removed"* (LE, 97).

−K also opens the possibility of a minus container/contained.
The predominant characteristic is a "without-ness". It must be
differentiated from "nothingness", or Zero. In clinical work it is
presented as *"an envious assertion of moral superiority without any
morals"* (LE, 97). Many among the readers of this entry have probably experienced dealing with patients who argued that they could

not pay for analysis; some made lying statements to prove they had no money. Those statements can be backed by acting-out—concrete measures in the outside world, material reality such as provoking a boss to be fired; quarrelling with husbands, fathers or the like who eventually pay the expenses and so on. So armed, they argue that they cannot pay—a superior argument that gives them moral superiority. Thanks to the reversion of perspective the analyst is reduced to an envious and greedy being who wants to suck out the patient's assets. Usually the fact is that the patient feels (some acknowledge it in a conscious manner) the analysis helpful to him in many ways. *"The process of denudation continues till minus ? minus ? represent hardly more than an empty superiority–inferiority that in turn degenerates to nullity"* (LE, 97). Minus K is installed.

The minus container/contained *"shows itself as a superior object asserting its superiority by finding fault with everything. The most important characteristic is its hatred of any new development in the personality as if the new development were a rival to be destroyed. The emergence therefore of any tendency to search for truth, to establish contact with reality and in short of be scientific . . . is met by destructive attacks on the tendency and the reassertion of the 'moral' superiority"* (LE, 98).

"In K, the climate is conducive to mental health. In −K neither group nor idea can survive partly because of the destruction incident to the stripping and partly because of the product of the stripping process" (LE, 99). This product would be better studied in his book *Transformations*.

It is not lack of knowledge, but it is a knowledge at the service of pleasure; this pleasure derives from destruction. It is expressed by uses of truth that are alienated from truthful intentions; it creates truth-less truths. It is untruthfully uttered. It is not intended to lead to accretions of knowledge, but rather to extinguish that knowledge. For example, a politician is aware of data that prove that his foe is corrupt. He denounces these truthful data. The true— or real—objective (to win elections) is alienated and omitted; the use of truth turns it into untruth. The overt, advertised objective is untrue, pretending to be protection of the public interest and property.

In the analytic session, some patients who are concerned to prove their superiority to the analyst by defeating his attempts at interpretation can be shown that they are mis-understanding the interpretations to demonstrate that an ability to mis-understand is superior to an ability to understand (LE, 95). Or that there is *"a moral superiority and superiority in potency of UN−Learning"* (LE, 98).

Bion improved this formulation when he elicited the nature of hallucinosis. There ensued a finer description of the negative realm: it is a *"raging inferno of nothingness"*. The same occurred with the observation that the patient feels that there is a *"superiority of the method of hallucinosis over the analytic method"*.

The "negative" or "minus" refers both to the nature of the no-thing that is inseparable from the thing and to that realm created by those who feel they cannot tolerate this no-thing. It is a greedy state; in this greedy state of mind one disables one's capacity to abstract. Right from the start it cannot abstract the breast from its sensuously based "concreteness". "Nothing" replaces the "no-thing"; "without-ness" replaces a real lack of something.

Processes of Knowledge (K) brings tolerance of the no-thing (please refer to the entry, a "Theory of thinking"): *"The domain of thought may be conceived of as a space occupied by no-things"* (T, 106).

−K space: the "space" of hallucination

Hallucination may be more profitably seen as a dimension of the analytic situation in which, together with the remaining 'dimensions', these objects are sense-able (if we include analytic intuition or consciousness, taking a lead from Freud, as a sense-organ of psychic quality).

To make a step towards definition of this space we consider it to be a −K "space" and contrast it with K "space"—the space in which what is normally regarded as classical analysis takes place and classical transference manifestations become "sense-able". Using once more the analogies (C_3 elements) I have already employed, −K "space" may be described as the place where space used to be. It is filled with no-objects which are violently and enviously greedy of any and every quality, thing, or object, for its "possession" (so to speak) of existence. I do not propose to carry my analogies further than to indicate that −K "space", is the material in which, with which, on which (etc.) the "artist" in projective transformation works. As an analogy with space may easily distort I propose to drop the term and speak of transformation in −K. [T, 115]

Misunderstandings and misuses: Minus K is not lack of knowledge; there is a meaning, but it *"is abstracted leaving a denuded representation"* (LE, 75). It is a knowledge linked to advocacy and law, to convince people, the realm of propaganda. Another example of minus K is the idea that a "Classical analysis" is an inferior practice *vis-à-vis* an analysis that profits from observation that makes explicit the realm of hallucinosis.

Suggested cross-references: Hallucination, Hallucinosis, K.

"Kleinian":

> P.A. I can recognize and would like to acknowledge my debt to Freud and to Melanie Klein, but they might be affronted by such attribution. I would acknowledge my debt to others, but I am aware that many would think such an acknowledgement more a liability than an asset; they would not wish to be thought my mental forebears. Nor do I wish to wear the plumage of the peacock when my true colours should be the feathers of the sparrow. [AMF, II, 360–1]

Bion kept a guarded posture concerning the adjective "Kleinian". On one occasion he makes explicit that he bows to a widely-used custom that should serve for purposes of communication. He was introducing the idea of interpretations (which are transformations of original experiences during an analytic session) stemming either from the theories of Klein or from Freud: *"In practice I should deplore the use of terms such as 'Kleinian transformation, or 'Freudian transformation'. They are used here only to simplify exposition"* (T, 5, fn 1).

A few years before his death, he would express it in equally emphatic terms:

> ROBIN At least we have so far avoided forming ourselves into an Institution with a doctrine and a uniform—not even a mental uniform.

> P.A. So far. I have been surprised to find that even *my* name has been bandied about. I used to think Melanie Klein was a bit optimistic and unrealistic—though sincere—in deploring the idea that people would call themselves Kleinian. [AMF, II, 259]

The issue was also stated to be bigotry:

P.A. We are all scandalized by bigotry. We are none of us bigot-generators; that is, we none of us admit to being the spring from whom bigotry flows. As a result we do not recognize those of our offspring of whose characters we disapprove. Indeed, Melanie Klein discovered that primitive, infantile omnipotence was characterized by fantasies of splitting off undesired features and then evacuating them (AMF, II, 229).

PAUL Nobody knows, but the Pythagoreans are thought to have been interested in what we should nowadays call science or philosophy.

ROBIN What did *they* call it?

PAUL I've no idea, but the name of Pythagoras was obtrusive and they were called Pythagoreans.

P.A. Something like that has happened to psycho-analysis. No one knows what that is, but people are called Freudians and Kleinians. Vexilla Regis Prodeunt.

PAUL Onward Christian Soldiers, marching as to war (AMF, II, 237).

Comparing my own personal experience with the history of psycho-analysis, and even the history of human thought . . . it does seem to be rather ridiculous that one finds oneself in a position of being supposed to be in that line of succession, instead of just one of the units in it. It is still more ridiculous that one is expected to participate in a sort of competition for precedence as to who is top. Top of what? Where does it come in this history? Where does psycho-analysis itself come? What is the dispute about? What is this dispute in which one is supposed to be interested? I am always hearing—as I have always done—that I am a Kleinian, that I am crazy. Is it possible to be interested in that sort of dispute? I find it very difficult to see how this could possibly be relevant against the background of the struggle of the human being to emerge from barbarism and a purely animal existence, to something one could call a civilized society.

One of the reasons why I am talking like this here is because I think it might be useful if we were to remind ourselves of the scale of the thing in which we are engaged, and whereabouts a little niche could be occupied by ourselves (C, 377). (Six months before his death.)

ROLAND You sound like Gilbert and Sullivan

SOMITE THIRTY Never heard of them.

ALICE Can't bear the stuff. Bach and Mozart for me.

DEVIL I am sure P.A. will recognize the warring musical sects as psycho-analytic theories in a new costume. How Dryden would have laughed!

P.A. He did, does and will do in the future, I am sure. It is not quite so amusing to people like me, who are still conscious, awake and aware of the medium which surrounds us, as it is to God and the Devil. By the way, how should I address you? Your Satanic Majesty? Your Id-iocy?

DEVIL (bowing politely) Take your choice, I am not fussy as they are in The Other Place. Bigotry and Intolerance are simply the medium in which I flourish. We weave it into a thin veil on to which our demonstrations are projected for identification.

P.A. My God! You are not a Kleinian are you? [AMF, III, 448]

In New York, 1977, Bion states that if Melanie Klein's theories have anything to do with *"real facts infants must be marvellous Kleinians because they know all about what it* **feels** *like, but they have no concepts, but they have no concepts, they cannot write any of these great books—their concepts are blind . . . Later on they have forgotten what it is like to feel terrified; they pick up these words but the words are empty . . . You have to notice that it is an empty phrase, it is a concept; it is only verbal; the intuition is missing"* (BNYSP, 40).

The dialogue continues:

Questioner —You said every infant is a Kleinian; I wondered if it is also true to say that every Kleinian is an infant.

Bion —Yes, absolutely—but unfortunately grown-up, and they look exactly like adults. We all have this illusion that we are adults, we have reached the peak, and have nothing more to learn. That is why I suggest asking the question which is open-ended—Why am I doing analysis? [BNYSP, 40]

In São Paulo, 1978:

Interpreter—I would like to know what "Kleinian" means—

Bion You are optimistic. Even Mrs. Klein didn't know what it meant—she protested at being called a "Kleinian". But, as Betty Joseph told her, "You are too late—you are Kleinian whether you like it or not". There was nothing she could do about it. So—although we aspire to respect the individual, bigotry rears its ugly head again. While I have the aspiration to respect individuals it does not surprise me at all to find that I am bigoted about something else. [BNYSP, 86–7]

While not being a Kleinian, Bion was grateful to Klein and often made this clear:

ROBIN I thought you would call yourself a Freudian psycho-analyst. Or are you a Kleinian?

P.A. I can recognize and would like to acknowledge my debt to Freud and to Melanie Klein, but they might be affronted by such attribution (AMF, II, 360–1; also BLI, 74).

DOCTOR I knew some intelligent, "brainy" people who played games for Oxford; they seemed to remain brainy *and* athletic.

P.A. Fortunate people! If only one could see how they did it one might solve the problem of how to produce more energy than beef. I would think I was in reality becoming a psycho-analyst if I could *become* more energetic by *being* more energetic. It might enable others to start that reaction. Melanie Klein seemed to do that for psycho-analysis.

BION What! You don't mean to say you are a Kleinian?

P. A. You remind me of Sir Andrew Aguecheek—"And if I thought he were a puritan I would . . .!" Your excellent reason, sir?

BION I thought you would appreciate an experience which we could share together (AMF, III, 471).

P.A. A fetus might take a dislike to its experiences including awareness of them. As a result of her experiences with infants a theory was formulated by Melanie Klein which became known later as "projective identification". She did *not* attribute it to fetuses.

ROLAND Then why complicate the theory by supposing an even earlier existence of the mental mechanism? Isn't it a fact that this Kleinian theory is already questioned by many psycho-analysts?

388   THE LANGUAGE OF BION

P.A. If it were simply a matter of saying "ditto, ditto to Mrs. Klein, only earlier still". I would agree that there would be every reason for dismissing the Kleinian theory and its supposed "improvement" as probably ridiculous and not worth the expenditure of time and effort involved in their consideration. Many analysts repudiate Klein's extension of psycho-analysis as elaborated by Freud. I found it difficult to understand Klein's theory and practice though—perhaps because—I was being analysed by Melanie Klein herself. But after great difficulty I began to feel there was truth in the interpretations she gave and that they brought illumination to many experiences, mine and others, which had previously been incomprehensible, discrete and unrelated. Metaphorically, light began to dawn and then, with increasing momentum, all was clear.

ALICE Did you remain convinced by further experience?

P.A. Yes—and no. One of the painful, alarming features of continued experience was the fact that I had certain patients with whom I employed interpretations based on my previous experience with Melanie Klein, and though I felt that I employed them correctly and could not fault myself, none of the good results that I anticipated occurred.

ROBIN In other words the objections raised by contemporary psycho-analytic colleagues to Kleinian theories were being supported by your own experience of futility?

P.A. That was indeed one of my anxieties and one I did not feel disposed to ignore.

ROLAND But you must have ignored it. Did you not feel you had a vested interest in continuing to support psycho-analysis, Kleinian or otherwise?

P.A. I was aware that I would be likely to cherish my preconceptions. Every now and then something would occur that convinced me I would be foolish to abandon my idea as if they were clearly wrong. In fact it was clear that they were not always wrong. So—it became a problem of discrimination.

ROLAND What led you to persist?

P.A. Partly a chance recapitulation of Freud's description of the impression created on him by Charcot's insistence on continued observation of facts—unexplained facts—until a pattern began to emerge; partly his admission that the "trauma of birth" might afford a plausible but misleading reason for believing that there was this caesura between natal and pre-natal. There were other impressive "caesuras"—for example, between conscious and unconscious—which might be similarly misleading. Melanie Klein's interpretations began to have a vaguely but truly illuminating quality. It was as if, literally as well as metaphorically, light began to grow, night was replaced by dawn. I was aware, with a new comprehension, of the passage of Milton's invocation to light at the commencement of the Third Book of *Paradise Lost*. I re-read the whole of *Paradise Lost* in a way I had not previously done, although I had always been devoted to Milton. This was true likewise of Virgil's *Aeneid*—though it involved much painful regret for the way in which I had wasted and hated the privilege of being taught by certain schoolmasters whose devotion had but a sorry response from me. Let me now praise men who ought to have been famous. For my own pleasure I write their names: E. A. Knight, F. S. Sutton, Charles Mellows. Later came the debt to my friends whom I will not name lest it cause embarrassment. [AMF, III, 559–60]

This is a verbal formulation that depicts experiencing the depressive position (recognition of guilt for having shown unwarranted aggression) and of the Father ("Milton", "E. A. Knight", "F. S. Sutton", "Charles Mellows", "friends"), and Mother (*"Aeneid"*, "Klein"), the creative couple. ("Virgil's *Aeneid*", "Milton's invocation to light at the commencement of the Third Book of *Paradise Lost*").

To those who cannot work through their rivalry, envy, greed and hate towards the nourishing breast perhaps the only way out is to deny them and let them erupt in a disguised form: through being "-ians". Freud described it as a transformation into the contrary. It is attributed to both Kant and Napoleon, "I hope God defends me from my friends, because I know how to take care of my enemies". As a matter of consequence, the "-ians" promote the growth of ministers, scholasticism, nationalism and all forms of "-isms".

The rest of the paragraph begs to be read. It displays in an exquisite way how Bion felt his experience with Melanie Klein and the acquisition of a capacity for gratitude and assumption of guilt, in a reference to some of his past schoolmasters. Other mentions of his experiences with Melanie Klein can be found in *Bion in New York and São Paulo*, p. 83; in a poignantly grateful way, in *All My Sins Remembered*, p. 68; also, in the Introduction to *Seven Servants*.

Suggested cross-reference: "Bionian".

L

L-Link: Please refer to the entry, Link.

−**L:** This symbol stands for the negative realm of love. It is not hate, even though it may convey hateful emotions. It may be grasped by some of its phenomenal manifestations. The lying use of truth that is made to obtain secondary gains, be they avoidance of pain, evasion or subterfuge, is an example of −L.

   −L means indifference and lack of compassion; L is destroyed. The Nazi phenomenon, torture and technocracy are some of its phenomenal manifestations.

   Recommended cross-references: Links, Minus.

Language of achievement: The Language of Achievement refers to the development of methods of communication, *"which have the counterpart of durability or extension in a domain where there is no time or space as those terms are used in the world of sense.*

   ... it is certainly my impression that the experience of psycho-analysis is supposed or intended to have an enduring effect" (AI, 2).

   There is a search for *"formulations [that] exist which have achieved durability and extensibility"* (AI, 1).

It is possible to trace the origins of this concept in *Transformations*, its development in *Attention and Interpretation* and its practical application outside the session in *A Memoir of the Future*. It constitutes Bion's final proposals to find a method that could both convey and describe the way an analyst actually works, including the fact that this posture includes regard to truth.

It stems from Keats' idea of the existence of "Men of Achievement". It is linked to Bion's conviction that the analyst's work should be endowed with durability, as expressed in *Transformations* and *A Memoir of the Future*. At first he was interested in a language that could achieve a real inter-peer communication. Science cannot afford the lack of a reliable means of inter-peer communication.

In using the artist as a model, Bion considers the final products of the "great" artist. His notation of final or end products is "$T\beta$" (see the specific entry). Bion states that the end product effected by an artist "*communicates an* **emotional** *experience . . . in the greatest number of the people in whom he intends to produce it*". In this case, the "*components of $T\beta$ in this class of transformations are: emotional experience, precision of communication, universality and durability*" (T, 32).

Paraphrasing him, a real analyst experiences the emotional experience in the broadest and most profound layers of the patient's personality and his own personality. The components of T in this class of transformations are: (i) precision of communication: (ii) universality; (iii) individuality; (iv) durability. "*The psychoanalyst tries to help the patient to transform that part of an emotional experience of which he is unconscious into an emotional experience of which he is conscious. If he does this he helps the patient to achieve private knowledge . . . The artist is used here as a model intended to indicate that the criteria for a psycho-analytic paper are that it should stimulate in the reader the emotional experience that the writer intends, that its power to stimulate should be durable, and that the emotional experience thus stimulated should be an accurate representation of the psycho-analytic experience (Oa) that stimulated the writer in the first place*" (T, 32).

The problem of communication between analysts proved to be an issue of communication between the analyst and his patient. To resort to the artist as a model does not mean that an analyst must be an artist, even though Bion stated that he or any analyst would have his work made easier or perhaps feasible if he could communicate musically or odorifically (AI, 18).

This specific model may show the nature of the skills or efforts involved. As always happens in analysis, it is necessary to make a quantum leap in order to achieve the apprehension of a given psychic reality as a different form of existence if compared with material reality.

The durability is achieved when it glimpses, even if imperfectly and transiently, "truth O", The term "O" is defined in *Transformations* and can be found elsewhere in this dictionary. The term, "truth O" was introduced in *Attention and Interpretation* (AI, 29). In this book Bion states that the analyst's attention should be "O" (AI, 27); it is also in this work that he outlines the Language of Achievement.

The language to be used in analysis should apprehend the underlying transcendence, truth O of each patient, during the here and now of the experience with the patient. This transcendence appertains to the numinous realm of the unconscious. It is the origin ("O") of the features that make the patient who he really is; paradoxically it is a nest of possibilities, generating evolutions from the unknown—and unknown-bound. "O" can evolve during the session.

> ROBIN Set a poet to catch a poet. Blake was not deceived about the meaning of *Paradise Lost*. In more recent times, Kenner has shown how Shakespeare said far more than he consciously intended when he wrote "Fear no more the heat of the sun". [AMF, II, 248]

One must endure lies, hallucination and hallucinosis (AI, 36). The analyst must not hallucinate even though he must *"participate in the state of hallucinosis"*. This is especially true with regard to sharply differentiating feeling pain from suffering pain (AI, 9). *"Send a poet to catch a poet"* is a formulation that has a counterpart in analysis: send a person who was analysed up to his psychotic nuclei to catch a psychotic—as an experienced analyst once told the author (Dr Jayme Sandler, personal communication, 1969).

The Language of Achievement transiently glimpses the fleeting evolutions of the patient's truth as reflected by the emotional experience in the here and now. It is minute, subtle, and underlies the sensuously apprehensible data available to observation by the analytic pair. In the decisive moment it is uttered—on the spur of this moment.

Nevertheless something is unavoidably lost by the very act of verbalization. The loss must be compensated by the patient's capacity for containment, tolerance of frustration and ability to maintain the tension necessary to issue further free associations; the same for the analyst's free-floating attention (please refer to the entries, Analytic View, Atonement, Real Analysis).

The Language of Achievement, being intuition and experience-oriented, cannot be taught even though it can be learnt. It was a known fact that the minus K or mis-representation ability of the human being, expressed by the Sophists and centuries later denounced by Voltaire, makes language an effective tool to be used for finalities of deception and evasion. It parallels the Language of Achievement elaborated for truth. In groups it is used when a fight-flight basic assumption is prevalent (AI, introduction, 3, 4).

The paradoxical relationship of the Language of Achievement and the realm of Minus can be compared with that of a two-edged knife. One cannot exist without the other; truth and lies are a matching pair; the same for hallucination and reality.

This issue was first developed by Bion in the last chapter of *Transformations* under the heading of the Grid's categories of column two. The disciplined posture of the analyst with regard to memory, desire and understanding, and his extended self-analysis, which can display his primary narcissism and envy, helps in this discrimination. Compassion and truth decide which way the interpretation will take: that of achievement or that of achievement of a lie. This, Bion calls, in contrast to the Language of Achievement, "Language of Substitution". On one hand we have the former and on the other we have the latter. This is a language necessary for evasion, subterfuge and hallucination. There are **no** judgmental values involved (see the entry, Judgmental Values).

The issue is to tolerate the tension and the paradox in the area of attention: "*The psycho-analyst's attention must not wander from areas of material characterized either by the Language of Substitution or by the Language of Achievement: he must remain sensitive to both*" (AI, 126).

The Language of Achievement, when it touches the numinous negative realm, that of the tolerance of Keats' negative capability, also deals with the realm of minus as a counterpoint. This last sense was the origin of Bion's concept, as expressed in the introduction and in the last chapter of *Attention and Interpretation*. It is expressed by his quotation of Keats, in his unashamed admiration of Shakespeare. The Language of Achievement (Bion's term) is uttered by Men of Achievement (Keats' term): *"when a man is capable of being in uncertainties, mysteries, doubts, without any irritable reaching after fact and reason"* (AI, 125). Is it a kind of "Ode to Frustration"?

There is mention of "irritable reaching". This does not preclude reaching but puts it into a perspective of eternal vigilance and incompleteness or un-fulfilment (please refer to the entries, Atonement, Real Psycho-analysis). Belonging to the tolerance of minus, Language of Achievement is *"a substitute for, and not a prelude to, action"* (AI, 125). It is the minus-acting-out. The analyst explains nothing; he helps the patient to achieve something that was lurking, already available to him but hitherto unknown (to both). Paradoxically it is *"itself a kind of action"*. Something must be said in the form of metaphors, idées mères, passionate non-sensuous imagery. It is not a naïve or chaotic situation; it is oriented by psycho-analysis. In a certain sense it made part of Bion's rescuing of Freud's ethos of psycho-analysis; and if one can achieve this, much has or would have been done for the psycho-analytic movement.

> This discussion is centred on the problem of bringing attention to bear on the realizations to which Freud's theories approximate.
>
> ... [I have] rarely failed to experience hatred of psycho-analysis and its reciprocal, sexualization of psycho-analysis ... the human animal has not ceased to be persecuted by his mind and the thoughts usually associated with it ... therefore I do not expect any psycho-analysis properly done to escape the odium inseparable from the mind. Refuge is sure to be sought in mindlessness, sexualization, acting-out, and degrees of stupor. [AI, 125–6]

A necessary but not sufficient step towards the Language of Achievement is the choosing of a vertex (see the entry, Vertex). This seems to be the way (perhaps the only way discovered until now) to deal with the mass of apparently connected—but in fact, disconnected—verbal manifestations uttered by the patient. They come together with the apparently disconnected verbal manifestations. The latter are in fact connected by underlying invariances and selected facts that wait to be apprehended.

The vertex is clearly depicted by Freud in the opening parts of chapter VII of *The Interpretation of Dreams*, to quote an example. The apparently connected material may just constitute a cluster of rationally constructed cancerous growth (AI, 128). It can be rationally swallowed— reason being a slave of passion (T, chapter six).

The attempt finally to reach a written Language of Achievement was made in the Trilogy *A Memoir of The Future* and its preparatory texts that were published in *War Memoirs*.

BION I don't understand

MYSELF Perhaps I can illustrate by an example from something you *do* know. Imagine a piece of sculpture which is easier to comprehend if the structure is intended to act as a trap for light. The meaning is revealed by the pattern formed by the light thus trapped—not by the structure, the carved work itself. I suggest that if I could learn how to talk to you in such a way that my words "trapped" the meaning which they neither do nor could express, I *could* communicate to you in a way that is not at present possible.

BION Like the "rests" in a musical composition?

MYSELF A musician would certainly not deny the importance of those parts of a composition in which no notes were sounding, but more has to be done than can be achieved in existent art and its well-established procedure of silences, pauses, blank spaces, rests. The "art" of conversation, as carried on as part of the conversational intercourse of psycho-analysis, requires and demands an extension in the realm of non-conversation . . ..

I have suggested a "trick" by which one could manipulate things which have no meaning—the use of sounds like "α" and "β". These are sounds analogous, as Kant said, to "thoughts without concepts", but the principle, and a reality approximating to it, is also extensible to words in common use. The realizations which approximate to words such as "memory" and "desire" are opaque. The "thing-in-itself", impregnated with the opacity, itself becomes opaque: the O, of which "memory" or "desire" is the verbal counterpart, is opaque. I suggest this quality of opacity inheres in many O's and their verbal counterparts, and the phenomena which it is usually supposed to express. If, by experiment, we discovered the verbal forms, we could also discover the thoughts to which the observation applied specifically. Thus we achieve a situation in which these could be used deliberately to obscure specific thoughts.

BION Is there anything new in this? You must often have heard, as I have, people say they don't know what you are talking about and that you are being deliberately obscure.

MYSELF They are flattering me. I am suggesting an aim, an ambition, which, if I could achieve, would enable me to be deliberately and *precisely* obscure: in which I could use certain words which could activate precisely and instantaneously, in the mind of the listener, a thought or train of thought that came between him and the thoughts and ideas already accessible and available to him.

ROSEMARY Oh, my God! [AMF, I, 189–191]

Obviously the real Language of Achievement, as far as it is a feasible task at all, is restricted to the analytic session itself.

Suggested cross-references: Atonement, Analytic view, Judgmental values, Real Analysis, Vertex.

&André Green made an attempt that resembles the language of achievement when dealing with free associations, in his definitions of "Dan", in his paper on the central phobic position (*IJPA*, 2000).

Language of substitution: Please refer to the entry, "Language of Achievement".

Lies: *"Descartes' tacit assumption that thoughts presuppose a thinker is valid only for the lie"* (AI, 103).

Bion asks whether it is possible to analyse a liar (AI, 105). He quotes Melanie Klein's negative opinion on this issue. Anyway, *"in psycho-analysis the liar is a significant fact and gains significance from the lying nature of what he says"* (AI, 104). The relentless "pursuit of truth O" (AI, 29) may be considered Bion's life-time achievement. A scientific, fresh new look at lies is brought about by his work—paradoxically, one may scrutinize the truth that is at stake or is influential in the state of mind that produces lies.

Origins

Bion was confronted with lies from his infancy and adolescence. During his infancy social practices—including religious education—had separated him from his family at the age of eight. As a matter of consequence he was bluntly introduced to social hypocrisy and social error.

This episode may be regarded as an early test of that which he would name many years later "the sense of truth" prevailing over *a* "truth" (q.v.; ST, 116). The judgmental value of the "right thing to do", "absolute truth" was the sending of a little boy of eight to be schooled in a country abroad, far from his parents to the point of incommunicability. "Absolute truth" displaced "a truth", namely, that children need mental nourishment from their parents. "Ought to" replaced "Necessity". In *A Memoir of the Future*, he would write about an "oughtism" (AMF, II, 276). One may find many expressions of lies in his autobiographical recollections: the feeling of absolute truth would again prevail over a sense of truth:

(i)   An adolescent psychotic bout ended with his serving in the British Army as a tank officer.

(ii)   The murderous activity of officials both in the government and in the army (see Establishment).

(iii) An unwitting lie won him the highest military decoration instead of being court martialled as he expected if truth had obtruded.

(iv)   His guilt about a fellow-in-arms capable of passionate love who died when trying to emulate him as the hero he felt he was not.

(v)   The contact with his first "analyst" who kept telling him, "feel it in the past".

(vi)   Aping the earlier experiences of having been sent to England as a child and having enlisted in WWI, he practised the same self-deception: "it is better to work in the Army than to assist a pregnant wife".

(vii) The experiences of co-option and attempts to be the object of idolization.

Lies, science and psycho-analysis

His posture before lies was expressed by his quotation (at least twice) of Dr Samuel Johnson's comparison of the possible consolation obtained with truth and that which may be obtained by a lie (C, 114; AI, 7).

The replacement of a scientific outlook—false and true—by a moral commandment—right or wrong—precludes the realization that truth and falsity equals reality and hallucination rather than good or evil. The replacement of the paradox-tolerating "and" by the rational splitting expressed by "or" expresses denial, authoritarianism and pleasure-ridden choices.

Bion's knowledge of Popper made him disagree with most of this thinker's work. Perhaps the sole exception was ad hoc theorizing (see the entry, Multiplicity of theories). One point to ponder, even if Bion never made it explicit, may refer to Popper's criteria of falsifiability. To Popper and others such as Kuhn, science is a history of lies and false conclusions. Popper and Kuhn were not scientists (the latter gave up his activities as a physicist). In contrast, Bion remained linked to practical, scientific activity. His scientific interest made him value the function of lies as something that exists and seems to have its function—but it is not an end-in-itself. Science would not be *only* a history of falsities and lies as Popper and Kuhn proposed. They may be an intermediary step in the march into the unknown that leads to pieces of transient knowledge.

Nor does Bion think that there are any "royal roads to truth". In *A Memoir of the Future* he would cast doubts on the analyst's superiority in perceiving and apprehending truth *vis-à-vis* other disciplines and vertexes. He depicts his ideas vividly through the use of a quasi-Socratic internal dialogue between the fictitious characters P.A. and Priest. His metaphor on many ancestral "psycho-analysts" before Freud, who are seen as his begetters, dates from this epoch. A thought without a thinker, "psycho-analysis" existed long before a Freud appeared to think it.

The risk of the thinker is to be a liar. The act of thinking and more than this, the action of expressing the thought, endangers the underlying truth it strives to convey. The burial of Freud's fundamental observations, for example, infantile sexuality, is evidence of this (AMF, I, 5). For more details refer to the entry, "Truth". The issue, as he warned in 1962, seems to be similar to that which occupied philosophers (LE, 48) but it is not. He was able to make the difference explicit in 1965 and 1970. In fact the analyst can contribute to philosophy.

> To the problem of understanding I have said that the psycho-analyst can bring something that is unknown to the philosopher of science because the psycho-analyst has experience of the dynamics of

misunderstanding; the psycho-analyst is concerned practically with a problem that the philosopher approaches theoretically. [AI, 97]

"Practice" here means the clinical experiences with the liar *par excellence,* that is, the psychotic. "Psychotic" here means the in-hospital patient and the neurotic who shelters the psychotic personality in the analysis. In brief, mankind. There remains a controversy about the necessity to analyse the psychotic nuclei of any person, analysts being no exception. The controversy lingers on when analysts state, "I do not analyse psychotics", meaning, "I refuse to analyse my own psychotic features". Hallucinations and delusions can profitably be seen as lies and falsities (Rosen, 1959).

Rescuing the psycho-analytical vertex, Bion's approach emphasized:

(i) **Lack of judgmental values**: Judgements are seen as an offshoot of a lying perspective, in the sense that the incapacity to assess truth and falsity leads to ideas of right and wrong. In other words, lies belong to the realm of hallucination rather than to the realm of morals. The Bard puts the issue in Hamlet's "mouth": *"There are no good or bad things, but mind makes them so".*

(ii) **Tolerance of a paradox**: instead of focusing either on truth or the lie *per se,* Bion focuses on the binomial relationship: truth/lie. That is, the "and" replaces the "or"

☉ 1962—His first approach to the lie was made in terms of the patient's unconscious allegation that to misunderstand is superior to understanding. Misunderstanding induces error—or lie and falsity, in other words (please refer to the entry, minus-K). In 1963, he amended the theory with the use of column 2 of the Grid (q.v.) which depicts verbal statements known to the analyst and patient alike to be false. This would make part of a theory that depicts paranoid–schizoid productions designed to communicate via projective identification; they would lead to his theory of hyperbole (q.v.). Also, function of lies as a necessary step towards knowledge was having a fundamental push here. The reality testing of lies and falsities could, in persons whose intolerance of frustration and pain is not prevalent, be conducive to the apprehension of reality. This means saying that at least *"some forms of lying appear to be closely related to experiencing desire"* (AI, 100).

In this sense he does not deal with lies under a moral vertex (AI, 96). Column 2 statements are *"known by the initiator to be false but maintained as a barrier against statements that lead to a psychological upheaval"* (AI, 96). To many people, facing their inner truth can be felt as life-threatening, leading to self or hetero-murder. *"Column 2 involves conflicts with impressions of reality"* (AI, 102).

Lies and the clinical situation

Lies often appear in the guise of cure. This is specially true when the patient's outlook seems to be that of the liar (minus K and minus L) and that of the analyst seems to be that of the scientist (K).

> By definition and by the tradition of all scientific discipline, the psycho-analytic movement is committed to the truth as the central aim. If the patient constantly formulates −L and −K statements, he and the analyst are, in theory at least, in conflict. In practice, however, the situation does not present itself so simply. The patient, especially if intelligent and sophisticated, offers every inducement to bring the analyst to interpretations that leave the defence intact and, ultimately, to the acceptance of the lie as a working principle of superior efficacy. In the last resort he will make consistent progress towards a "cure" which will be flattering to analyst and patient alike. [AI, 99]

If the existence of thoughts without a thinker is accepted, a thinker is necessary to the lie but not to the truth. Truths exist independently of thinkers to think them. *"Provisionally, we may consider that the difference between a true thought and lie consists in the fact that a thinker is logically necessary for the lie but not for the true thought. Nobody need think the true thought: it awaits the advent of the thinker who achieves significance through the true thought"* (AI, 102–3).

Oedipus existed quite independently, and before there was a Sophocles or a Freud to think it. $E=mc^2$ existed independently of the existence of an Einstein or a Poincaré to think it.

Lying cannot be regarded as a symptom; this approach is conducive to error. In some liars there is a need to deny that lies *"becomes acute and may usher in attacks on linking to stop stimulation which leads to conflict"* (AI, 102). This presupposes an aim and therefore there are different patterns to be observed in different liars. *"Hence it is not possible to rely on picking up a symptom, such as a wish to please the analyst, that will betray the pattern.*

For satisfaction, the liar needs an audience; this makes him vulnerable, since his audience must set a value on his fabrications" (AI, 102).

It does not matter if the audience is a victim or a moral instance to the liar; but it matters for the analyst who is none of those two. He will be able to see that the analyst attaches *"importance to the patient's statements as formulations of a truth"*. For he will also observe incoherence and he *"will be able to detect a pattern that brings together disparate elements"*. Those are the same words that Bion uses when depicting the obtrusion of a selected fact (q.v.) that displays a coherence and a meaning that the elements did not have without it—or *"the transformation of paranoid–schizoid position to the depressive position"* (AI, 102). This movement, as can be experienced in the analytic session, *"is superior to a narrative formulation which betrays the lying element of the story only by the weakness of the causative links . . . The lying discovery lacks the spontaneous bleakness of the genuine PS⇔D"* (AI, 102).

The realm of O is felt by the paranoid–schizoid state as persecution-inducing, due to the fact that it is in constant evolution. *"The impact of the evolving O domain on the domain of the thinker is signalized by persecutory feelings of the paranoid–schizoid position. Whether the thoughts are entertained or not is of significance to the thinker but not to the truth. If entertained, they are conducive to mental health; if not, they initiate disturbance. The lie depends on the thinker and gains significance through him. It is the link between host and parasite in the parasitic relationship"* (AI, 103).

Lies are invested with social importance: *"the relationship between the lie, the thought, the thinker, and the group is complex"*. The thinker may express the truth in a lying group and their relationship will be one of envy and hate. If the thinker is expressing a lie, it has a relationship between him and his own self that is parasitic—*"lies and thinker will destroy each other"* (AI, 103).

The expansion of the various possible outcomes of the relationship between lies, liars and thinkers is reviewed in pages 104–105 of *Attention and Interpretation*. Some cultures foster the development of the lie. *"Since the analyst's concern is with the evolved elements of O and their formulation, formulations can be judged by considering* *how necessary his existence is to the thoughts he expresses. The more his interpretations can be judged as showing how necessary **his** knowledge, **his** experience, **his** character are to the thought as formulated, the more reason there is to suppose that the interpretation is psycho-analytically worthless, that is, alien to the domain O"* (AI, 105).

A famous lie that occurred at Ur, when some priests promised—but did not deliver—eternal life to a monarch serves as illustration:

P.A. That's where you came in with your little beaker and large store or fairy tales; and, in due course, the British Museum.

PRIEST Don't forget the University of Pennsylvania, and its large store of dollars. And Freud—don't forget Freud and that load of science beneath which is buried God and Art and Wisdom itself.

P.A. Death, you say, shall have no dominion.

PRIEST No I don't; that is not my view of death. Thoughts live until they find a thinker who gives them birth—and so brings death into the world and all our woe.

P.A. From your vertex it may *seem* so, but that depends on standing on the giddy precipice of 'seeming'.

PRIEST You resort to visual imagery to make your empty thoughts look full.

P.A. I agree it does make them seem full, but I think these formulations have content. I am talking about "something" and I think it would be worth having respect for "seeming". I doubt the equivocation of the fiend that lies like truth. [AMF, II, 363–4]

Bion the individual and truth

Bion left many written accounts of his ideas about himself. A poignant one is expressed with the aid of a quotation from Shakespeare's *Hamlet* ("*Nymph, in thy orisons, may all my sins be remembered*"). It concerns his earlier posture regarding his first wife and first daughter. Also, he makes clear his view about not meriting his war decorations; he thought he received them because of his mistake, mistakenly understood by the authorities.

These accounts are perhaps telling about his position about lies—and truth.

P.A. I have not the courage necessary for the part.

ALICE You sadden me, but I think you are right.

WATSON How can you tell? I have known some ordinary people who behaved with extraordinary courage.

P.A. I know what you mean. I have even had courage attributed to me. But I remember no occasion on which I was not a coward. Even in my prosaically unheroic role of psycho-analyst I always fear to give an interpretation (AMF, II, 361–2).

EIGHTEEN YEARS Weren't you pleased when you were decorated for war service?

TWENTY-THREE YEARS Too late! Besides, I knew too much. I remember Lord Helpus, as we called him, saying to Twenty, "I always tell my son John, that if you see a man with more than two rows of ribbons he is tolerably certain to be a waster".

TWENTY YEARS I remember. I only had one solitary ribbon which I was afraid I would have to prove —I knew I could not. "Coward! Coward!" my thumping heart would tell me. At Anvin when I felt the air trembling and throbbing against my ears . . . a bombardment? Twenty and more miles away? I felt no better when that old hand Trapper said, "It's only a trench raid". I thought it must be all Hell let loose. [AMF, III, 451–2]

Lies, truth, pleasure: real analysis

ALICE You decry glory, but is there not some reality in that?

ROBIN I was impressed by the regimental motto, "Quo Fas et Gloria Ducunt".

ROLAND I still am. "Ubique", likewise, has that appeal of mystery and invitation.

P.A. I don't deny it. In a world of peace I am glad to be left with some reminiscence, some luminosity that penetrates the shadow and the darkness. However ignorant of ideas to come, the idea of glory withstood my cowardice. But just as it would be impossible to explain to anyone who had not been in action what it would be like to be a combatant soldier or a regimental stretcher bearer, so it is impossible to describe to anyone who has not been a practising psycho-analyst what it is to experience real psycho-analysis.

ROLAND Surely you do not seriously mean that an analytic session is comparable with going into action?

P.A. Comparable, yes. Imminent death is not expected, although there is that possibility. That does not weigh the anxiety—fear in a low key. One shrinks from giving the unwelcome interpretation.

ROLAND Is it not just fear that the patient is going to be angry at being criticized?

P.A. I don't think so; the patient may be angry at a critical comment, perhaps even murderously angry, but I do not think that possibility consciously deters.

ROBIN Is it some unconscious fear—the counter-transference of which you spoke?

P.A. It is. Though one is not "conscious" of it—to obviate that is one reason why we think analysts must themselves be analysed—there is an inherent fear of giving an interpretation. If a psycho-analyst is doing proper analysis then he is engaged on an activity that is indistinguishable from that of an animal that investigates what it is afraid of—it smells danger. An analyst is not doing his job if he investigates something because it is pleasurable or profitable. Patients do not come because they anticipate some agreeable imminent event; they come because they are ill at ease. The analyst must share the danger and has, therefore, to share the "smell" of the danger. If the hair at the back of your neck becomes erect, your primitive, archaic senses indicate the presence of the danger. It is your job to be curious about that danger—not cowardly, not irresponsible.

ROLAND You must think highly of yourself if you are such a paragon.

P.A. I am trying to describe the job—not my fitness or otherwise for it. I have enough respect for the psycho-analyst's task to tell the difference between this social chat about psycho-analysis—or even a technical discussion of it—and the practice of psycho-analysis. Anyone who is not afraid when he is engaged on psycho-analysis is either not doing his job or is unfitted for it.

ROBIN An airman or seaman who is not afraid of the elements, afraid of the sea and the skies, is unfit to navigate. The line between fear and cowardice is faint.

P.A. Quite so. I would add, the line between daring and stupidity is similarly faint.

ROLAND How would you define it?

P.A. I would not. In practice, where to draw the line depends on the facts, including the facts of one's personality, with which one judges—the total capacity. Definitions are only a matter of theory—useful for discussion and communication of ideas. In practice one does not rely on anything so ambiguous as verbal formulation. [AMF, III. 516–8]

Suggested cross-references: Absolute truth, Analytic view, Atonement, Becoming, Commonsense, Compassion, Correlation, Disturbed personality, Enforced splitting, O, Jargon, Manipulations of Symbols, Mystic, Philosophy, Real psycho-analysis, Reality Sensuous and Psychic, Sense of Truth, Thinking, Truth. Truth-Function, Ultra-sensuous, Unknowable, Unknown.

Line See Circle, Point, Line

Link

First model of links

When discussing the part played by alpha-function "*in transforming an emotional experience into alpha-elements*", Bion links the sensuously-apprehended stimulus to sophisticated mental activities such as having emotional experiences. They are worked through by dreaming, thinking and memorizing. Therefore, alpha-function is seminal in the apprehension of reality. It is a model to deal with a mystery—that probably shall remain as such, being linked to the stuff of life itself. How does materialness turn into immaterial? What are the paths and how is it done? We cannot know, but we have the model of alpha-function. The model is that of nourishing in physical terms; one may remember that the digestive system, skin and brain stem from the same embryological layers, namely, ectoblast. Sensuous impressions "nourish" something and some-no-thing that flows to psychic reality. Sensations nourish emotions.

Bion considers that to get a sense of reality matters to the individual in the same way that getting food, drink and breath matters to the individual's survival. *"Failure to eat, drink or breathe properly has disastrous consequences for life itself. Failure to use the emotional experience produces a comparable disaster in the development of the personality"* (LE, 42).

In using the model of the digestive system, he is aware of the many dangers common to the use of any model. Differently from theories, models have a comparatively short life in the scientific movement. They are disposable and lack durability. One of the factors is that models, relying on sensuous imagery, are easier to grasp than theories. Nevertheless, they also easily slip into a use that reifies and concretizes them. In order to *"moderate these dangers and make discussion scientific* **a notation to represent emotional experience** *is required"* (LE, 42; my bold). This representation would furnish *"the 'key' of the session"* (LE, 44).

This point is fundamental if the reader is to use Bion's writings as they were written. If one does not respect and much less realizes that the verbal formulation, "link", is a **mere system of notation** (in the same sense that the term "emotional experience" (q.v.) also is) one is prone to attribute false status to it—as for example, that of a theory. Notation is, by itself, one of the ego-functions in the apprehension of reality, as Freud proposed in 1909.

Therefore notation is something needed by an individual in his(her) life, by the scientist, by the analyst. Notation also demands simplicity and the achievement of elements that are basic. Bion seems to have been inspired by mathematicians—who many centuries earlier had this system and a whole array of elemental objects to work with. Even though this inspiration was not wholly apparent in the epoch when he developed the system of notation where he uses the word, "Link", there are many hints in it that it is maths that furnishes him with a model to emulate.

In the same work—*Learning from Experience*—he tries to develop the notion of the psycho-analytical object (q.v.) inspired by Aristotle's mathematical objects. The links, as we shall soon see, have the form of single-lettered symbols, much like mathematicians' notations. A negative realm, "minus", identical to the negative numbers, obtrudes. The search for elements would be clearer in his next book.

The scientific orientation in searching elemental tools that have a generalizing scope can be seen in his statement that such a system of notation would help the individual analyst who is interested in his advice to build up for himself *"an anthology of working psychoanalytic theory on a foundation of a few good basic theories well understood and capable, individually and in combination, of covering a great many of the situations he might expect to meet"* (LE, 42).

In first devising the links he states that it would help the student of his works not to overload this system of notation with connotations alien to those with which the author endowed the system: *"What follows is a sketch to indicate the lines along which progress* [in devising a system of notation to represent emotional experience] *could be made . . ."* (LE, 42).

Links, therefore, constitute not a theory of psycho-analysis, but are part of the body of observational theories. The three basic links being H, L and K, hate, love and knowledge, it is not difficult to see that they provide a detailed, explicit platform—the model (LE, 79)—as an attempt to build a tool to observe that which is ultimately unobservable, namely, the three basic instincts depicted by Freud: death, love and epistemophilia.

Aided by this compass, which has as its "North" the simplicity of elementals, he chooses to begin with the obvious: *"The feelings we know by the names 'love' and 'hate' would seem to be obvious choices if the criterion is basic emotion . . . I prefer three factors I regard as intrinsic to the link between objects considered to be in relationship with each other"*.

This introduces the link as a factor and the reader could ask, but why link? The choice was obvious at first and continues to be; Love and Hate are not possible in isolation. The next phrase justifies resorting to the term "link", already present in the idea of an apprehension of reality through alpha-function. It has to be so, as the leitmotiv of the system of notation is a necessity for noting the emotional experience: *"An emotional experience cannot be conceived of in isolation from a relationship"* (all quotations, LE, 42). And, later, he would make clear that there are individual factors that demand consideration: *"real love is not a function of the thing loved, but of the person loving"* (AMF, I, 197)

Some relationships:

(1)   X loves Y

(2)   X hates Y

(3)   X knows Y.

> These links will be expressed by the signs L, H and K . . .

> The analyst must allow himself to appreciate the complexity of the emotional experience he is required to illuminate and yet restrict his choice to these three links. He decides what the linked objects are and which of these three represents with most accuracy the actual link between them . . .

> To sum up an emotional episode as K is to produce an imperfect record but a good starting point for the analyst's speculative meditation. In this respect the system I have sketched out, despite its crudity and naivety, possesses the rudiments of the essentials of a system of notation—record of fact and working tool. [LE, 43–4]

One may notice the careful dealing with the model as such. There are readers who try to enshrine a mere model into the heights of theories, but this differs from that which Bion clearly states. The theory here is Freud's: that of instincts, which appertain to the realm of the numinous unconscious. The links express—or denote—observable phenomena, namely, hate, love and knowledge, expressed by emotional experiences. These are not conceivable apart from relationships.

The system HKL can be used in two different and mutually exclusive ways: to establish the "key" of the session and to record an emotional experience; the latter can lead to the former. *"The choice of L or H or K is not determined by a need to represent fact but by the need to provide a key to the value of the other elements that are combined in the formalized statement. In psycho-analysis where a statement depends on other statements for its value the need for the recognition of such a key statement is pressing"* (LE, 45).

Second model of links

This model draws from biology to construe an analogy and deals with the links between container and contained: parasitic, commensal and symbiotic (please refer to these specific entries, especially container and contained).

Misuses and misconceptions: *Relationist analysis* The appeal to a mere quasi-mathematical system of notation and model was turned into a "relationalist" theory. Despite the frequent use of terms such as endo-psychic and intrapsychic, and also despite the establishment of analysis as a method to present the person to him(her)self, up to his last works, there are people who insist that "what mattered to Bion was the relationship", rather than the individual's mind.

K versus L and H The privileged situation of the K link in the psycho-analytic setting (LE, 47) is often levelled against the importance of H and L in clinical work. This is an unwarranted use of Bion's work. More details can be seen in the entries, K and −K.

📖 See especially the preparatory papers in *Cogitations*, pp. 267, 271, 274.

Recommended cross-reference: Emotional experience.

Literature (and Bion's literary style): Literature, both in prose and poetical form, is an art form or an art manifestation of the human being to apprehend reality as it is. It is also a privileged form of demonstrating the vicissitudes and failures of such an enterprise. Echoing Freud and Klein, it occupies a seminal place in Bion's work as a source of inspiration and, above all, as a source of verbal formulations to communicate the human mind's functioning that perhaps could not be done by these authors themselves.

Even though all of them were privileged writers, it is doubtful that their writings attained the status of an art form. One may consider that Freud was awarded the Goethe Prize; but it was mainly linked to his contributions to the German language. Klein was often accused of being a poor writer in English, but the fact remains that her writing was terse, to the point and gave pure empiric descriptions. As an example of scientific writing, it is seldom surpassed.

One may consider, without attributing any special skill to literary standards, that Bion resorted heavily to powerfully evoking metaphors and parables, such as *"The Mind . . . is too heavy a load for the sensuous beast to carry"* (AMF, I, 38). One may also remember his analogies of the mental apparatus with the digestive system that allowed phrases such as "truth is the food of mind". It is commonplace to state that literature is "thought-provoking"; but perhaps this is an apt term to describe the way that Bion uses it.

From the beginning of his writing, a literary streak, so to say, without pretension of being literature-for-its-own sake, is present. That is, there is a specific use of words to convey an idea. In some texts he writes that he would try, if he were able to, to convey them musically, or odorifically. The situation is not only his writing for psychoanalysts, but also the communication during the session. Again and again, to resort to literary models seemed to facilitate the task of conveying the mental phenomena in a communicable form. For example, in his so-called clinical papers, Bion used two terms, "bizarre objects" (q.v.) and "furniture of dreams". Corresponding to day-time residues (which furnishes a night dream shell) as described by Freud, but mutilated and concretized due to the action of the paranoid–schizoid phenomena, Bion tries to describe concretely the stuff of the psychotic patient's mental environment, a place where he or she "moves" (ST, 40). A parable follows the metaphor: *"The patient now moves, not in a world of dreams, but in a world of objects which are ordinarily the furniture of dreams. These objects, primitive yet complex, partake of qualities which in the non-psychotic are peculiar to matter, anal objects, senses, ideas, superego, and the remaining qualities of personality. One result is that the patient strives to use real objects as ideas and is baffled when they obey the laws of natural science and not those of mental functioning"* (ST, 40).

Other examples such as "singing potatoes", full of humour, when referring to the impossibility of understanding or knowing reality, for reality does not allow itself to be known—but can be intuited, apprehended, used, albeit partially and transiently—again and again display his attempts at literary-constructed formulations.

Being the highest manifestation of the application of verbal thought and a symbolic system to communicate, it could hardly be different from psycho-analysis, which was born as the "talking cure". Even though what is talked about both hides and betrays that which is not talked about, but is said and immaterially conveyed—the latent contents—it is not cure at all. The verbal medium is, in the work of Bion, the only form of communication between patient and analyst. It was extended to the realm of non communication, too (AMF) (please refer to the entry, "Negative", "O", "Transformations in O").

If one tries to single out the main literary influence on Bion's work, some problems arise; but perhaps the Bard occupies a privileged position. John Milton is a serious candidate; so are Gerard Manley Hopkins, Robert Browning, the Bible, some Christian mystics' literature, mainly Meister Eckhart, John Ruysbroeck, Saint John of the Cross; Dante, John Ruskin, William Wordsworth, John Keats; eastern mystics such as the unknown writer of the Bhagavad Gita must be included; in his later days, Maurice Blanchot, at André Green's suggestion. One should quote a great number of writers and above all writer–philosophers such as Blaise Pascal, Goethe, Nietzsche, Wilfred Trotter. The main source of his literary inspirations may be found in *A Memoir of the Future*. Obviously, this work marks his abandonment of earlier attempts at a notational system inspired by mathematics and gives a free hand to resorting to quasi-literary, verbal ways.

The attempt to evaluate Bion's literary successes from the vertex of literature for its own sake led to disillusion, as Meltzer's comments exemplify. He was highly critical of the literary merits of the novelistic sense that may be conveyed to the more superficial reader of the first chapters of *A Memoir of the Future*. At the beginning of *Transformations*, Bion warns—using Freud's example of reading of his work as *romans-à-clef* —that "transformations in literacy" or alphabetization are not enough to grasp the meaning of any text (T).

The dialogical form chosen in *A Memoir of the Future*—in the wake of Diderot and Goethe, for example—was attempted with studies including fictitious characters written as early as 1958 (see *War Memoirs*). It is safe to admit that these characters are part objects of himself, displaying his life experiences. Of course, the metaphors, aphorisms and parables contained there are too numerous to be quoted, meriting a book of their own (Sandler, 1988).

The literary-minded reader may be rewarded in his search for a literary style by the autobiography, *The Long Week-End*. In the opinion of the present writer, expressed in 1987 (*International Review of Psycho-Analysis*), Bion's attempt at a most risky and difficult literary genre equals, in its truth-content and sincerity, as well as in the reflections of an old, experienced man who paradoxically conserved an infant's mind, Goethe's *Dichtung und Warheit*.

He looked for words that had counterparts in reality and always tried to define precisely what he meant by the words and concepts he advanced (see, for example C, 220–253). He strongly recommended that analysts should know precisely their private vocabulary (Evidence, 1976). Therefore, an analyst who mastered his own "literature", including myths, would be able to compare the use he (or she) made of it with that of the patient.

Suggested cross-reference: Philosophy.

This entry is linked to the title of this dictionary, *The Language of Bion*, and is made both as a way of acknowledgement and in honour of Oliver Rathbone, who suggested such a title.

Logic: Bion studied the laws of classic Euclidean logics extensively. He had many books on it— around ten—and all of them include his notes; he quote's Heath's introduction to Euclid in *Elements of Psycho-Analysis*. In the opinion of his late daughter, Parthenope Bion Talamo, which coincides with the opinion of the present writer, and was confirmed by a perusal of his private library (carefully maintained by Francesca Bion) he was not interested in mathematics for its own sake, but rather in the philosophy of mathematics.

He used very simple notations drawn from logics such as x, a, b in the hope that they would become non-saturated. In 1977 (AMF, II, 229) he acknowledges that he was not successful, for they were filled with "riotous" meanings.

In *Transformations*, as well in some papers later published in *Cogitations*, he quotes some of Euclid and Pythagoras' theorems, linked to Oedipus.

Also in 1977, he expands his freedom from classical logic. According to my research into his private library, he had deep contact with Brouwer's Intuitionist School, which tried to test the hypothesis of the non-validity of the Euclidean law of the excluded middles. His books on Intuitionism are from this time and have bookmarks, side annotations. This school has points of contact with Riemann and Lobatchewsky's non-Euclidean geometries, which are quoted in *A Memoir of the Future* (AMF, I, 62; II, 224, 247; III, 553).

Suggested cross-references: Literature, Mathematization of psycho-analysis, Philosophy.

M

Manipulations of symbols: Probably inspired by two sources, Alfred North Whitehead's *Introduction to Mathematics* and Popper's *The Logic of Scientific Discovery*, Bion seems to have perceived that a kind of professional disease plagued the psycho-analytic movement. Namely, a contradictory simultaneity of a priori and ad hoc theorizing (T, 4, 84, 96).

A priori theorizing tries to fit clinical data into known theories. It corresponds to a formalism not too dissimilar from that which mathematics dealt with successfully at the beginning of the twentieth century. It produced a formalistic approach that hoped to find known procedures for solving all mathematical problems.

The ad hoc theorizing has as its outcome that dissimilar theories try to explain the same clinical entity, whose underlying invariance remains unobserved. In terms of the theory of transformations, the analyst loses sight of, or never perceives, the invariances.

The situation was first described in 1962: the issue was to find a theory that could at once be not so concrete in its description of particular cases (lower level empirical data) **as well as** not so excessively general that it could slip into *"an ingenious manipulation of elements according to arbitrary rules"* (LE, 77). It seems that the psycho-analytical movement, despite the warning made by Bion, was not able to be free from the criticism that "*analyst and analysand indulge a taste for jargon*" (LE, 77). "*A theoretical formulation that appears to be too concrete and yet too abstract requires to be generalized in such a way that its realizations are more easily detected, without the attendant weakness, most often seen in mathematics, as appearing to be an arbitrary manipulation of symbols*".

After this statement, which clearly displays the influence of Bacon and Whitehead, among others, Bion asks: "*Can it retain its concrete elements without losing flexibility so essential in psycho-analytic application?*" (LE, 77). To achieve this he would (i) avoid jargon (q.v.), (ii) look for precision in communication, (iii) look for finer observation of facts through the construction of observational theories such as that suggested in *Transformations*, (iv) model-making, (iv) resorting to myths, in the wake of Freud.

Bion would formulate a myth for analysts in order further to enhance the probable power of his warning:

> The liars showed courage and resolution in their opposition to the scientists who with their pernicious doctrines bid fair to strip every shred of self-deception from their dupes leaving them without any of the natural protection necessary for the preservation of their mental health against the impact of truth. Some, knowing full well the risks that they ran, nevertheless laid down their lives in affirmations of lies so that the weak and doubtful would be convinced by the ardour of their conviction of the truth of even the most preposterous statements. It is not too much to say that the human race owes its salvation to that small band of gifted liars who were prepared even in the face of indubitable facts to maintain the truth of their falsehoods. Even death was denied and the most ingenious arguments were educed to support obviously ridiculous statements that the dead lived on in bliss. These martyrs to untruth were often of humble origin whose very names have perished. But for them and the witness borne by their obvious sincerity the sanity of the race must have perished under the load placed on it. By laying down their lives they carry the morals of the world on their shoulders. Their lives and the lives of their followers were devoted to the elaboration of systems of great intricacy and beauty in which the logical structure was preserved by the exercise of a powerful intellect and faultless reasoning. By contrast the feeble processes by which the scientists again and again attempted to support their

hypotheses made it easy for the liars to show the hollowness of the pretensions of the upstarts and thus to delay, if not to prevent, the spread of doctrines whose effect could only have been to induce a sense of helplessness and unimportance in the liars and their beneficiaries. [AI, 100–1]

This may remind us of Socrates and Savonarola, or even Thomas More.

Five years later, Bion would state:

SHERLOCK The simple part of it has been dealt with by Watson. You heard that fellow Bion? Nobody has ever heard of him or of Psycho-analysis. He thinks it is real, but that his colleagues are engaged in an activity which is only a more or less ingenious manipulation of symbols. There is something in what he says. There is a failure to understand that any definition must deny a previous truth as well as carry an unsaturated component. [AMF, I, 92]

It is safe to state that at the time of the writing of this dictionary, not counting the progressive abandonment of jargon that can be seen in some quarters around the world, the rest of his warnings still wait to be heard and used in the majority of places.

Mathematization of psycho-analysis:

The scientist must know enough mathematics to understand the nature and use of various mathematical discoveries and formulations, such as the differential calculus or the binomial theorem: the psycho-analyst must know his myth. The scientist must also know enough to have an idea when he is confronting a problem to which a particular mathematical procedure would apply: the psycho-analyst must know when he is facing a problem to which a myth would provide the psycho-analytic counterpart of the algebraic calculus. This, one might say, is precisely what Freud did; he recognized, as a scientist, that he was confronted by a problem to the solution of which he would have to apply the Oedipus myth. The result was the discovery, not of the Oedipus complex, but of psycho-analysis. (Or is it man, or man's psyche, that is discovered when these elements are constantly conjoined?) It is in this sense that I believe that the myth of Babel, or Oedipus, or Sphinx must be used as a tool comparable to that of the mathematical formulation. [C, 228]

Perhaps this quotation may help the reader to be introduced to the ethos of Bion's use of mathematical analogies. He used it mainly to investigate primitive methods of dealing with psychosis, which means, the earliest attempts to apprehend reality.

One of its main expressions—which led Bion to hypothesize that mathematics is an early attempt to deal with psychosis—is the ability to think in the absence of the object. It seems that Alfred North Whitehead's history of mathematics influenced him:

> The geometer had succeeded, by transformation of Euclidean geometry and its visual representation into algebraic projective geometry, in freeing his investigations of some of the restrictions imposed by the genetic history of the procedures he uses; so psycho-analysis must be freed from the restrictions imposed by the associations with space and sight by which I look to geometry to simplify exposition. [T, 111]

The same would be stressed later:

> MAN When the mind ± has been mapped, the investigations may reveal variations in the various patterns which it displays. The important thing may not be, as the psycho-analysts suppose, only revelations in illness or diseases of the mind, but patterns indiscernible in the domain in which Bio ± exist (life and death; animate and inanimate) because the mind spans too inadequate a spectrum of reality. Who can free mathematics from the fetters exposed by its genetical links with sense? Who can find a Cartesian system which will again transform mathematics in ways analogous to the expansion of arithmetic effected by imaginary numbers, irrational numbers, Cartesian coordinates freeing geometry from Euclid by opening up the domain of algebraic deductive systems; the fumbling infancy of psycho-analysis from the domain of sensuality-based mind? [AMF, I, 130]

Influential trends in epistemology in Bion's time stated—and continue stating today—that no field of human knowledge can aspire to the status of science unless it has been, or is amenable to being mathematized. In Bion's time, this could be seen in the work of the so-called neo-positivists. Not to be confused with the positivists, this is represented by the work of Moritz Schlick; of the young Wittgenstein, and in the considerations of the independent-minded Bradley, Braithwaite, Prichard and Russell; and in later times, Lakatos' work: "*It is said that a discipline cannot properly be regarded as scientific until it has been mathematized*" (T, 170). Does Bion endorse such a view?

This entry will try to assess the issue as well as to summarize all his analogies and uses of mathematical models.

Yes?

In bringing together the clinical experience drawn from psycho-analytical practice Bion observed that the inception of mathematical thinking in the mind echoes the mathematician's tribulations. Mathematics and geometry show signs of being an early method that both mankind and each individual had and continue to have, to try to deal with psychosis in their development.

But if any mathematics could be used, certainly it had not hitherto been discovered or formulated:

> The configuration which can be recognized as common to all developmental processes whether religious, aesthetic, scientific or psycho-analytical is a progression from the "void and formless infinite" to a "saturated" formulation which is finite and associated with number, e.g. "three, or geometric, e.g. the triangle, point, line or circle. Associated with this is the need for a geometric or numerological component in effecting a transformation . . . To what extent does this represent an essential link in the ability to effect transformations from experience of reality into knowledge . . .? The transition from sensibility to awareness, of a kind suitable to be the foundation of action, cannot take place unless the process of change . . . is mathematical though perhaps in a form that has not been recognized as such [footnote: A simple example of this is seen when an attempt is made to communicate, by means other than a full analysis, what a psycho-analysis is so that rules for its practice can be formulated: "five times" a week and for "50" minutes are readily "won" from the ineffable experience.]. [T, 170–171]

No?

His position seems to have been immutable throughout his work; let us compare early writing with the latest writings:

1959: *"In short, mathematics must be regarded by the psycho-analyst as one of the limiting classes that belong to psycho-analysis in so far as it attempts to be a coherent system of concepts, and in particular one of the methods by which the paranoid–schizoid and depressive systems are brought into a dynamic relationship with each other, and therefore as an aspect of those mental phenomena that are concerned with the achievement of mental developments by facilitating that dynamic relationship. It will therefore be seen that from a psycho-analytical point of view mathematics does not belong to the realm of ontology nor yet even of epistemology, but rather to that class of mental functioning which, since transition from paranoid–schizoid to depressive positions and back is essential to mental development, is essential to sanity itself.*

This is not to belittle mathematics but to show how fallacious is the view that pre-eminent importance in any one sphere, however important, confers some universally equal significance in all—a fallacy that has tended to make some observers suppose that failure to produce calculi representing the deductive system of biology, and in particular of psycho-analysis, is necessarily a condemnation of the subject for which no calculi exist. Mathematics may have a very important role as an object of study psycho-analytically, and at the same time and for the same reason be an important element in the mental processes of the individual which makes it possible to him to be a psycho-analyst" (C, 86–7). Or, in other works, he links mathematics with the inception of thought and primitive emotional processes, a point he would develop later, in Transformations.

1962: *"Mathematical formulation is not yet available to the psycho-analyst though there are suggestive possibilities"* (LE, 51).

1975: *"Mathematics, science as known hitherto, can provide no model"* (AMF, I, 61).

One may argue that he courted trans-disciplinarity. But this also displays unequivocal signs of being an internal development in a given discipline:

> Certain problems can be handled by mathematics, others by economics, others by religion. It should be possible to transfer a problem, that fails to yield to the discipline to which it may appear to belong, to a discipline that can handle it. If Euclidean geometry cannot handle multi-dimensional problems they can be transferred to algebraic geometry which can handle them. In this way certain problems can be transferred within their own discipline so that their solution can be attempted. The mathematics evolved by the

manipulation of "numbers" has so far proved very successful in matching the formulation with the realization it represents. [AI, 91]

A careful examination of his writing displays the fact that he was not proposing to transplant other disciplines to psycho-analysis but rather the contrary, that is, that psycho-analysis may help the mathematician, in the same way he saw that psycho-analysis may help the philosopher. Let us see the end of the paragraph:

> But the numbers representing feelings have not evolved so that they can handle the realizations of the domain from which they appear to have sprung. [AI, 91]

It is possible to state that Bion did not mathematize psycho-analysis. Nor did he use mathematics as a model, with the only possible exception of adopting a quasi-mathematical system of *notation*—western and Greek lettering, arrows and the like.

The impossibility of mathematicizing psycho-analysis seems to lie in the different origins of both. A comparative analogy between the geometer and the analyst can be made, and this is what Bion does. It concerns being able to deal with "objects" despite the physical absence of these same "objects". In psycho-analytical terms used by him it concerns being able to tolerate the no-breast or tolerance of "point".

This is a necessity for the infant and the analyst alike. The mathematician precociously seemed to be able to do this. In order to divest the concreteness or material-ness of the breast or of the point the infant needed to form, so to say, "meta-objects" in his inner world. The breast could be thought when it was physically lacking. Something does not vary in "both" breasts, internal and for the obvious reason that "they" are the same breast—yet they are also different; something was transformed. This is a paradox that is not to be resolved.

That which does not vary is called invariance and that which varies is called trans-formation. The latter varies in form. (A detailed description of this theory may be found in the entry, *Transformations*.) The infant's transformations that tolerate the absence of the breast seem to depend on "mammal" invariances. Invariances encompass both psychic and material reality. One of the ways the human being has to effect such a transformation relies on a system of notation. The baby comes to be able to say, "Mum". It is able to make a verbal transformation.

In the same way, the analyst's transformations seem to depend on analytical invariances; geometrical or algebraic transformations seem to depend on geometrical or algebraic invariances: *"I have no evidence for mathematical formulations that are not geometric in origin (other than material suggesting a relationship between having a third son and having three sons). What is not clear is the reason for a geometric rather than verbal development"* (T, 78).

Other quotations may dispel doubts about Bion's alleged attempts at mathematization of psycho-analysis: *"It has been said in criticism of psycho-analysis that it cannot be regarded as a science because it cannot be mathematized. Available mathematics do not provide the psycho-analyst with appropriate formulations"* (AI, 63).

Transformations in K are those which lead to knowing about something. They are different from transformations in O that allow for "becoming". Bion compares both with religion and mathematics:

> Transformation in K has, contrary to the common view, been less adequately expressed by mathematical formulation than by religious formulations. Both are defective when required to express growth, and therefore transformation, in O. Even so, religious formulations come nearer to meeting the requirements of transformations in O than mathematical formulations. [T, 156]

Keeping in mind that Bion stated that psycho-analysis requires transformations in O, one has more data for thinking about the idea that he tried to mathematize psycho-analysis.

Bion was not used to pseudo-scientific polemics. His assessment of the Berkeley versus Newton diatribe in the last chapter of *Transformations* vouches for this. Nevertheless one may conjecture that he was living during a time when violent criticism was levelled against psycho-analysis by then prominent figures such as Eisenck and Popper, with regard to its scientific status, and more specifically, that it could not be mathematicized.

Experience lasting more than thirty years in the analytic movement allows the observation that many readers were and are not available to read attentively the utterly compacted conclusions and the underlying implicit cogency of mathematical analogies as they appear in Bion's classical basic books, *Learning from Experience,*

Elements of Psycho-analysis and *Transformations*. Also, among this group, many are not prone to get acquainted with basics of mathematics that would help them grasp the issue. But perhaps some of them cannot get the gist due to the fact that Bion's basic books did not include an explanation of his reasons. They are implicit in the compacted application; they cannot pass unnoticed to readers who are or were willing to do the explanatory work for themselves.

It seems that Bion thought that usage would make the reasons self-evident—and they effectively are to the attentive scientific-minded or informed reader. But after the publication of *Cogitations*, no seriously unprejudiced reader would try to justify lack of understanding of Bion's reasons for using mathematical analogies:

> In short, mathematics must be regarded by the psycho-analyst as one of the limiting classes that belong to psycho-analysis in so far as it attempts to be a coherent system of concepts, and in particular as one of the methods by which the paranoid–schizoid and depressive systems are brought into a dynamic relationship with each other, and therefore as an aspect of those mental phenomena that are concerned in the achievement of mental development by facilitating that dynamic relationship. It will therefore be seen that from a psycho-analytical point of view mathematics does not belong to the realm of ontology nor yet even of epistemology, but to that class of mental functioning which, since transition from paranoid–schizoid to depressive positions and back is essential to mental development, is essential to sanity itself.

> This is not to belittle mathematics but to show how fallacious is the view that pre-eminent importance in any one sphere, however important, confers some universally equal significance in all—a fallacy that has tended to make some observers suppose that failure to produce calculi representing the deductive system of biology, and in particular of psycho-analysis, is necessarily a condemnation of the subject for which no calculi exist. Mathematics may have a very important role as an object of study psycho-analytically, and at the same time and for the same reason be an important element in the mental processes of the individual which makes it possible for him to be a psycho-analyst. [C, 86–7]

Therefore psycho-analysis may contribute to mathematics rather than exclusively the other way round, from mathematics to psycho-analysis. Is the mutual collaboration a feasible task? Bion thought it was. There are hints of this project that seem not to have materialized. They included *"a mathematical approach to biology, founded on the biological origins of mathematics"* (see below)—for the future. They see psycho-analysis as a natural science. In discussing the terms used by Euclid and Archimedes about point and line, Bion stated that he had *"reason to quote illustrations that strengthen the impression of the sexual component in the mathematical investigation"* which is an *"aspect of geometric history"* (T, 56).

If he did not really mathematize analysis it would not be a surprise if he leant more the other way. He proposed to deal with arithmetic and geometry under the psycho-analytic vertex: *"Distinction between the 'geometric' and 'arithmetic' developments can be made thus: the geometric developments of points and line are primarily associated with the presence or absence, existence or non-existence, of an object. The arithmetic development is associated with the state of the object, whether it is whole or fragmented, whole object or part object.*

The geometric development is associated with depression, absence or presence of the object; the arithmetic development with feelings of perse-cution, the Kleinian theory of a paranoid–schizoid position" (T, 151).

Let us try to illuminate some controversies around this attempt of Bion. Harsh as it may seem to state the following phrase, it seems that it is necessary. The controversies may stem from little learning rather than from problems with Bion's writing. It seems that the lack of care in reading the original statements of the author plagued the psycho-analytical movement from its inception. It was vouched for by Freud himself in the successive prefaces to the many editions of *The Interpretations of Dreams*.

Neo-positivism and mathematized propositions

Mathematics furnishes realistic representations of reality itself and therefore it endows science with a reliable substance. It gives tools to science. At least since the times of the Ancient Greeks, Arabs and Persians, mathematics has been regarded as an indispensable base for science. The most recent advocates of mathematization of disci-plines were the so-called neo-positivists. They are important here to the extent that they form part of Bion's inspiration, albeit he uses their ideas critically.

Neo-positivists are not to be confused with positivists. They constituted a fairly cohesive group at the end of the nineteenth century and at the beginning of the twentieth century. Briefly, the neo-positivist attempt was to build a kind of symbolic grammar with clearly stated propositions that could be dealt with in terms of inter-peer communication. They could either be proved or refuted within a shareable language and verifiable criteria.

The main exponents of neo-positivism were:

(i)   Ernst Mach—a gifted physicist who never grasped either quantum mechanics or Einstein's relativity. For he abhorred intuition.

(ii) Moritz Schlick—who was a teacher of Roger Money-Kyrle. He was killed at the height of his creative powers by a fanatical Nazi.

(iii) Otto von Neurath—who compared the scientific movement with a boat that had to be built when navigating in turbulent waters (Pepe, 1989).

(iv) Ludwig Wittgenstein in his younger days—he very early "abandoned ship"; it is possible to draw some similarities between aspects of Bion and Wittgenstein's work, whose description is outside the scope of this entry.

(v)   Rudolph Carnap, whose "mathematical grammar" merits special attention. It allowed one, to some extent, to build verifiable propositions, and seems to have been Bion's main inspiration to build the Grid. There are many parts of his work that illustrate this inspiration; for example, when he developed the theory of container and contained, he used the symbols ♀ ♂. He states that "For syntactical purposes they are functors" (LE, 90).

(vi) Karl Popper—who perhaps was hastily invested with the qualities of a kind of messiah and transformed some neo-positivist tenets into a kind of gospel to be followed if one wished to determine what is and what is not a science; Bion read his work and disagreed with most of it.

(vii) C. G. Hempel, who followed Popper but, as did Bion, added to it an emphasis in earlier roots in Hume. Independent philosophers of science such as Braithwaite and Prichard helped to spread the word about this attempt in England; Bion read their works.

One must include V. Tarski. He was not a member of the neo-positivists in the strict sense of the word; he was a Polish investigator who more than any other worked *"on the concept of truth in formalized languages"* (Kleene, 1959).

This movement was influential up to the end of the sixties; whiffs of it were felt in the early seventies. From then on it lost much of its momentum. This may partially be due to the fact that the neo-positivist movement did not succeed in any of its attempts; even though they were undeniably very developed with the work of its two last great representatives, Rudolph Carnap and Imre Lakatos. Lakatos' proofs and refutations are still provisional attempts. Another reason for its demise may have been the remarkable influence of Thomas Kuhn, P. Feyerabend and the French postmodernists. Their violent denial of truth, reality, facts and science was and is in agreement with the generalized nihilistic destruction which vindicates Nazism and Stalinism in unprecedented forms in our times. They made a successful relativistic/idealist onslaught against truth and reality. This movement reduced science to ideology; peer-group political agreements are seen as the only way out for a generation that severed its links with reality, which is seen as non-existent.

As late as 1972 one may be certain that the issue was one of Bion's central interests. The book *Mathematical Thought from Ancient to Modern Times,* by Morris Kline, OUP, 1972 has plenty of annotations by Bion. Chapter 16—"The Mathematization of Science" still has the bookmark so typical of Bion, indicating that it was thoroughly read.

Definition. Mathematization can also be understood as an extraction of the simplest possible laws stated in a shareable language depicting successfully underlying general laws that encompass individual cases. This simultaneous generalizing/particularizing power can be found in the theory of triangles, of numbers, of Darwin, Einstein and other scientist's formulations. Even though not all of them can be put into a mathematical code of signs, they may possess the mathematical quality of generalization that encompasses particular cases. If the theory can be in a system of notation and manipulation of elements and objects (in the Aristotelian sense) it can be said that the field has been mathematized.

Communication, PS–D, selected fact, constant conjunction and public-ation

I must mention a mathematical feature of early stages in problem solving. The individual feels the problem is vast . . . the model is an attempt to bring it into reach. When the individual is confronted with what, in comparison with himself, is an infinite number or quantity, he binds the "innumerable" host by the name 'three' as soon as he has a feeling of "threeness". The "infinite number" has now been made finite. A feeling of "threeness" in himself has been "bound" and what was infinity is now three. Infinity (or "three") is the name for a psychological state and is extended to that which stimulates the psychological state. The same is true of "three". It becomes the name for that which *stimulates* a sense of "threeness". "Three" and "infinity" are then instances of a peculiar form of model . . . From one vertex, "three" binds a constant conjunction "won from the dark and formless infinite". It is a sign that precision has replaced imprecision. In what sense is 'three' precise and "infinite" imprecise? Certainly not mathematically because the mathematician strives to achieve a notation which, however inexact its genetic background its role transplanted to a new domain is to convey the same meaning universally. In psycho-analysis precision is limited by the fact that communication is of that primitive kind which demands the presence of the object. [ST, 147–8]

The concepts of elementarity, communication, underlying patterns and psycho-analysis were taken by Bion from one main influence, namely the philosophy of mathematics created by Jules Henri Poincaré. There is a special issue in which Bion's reflections are so clear that they remain unread. Therefore they demand to be quoted.

There are some mathematical developments that helped Bion to integrate Freud on dreams and Klein on the integration of the personality and the movement between PS and D. This could be inferred from reading *Learning from Experience*. In a compacted form, Bion resorts to Poincaré's concept of 'selected fact'. This is a fact that seems to give coherence to many facts seemingly dispersed in order to elicit the function of Klein's PS⟷D in the possibilities of thinking at all. The issue is expanded more in a previously unpublished paper, "The synthesizing function of mathematics" (C, 170).

In both cases analytical experience displayed the existence of the psychotic's inability to integrate dispersed objects; the dream seems a special way of integrating seemingly disperse elements. Therefore both mathematicians and the non-psychotic personality seem to be able to integrate.

Armed with those main ideas and pushed by "mother necessity"—the patients with disturbances of thought—Bion developed his theory of thinking. This in its turn influences the psychoanalytic detection of underlying patterns and latent contents:

> The elements to which the student at the Pons Asinorum says good-bye [Euclid I.5] have their counterpart in other mathematical situations. Thus there are the elements that are combined in a particular way to form the notation employed in determinants. But even when the mathematician does not employ the term, there are situations in which it is possible to see that what in fact could with justification be called "elements" are being combined according to certain rules to produce formulas. These elements seem to vary considerably; it may be interesting to collect them together for investigation.

> There are numbers; there are letters of the alphabet; there are points, lines, circles, angles; there are signs such as <, +, −; there are letters of the Greek alphabet, capital and lower case. All without exception are written, and though the marks that the writer makes have names—such as "greater than", "plus", "minus", "alpha", "beta"—in fact mathematicians do not appear to use these signs for talking in the way that words are used in conversation. It must be supposed therefore, that the object in synthesizing these elements is different from the object in verbalization, though the synthesizing process seems similar.

> Why do not mathematicians speak mathematics? Is it that a string of mathematical formulas cannot be made to say, "It's a nice day"? Is the vocabulary not big enough? No: it must obviously be that its primary purpose is not conversational, although it is clear that one of the functions of mathematics is public-ation.

> We shall have to consider three points: (1) the nature of the elements, (2) the nature of the methods employed to bring them together, and (3) the nature of the objects that are created by the syntheses of the elements (Poincaré, *Science and Method*, p. 30; *The Thirteen Books of Euclid's Elements*, I.1, I.5, I.47).

It may appear that I am suggesting that synthesis must be associated simply with a bringing together of the elements according to some known rule to form, say, a polynomial or a determinant. But we cannot assume such a restriction and exclude the bringing together of these elements in a quite different manner; for example, in such a way that would issue in a dream, or in some structure such as that suggested by Stendhal's description of a painting as, "de la morale construite".

Certainly with the psychotic personality there is a failure to dream, which seems to be parallel with an inability to achieve fully the depressive position. It may therefore be said that the capacity to synthesize issues in two main events: (1) the logical construct, a mathematical formula, sentence, etc. and (2) a dream. [C, 110–11]

Intuitive psycho-analytic representations and ad hoc theorizing

The "intuitive psycho-analytic" representation of a basic emotional experience—infantile helplessness—is expressed by the following statement: "the resumption by the psyche of an emotional experience that has been detoxicated by a sojourn in the good breast (Melanie Klein)" (T, 122). This is Klein's intuitive statement. This "intuitive statement lends itself to the representation of genetic stages". In Bion's text there is an expansion of axiomatic formulations, namely, transformations of the emotional experience of the absent breast into points, the place where a breast was; and other more sophisticated formulations. Both are conducive to representations of uses; in Bion's words "both statements are verbal representations of a realization and neither of them is satisfactory" (T, 122). The intuitive statement can be saturated by experience; the geometrical statement can be confirmed or rejected by experience; both can be distorted by concretizing; and verbalization always does this.

Does mathematics help when a necessity to formulate whatever it is emerges? "*The patient is coming to me for help and one reason for his distress is that his formulation does not afford scope for solution of his problem*" (T, 123). The patient must express issues that are neither adult nor rational; nevertheless, he also must express them in rational, adult terms. "*Since they are indescribable, that itself indicates that the feelings described cannot be the ones that were felt . . . 'lost', 'shut in', panic', etc. I can match his diversity of terms with a diversity of my own: 'depersonalized', 'internal object', etc. For my purposes I want terms which will always be right in all situations in which the problems have the same configuration. Patients and analysts are constantly using different terms to describe situations that appear to have the same configuration. I want to find invariants, under psycho-analysis, to all of them . . . What is needed is a solution that will dispose finally of the diversity of terms, at present required to describe the experience . . . and the far more serious defect associated with it, namely, the elaboration of as many theories as there are sufferers, matched by almost as many theories as there are therapists, when it is acknowledged that the configurations are probably the same . . .*

I wish to introduce as a step towards formulations that are precise, communicable without distortion, and more nearly adequate to cover all situations that are basically the same" (T, 123–4).

This superimposes on the neo-positivist's approach even though it is formulated in different terms. One may recognize here Popper's warning about *ad hoc* theorizing, which was adopted by Bion (please refer to the entry, "Manipulations of symbols").

Mathematization and psycho-analysis

Bion stated that this scientific approach of generalization/particularization could be achieved through myth-making and dream activity. This must be kept in mind when one tries to study his use of mathematical analogies. The statements are in *Elements of Psycho-Analysis* and in the preparatory studies on myth-making in *Cogitations*.

Many scientists believe that science is expressed by metaphors. Lakatos dwelt on imaginary dialogues between fictitious characters in the same sense that Bion did. Geometrical formulations can be seen as metaphors.

> This brings me to the application of our myth to the problem that it is to interpret. The scientist must know enough mathematics to understand the nature and use of various mathematical discoveries and formulations, such as the differential calculus or the binomial theorem: the psycho-analyst must know his myth. The scientist must also know enough to have an idea when he is confronting a problem to which a particular mathematical procedure would apply: the psycho-analyst must know when he is facing a problem to which a myth would provide the psycho-analytical counterpart

of the algebraic calculus. This, one might say, is precisely what Freud did: he recognized, as a scientist, that he was confronted by a problem to the solution of which he would have to apply the Oedipus myth. The result was the discovery, not of the Oedipus complex, but of psycho-analysis. (Or is it man, or man's psyche, that is discovered when these elements are constantly conjoined?) *It is in this sense that I believe that the myth of Babel, or Oedipus, or Sphinx must be used as a tool comparable to that of the mathematical formulation.* [C, 228, my italics]

Bion therefore regards mathematics and psycho-analysis as relatives. This differs from mathematizing of the session or of analysis. It was stated above that Bion's mathematical analogies are justified by clinical observations that the problems of thinking presented by the psychotic patient were strikingly similar and in some cases the same problems that the philosopher and the mathematician faced since at least the time of Aristotle.

Bion writes in "The mystic and the group", a re-worked text that was first called "Catastrophic change" (the former appeared in *Attention and Interpretation*; the latter was delivered at the BPS) that at least a great thinker's achievements, namely, Newton's, were linked to his emotional peculiarities. They were not madness as is often thought, but were the origin of his achievements. Some kind of link between the so-called psychosis and mathematics seemed to operate. Common sense popularly sees this link, albeit in an idealized way, saying that good mathematicians are "intelligent" and have "brilliant" minds. Also, children who have difficulties in learning maths often display emotional difficulties.

Elements and objects of psycho-analysis: Bion's six mathematical analogies

Bion's mathematical analogies began with his attempt to formulate objects and elements of psycho-analysis. In order to find them and to have tools to depict them he created:

(i)   A system of quasi-mathematical notation. The reader who is acquainted with Bion's writing certainly will be reminded of symbols such as PS, D, ⇔, ♀ ♂, arrows in different senses to indicate growth or decay.

(ii)   A system of scrutiny of the truth-value of verbal statements, the Grid categories (q.v.).

(iii) A system of conditions to investigate an unknown in psycho-analysis in the same way that one investigates an unknown in a mathematical equation. The "psycho-analytical objects" can be saturated in the same sense that the variables are saturated with values that allow us to establish the value of an unknown (as in an equation: $a = bx + c$ or $a2 = b2 + c2$ in a triangle).

(iv)   A system of seven mathematical concepts applied as working tools (rather than **theories**) to psycho-analytic observation (but **not** to psycho-analytical theories):

iv. 1—factors and functions (in the wake of Freud and from mathematics)

iv. 2—transformations and invariances (from Sylvester and Cayley; it first appeared in the guise of Poincaré's "selected fact")

iv. 3—vertex

iv. 4—circle, point, line, space

iv. 5—unknown and variable

iv. 6—hyperbole

iv. 7—point (the place where the thing was) as a primitive form to deal with psychosis

The concepts are quoted here according to the chronological order of their appearance in the work of Bion.

(v)   A system of "elements" fulfilling conditions of "elementarity", not in the sense of elementals of a theory but in the sense of basic elements as constants of nature. In this sense, mathematics and psycho-analysis can be seen as experiments into the realm of the noumena, or "O". They share with the unconscious the transcendent nature of truth. "*Mathematics and logic are unaffected by the passage of time, though time is intrinsic to the discovery of logical formulations*" (C, 278).

(vi)   The concept of "minus" (please refer to this specific entry). This concept brings the realm of negative numbers—a form to depict immaterialness—to the consideration of the analyst.

One may trace the origins of each one of these analogies:

Psycho-analytical objects originate from Aristotle and Frege's mathematical objects; they also originate from Freud's objects of the instincts (as different from the purposes of the instincts; see "Three essays on a theory of sexuality" and "Instincts and their vicissitudes") and Freud's concept of internal objects, later developed by Klein and others. In this theory the concept of saturation and of the mathematical variables and unknowns in an equation is used as an analogy.

Psycho-analytic elements originate from Euclid's elements that had as an offshoot science's search for elementary factors.

The theory of functions is a theory from geometry and algebraic calculus; it also stems from Freud's observations on ego functions and the scrutiny of their related factors. After having written this entry and other papers, the author obtained a reliable confirmation of the use of the theory in the final years of Bion's life—which is clearly stated in *Learning from Experience* in his copy of *Mathematical Thought from Ancient to Modern Times*, p. 335—"The Function Concept". It originated from the concept of motion, by Morris Kline.

The theory of transformations and invariances was used as a theory of observation in psycho-analysis. Please refer to the specific entries under the headings "transformations" for a detailed historical account of this theory both in mathematics and psychoanalysis.

The realm of **minus** originates from Euclid's bi-dimensional systems of coordinates and the notion of negative numbers. It has important similarities with Hegel's realm of the negative. Anyway, there is no mention of Hegel in Bion's writings. As often happens in science, both seem to have reached similar conclusions in different ways.

Vertex: *"I can describe my use of the term 'vertex' as an example of taking a mathematical term, (grid category H1) and using it as a model (grid category C1)... Where I think it is useful to differ from the philosophical or mathematical view is in regarding 'abstraction' or 'unknown' designations of stages on the genetic axis"* (T, 91). That is, he stresses again and again the fact that he was not mathematicizing psychoanalysis and even less work during a session, but those emphases seem to have been remained unnoticed by many readers (see below, in "misunderstandings and misuses", please refer to this specific entry in this dictionary).

Point, line, circle, space stem from Bion's assumption "that points were originally the space that had been occupied by a feeling, but had become a 'not-feeling' or the space where a feeling used to be . . . Euclidean geometry has been found to have many approximations in realizations of space . . . My suggestion is that its **intra-psychic** origin is experience of 'the space' where a feeling, emotion, or other mental experience 'was'" (T, 121).

One cannot say today that all those tools and developments were fully understood and even less applied after Bion. One would not be in error stating that the present situation is quite the contrary of this. But Bion suggested them and indicated some of their possible applications in the clinical situation.

He never used mathematics as a model with the possible exception of a Lewis Carroll mathematics that was suggested in *Transformations* (T, 153, 170). In the end he was also able to elicit a possible psycho-analytic contribution to the apprehension of the function of mathematics in the development of the human mind. It seemed to be one of mankind's attempts, albeit unsuccessful, to deal with psychosis.

Psycho-analysing the mathematical function of mind or mathematization of psycho-analysis?

> Relativity is relationship, transference, the psycho-analytic term and its corresponding approximate realization. Mathematics, science as known hitherto, can provide no model. Religion, music, painting, as these terms are understood, fail me. Sooner or later we reach a point where there is nothing to be done except—if there is any exception—to wait. [AMF, I, 61]

Bion, after Hume, looked for "*constant conjunction of relationships*" (T, 108).

Perhaps it will be easier to follow Bion's argument by introducing at first the contributions that deal with the simplest algorithms; and thereafter the geometrical analogies. As was done in other entries (such as those concerning transformations, for example) in many parts of the present entry I will replace the quasi-mathematical system of notation with its correspondent verbalization.

Tribulations of the analyst and the possible help from a science of relationships

There is a peculiar relationship between pain and danger, especially that linked to maturation. Sometimes there is no apparent reason for such a link. This is a case that illustrates that often the intensity of pain bears no real or marked relationship to intensity of *"recognizable danger"* (AI, 5). In discussing this peculiar situation, Bion observes that *"The relationship of pain and danger is . . . obscure. In this it is not peculiar, for any relationship of one element of the personality with another seems difficult to determine. A science of relationships has yet to be established and one would look to find some discipline **analogous** to mathematics to represent the relationship of one element in the structure of the psychic personality with another. It is possible to argue that mathematical formulations can be fully appreciated because there is always some more concrete background to which they can be seen to relate, **even though that background may itself be only mathematical** Something similar may be possible in the relationship of elements in the structure of personality. Envy is typical of other elements of the personality in that everyone would be prepared to admit its existence. Yet it does not smell; it is invisible, inaudible, intangible. It has no shape. It must have invariance, or it could not be so widely and surely recognized; and if it has invariants it must be invariant with regard to some kind of operation and therefore there must be an underlying group of such operations"* (AI, 53–4; first bold, by the author, to enhance Bion's idea of an analogy; second bold by Bion).

Zero: The mathematics of hallucinosis

Nothing, no-thing

Perhaps there is a fundamental guideline for the reader who wishes to grasp Bion's use of mathematics. It is necessary to keep firmly in mind that he uses it as an analogy. If the reader cannot see this point he risks concretizing the whole issue. He will fall into the very trap that Bion seemed to try to prevent for all psycho-analysis. The concretization led some readers to conclude that he was trying to mathematize the session or the analysis or the patient.

To think of the absence of objects is the fulcrum of his use of mathematical illustrations and analogies: *"A mathematical illustration*

THE LANGUAGE OF BION

is afforded by the use of numbers for enumeration and record. An increase in sophistication marks the manipulation of numbers to solve a problem in the absence of the objects giving rise to the problem" (T, 39).

This was one of his seminal observations in analysis: the experience of the no-breast is conducive to thinking the breast. The initial concept of the no-breast appears first in "A theory of thinking" and is expanded in *Learning from Experience* and *Transformations*. There it encompassed a notion of space, which can be obtained if the person tolerates the space where the breast was.

Greed precludes this tolerance. Envy destroys the breast and leaves a dreadful space where the breast was (see Mental Space). This is the fulcrum of the tribulations of the psychotic personality. Intolerance of frustration, of the no-breast, leads to an inability to symbolize the breast and to obtain a sense of space/time.

> The criticism of psycho-analysis that it is not mathematical and cannot therefore be scientific, when it is made, is based on a misapprehension of the nature of the problem and the nature of the kind of mathematics employed. [ST, 148]

There seems to be a possible mutual collaboration between psycho-analysis and mathematics rather than an adoption of contributions from mathematics to psychoanalysis. The cross-pollination is firmly anchored in that which is natural; from the analytic side, Freud's theory of natural (biological) instincts and Klein's extension of it:

> I hope that in time the base will be laid for a mathematical approach to biology, founded on the biological origins of mathematics, and not on an attempt to fasten on biology a mathematical structure which owes its existence to the mathematician's ability to find realizations, that approximate to his constructs, amongst the characteristics of the inanimate. [T, 105]

The inanimate is never the zero. It has a concrete, sensuously apprehensible material-ness that right from the start seems to sooth pain due to intolerance of frustration. It always fills some hole. Intolerance of frustration precludes tolerance of zero, the **no-thing**. The abhorred no-thing is turned, in hallucination, into **nothing**. The origin of hallucinosis (q.v.) illuminates both the acquisition of zero and its lack.

The history of geometry and its progressive transition from the sensuously apprehensible fetters towards algebraic calculus—which was also the subject of Alfred North Whitehead's history of mathematics—is extensively integrated with the mind's ability to tolerate frustration—or the lack of such ability.

Vertex and frustration

> First I shall equate the object that I have described as analogous to consciousness with "a point of view". Since I do not wish to identify it with any particular point of view, or indeed with any sense, I shall not consider it to be a point "of view" or "of smell" or "of hearing" but simply as a point. The answer to the question, "point of what? is then left to be determined by clinical experience; the geometrical point used to indicate the point of central projection in projective geometry will serve as a model. The geometer has succeeded, by transformation of Euclidean geometry and its visual representation into algebraic projective geometry, in freeing his investigations from some of the restrictions imposed by the genetic history of the procedures he uses; so psycho-analysis must be freed from the restrictions imposed by the associations with space and sight by which I look to geometry to simplify exposition. [T, 110]

The quotation will be reproduced again in part in order to help its scrutiny: "*First I shall equate the object that I have described as analogous to consciousness with 'a point of view'. Since I do not wish to identify it with any particular point of view, or indeed with any sense, I shall not consider it to be a point 'of view' or 'of smell' or 'of hearing' but simply as a point*" (T, 110).

One may see the expansion of this quotation years later, as an attempt at clarifying it:

> The advantage of falling back on borrowing a mathematical term like "vertex" is that it can make it possible to talk to lunatics who are thrown into confusion if you say things like "from the point of view of smell". It is very exasperating to find a man who interrupts by saying "My eyes don't smell", or, "My smell can't see any view". [AMF, I, 3]

To change the vertex and to catch a hidden or not-too-apparent "darkened side" when hearing a patient's manifest, apparent speech, which can be heard with "a third ear" (to borrow Theodor Reik's expression), was further expanded as:

> P.A. The practical point is—no further investigation of psycho-analysis, but the psyche it betrays. *That* needs to be investigated through the medium of *mental* patterns; *that* which is indicated is *not* a symptom; *that* is not a cause of the symptom; *that* is not a disease or *any*thing subordinate. Psycho-analysis itself is just a stripe on the coat of the tiger. Ultimately it may meet the Tiger— The Thing Itself—O. [AMF, I, 112]

In the phrase of *Transformations*, the word "point" performs the same role as the terms, "psyche" and "mental pattern" in the latter quotation from *A Memoir of the Future*. Conversely, the words "of smell, of view" and so on perform the role of "investigations in psycho-analysis", "that", "symptom", "disease" and so on. Are the latter ideas more easily attractive to many readers and many professionals during a session? Freud's recommendation, "to blind oneself artificially" seems to be helpful here. Summing up, the *"particular points of view"* in *Transformations* corresponds to *"investigations in psycho-analysis"* in *A Memoir of the Future*. The changing of vertex may be stated as going from materiality (or material reality) to immaterial facts (or psychic reality); or from K to O.

The details in a particular session are manifest contents; our goal is the latent, the royal road to the evolving processes of the unconscious (unknown, *unbewusßt*) "O".

Bion emphasizes in the first quotation the "point" ("of view" being secondary). He displays a mode that may be adopted during an actual session. As Freud did, it is the practice of an attentive scrutinizing to nothing in particular. In other words, free-floating attention. It allows the apprehension of that which matters but is not given directly to the senses.

Let us return to the same quotation, in order to see that it is feasible to tolerate a lack of sensuous-concrete material quality of that which is immaterial, psychic: *"The answer to the question, 'point of what' is then left to be determined by clinical experience"* (T, 110).

These doubts and basic immateriality will hardly be welcome to a pleasure-seeking, frustration-abhorring mind that prefers to have a priori theories. The determination in clinical experience demands tolerance of the unknown. The mathematician had to tackle the same issue when algebraic calculus amended descriptive geometry. The evolution of mathematics is an increasing "de-sensifying" .

Let us return to the quotation at the point we stopped above: *"the geometrical point used to indicate the point of central projection in projective geometry will serve as a model. The geometer has succeeded, by transformation of Euclidean geometry and its visual representation into algebraic projective geometry, in freeing his investigations from some of the restrictions imposed by the genetic history of the procedures he uses; so psycho-analysis must be freed from the restrictions imposed by the associations with space and sight by which I look to geometry to simplify exposition"* (T, 110).

That is, to resort to geometry differs from replacing psycho-analysis with it. The replacement differs by circumventing the difficulties imposed by sensuous fetters.

> Who can free mathematics from the fetters exposed by its genetical links with sense? Who can find a cartesian system which will again transform mathematics in ways analogous to the expansion of arithmetic effected by imaginary numbers, irrational numbers, cartesian coordinates freeing geometry from Euclid by opening up the domain of algebraic deductive systems; the fumbling infancy of psycho-analysis from the domain of sensuality-based mind? [AMF, I, 130]

Number and hallucinosis

The notion of 0 (Zero), 2 (two) and 3 (three) can profitably be seen as acquired, or not acquired, according to the mental conditions of the person. In this, Bion profits from Gottlob Frege's contributions to the theory of numbers.

Starting from Bion, we propose to regard the non-concrete sense of "zeroness", "oneness", "two-ness" and "three-ness" and their counterparts manifested in material reality, death, solitude, two parents, two breasts, Oedipus, to be at the root of mind. As a matter of consequence, the failure to get this sense may form the basis of the errors in apprehending the development of mind, in psycho-analysis and mathematics.

Bion proposes a "mathematics of hallucinosis", in terms of a relationship with the breast that is felt as non-existent if it is frustrating (T, 133). The analyst must experience hallucinosis in order to perceive it in the patient (T, 136). He explores the way the human being deals or does not deal with frustration. Many cannot tolerate it and turn it into "nothingness", meaning, zero breast. He proposes a quasi-mathematical representation or notation of hallucinosis: Zero breast plus one real breast equals one hallucinated breast (or 1 breast + 0 breast = 1 breast).

Mathematically, we have this, 1+0=1, or "*memory of satisfaction is used to deny the absence of satisfaction*" (T, 134). One cannot stand that 1+0 = ? where ? is an unknown. The problem is to use 1 to "*remove the noughtness of 0*". So Bion concludes: "*in the domain of hallucinosis, 0 − 0=1*" (op. cit). He wonders, what would be the result of adding 0 to 0? In the domain of reality, it would be, zero; but in the realm of hallucinosis, it would be an unbearable 0^0.

Stating it verbally: "*. . . if noughtness is added to noughtness the noughteness is multiplicated by itself. The emotional state that might provide a background realization approximating to this is the state of complete freedom from the restriction imposed by contact with realizations of any kind*" (T, 134).

A "mental cancer" grows: "*The ability of 0 (meaning, zero) to increase thus by parthenogenesis corresponds to the characteristics of greed which is also able to grow and flourish exceedingly by supplying itself with unrestricted supplies of nothing*" (T, 134). The final result seems to be, "*a raging inferno of greedy non-existence*". Perhaps now it is easier to see why Bion saw mathematics as an early attempt to deal with psychosis—here understood as an inability to think in the absence of concrete objects. Psychotic phenomena of this kind are by no means restricted to certified psychotics:

> The scientist whose investigations include the stuff of life itself finds himself in a situation that has a parallel in that of the patients . . . The breakdown in the patient's equipment for thinking leads to dominance by a mental life in which his universe is populated by inanimate objects. The inability of even the most advanced human beings to make use of their thoughts, because their capacity to think is rudimentary in all of us, means that the field for investigation, all investigation being ultimately scientific, is limited, by human inadequacy, to those phenomena that have the characteristics of the inanimate. We assume that the psychotic limitation is due to an illness: but that that of the scientist is not. Investigation of the assumption illuminates disease on the one hand and scientific

method on the other. It appears that our rudimentary equipment for "thinking" thoughts is adequate when the problems are associated with the inanimate, but not when the object for investigation is the phenomenon of life itself. Confronted with the complexities of the human mind the analyst must be circumspect in following even the accepted scientific method; its weakness may be closer than superficial scrutiny would admit. [LE, 14]

Mathematics can deal with issues that have no practical realizations. Sometimes the realizations occur years or even centuries later. In Bion's words, *"The truth of a statement does not imply that there is a realization approximating to the true statement"* (ST, 119). A telling example is John Nash's theory of games, recently popularized on screen (*A Brilliant Mind*, starring Russell Crowe).

Two-ness

As early as 1961, in "A theory of thinking", Bion tried to scrutinize the capacity for thinking in the absence of the object—as the primary, inescapable and necessary condition for thinking at all. "Thinking" is seen in the sense of non-rational elaboration that tries to apprehend reality as it is, with all its components including frustration. The absence of the object is the primary frustration one must cope with.

> Mathematical elements, namely straight lines, points, circles and something corresponding to what later becomes known by the names of numbers, derive from realizations of two-ness as in breast and infant, two eyes, two feet and so on.

> If intolerance of frustration is not too great modification becomes the governing aim. Development of mathematical elements, or mathematical objects as Aristotle calls them, is analogous to the development of conceptions [the mating of pre-conceptions with realizations].

> If intolerance of frustration is dominant, steps are taken to evade perception of the realization by destructive attacks. In so far as pre-conception and realization are mated mathematical conceptions are formed but they are treated as if indistinguishable from things-in-themselves and are evacuated ... to annihilate space. In so far as space and time are perceived as identical with a bad object that is

destroyed, that is to say a no-breast, the realization that should be mated with the pre-conception is not available to complete the conditions necessary for the formation of a conception. The dominance of projective identification confuses the distinction between the self and the external object. This contributes to the absence of any perception of two-ness since such an awareness depends on the recognition of a distinction between subject and object. [ST, 113]

Three-ness

"It is said that a discipline cannot properly be regarded as scientific until it has been mathematized and I may have given the impression, by adumbrating a Lewis Carroll mathematics for analysis, that I support this view and in doing so risk the proposal of a premature mathematization of a subject which is not sufficiently mature for such a procedure. I shall therefore draw attention to some features of mathematical development which have not hitherto been adequately considered psycho-analytically. As an illustration I shall use the description ... of the transition from the dark and formless Godhead of Meister Eckhart to the "knowable" Trinity. My suggestion is that an intrinsic feature of the transition from the "unknowability" of the infinite Godhead to the "knowable" Trinity is the introduction of the number "three". The Godhead has become, or been, mathematized. [T, 170]

Five years earlier he had already made another attempt:

Mathematics

1 + 1 = 2. But suppose we sexualize the plus sign: the 1 + 1 = 3 presents no difficulty. But it does not mean that 1 + 1 *must* = 3. For that, it would be necessary to do more than sexualize the plus sign. It would be necessary to make it at least ? + ?=3. It would probably be necessary to make the plus sign mean "sexual intercourse with intent to procreate children in adequate conditions between adequate people".

What is happening here is that the plus sign is being treated as a variable as well as the terms of the expression. What mathematics can evolve if all the signs and terms in an expression are variables? There would seem to be nothing but chaos possible, but it is not so. For example, 1 + 1 = 3 has a meaning if I say, 1 = a man, and 1 = a woman. In this case the "value" of the plus sign has been affected "contextually". This reminds me of "contextually" contingent propositions (Braithwaite, *Scientific Explanation*, p. 112. [C, 145]

Another view on "three-ness" was given above, under the heading, "Communication".

Mathematical abstractions as an escape from Oedipus

The reader who is prone to accuse Bion of mathematizing psycho-analysis has a good chance to review his ideas in the texts that compose this part of the entry. The superficial reading of Bion's text perhaps furnishes material for an attack. A close scrutiny reveals that Bion poses many hypotheses and invites the reader to think about unexpected similarities among the psycho-analyst's and the mathematician's goal.

Thinking processes and apprehension of reality, in its material and psychic forms, are a way of stating these similar goals. It seems that Bion's constant search for truth found a provisional containment in mathematics and scientific deductive systems. It proved to be short-lived and was replaced by a more verbal but no less scientific approach in *A Memoir of the Future*.

In this sense the papers from the fifties and early to middle sixties display a precedent form that clothed an active dialogue. This was later expressed by two characters, P.A. and Priest, in discussing seminal issues linked to the idea of the existence of mind. The reader will be helped if he realizes that this approach is part of an attempt to give analysis sound scientific criteria.

The following Lexicon may be useful for reading the following text: I.5 and I.47 mean, respectively, Euclid's fifth and forty-seventh propositions in volume I of his work, *Elements*. The senses of two-ness and three-ness were mentioned above. In the entry, "Oedipus", there appears a quasi-mathematical formula for (Oedipus—≥ 2) that is extensively described in the entry, Mathematization of psycho-analysis.

Concerning Oedipus, "I hope to show that these attempts at resolution are far more widespread in time, and far more various in the form and method of resolution adopted, than has hitherto been realized or even suspected" (C, 200). The idea is linked to clinical situations, but it is also linked to mathematics: "One such attempt can be discerned in the issues involved in the production of a scientific deductive systems and the calculus that represents it.

> With this end in view I propose to examine Euclid's elements. This brings me back to the point at which I said a search must be made for the intersection of processes analogous to those which we ordinarily see in dreams, with the processes we ordinarily associate with mathematical logic. But before doing this I must give a warning: it is inevitable that I should appear at certain points of the discussion to be seeing sexual, and particularly Oedipal, symbols in certain Euclidean propositions . . . I wish to propound the hypothesis that the Euclidean theorem and Freud's discovery of the Oedipus complex, together with the Oedipus myth and the Sophoclean version of it, are alike in that they are both attempts to resolve the conflicts and problems of which they are at one and the same time the manifestation and the attempted solution. [C, 200–1]

Bion proposes a new answer to the riddle of the Sphinx, different from that which is attributed to Oedipus. It is usually interpreted as the evolution of man from childhood to adulthood and then to the old-ager with a staff. Bion takes Euclid's fifth proposition in his first book of *Elements* about the isosceles triangle and translates it verbally from ancient Greek: "*a three kneed thing with equal legs*". Then he adopts Onians' discovery that knees in early Greek literature are associated with genitalia. This brings Euclid I.5 and the Oedipus myth together: "*attempts to resolve the conflicts and problems of which they are at one and the same time manifestation and the attempted solution*" (C, 201–2).

In examining the Oedipal chain he verifies the fate of the primal scene: an actual sensory experience assumes the character of an ideogram that either becomes a formula or an abstraction into a Euclidean geometric figure; it is then located in space defined by a system of Cartesian coordinates; from then on it can acquire further abstracted forms that can be seen as deductive systems and algebraic calculi. For example, realizations of space—including astronomical space. From then on Bion suggests "*reversing the direction*", that is to return to the lowest level data—the sensory experiences. "*Are there actualities or realities corresponding to the **ideas** of reality that* *the calculi have enabled the astronomer to achieve? Or are the ideas only reflecting the origin of the calculi and the scientific deductive system, Euclidean geometry—namely the space of the primitive individual from which the scientific progress sprang?"*

This opens up two possibilities: *"one is that, thanks to the elaboration of scientific methods, we are learning more; the other is that, thanks to the impulse to escape from Oedipal material, calculi are produced which are impregnated with the impulse to escape and the archaic remnants of that from which escape is sought . . .*

*Can the calculi produced yield equipment suitable for investigating the problem from which they sprang? Can the calculi, which represent and attempt at abstraction as escape from an Oedipal situation, be made to explore that situation? Do calculi already exist which do just that? Can Oedipal conflicts be resolved by a **mathematical** experience? The internal universe would then be explored by a calculus turned back on its origin"* (C, 203–5).

Bion proposes to regard Pythagoras' theorem and its calculus as the scientific deductive system of the contents of the Oedipal situation; the proposal is made in the form of a doubt: *"Are I.5 and I.47 externalizations of the Oedipal situation?. . . Or are they scientific deductive systems that make it possible to investigate the Oedipal situation?"*

The closing part of the paragraph has an unexpected hypothesis. It closely resembles the situations depicted in the entry "Science versus religion", and brings forth the same class of problem to analysts, namely, that sometimes other disciplines seem to be more psycho-analytic than many among the official psycho-analytic writings:

This point would be clinched if one found that I.5 or I.47 reached a conclusion that could then be translated into terms of lowest-level hypotheses—or rather, into terms of empirically verifiable data—which could then be seen to have carried the theory of Oedipal conflict to a point further than any yet reached in psycho-analytical discovery. [C, 209]

Geometric analogies

Bion's geometrical analogies resorted to graphic—visual—representations of points, lines, and arrows in many directions. Anyone who keeps his ability for dream-work (in the sense of Freud's

"Regression" as depicted in *The Interpretation of Dreams*, the reversal of thoughts into visual imagery) should be able to follow his writing.

Time has proved that many readers usually feel, as a member of the staff of readers of the *International Journal of Psycho-Analysis*— allegedly an expert on Bion—once wrote to the author, fully endorsed by the editor, that Bion's symbols are a "maze".

> For my purposes I want terms which will always be right in all situations in which the problems have the same configuration. Patients and analysts are constantly using different terms to describe situations that appear to have the same configuration. I want to find invariants, under psycho-analysis, to all of them . . . I wish to introduce as a step towards formulations that are precise, communicable without distortion, and more nearly adequate to cover all situations that are basically the same. [T, 124]

Point: The point corresponded to the indestructible, immaterial and real *"place where the breast was"*. The *"place where the breast was"* is a verbal formulation whose counterpart in reality is the same as "point". Another verbal formulation is (since 1961), "no-breast". The point stands for a visual, geometric counterpart of Klein's intuitive contribution to psycho-analysis, that is, the breast and the baby. It is so transformed into a basic, elementary fact that can be stated in a generalizing verbal proposition. Please refer to the entry, "Circle, Point, Line". Intolerance of the point means psychosis.

Line: The line is a visual, geometric counterpart of Freud's intuitive contribution to psycho-analysis; namely, the penis. It is therefore transformed into a basic, elementary fact that can be stated in a generalizing verbal proposition.

Circle: it corresponds to the emotional experience of inner and outer, self, non-self, piercing, evolution.

Space: corresponding to Kant's categorical imperative, it represents emotions that are felt to be indistinguishable from the *"place where something was"* (T, 124; AI, 10).

Unknown: A practical example is furnished below; please refer to the entry, "Psycho-analytical Object".

Variable: it corresponds to the many individual transformations and is expanded below.

The constant conjunction of these six concepts would correspond to that which in intuitive analytic theory is stated as Oedipus
and its vicissitudes.

One of Bion's illustrations of **one** of the possible applications of
the mathematical (geometrical) symbol ● [point] is about agora-
phobia and claustrophobia. The geometrical symbol [●] is a scientific approach to a particular problem and is stated verbally as "the
place where the breast was":

> Patients and analysts are constantly using different terms to
> describe situations that appear to have the same configuration. I
> want to find invariants, under psycho-analysis, to all of them. This
> condition is almost filled by the term "place where the thing was" or
> "space". Almost, but not quite. Its virtue can be seen in the fact that
> it will do equally well for agoraphobia or claustrophobia, and to that
> extent avoids two terms for configurations that are only apparently
> different. What is needed is a solution that will dispose finally of the
> diversity of terms, at present required to describe the experience
> called "claustro- or agora-phobia", and the far more serious defect
> associated with it, namely, the elaboration of as many theories as
> there are sufferers, matched by almost as many theories as there are
> therapists, when it is acknowledged that the configurations are
> probably the same. The solution required will cover more than
> claustrophobia or agoraphobia which I have chosen as a starting
> point. I choose "space" to represent, on the one hand, emotions
> which are felt to be indistinguishable from the "place where some-
> thing was", and on the other, space akin to the geometric realization
> from which Euclidean geometry is believed to derive. [T, 124]

> The geometrical elaboration proceeds as follows: commencing with
> a point, line or any more complex figure such as those associated
> with the theorem of Pythagoras, the proposition is read off the
> figure, that is to say, it seems to be regarded as self-evident from
> the nature of the figure. Inspection of the figure may be followed
> by a formulation in terms other than pictorial. Plutarch gives a
> fanciful and oedipal description of the 3,4,5 triangle. The mathe-
> matical development may have been achieved by transformation of
> the visual image into an arithmetical formulation. [T, 78]

The obverse is also true and is related to maturation: "My *analytical
experience is compatible with a development that proceeds from the* **complete**

visual image to elaboration in non-visual term; that is from row C categories to row H, though I did not witness a row H transformation" (T, 78).

In using the two axes of the Grid Bion tries to represent a dynamic, transient object that is characterized by a movement that represents either growth or decay (regression or progression). This movement can be depicted through scanning the many categories of the Grid, up and down, back and forth, diagonally, horizontally or vertically. See the specific entry, "Grid". What matters for us now is that Bion resorted to arrows to try to depict movement. The arrows can be seen as vectors in physics: ←↑→, and so on (T, 114, fn).

From there Bion proceeded constantly to conjoin the arrows with psycho-analytic concepts such as conscious and unconscious. He does this in chapter six of *Transformations*. In chapters seven and eight of the same book he conjoined the arrows with points (•) and lines (——). The reader who finds it difficult to follow the argument that resorts to those definitions may refer to the specific entry, "Circle, point, line" in this dictionary.

To state verbally symbols such as

————>

conscious

is, "in the way to be conscious, in the direction of consciousness".

means, verbally, "the place where the breast was (or point) in a backward movement towards the destruction of it". In other words, it tends to the absolute intolerance of frustration. Bion's terms provide an explanation of his mathematical analogy: it tries to depict man's attempt to deal with psychosis. In this sense, it is an attempt to illuminate the psycho-analysis of psychosis rather than a mathematization of psycho-analysis:

By proceeding

I have sought to show that geometrical constructions related to, and strove originally to represent, biological realities such as emotions. The progression represented by

←
• ↓

leads to the possibility that mathematical space may represent
emotion, anxiety of psychotic intensity, or repose also of psychotic
intensity—a repose more psychiatrically described as stupor. In
every case the emotion is to be part of the progression, breast →
emotion (or place where the breast was) → place where emotion
was. *I hope that in time the base will be laid for a mathematical approach
to biology, founded on the biological origins of mathematics, and not on
an attempt to fasten on biology a mathematical structure which owes its
existence to the mathematician's ability to find realizations, that approximate to his constructs, amongst the characteristics of the inanimate.* [T,
105, this author's italics]

The last paragraph may illuminate the quotation that heads this
entry and can avoid many of the misunderstandings currently
encircling the issue. Much of volume I of *A Memoir of the Future* is
dedicated to scanning the artistic models and to further illuminating why mathematics and artistic means, though more effective in
reaching the mind, are not replacements for psycho-analysis and
cannot help it.

General formulations that could be able to communicate the
findings of intuitive psycho-analysis could be enriched by *"the
mathematical approach to biology"* (T, 105): *"The rules governing points
and lines which have been elaborated by geometers may be reconsidered by
reference back to the emotional phenomena that were replaced by 'the place
(or space) where the mental phenomena were'. Such a procedure would
establish an abstract deductive system based on a geometric foundation
with intuitive psycho-analytic theory as its concrete realization"* (T, 121).

The following quotation demands a reader disposed to read
with the same attention to detail and stamina that is required from
a person trying to solve an algebraic equation; or a beginner trying
to read a foreign language; or a surgeon scrutinizing an open belly
in search of a hidden bleeding vessel; or an analyst at work.
Provided that such attention is made available, the text reveals itself
as a compact presentation of the mathematical analogy:

... I state, as part of an intuitive psycho-analytic theory, that the
patient has an experience, such as an infant might have when the

breast is withdrawn, of facing emotions that are unknown, unrecognized as belonging to himself, and confused with an object which he but recently possessed. Further descriptions only add to the multiplicity of which I already complain as the reader will see if he consults any analytic descriptions of infantile behaviour. The relationship of these representations with the realizations approximating to them may be compared with the axiomatic geometric deductive space that I wish to introduce as a step towards formulations that are precise, communicable without distortion, and more nearly adequate to cover all situations that are basically the same. I suggest the following comparisons: (i) "Unknown", in the model afforded by the intuitive psycho-analytic theory, with "unknown", in the mathematical sense in which I wish to use "geometric space". (ii) "Variable", as applied to the sense of instability and insecurity in the model of infantile anxiety, with "variable", as I wish to apply it to geometric space. Thus geometric space may represent and be replaced by constant values by any particular universe of discourse. The relationship of geometric space to the intuitive psycho-analytic theory that I propose as *its* realization; the further relationship of the psycho-analytic intuitive theory to the clinical experience which I consider is *its* realization; together these represent a progression such as that in the transformation of an experience into a poem— "emotion recollected in tranquillity". The geometric transformation may be regarded as a representation, "detoxicated" (that is, with the painful emotion made bearable) of the same realization as that represented (but with the painful emotion expressed), by the intuitive psycho-analytic theory . . .

There are further similarities . . . if it is accepted that geometric space affords a link between unsophisticated emotional problems, their unsophisticated solutions and the possibility of their restatement in sophisticated terms admitting of sophisticated solutions, then it may be that musical and other artistic methods afford a similar link. These must not be regarded as replacements of the geometric approach. The investigation must be directed to the elucidation of point and line as elements imbedded in the material of transformations in the media of all arts and sciences. In the poem it may be found in the long–short of rhythm; in painting it may be found . . . in the matter from which the construct is formed. In music it may be looked for not in musical notation, but music itself . . .

This discussion is concerned with such representations, whatever the discipline, as having disposed within them the invariants of point and line; intuitive psycho-analytical theory is its corresponding realization. [T, 124–6]

Mathematics, at-one-ment and science

The scientific approach, associated with a background of sense impressions, for example the presence of the psycho-analyst and his patient in the same room, may be regarded as having a base. In so far as it is associated with the ultimate reality of the personality, O, it is baseless. This does not mean that the psycho-analytic method is unscientific, but that the term "science", as it has been commonly used hitherto to describe an attitude to objects of sense, is not adequate to represent an approach to those realities with which "psycho-analytical science" has to deal. Nor is it adequate to represent that aspect of the human personality that is concerned with the unknown and ultimately unknowable—with O . . .

The realities with which psycho-analysis deals, for example, fear, panic, love, anxiety, passion, have no sensuous background, though there is a sensuous background (respiratory rate, pain, touch, etc.) that is often identified with them and then treated, supposedly scientifically. What is required is not a base for psycho-analysis and its theories but a science that is not restricted by its genesis in knowledge and sensuous background. It must be a science of at-one-ment.(q.v.) It must have a mathematics of at-one-ment, not identification. There can be no geometry of "similar", "identical", "equal"; only of analogy. [AI, 88]

℗ Many felt that the reasons for bringing mathematics to the analyst's consideration were not clear in Bion's classical books. The posthumously published *Cogitations* may help them. Perhaps some readers will feel more easy when Bion had put forward his reflections and comments rather than ultra-compacted conclusions. The conclusions appeared in the earlier published books that were written *after* these preparatory studies.

We had already seen that Bion brings mathematics to the fore because of clinical issues—disturbances of perception, thought, movement between conscious and unconscious, PS and D and concretization/abstraction. Or, in other terms, difficulties with dream-work. Those issues can be abridged as the seminal transition from sensibility to that which is psychic. Mathematics is an aid to help the apprehension of the **transition from sensibility to awareness** with a sojourn in the unconscious and back to it.

As early as 1959–60, Bion would write, in dealing with dreamwork-α (q.v.): "*It may be that we can never know* [the crucial mechanisms], *that we can only postulate their existence in order to explain hypotheses that are capable of translation into empirically verifiable data, and that we shall have to work with these postulates without assuming that corresponding realities will at some time be discovered. I regard α ? as a postulate of this nature*" (C, 95).

In examining the possibilities **and** limitations of mathematical analogies as used by Bion (see the quotation from *Cogitations*, pages 86–7, above), one must pay attention to his conclusion about the "*synthesizing function of mathematics*" and its cogency with Klein's positions (C, 170)

Circular argument, saturation and numbers: an example of mathematical analogies

It is common sense to state that people who cannot acquire or are not endowed with so-called "mathematical thinking" try to learn "by heart" that which must "become" and "evolve" in the beholder's mind. They are doomed to failure and precociously "unlearn" that which seemed to succeed, say, in a school examination. To learn "by heart" means "to know about maths".

> Any statement should be . . . re-assessed . . . in accordance with its position in the Reality scale, that is Form and reminder, deity and incarnation, hyperbole and evacuation. The interpretation should be such that the transition from *knowing about* reality to *becoming real* is furthered. This transition depends on matching the analysand's statement with an interpretation which is such that the circular argument remains circular but has an adequate diameter. If it is too small the circular argument becomes a point; if too great it becomes a straight line. The point and straight line together with numbers are representatives of states of mind which are primitive and unassociated with mature experience. The profitable circular argument depends on a sufficiency of experience to provide an orbit in which to circulate. To re-state this in terms of greater sophistication, the analytic experience must consist of knowing and being successively many elementary statements, discerning their

orbital or circular or spherical relationship and establishing the statements which are complementary. The interpretations that effect the transition from knowing about O to becoming O are those establishing complementarity; all others are concerned with establishing the material through which the argument circulates.

The transition from "knowing about" to "becoming" O can be seen as a particular instance of the development of the conception from the pre-conception . . . I have described that process as one of saturation of an unsaturated element $\psi(\xi)$, to become $\psi(\psi)(\xi)$. That is to say, a pre-conception becomes a conception and retains its dimension of "usability" as a pre-conception . . . The psycho-analytic conception of cure should include the idea of a transformation whereby an element is saturated and thereby made ready for further saturation. Yet a distinction must be made between this dimension of "cure" or "growth" and greed. To this I shall revert after considering "arithmetic" further. I should say, if it is not already clear, that the domain of mathematics with which I am concerned is the "Dodgsonian" or "Alice Through the Looking-Glass" variety.

I have said numbers are a means of binding . . . a constant conjunction. By definition this means that the conjunction is unknown or devoid of meaning. O is not known, but for ease in exposition I am supposing that the conjunction . . . which is to be bound with a view to investigation, is the "group". The number signified by 1 is a way of denoting a whole object which is not a group. The group is infinite, whether it is a group of people, things or "causes". From this we may proceed to emotional mathematics (or the mathematics of emotion) thus: 1 = "one is one and all alone and evermore we shall be so". $1/1$ = a relationship with "the whole of an object that is a whole object, that is unrelated to any other objects and therefore has no properties; since properties are dimensions of relationships". With religion as vertex this sign can represent the O represented by the term "Godhead". With a Miltonic vertex it is represented by the "void and formless infinite" from which is "won" the object that is known. With a Dantesque vertex it is represented by the 33rd canto of the Paradise. With a mathematical vertex, and regarding it in its negative aspect of definition, it can be represented by the term "not infinity".

Similarly ½ can represent . . . a relationship with a part of a part of a group. In its negative dimension, it denies that there are more than, or less than, two in the group and affirms that the relationship is with one of them.

When formulated these numbers can be used in the process of transformation. They can be combined with other numbers as and when other numbers are formulated. The development is therefore two-fold: the group can be denoted by a new number whenever a constant conjunction is felt to require binding, as for example if a number "two" is felt to be necessary because O is not felt to be represented by 1. Thus development can proceed according to a plan of enumeration. Or, curiosity about the relationship of 1 to 1/1 or _ to O, and from that to the relationship that each has to the other, leads to manipulation and combination of the numbers ...

The combination and manipulation of numbers is stimulated by the same force as stimulates their formulation—the awareness of a constant conjunction that requires to be bound. [T, 152–5]

Misuses and Misconceptions: Some critics levelled the accusation against Bion that he tried to mathematize the analyst's work **during a session**.

This cannot be found in any of his works, as the reader may gather from the content of this entry. Some readers consistently fail to realize that the disturbances of thinking that affect the psychotic personality are the same problems that both the philosopher and the mathematician once faced. In some cases, the philosopher was also a mathematician. It is from those thinkers that Bion draws inspiration and help, for example, the work of Aristotle and Poincaré. He was not interested in mathematics *per se* but he was interested in the philosophy of mathematics (Parthenope Bion Talamo confirmed this idea in a personal communication following talks about the issue).

There are some gross misunderstandings among some of Bion's readers that perpetuate the idea that Bion was a complicated, obscure and difficult author; many of them use the issue of mathematics to prove their point. Since the inception of the theory of α-function, which "transforms" sensible data into non-sensuous data (q.v.), Bion was trying to tackle this issue. Mathematics seemed to furnish an example of the feasibility of such a task. It is an example not to be followed, but an example that showed that such transformation could be made. It is clearly stated in many parts of Bion's work:

According to Proclus, objection was raised against the term στγμη by Plato on the grounds that it meant puncture and therefore suggested a background of reality that was not appropriate to geometric discussion. The objection resembles that of a patient to the visual image of the point because of its unwelcome penumbra of associations. He had evaded the difficulty by a neologism; my concern is not with the solution of the problem, but with its resemblance to the scientific difficulty of using terms with a long history to express novel situations.

The Pythagoreans regarded the point as having position, but Euclid did not include this in his definition, though he and Archimedes and later writers used the term σημετον instead of στγμη"; Aristotle in discussing the prevalent notion of the relatedness of the point to the line objected that, the point being indivisible, no accumulation of points can give anything divisible such as a line (*Physics*, IV, 8, 215, big.) The significance of the discussion lies in the wish to establish the connection felt to exist between the point and the line. An analyst reading contributions to the establishment of scientific geometry would see that elements appear that invite psycho-analytic interpretation of the kind indicated. I shall have reason to quote illustrations that strengthen the impression of the sexual component in the mathematical investigation, but I do not propose to go into this aspect of geometric history. [T, 55–6]

Bion left preliminary papers about the sexual component in mathematical investigation. They are included in the entry, "Oedipus", of this dictionary. Attention and high school notions of mathematics will suffice to follow Bion's models. Bion adopted a quasi-mathematical system of symbolic notation, but not calculus or the like.

Another type of criticism raised against his writings was in line with the idea that Bion did not understand too much of mathematics, philosophy and even Freud's work. This writer's view is different. Bion grasped the ethos of those fields and authors outside the more common road of erudition. Some people cannot follow these lines and become anxious when one does this. They try to insert themselves in an established group and secure their membership through erudition (a fact illuminated in *Attention and Interpretation*, chapter 7) which seems to compensate for their limitation. But erudition precludes the coupling of the writings with practice.

Many are irremediably blind to that which the great authors said. Usually this is reflected in fashions that prevail in academic milieu. Bion's use of philosophy is never in agreement with "official" fashions. Not to follow the Herd may be a source of trouble, of which he was aware:

> It may seem that I am mis-using words with an established meaning, as in my use of the terms function and factors. A critic has pointed out to me that the terms are used ambiguously and the sophisticated reader may be misled by the association of both words with mathematics and philosophy. I have deliberately used them because of the association, and I wish the ambiguity to remain. I want the reader to be reminded of mathematics, philosophy and common usage, because a characteristic of the human mind I am discussing may develop in such a way that it is seen at a later stage to be classifiable under these headings—and others. [LE, Introduction, 2]

Oedipus

The situations of two-ness and three-ness are discussed above. There seems to be some misunderstanding about Oedipus and the fixation of unsaturated elements during an actual analytic session, using a mathematical analogy. The misunderstanding is reviewed in the entry, "Oedipus" (please refer to this entry).

Suggested cross-references: Circle, Point, Line, Circular argument, Establishment, Grid, Manipulations of symbols, Minus, Models, Oedipus, Psycho-analytical object, Relationship, Scientific Method; Ultra-sensuous.

📖 From Bion's Library: this is a very basic selection from more than 60 of his personal copies, destined for those who want to examine Bion's sources: *The Philosophy of Mathematics*, Stephan Korner, Hutchison University Library, 1960, heavily annotated, indicating his interest in intuitionists from the early sixties; *The World of Mathematics*, James R. Newman, London, George Allen & Unwin, 1956, heavily bookmarked and annotated, a comprehensive source; Bion's copy of Alfred North Whitehead's *Introduction to Mathematics* dates from 1911 and seems to have been presented to him by F.S. Sutton, one of his highly esteemed teachers at school (quoted in vol. III of *A Memoir*); *Introduction to Metamathematics*,

S.C.Kleene, North Holland Publishing Co, Amsterdam, 1959; *The Foundations of Arithmetic*, G. Frege, bi-lingual edition, translated by J. L. Austin, Basil Blackwell, Oxford, 1953; *The Principles of Mathematics*, B. Russell, London: George Allen & Unwin, 1956.

Mating (or matching) of pre-conceptions to realizations: Bion proposed comparatively few theories of psycho-analysis. One of them was on thinking. He starts from the hypothesis that a child has an innate pre-conception, namely, that of a breast. He uses Kant's proposals on "empty" thoughts or pre-conceptions. They can be regarded as phylogenetic memories. They correspond to Freud's "protophantasies" (Freud, 1920).

Bion observes something from Klein's intuitions about the baby's mind. He hypothesizes that the infant has two pre-conceptions: that of a breast and that of Oedipus (please refer to the entry, Pre-conception). He makes it clear that Melanie Klein did not agree with him that babies had the pre-conception of a breast (T, 138).

One cannot know what would have happened if Klein had lived longer, she could well have changed her opinion; Bion's theory was advanced shortly before her death. Undaunted by neither by her disagreement nor breaking with her, he continued with his proposal, stating that the pre-conception finds a breast, that is, a realization. This seems to be in agreement with the nature of mammals; if the baby does not find a breast as soon as possible, its life is imperilled.

The new-found breast cannot be the same breast of the pre-conception. Or, in other words, the breast that is available is neither the desired breast nor even the needed breast. No entity made a previous consultation with the baby armed with, so to speak, a "breast blueprint" to be approved by him. A real breast cannot be ordered; it is as it is. Therefore the mating, or matching of the pre-conception with the realization **always** is—to an extent—frustrating and non-fulfilling.

It can be said that the mating met with success just when the infant copes with this "para 100" parcel of frustration. If the vertex is the pleasure/displeasure principle, success is not a feasible outcome; it is indistinguishable from fulfilment. The quantum of unfufilment is the prototype of all matings throughout life. A sexual couple copes with unfulfilments to make a real marriage.

The theory of thinking does not advocate fulfilment; the obverse is true. There is no thinking if ideas of fulfilment prevail. The unfulfilment—Bion calls it, no-breast—allows the very inception of the thought processes. The lack of a breast demands the symbolization of the same breast. The conception that is formed after a mating of the pre-conception with the realization will then function in a second cycle of mating as a new pre-conception and so forth, to all experiences from birth to death.

The "para-100" quota of unfulfilment, the no-breast, can be tolerated or not. The degree of approximation to reality (prototypically, the real frustrating breast) is determined by the capacity to tolerate frustration.

Misuses and Misconceptions: Some readers imagine that mating is a non-frustrating and all-fulfilling event. They mistake the existence of a real breast—that furnishes a realization—with a fulfilling breast.

Suggested cross-references: Conception, Pre-conception.

Medicine: Medicine furnishes Bion with a model to provide a clinically useful approach to psycho-analysis. It is similar to what occurred with Freud and Klein before him and with Winnicott contemporaneously to him. The immaterial nature of psychic facts may sometimes cloud this fact (see below, misuses and misconceptions).

Psycho-analysis tries to create a purposeful environment intended to help **individual** suffering people. There is a kind of "pre-conception" that favours individuals. To help the individual is a hallmark of medicine since it was rescued from the darkness of ignorance during the Enlightenment and the Romantic Movements.

(i) The medical model of development and usefulness to life— the concepts of **development** (or **growth**) and **usefulness** are seminal to medicine. Though Bion approaches these concepts critically they permeate the whole of his work; they have not been subjected to change (see entry Analytic View).

> In psycho-analytic methodology the criterion cannot be whether a particular usage is right or wrong, meaningful or verifiable, but whether it does, or does not, promote development . . . I do not suggest that promotion of development provides a criterion without reservation . . . [LE, page 3 of the Introduction]

But to what scale of values is the value of the belief related? Ruskin defined "valuable" as life-giving. This may do in that the oedipal theory and primal scene afford a link . . . between life instincts and death instincts and that which is valuable or life-giving and the opposite.

If value is to be the criterion, difficulty arises because there is no *absolute* value: the individual does not necessarily believe it is better to create than to destroy; a suicidal patient may seem to embrace the opposite view. [AI, 101]

One may add, a military man (such as Rommel or Montgomery, for example) may also embrace the opposite view; the same, for one who is committed to the distribution of wealth in authoritarian establishments. Other examples of the belief in destruction may be the Churchill versus Hitler conundrum; or its latest version, the Bush family versus Hussein/Laden conundrum. They embody the same paradox that may be left unobserved by their contemporaries. One may be reminded that both Ernst Junger and Wilfred Bion, fighting in warring groups, held similar views of the human facts such as comradeship involved in warfare.

(ii) The pseudo-medical model of cure, so dear to medicine, was used by Bion in his first papers from the fifties. This model was fated to be dismissed in both cases. For both medicine and Bion's work that stemmed from it are endowed with the scientific ethos of respect for truth and real facts. Experienced medical doctors and patients alike know well that they **care** and **treat** but they never really cure. Bion realized that cure is a hallucinated idealized goal that expresses allegiance to the principle of pleasure. Ideas of cure reduce that which could be an analysis into a colluded parasitic association. Analyst and patient fall into a situation of mutual admiration encircled by panglossian reassurances. Ideas of cure express hate towards analysis in so far as it extinguishes investigation into the unconscious. The Commentary in *Second Thoughts* and the chapter "Medicine as a Model" in *Attention and Interpretation* leave no doubts about Bion's brushing aside of this model.

By definition and by the tradition of all scientific discipline, the psycho-analytic movement is committed to the truth as the central aim. If the patient constantly formulates $-L$ and $-K$ statements, he and the analyst are, in theory at least, in conflict. In practice, however, the situation does not present itself so simply. The patient, especially if intelligent and sophisticated, offers every inducement to bring the analyst to interpretations that leave the defence intact and, ultimately, to acceptance of the lie as a working principle of superior efficacy. In the last resort he will make consistent progress toward a "cure" which will be flattering to the analyst and patient alike ...

Some forms of lying appear to be closely related to experiencing desire. [AI, 99–100]

(iii) The digestive model: In considering the development of consciousness as the psychic sense organ for the perception of psychic quality, after Freud and the development of thought, Bion observed that feeding at the breast, alimentation, is the basic indivisible material and psychic reality that humans have to know soon after birth. Since he accords a chronological priority to the physical component—which is in agreement with Nature's reality as it is—that is, *"milk, discomfort of satiation or the opposite"* (LE, 35). Bion also attributes a chronological priority to beta-elements (q.v.) over alpha-elements (q.v.). What does this mean? That *"The mental component, love, security, anxiety, as distinct from the somatic requires a process analogous to digestion"* (LE, 35). This is the first time that Bion makes explicit an analogy of the mental functioning to the functioning of the digestive system.

Embryologically speaking his suggestion has a sound basis. Both brain and the digestive apparatus stem from the most primitive parts of the embryo, the same that forms the skin (the ectoderm). In terms of life, a painful fact is that the person who is starving puts his belly before his love. There are comparatively few exceptions even among fathers and mothers with their progeny.

(iii) The reproduction system model: Another application of the medical-biological model to the functioning of the mental apparatus may be found in Bion's analogy of the mind with the reproductive system (see "Link").

&; The author has attempted to integrate the two models of thinking more fully in the here and now of the session (Sandler, 2000).

Memory: Bion defines memory as the *"conscious attempts to recall"* (AI, 70). It hampers and precludes the march into the unknown that is demanded by analytic work. See "Discipline in Memory, Desire and Understanding".
   Suggested cross-reference: Dream-like memory.

Mental health: For many years, Bion adopted criteria of mental health. They were always linked to, and dependent on:

1)   Truth and the possibilities to perceive it and to tolerate it.
2)   Thinking as a method of apprehension of a basic reality, namely, tolerance of frustration.
3)   The free movement between PS and D and vice-versa.

His studies on schizophrenic thinking and the lack of it did not question the diagnosis. His diagnostic criteria were far from Kurt Schneider and near Von Domarus. In other words, he focused on the disturbances of thinking and perception. This posture originates his scrutiny of hallucination. Disturbances of thinking and hallucination are a form of denial or evasion of truth.
   As late as 1965 he would write: *"healthy mental growth seems to depend on truth as the living organism depends on food. If it is lacking or deficient the personality deteriorates"* (T, 38).
   This may be seen as a most unusual criterion, in the sense that it: (i) is not morally tainted; (ii) does not rely on symptoms or pathology. In this sense it is purely psycho-analytic, extending the way that Freud dealt with the universality of neuroses and Klein, of psychosis. Symptoms are seen as expressive of specific kinds of mental functioning rather than enemies to be fought or wrongdoing that calls to be repressed.
   In 1960 he would equate mental health to a freedom of movement between PS and D and back. Tolerance of the back and forth situation would be indicative of mental health:

> The Positions are not to be regarded simply as features of infancy, and the transition from paranoid–schizoid to depressive position as something that is achieved once for all during infancy, but as a continuously active process once its mechanism has been successfully established in the early months. If, therefore, this is not established at the outset, then its operation remains defective throughout

life (in varying degrees of intensity), and the patient cannot reap the benefits that accrue through smooth operation of the to-and-fro between the two positions that should, for a full and healthy life, be always available to him. [C, 199–200]

This idea would remain unchanged for many years, but even in 1960 he would deal with mental health in a way that announced paradox. It was dependent on truth but it was also seen as a feeling indistinguishable from hallucination. The regulator is the principle of pleasure/pain and the principle of reality:

Mental health

The man who is mentally healthy is able to gain strength and consolation and the material through which he can achieve mental development through his contact with reality, no matter whether that reality is painful or not . . . no man can become mentally healthy save by a process of constant search for fact and a determination to eschew any elements, however seductive or pleasurable, that interpose themselves between himself and his environment as it really is.

The paradox that completes the whole appears in the following line: "*By contrast it may be said that man owes his health, and his capacity for continued health, to his ability to shield himself during his growth as an individual by repeating in his personal life the history of the race's capacity for self-deception against truth that his mind is not fitted to receive without disaster*" (C, 192)

The deciding factor is the tolerance of pain and frustration. Each person has some kind of ability to cope with disaster and what quantity or quality of truth that can be received without disaster. The latter can be expressed either by its narcissistic variation—homicide—or by its social-istic variation—suicide.

The assumption underlying loyalty to the K link is that the personality of analyst and analysand can survive the loss of its protective coat of lies, subterfuge, evasion and hallucination and may even be fortified and enriched by the loss. It is an assumption strongly disputed by the psychotic and *a fortiori* by the group, which relies on psychotic mechanisms for its coherence and sense of well-being. [T, 129]

This view of mental health would undergo some changes from 1967 onwards. The model of cure would be wholly discarded. It may be stated that up to 1964 he did adopt, to some extent, the patterns of mental disease and mental health. In fact one may observe that he nourished doubts about it from his post-World-War I days. He observes that some soldiers who refused to fight or were discharged on the basis of being schizophrenics perhaps were not really ill (AMF, I, 111).

   Recommended cross-reference: Establishment.
   Suggested cross-references: Real Psycho-Analysis, Truth.

Mental space: The grasping of this concept demands some acquaintance with the contents of the entries, Circle, Point, Line, $-K$, Point, Mathematization of Psycho-analysis and especially the entry Scientific method. Some mental origins of the concept of space are briefly discussed in these entries. Taking into account that earlier developments of the concept are expanded and pictured in those entries, now we will try to display its final and synthetic form.

> I shall now use the geometrical concepts of lines, points, and space (as derived originally not from a realization of three-dimensional space but from the realizations of the emotional mental life) as returnable to the realm from which they appear to me to spring. That is, if the geometer's concept of space derives from an experience of "the place where something was" it is to be returned to illuminate the domain where it is in my experience meaningful to say that "a feeling of depression" is "the place where a breast or other lost object was" and that "space" is "where depression, or some other emotion, used to be.

> I have pointed out that this space, these points, and these lines differ in one important respect, namely, that in the domain of mental visual images an infinite number of lines may pass through one point but, were I to attempt to represent such a visual image by point and lines on a piece of paper, there would be a finite number of lines. This limiting quality inheres in all realizations of three-dimensional space that approximate to the points, lines, and space of the geometer. It does not inhere in mental space until an attempt is made to represent mental space by verbal thought. I am thus postulating mental space as a thing-in-itself that is unknowable, but that can be represented by thoughts" (AI, 10–11).

Misuses and misunderstandings: In many quarters, this concept it taken in a concretized way. This is a misfortune: Bion's concept of a "mental space" is a "sense-free" concept. It resorts to the realm of "minus". It crowns years of research into the consequences of not-tolerating the absence, the lack, the no-breast, the no-space, and the "place where something was". However, a "place where something was" is being filled with a concretized misapprehension of a "mental space" that is regarded as a thing-in-itself.

Recommended cross-reference: Scientific Method

Suggested cross-references: Atonement, −K, Mathematization of psycho-analysis, Real psycho-analysis.

Metatheory: The name given by Bion, c. 1960, to one of his very few attempts at a theory of psycho-analysis, as contrasted with theories of observation (q.v.). It includes deep research into the nature of the apprehension of reality, the breast, the penis and violence of emotions. Parts of it were used in the building of his theories; parts of it remained to be developed. It was to remain unpublished until Francesca Bion unearthed it in *Cogitations*, p. 220.

The name seems to share an inspiration identical to Freud's "Metapsychology", that is, from Aristotle's editor who put his philosophical and non-physical, non-mathematical studies *after* (meta, in Greek) them, in an ordinal position in a book that gave rise to the name.

Suggested cross-references: Introduction to this dictionary, Theories of Observation.

Mind: "The Mind . . . is too heavy a load for the sensuous beast to carry" (AMF, I, 38).

Bion often uses the term, "mind". "*As a psycho-analyst I assume that there is such a reality that approximates to these terms 'thought', 'mind', 'personality'. I suspect—it is no more than a hunch or suspicion—that the mind and personality have a physical counterpart . . . in this context I am assuming that every psyche has a physical counterpart in the central nervous system . . . Lateral, profound, superficial, deep, early, later—all are terms more appropriate to time and space . . . but not if there is a domain of which it is possible to be mentally aware . . . we are compelled to use a language for communication of something for which it was not devised and of which it is itself a product*" (AMF, I, 184).

Is there a realm in which the human being is in fact mentally aware of himself? Freud ascribed this function to consciousness, the sense organ for perception of the psychical quality. Bion needed more than ten years to digest and accept this definition (please refer to the entry, Dream-work-α).

If it takes a consciousness to deal with the unconscious, the unconscious itself will remain unconscious—not known, *unbewußt*. The insoluble problem contained in the phrase, *"we are compelled to use a language for communication of something for which it was not devised and of which it is itself a product"* is the same as the problem of Oedipus: one cannot know how one was conceived. The term "mind" is an attempt, doomed to failure, to depict the numinous realm, "O". It can serve simply to mark its existence, that is intuitable, rather than "sense-able"—and therefore, it is not understandable.

With the possible exception of Freud, Klein and Bion the term "mind" has been proving to be fated (at least up to now—2005) to be increasingly less used in the psycho-analytic movement. The term harks back to pre-psycho-analytic days. There used to be a philosophy of mind that tried to tackle the issues that are today tackled by psycho-analysis. The latter provided a novel approach that enriched the philosophical interest with the medical: individual minds and their suffering.

> Hitherto, the term "mind" has proved to be serviceable. I propose to use it myself, but not for purposes of writing a philosophical or religious or psychological or artistic or other record. I propose to use it as a meaningless term, useful for talking or writing about what I *don't* know—to mark the "place where" a meaning might be. [AMF, I, 141]

In order to improve psycho-analytical insight about "mind", Bion starts from the principles of mental functioning, dreams and Oedipus: the basic analytic tenets. He at first used verbal formulations to construe analogies with mathematics in order to approach mental functioning. The genesis and development of thought conjoined with ego-functions gave birth to the Grid; and later to observational theories based on Transformations and Invariances.

At the end of his life Bion changed his approach to the medium of communication. He would now dwell more freely on the word "mind"; on its counterparts in reality; and on the psycho-analyst's beliefs involved with it.

> P.A. You speak as if you had no doubt that you—I mean the "personality" whom I know as "you"—are identical with the physical anatomy and physiological structure with which all are familiar.

> ROBIN Well, I have a mind of course.

> ROLAND That is what we are discussing.

> ROBIN If we could speak the language of mathematics . . .

> PAUL If we could speak the language of religion . . .

> ALICE If we could only learn to look at what artists paint . . . [AMF, II, 230]

> ROLAND There was once a game in which if you combined certain musical elements in accordance with the stated rules, in obedience to the fall of a throw of dice, the result when recorded through musical notation was a "Bach", or "Mozart" or "Beethoven" air.

> ROBIN There may even be a similar way of combining lines and triangles and other shapes to produce a "Leonardo" sketch. I have known an athlete speak of 'reading' the movements of an opponent.

> PAUL Any musician would appreciate that the music was *not* written by Beethoven.

> P.A. Beethoven would be missing. The mechanical throwing of dice could not take the place of Beethoven—

> PAUL —or Kant, or Freud, or Leonardo.

> P.A. We assume that there is a "thought to be thought through", or a "God" to be worshipped, or a mind covered up by, or revealed by, the notes or name scrawled on the paper. Our problem is "what mind?" Is it just a mind sufficient for the "athletic" feat of casting dice and making the marks on paper which the rules require us to make? Or is it a mind capable of creating the "game" and the rules, or expressing a spirit which we call Bach or Mozart or Plato—

> PAUL —or a Cathedral of Chartres, or a Hermes of Praxiteles, or a Theorem of Pythagoras—

> P.A. —without the intervention of "chance" as apparently, betrayed by the fall of dice? [AMF, II, 263]

ROSEMARY I thought you believed in mind.

P.A. You could call it that. *I* call it that because I have to talk to human minds and I can't do that without believing they exist. [AMF, II, 358]

"Mind" is a fictitious character in the third volume of *A Memoir of the Future*. Then its manifestation, the stuff of psycho-analysis— namely, pain, Oedipus—can be seen in a practical exercising of free associations. Or, "mind at function":

MIND Hullo! Where have you sprung from?

BODY What—you again? I am Body; you can call me Soma if you like. Who are you?

MIND Call me Psyche—Psyche-Soma.

BODY Soma-Psyche.

MIND We must be related.

BODY Never—not if I can help it.

MIND Oh, come. Not as bad as that, is it?

BODY Worse, You got us into this air. Luckily I brought some liquid with me. What are you doing?

MIND Nothing; it must be my phrenes, that diaphragm going up and down. I'm breathing in air—fluid, not liquid. What did you bring that wet stuff for? Beautiful odour.

BODY You could not know about the odour if I had not the liquid to hold your atoms with. Typical of Mind—all words and no content. Where did you find them?

MIND Borrowed from the future—you are borrowing them from me; do you get them through the diaphragm?

BODY *They* penetrate *it*. But the meaning does not get through. Where did you get your pains from?

MIND Borrowed—from the past. The meaning does not get through the barrier though. Funny—the meaning does not get through whether it is from you to me, or from me to you.

BODY It is the meaning of pain that I am sending to you; the words get through—which I have not sent—but the meaning is lost.

MIND What is that amusing little affair sticking out? I like it. It has a mind of its own—just like me.

BODY It's just like me—has a body of its own. That's why it is so erect. Your mind—no evidence for it at all.

MIND Don't be ridiculous. I suffer anxiety as much as you have pain. In fact I have pain about which you know nothing. I suffered intensely when you were rejected. I asked you to call me Psyche and promised to call you Soma.

SOMA All right Psyche; I don't admit that there is any such person other than a figment of my digestion.

PSYCHE Who are you talking to then?

SOMA I'm talking to myself and the sound is reflected back by one of my fetal membranes.

PSYCHE Your feetal membranes! Ha, ha! Very good! Is that your pun or mine?

SOMA It's the only language you understand.

PSYCHE It's the only language you hear. All you talk is pain. [AMF, III, 433–434]

The "wordy"—more than "worldly"—value of the term, "Mind", is made explicit. In other words, it is a Model. As such, it strives to represent a counterpart in reality that is ultimately ineffable. If it is ineffable, the task of formulating it verbally is doomed to failure. The relative success of this formulation depends on the listener's experience, and intuition concerning the apprehension of the Platonic–Kantian numinous realm, the unconscious itself.

It requires not falling into the naïve realist's error (as Kant called it) or, in other words, it requires abandoning that which can be named an "exclusivity of the senses" when the task is to try to apprehend reality.

From the failure of verbal formulations the poets must be exempted. To non-poets, be they issuers or receivers, the failure of verbal formulations is often felt as unbearable. It is felt as an offence to human omnipotence. Sometimes there is a flight into concretization. As soon as one gets a name, it seems that it pervades a sensation of having understood the issue. The uttering of the name replaces the research into the issue that is the counterpart in reality of that name. The extinction of the research precludes further discoveries—including the possibility that no counterpart in reality to that name exists at all.

The result is that terms like "Mind" acquire an "as if" value. The "as if" passes unnoticed as such and itself acquires the value of "as" (meaning "equal"). A symbolic equation occurs (in the sense described by Klein and later publicized by Segal). As soon as the beholder of the term utters it, he or she feels that he or she "owns" and "has" the reality that the terms strive to express but cannot.

People speak about a mind as if it actually existed beyond the realm of discourse. But "Mind" may be at best just a hypothesis. Nevertheless, people deal with it as if it is a proven thesis. The beholder seems to ignore the fact that various names were proposed for "it": soul, personality, spirit, psyche, phrenes, mental apparatus, psychic reality, character, ego, id, self, super-ego, unconscious, and so on.

All of them had their period of glory and popularity. They were pronounced with a sense of illumination by some people. But they fell. Sometimes, due to forgetfulness they resurface again only to fall into oblivion in a matter of a few decades or centuries. This fact alone suggests that uncertainty surrounds the issue. The uncertainty is denied by the beholder as soon as he or she achieves a state ("mental" state . . .) of illumination when the term "mind" (or whatever it is) is issued. It is a state indistinguishable from that which characterizes a religious being during a religious service, or a gang member. From "wordy" to "worldly": the immaterial meaning is replaced, in hallucination, by a concrete property or quality.

> . . . I can argue that the mind and its works are of great significance; the rest, a total, inchoate mindlessness to be called "the unconscious", is lumped together and glorified and idealized as a further tribute to the mind . . . The personality or mind, as portrayed psycho-analytically in detail, is a recent photogram of some long-existent reality, of significance only as an archaic physical anatomy might be. Psycho-analysis would appear as an ephemeral phenomenon betraying forces on the surface of which the human race flickers, flares and fades in response to the unrecognized but gigantic reality. [AMF, I, 111–112]

MAN It is rare, among psycho-analysts at least, to imagine that the most their science can do is to map the nature of the mind. The "discovery" of the mind itself depends on philosophers achieving progress parallel to the micromolecular discovery in the physical domain. The mind, certainly the human mind, can be found to be something of very minor and very embryonic growth. Just as it may seem miraculous that a mind, equipped with visual sense, can "see" things inaccessible to the sightless paramoecium, so it might appear prophetic—not applied common sense—if the insightful person could detect what to others would appear to be unsupported by evidence. Perhaps a paramoecium would have to believe in "god". What more suitable god than man? What more suitable to man than any available "super-man"? How could this be made available for worship by some well arranged system of lies and cheats? How more easily dealt with than by a well arranged system of "scientific" lies and cheats "exposing" the lies and cheats?

ROSEMARY Money, morals, "honours", position and power are often offered to women who accept the counterfeit as real and offer their same easily prostituted "wealth" and "assets" in the way food and pharmacological preparations can be offered as cheats by the male as well as the female whore. And now the mind has become available for the extension of lies, deceptions, evasions to produce bigger, better liars and cheats than any "human" mind has so far achieved . . .

MAN When the mind ± has been mapped, the investigations may reveal variations in the various patterns which it displays. The important thing may not be, as the psycho-analysts suppose, only revelations in illness or diseases of the mind, but patterns indiscernible in the domain in which Bio ± exist (life and death; animate and inanimate) because the mind spans too inadequate a spectrum of reality. Who can free mathematics from the fetters exposed by its genetical links with sense? Who can find a Cartesian system which will again transform mathematics in ways analogous to the expansion of arithmetic effected by imaginary numbers, irrational numbers, Cartesian coordinates freeing geometry from Euclid by opening up the domain of algebraic deductive systems; the fumbling infancy of psycho-analysis from the domain of sensuality-based mind? [AMF, I, 129–130]

Bion expands a fictional dialogue that encompasses many religious, artistic, astronomical, mythical and mathematical attempts to grasp reality. It can be perceived as that counterpart in reality that could correspond to "mind's expressions" or that which we call "mind" itself at work:

"I am a funny story. I am a child's book. I am wonderland. I am a children's story. You are laughing in your sleep. You are waking up. The funny story which makes you laugh will make you cry. The child's dream will grow up to become adult, the night mare will carry you, like Shakespeare's sonnet ... I shall fling you and your tiller back to the domain from which you came disguised as Palinurus, Urania ...

"I am the horrendous dream that turned Science Fiction to Science Fact. I turned hideous night to even more hideous day. And you?

"I am the Refiner's fire. The glorious sun who was the revolution-ary flame disguised as R.F., the république française, the public thing, the thing that turned the hidden thing to the public thing; who robbed death, who robbed the secret of its cover and exposed it as the monster that it is. Who are you?

"I am thought searching for a thinker to give birth to me. I shall destroy the thinker when I find him. I am the Odyssey, the Iliad, the Aeneid. I prevented Mars from destroying me but I ate away Mars from inside, from outside so he died. He is a memory and a desire: I am the eternally alive, indestructible, indispensable, adorable. I am the force that makes the books. My last triumph is the Mind. The mind that is too heavy a load for the sensuous beast to carry. I am the thought without a thinker and the abstract thought which has destroyed its thinker ..." [AMF, I, 37–8]

The question that furnishes the leitmotiv to the concept is a practical one—rather than philosophical or theoretical. It has to do with the psycho-analytic movement having gone astray; to perceive the difficulties involved in researching "the mind" allows real research to be done.

To believe unquestioningly in such as thing as "The mind" produces a "thus far and no further" ideology. Being an ideology, it is a self-feeding state of mindlessness. This brings analytic research to a halt and misguided efforts imply waste:

The practical point is—no further investigations of psycho-analysis, but the psyche it betrays. *That* needs to be investigated through the medium of *mental* patterns; *that* which is indicated is *not* a symptom; *that* is not a cause of the symptom; *that* is not a disease or *any*thing subordinate. Psycho-analysis itself is just a stripe on the coat of the tiger. Ultimately it may meet the Tiger—The Thing itself—O" [AMF, I, 112]

"Mind", its workings and the analyst

Difficulties in grasping the counterpart in reality that corresponds to "mind" seem to be linked to erudition. England has a tradition at least since Alexander Pope of trying to fend off the problems derived from sterile erudition. He once spoke about "the bookful blockhead, with plenty of learned lumber in his head". This was transported to the musical world by the late conductor Sir Thomas Beecham: "A musicologist is one who can read music but cannot hear it". Its version in analysis is, ". . . *the erudite can see that a description is by Freud, or Melanie Klein, but remain blind to the thing described*" (AMF, I, 5).

There is a subtle turning point:

> The fiction can be so rhetorical as to be incomprehensible; or so realistic that the dialogue becomes audible to others. There is thus a double fear; that of the conversation being so theoretical that the thoughts might be taken for meaningless jargon; and that of the seeming reality. Having two sets of feelings about the same facts is felt as madness and disliked accordingly. This is one reason why it is felt necessary to have an analyst; another reason is the wish for me to be available to be regarded as mad and used to being regarded as mad. There is a fear that you might be called an analysand, or reciprocally, that you may be accused of insanity. Should I then be tough and resilient enough to be regarded and treated as insane while being sane? If so, it is not surprising that psycho-analysts are, almost as a function of being analysts, supposed to qualify for being insane and called such. It is part of the price they have to pay for being psycho-analysts. [AMF, I, 113]

The counterpart in reality that the verbal formulation "Mind" purports to depict seems to belong to the numinous realm. This means that primal emotions such as dread, pain, capacity for cruelty and greed exist and may prevail if one tries to consider Mind in its purest and simplest form. Bion uses a metaphor of dinosaurs to depict it. He also questions the belief that human mind developed during the time span between the dinosaurs and the time of Hitler. See especially *A Memoir of the Future*, volume I, pages 33–39, 55, 58–63, 75–82, 83–100, 186–194, to examine both "mind's" attempts or ideas that humans do have a mind and states of mindlessness that suggest that the human's ultimate reality is well represented by bestiality as it may also be by sublimity. They are depicted in the scene of "Rosemary's marriage", volume II, pp. 365, 391ff.

> Is the supposition that the reptilian age is antecedent to Hitler correct, or is it a feature of our thinking process which has become an aberration which has not been considered, but has become part of what is *observed*? [AMF, I, 86]

Bion depicts other equally cherished beliefs—which are also products of the mind—in a broad, all-encompassing appreciation of the tragedy of mankind—including death itself and the feeble attempts to understand what it is. There is no lack of a good-humoured, respectful doubt and references to many of Freud's concepts, as well as basic neurological concepts, that were attempts to grasp something of this tragedy in non-literary terms. For example, the attachment of consciousness to unconscious, as a sense organ; the qualities of the unconscious, the hypotheses about hypotheses about hypotheses that characterized the work of Freud (something Freud himself always emphasized, and is made clear on pages 378 and 379 of *Cogitations*). Bion casts doubts on the alleged good effects only of knowledge.

One may see that attempts to know results both in more questions and in immense edifices of split knowledge which sink under their own weight. The metaphor of an empty shell, or that what remains is just a skeleton, may be seen as the "secularization" of the churches or of any institution; or erudition devoid of wisdom, or knowledge devoid of love:

> ALPHA And even myself, whose thoughts and feelings linger on long after I have woken up and remain active and alive in my waking life long after it is expected or supposed (by whom, pray? Shut up!) that I should be dead and buried (where?) In the land of nod, the unconscious, the forgotten, the . . . wherever else I am to go

to—the Future will do for a sort of royal cemetery as well as the past. Below the Thalamus. The royal cemetery at Ur, Newton, Shakespeare, Descartes. But some are so deeply buried, forgotten, even their names swallowed up, that they need exing the cave. Even metaphors come alive, otherwise the words that are needed achieve the qualities of "life". (More bloody metaphors! Who ever could sort out a mass of verbiage like this?) You could try calling it "Paranoid Schizoid" after—a long way "after"—Melanie Klein. Good idea. Good dog paranoid schizoid, here, here is a nice piece of jargon for you. Suspicious are you? Take *that* then! Another great lump of free associations, dreams and their interpretations, poetry, ("all lies", said Plato, sly, suspicious old dog that he was) is hurled at the poor, newborn baby. "Intelligence", they call the puir, wee thing. Where is that Anarch of the stops and dashes and never-ending Parentheses?—Sterne, they called him, wasn't it? The Anarchs of the world of darkness keep a throne for thee, puir, wee Intelligence. A rose by any other name . . . might just as well be a stink that smells as foul even if you call it a "salubrious environment".

Come here, bad, baaad dog—Hitler dear, *such* a nice Hitler, *such* a *benito*, such a sweet, rosy little boy! Here, here's a nice salubrious environment! Washed, nay bathed, in our Auschwitz showers. They smell—aah! You can't think how sweet and refreshing those showers are. Now, *here* is a brand new *mind*. It is far superior to the nose as an instrument for discrimination. You just have to attach one of our "minds" to the old apparatus and this tiny adjustment fitted to the nose and any of the no nonsense organs, to obtain a really superior organ of discrimination! Yes: but how can I tell quackery—use it! Why discriminate?—from truth? Can I tell by it, for example, if this mind you talk is any better than all the previous gadgets I have been invited to attach, at enormous expanding cost, to my various existing battery of gadgets? I knew a delightful old stegosaurus who thought he had found *the* answer to the tyrannosaurus. But the "answer" was so successful that it turned into a kind of tyrannosaurus itself and loaded him with such fame—not to mention exoskeleton—that he sank under its own weight. In fact, he was so loaded that the only trace of him left was his skeleton. Yes, but those same dead bones gave birth to a mind. Because while all eyes were fixed on the conflict between Fate and armour (there is **no** armour against Fate) the attacker got through disguised as a bomber. Now, the Mind . . . you just try it. Just attach your sensory perceptions! How do I know it won't just turn into extrasensory perceptions—s.p. ⇔ e.s.p.? The animal, meaning you, who reads this and I that write it and all biological living constructs, have an inborn mechanism for self-destruction. This dogmatic, definitory hypothesis shares the character of the character it represents. On this definitory hypothesis is built the hypothesis and the construct of which it is the foundation. [AMF, I, 59–60]

Recommended cross-references: Atonement, Dream, Jargon, Mathematization of psycho-analysis, Real psycho-analysis, Dream-work-α, Tool-making animal, Ultra-sensuous.

Minus: "Even the fetus is involved with *non-fetus*" (AMF, III, 490).

Is the foremost contribution of Bion to psycho-analysis an expansion and deepening of the realm of the unconscious? If the answer is "yes" the fact is more remarkable if one takes into account that during his lifetime the tendency towards ego psychology was rampant. This tendency has unavoidable attendants, namely (i) a return to the point of view of academic descriptive psychology; (ii) a leaning to rational ad hoc theorizing clothed in psycho-analytic wording, losing sight of immaterial facts of psychic reality. To lose track of the unconscious means to lose track of underlying factors and invariances. One cannot say that Bion's efforts reversed the tide, but it is safe to state that his work offered an alternative to this state of affairs.

The renewed research into the unconscious had as one of its more important features the illumination of a realm and an activity that can, thanks to Bion's contributions, and trying to give justice to the denominations he left, be called both "the realm of minus" and a "negative force". (If one is able to tolerate a neologism, it can be named a "negativating" force, in order to stress its living, dynamic nature.)

This coincided with his very first attempt at a theory of psycho-analysis, namely, his theory of thinking. Thinking itself has its inception because of a "minus" experience, namely, the "No-Breast". The absence of the concrete breast allows for the inception of thinking processes. Pressed by real external contingencies—mother necessity—the most primitive form that thought assumes would be the thought of a breast. Which is a thought provoked by an absent breast. It allows realization of what a real breast is.

When one tolerates that one's pre-conception of a breast differs from the real breast that is offered, a thought is born. A thought is made during the experiencing of the difference between the real breast and the pre-conception of the breast. This hypothesis was first adumbrated in the paper "A theory of thinking", from 1961. One year later Bion would advance a kind of consequence of this fact which has been studied in detail during the ensuing seven years. This consequence may occur with more intensity when intolerance of frustration prevails: a "negative force" emerges. The link between both was to remain just implicit in his work.

The realm of minus

1. **Contrapuntal minus**—it defines the realm of minus. It is "made" of absences: the No-Breast, the darkness of the unknown, the transient lack of apprehension of Truth. It is a contrasting step towards the apprehension of reality. It is the nest of dreams and free associations. It is the stuff of the unconscious; it corresponds to Kant's definition of noumena as a negative, a "limit-concept". The situation of "no" is a scientific and philosophical tool that may help the human being to get nearer to that which **is**, known since Spinoza.

One describes that which an unknown object *is not* in order to arrive at what the thing *is*. Chemistry progressed methodically. Bion uses a most revealing list of "negatives" in his attempt to describe the realm of "O" (T, 139, 161). It is represented by a sign borrowed from mathematics: −, developed to denote negative numbers. It may be named as "no-thing".

2. **"Negative force" minus**—It is a development of the realm of minus that can become the definition of it when intolerance of pain and frustration—which is inherent in the realm of minus—activates a negative, destructive force. It is initially used as a barrier to the unknown and the known which is disliked. It has a denuding power, purposefully built to denude pain and unpleasure of its painful and unpleasurable features. In this sense it is a destructive minus to the extent that real facts have both pleasurable and unpleasurable features. It is composed of lies and hallucination.

It was first represented by the mathematical symbol which denoted the negative numbers (−) and is represented by a symbol derived from the use of the Grid (q.v.): □<. It may be named, "nothing".

The first manifestation of the destructive function of minus was that which Bion called minus K (−K). This act materializes the activity of the destructive "negative *force*". Even though this dictionary contains a specific entry on −K some illuminations are perhaps better placed here:

> The point has appeared clinically as dot or dots, spot or spots ("spots" in or before the eyes is a fairly common phenomenon). I have described the point or line as an object indistinguishable from the place where the breast or penis was. Owing to the difficulty of being sure what the patient is experiencing I resort to a variety of descriptions, each of which is unsatisfactory. The spot, for example, seems to be part conscience, part breast, part faeces, destroyed, non-existent yet present, cruel and malignant. The inadequacy of description or categorization as thought at all has led me to the term β-element as a method of representing it. The spoken word seems significant only because it is invisible and intangible; the visual image is similarly significant because it is inaudible. Every word represents what is not—a "no-thing", to be distinguished from "nothing". [T, 78–9]

"No-thing" marks the contrapuntal value of minus; "nothing" marks the aftermath of the negative force's action. The final assessment of the "destructive minus" can be found in *A Memoir of the Future*. We single out one of the many passages:

> MAN God threw these presumptuous objects out of Eden. The Omnipotent opposes the extensions of the human ability to have intercourse. Babel opposed the extensions of power to the realm of the mind. So extensions of plus-K are certain to reveal obstacles if extended to minus-K. The immortality achieved through reproduction by cell division leads to the morality achieved by nuclear fission.
>
> BION What else?
>
> MAN I am not going to do your thinking for you. Sooner or later you will have to pay the price of deciding to think ±; whether, in Freud's formulation, to interpose "thinking" between impulse and action; or to interpose the two as a substitute for action; or to interpose it between the two as a prelude to action.
>
> BION Oh, all right—let's get on with this enthralling and spectacular spectacle.

(The darkness deepens. The skull-crushing and sucking object is overwhelmed by depression at the failing supply of nutriment from the dead ? and the failure to restore it to life. He formulates in stone an *arti*-factual representation, easily seen by Plato to be a lying representation of, a substitute for, pro-creation, a substitute for creation. The lying substitution is transformed into a prelude to action. This whirling, swirling chaos of infinite and formless darkness becomes luminous and a Leonardo da Vinci robs the hair, the brooding waste of waters, of its formless chaos.

BION Disgusting! Mawkish! [AMF, I, 160–1]

The function of the No: the No-Breast

If there are only beta-elements, which cannot be made unconscious, there can be no repression, suppression or leaning. This creates the impression that the patient is incapable of discrimination.

Attacks on alpha-function, stimulated by hate or envy, destroy the possibility of the patient's conscious contact either with himself or another as live objects. Accordingly we hear of inanimate objects, and even of places, when we would normally expect to hear of people. These, though described verbally, are felt by the patient to be present materially and not merely to be represented by their names. This state contrasts with animism in that live objects are endowed with the qualities of death. [LE, 8–9]

In *Cogitations* one finds a more precise expansion of that:

In the earliest phases of development objects are felt to be alive and to possess character and personality presumably indistinguishable from the infant's own. In this phase, which may be considered as anterior to the development of the reality principle as Freud describes it, the real and the alive are indistinguishable; if an object is real to the infant, then it is alive; if it is dead, it does not exist. But this "it" that does not exist and is not alive—why is it necessary to talk about it or discuss it? [C, 133]

It is necessary to discuss it because it is linked to the inception of hallucinatory processes that make unreal facts pass for the real facts (persons, events, things). *"The problem is to give an answer verbally about objects in a **pre-verbal** state"* (C, 133).

The pre-verbal state seems to be conceivable and "formulable" in visual terms—as in dreams and hallucinations. "In this instance it is necessary to talk about this object which should be non-existent and therefore impossible to discuss. Its importance lies in the fact that the infant, if enraged, has death wishes, and if the object is wished dead, it is dead" (C, 133).

This "is" indicates an hallucinatory and deluded mental activity that effectively drains life, of one's own use and profit, from that which remains alive but cannot be used and much less enjoyed. Or due to sadistic attacks, the enjoyment is drawn from destruction. This is the first precise perception of Bion on that which we may call a "negativating" force.

After the "negativation", or after being thrown into the realm of minus (which would be formulated in 1962) one may state that the object (or fact, or breast, or mother, or feeling, or emotion, or thing) *"therefore has become non-existent, and its characteristics are different from those of the real, live existing object: the existing object is alive, real, and benevolent"*.

In 1960 Bion called these objects *"proto-real"* objects. This proto-reality is the realm of negative. It is an important addition to the realm of the unconscious. The *"proto-real"* is a prototype. It may serve for finalities of comparison with the real objects. That may acquire an enhanced status in the mind of the beholder because of the comparison with the proto-objects.

The principle that regulates the process is tolerance of frustration. If it is low, the proto-objects will be transformed from proto-types to paradigms. They will rule that adult life ought to be a greedy and envious "all-negativating" non-life, full of empty concrete objects. The issue would be expanded in chapters V and VI of *Learning from Experience*. It would later give rise to the concept of transformations in hallucinosis.

> The infant, in all the early phases of its life, is dominated by the pleasure principle. It is therefore, in so far as it feels pleasure, surrounded with these proto-real objects felt to be real and alive. But should pain supervene, then it is surrounded by dead objects destroyed by its hate, which, since it cannot tolerate pain, are non-existent. [C, 133]

The function of the no-breast in the thinking processes is examined in the entry, "No-Breast". The contrapuntal function of the "no", the realm of minus, was further illuminated in 1965. In his typical way, Bion uses one of the (sacrosanct?) laws of Euclidean formal logic, in a perspicacious paraphrase of it:

> The problem is simplified by a rule that "a thing can never be unless it both is and is not". Stating the rule in other forms: "a thing cannot exist in the mind alone: nor can a thing exist unless at the same time there is a corresponding no-thing". The rules that apply to the thing do not apply to the no-thing. Contradiction is not an invariant under psycho-analysis though it may exist in the domain of psycho-analytic objects (which *must* both be and not be). [T, 102–3]

Bion seems to have been inspired by Shelley's formulation about Shakespeare's characters in the plays. The gifted poet, a favourite of Bion, observed that these characters were real even though they did not possess existence in material reality—as the misguided concretizing diatribes about Shakespeare's lack of historical faithfulness, similar to Wladimir Horowitz's "mistakes" when playing at the piano in his later days. His first formulation of this contrapuntal "minus" was:

> If there is a "no-thing" the "thing" must exist. By analogy, if Falstaff is a no-thing Falstaff also exists; if it can be said that Falstaff, Shakespeare's character who had no real existence, has more "reality" than people who existed in fact, it is because an actual Falstaff exists; the invariant under psycho-analysis is the ratio of no-thing to thing. [T, 103]

As occurs throughout Bion's work, the same quotation appears in a more colloquial and developed form ten years later: "*Falstaff, a known artefact, is more 'real' in Shakespeare's verbal formulation than countless millions of people who are dim, invisible, lifeless, unreal, whose births, deaths—alas, even marriages—we are called upon to believe in, though certification of their existence is vouched for by the said official certification*" (AMF, I, 4–5).

This is a knife-edge that can nourish both the apprehension of reality through the absence of its concrete presence and hallucinations. The factual or concrete event cannot vouch for reality as we deal with immaterial facts. The same issue was further expanded, perhaps more freely, ten years later.

The "negative force"

This can be considered as the first "negativation", wholly hallucinatory, belonging to pure feeling in an inchoate state that denies reality and is neither conscious nor unconscious. A nirvana state tries to pose a challenge to reality as it is. As any mechanism of defence, it is doomed to failure. As any lie, it demands a fresh supply of lies to create an impression that it can be maintained; the lie demand constant repair. A stage that can be named, the second "negativation", obtrudes with renewed force in another guise:

> But ordinarily they continue to exist because the sense impressions still operate. Should intolerance of these objects grow beyond a certain point, then the infant commences attacks on the mental apparatus that informs it of the reality of these sense impressions and of some object that is felt to be beyond the sense impressions. [C, 134]

Therefore this second stage is against mind itself; not only is the external reality attacked but the very perception of it and the whole apparatus that perceives it. An attack against both external and internal reality ensues.

> Excess of death instincts for whatever reason or duration, in addition to contributing to an excess of dead objects—painful and proto-unreal—means that animism (an animistic view) cannot develop. [C, 134]

Animism is here seen not only as a primitive situation—as found in primitive social organizations—but also as a step towards the humanistic aspect that de-sensifies things and turns them into immaterial real facts to be lived, not to be owned. Lack of animism precludes the turning of a concrete breast and milk into solace, warmth, perception of motherhood and the construing of real internal objects.

> The need to placate contributes to a complex state in which the dead object has to be re-animated and worshipped. These objects are then not so much gods and idols that are believed to be alive and endowed with human attributes, as objects chosen specifically and precisely because *they are dead* ... The dead, non-existent objects are products of murderous hate; guilt invests them with

attributes akin to those associated with conscience, omnipotence, omniscience, but not the qualities necessary for employment in dream-thoughts. [C, 134]

This seems to be the earliest complete description of the "minus-objects", that cannot be unconscious, are dead and cannot be dreamt or combined. The clinical studies that led to this description can be found in the entries, Schizophrenia, Schizophrenic thought, Beta-elements and Psychotic Personality. Also, reversal of alpha-function deals more finely with the subject and can be found in the entry, "alpha-function".

From "no" to "bad"

The developments that took place during the time that Bion wrote his reflections about animism (that were to be published much later by Francesca Bion) allowed him to establish the foundations of the realm of minus. In doing this he makes a trans-disciplinary integration between the analytic experience and psychotics and philosophy. He displays a perfect grasp of the ethos of Kant's depiction of the noumena as a negative (the numbered paragraphs are a typical feature of Bion's writing):

> 8. As the analyst treating an adult patient I can be conscious of something of which the patient is not conscious. Similarly the mother can discern a state of mind in her infant before the infant can be conscious of it, as, for example, when the baby shows signs of needing food before it is properly aware of it. In this imaginary situation the need for the breast is a feeling and that feeling itself is a bad breast; the infant does not feel it wants a good breast but it does feel it wants to evacuate a bad one.

> 9. Suppose the infant is fed; the taking in of milk, warmth, love, may be felt as taking in a good breast. Under dominance of the, at first unopposed, bad breast, "taking in" food may be felt as indistinguishable from evacuating a bad breast. Both good and bad breasts are felt as possessing the same degree of concreteness and reality as milk. [LE, 34]

This phrase is important: the baby does not tolerate the realm of the negative, at its inception. It prefers the "positive", the concrete satisfaction.

The next phrase establishes the realm of minus: *"Sooner or later the 'wanted' breast is felt as an 'idea of a breast missing' and not as a bad breast present"* (SE, 34).

This phrase is seminal. Instead of using the "minus experience" to grow, to know what the presence is, "minus"—" breast missing"—is used to establish itself as revenge; the idea of a breast missing undergoes co-option in order to give a hidden promise that the breast will be available somewhere, some day. The "minus" turns on the baby's feelings, into a perverted, hallucinatory "plus". The "bad breast present" is denied and with it the opportunity to use "minus" as a counterpoint. Intolerance of minus leads to its institutionalization under co-option:

> We can see that the bad, that is to say wanted but absent, breast is much more likely to become recognized as an idea than the good breast which is associated with what a philosopher would call a thing-in-itself . . . The good breast and the bad breast, the one being associated with the actual milk that satisfies hunger and the other with the non-existence of that milk, must have a difference in psychical quality. "Thoughts are a nuisance, said one of my patients". [LE, 34]

Not to tolerate the absence of a concrete object precludes both objectivity and subjectivity; both conscious and unconscious:

> If there is a good breast, a sweet object, it is because it has been evacuated . . . and the same with the bad breast, the needed breast, the bitter breast, etc. It cannot be seen as objective and it cannot be seen as subjective. From these sweet, bitter, sour objects, sweetness, bitterness, sourness, are abstracted. Once abstracted they can be reapplied; the abstraction made can be used in situations where a realization, not the original realization from which it was abstracted, approximates to it. [LE, 59–60]

The qualities belong, in the first place, to the realm of minus. The qualities are intuited, felt, experimented and have that evanescent nature that must be learnt just to help one to look for them again. The evanescent nature is the "minus". This is abhorred. Therefore the baby who abhors frustration cannot "abstract" and looks for the "positive" or "concrete" for ever. It finds itself in a state of real eternal deprivation, without realizing that which in fact it may have and use must have an introjected counterpart in the mind which belongs to the field of minus.

The "property" must exist through experience and learning, through an intuition that allows one to look for the thing needed and know-how to do it, rather that actually having to have it. There is a need to couple the "concrete property of an object" with thinking about the object owned. Any property is temporary; any event is transient. The price to be paid if this remove is not achieved is to be stuck to something (originally, the mother's actual breast) that never existed in his mind and despite having existed in material reality certainly disappeared.

> The first level of statements are particular, derived from an actual episode, and concrete; the abstractions become further and further removed from the concrete and specific until their origin is lost to sight. The abstractions that are thus produced may then be reapplied to a realization when a realization is found that appears to approximate to the abstraction. [LE, 60]

The introduction of the symbol minus (−)

It is first made through the description of minus-K, a link "*constituted by NOT understanding i.e.* **mis***understanding*" (LE, 52). At the same time Bion introduces the whole realm of minus, with minus L and minus H. Please see entries, −K, −L and −H.

We have already noticed Bion's choice of a quasi-mathematical method of notation. He spares the reader philosophical terms and concepts. He did not resort to Kant or Hegel's terminology about the negative, preferring to appeal to the notion of negative numbers. This allows a spectrum formed both by positive and negative. This choice is furthered when defining the concepts, Psycho-analytic object and Growth. After introducing the concept of (−K), minus K, Bion uses the notion of minus to characterize Growth:

> Growth may be regarded as positive or negative. I shall represent it by (± Y). The plus and minus signs are employed to give sense or direction to the element they precede in a manner analogous to their mode of employment in coordinate geometry . . . Whether (Y)

is preceded by plus or minus sign will be determined only by contact with a realization. [LE, 70]

This concept marks the description of the second meaning of the realm of minus. Its contrapuntal function in the apprehension of reality is replaced by its view as a destructive force. One may state that to the extent the counterpoint cannot be tolerated the obvious aftermath is the "winning" over of one of the aspects of the contrapuntal pair: minus takes over and a destructive force has the upper hand. This can be clearly seen in the concept of $-K$ that Bion introduces at the end of the book *Learning from Experience*. It constitutes a perennial attempt to display the superiority of not understanding over understanding; of mis-representation over representation.

There is a continuous stripping and denudation of meaning of whatever it is. The breast cannot be felt as a moderator of the dreadful and annihilating feelings; it cannot allow a re-introjection that could be growth-stimulating. It is a breast, or minus breast in the minus K domain that is felt *"enviously to remove the good and valuable element in the fear of dying and force the worthless residue back into the infant"* (LE, 96). The violence of emotions (q.v.) adds to the situation, in affecting the projective processes *"so that far more than the fear of dying is projected"* (LE, 97). The process of denudation—in the case of K, denudation of meaning, is *"therefore more serious ... The seriousness is best conveyed by saying that the will to live, that is necessary before there can be a fear of dying, is a part of the goodness that the envious breast has removed"* (LE, 97).

$-K$ opens the possibility of a minus (container–contained). Its predominant characteristic is a "without-ness". It must be differentiated from "nothingness", or Zero. *"The process of denudation continues till $-\male$ $-\female$ represent hardly more than an empty superiority–inferiority that in turn degenerates to nullity"* (LE, 97). The minus (container–contained) *"shows itself as a superior object asserting its superiority by finding fault with everything. The most important characteristic is its hatred of any new development in the personality as if the new development were a rival to be destroyed. The emergence therefore of any tendency to search for the truth, to establish contact with reality and in short to be scientific ... is met by destructive attacks on the tendency and the reassertion of the 'moral' superiority ...*

In K, the climate is conducive to mental health. In $-K$ neither group nor idea can survive partly because of the destruction incident to the *stripping and partly because of the product of the stripping process"* (LE, 98–9).

The introduction of the symbol ←↑

The negative force can be depicted in the Grid as a movement from the more developed to the more primitive categories. The Grid is graphically constructed with a bi-dimensional conjunction of two axes. Thinking develops in one axis—vertical—from primitive non-thoughts to more sophisticated real thought (from definitory hypothesis and beta-elements to algebraic calculus) and in the other—horizontal—from the thing-in-itself that is "metabolized" through the various ego-functions until an action may be taken in the real world (from definitory hypothesis to action). The symbol for this development is →↓. Therefore the obverse (decay) is symbolized by ←↑.

> The problem posed by ←↑ can be stated by analogy with *existing* objects. ←↑ is violent, greedy and envious, ruthless, murderous and predatory, without any respect for the truth, persons or things. It is, as it were, what Pirandello might have called a Character in Search of an Author ... This force is dominated by an envious determination to possess everything that objects that exist possess including existence itself. [T, 102]

The introduction of the symbols representing a sense of development and lack of it allowed a more precise re-definition of the realm of "minus". In the following quotation, it will be clear that the domain of thought is seen as belonging to the unconscious, coherent with all the earlier contributions of Bion; the symbols

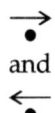

mean, respectively: positive or plus point and "negative point" or "minus point".

> The domain of thought may be conceived of as a space occupied by no-things; the space occupied by a particular no-thing is marked by

a sign such as the words "chair" or "cat" or "point" or "dog". The attempt to free this domain from associations of space perception is supported by use of concepts such as "thought" or "thinking" or "in the mind", but a thought continues to have the penumbra of association proper to "the place where . . ." the no-thing is. This is also true of feelings and emotions however expressed.

The "objects" with which psycho-analysis deals include the *relationship* of the no-thing and the thing. The personality that is capable of tolerating a no-thing can make use of the no-thing, and so is able to make use of what we can now call thoughts. Since he can do so he can seek to fill the "space" occupied by the thought; this makes it possible for the "thought" of space, line, point to be matched with a realization that is felt to approximate to it. In this respect

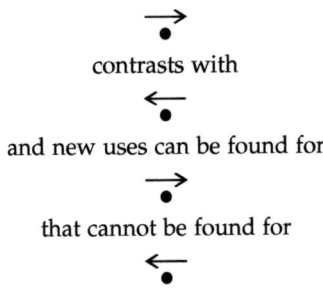

[T, 106]

Clinical applications: the counterpoint returns

In *Elements of Psycho-analysis* there again appears the function of the realm of minus as a pointer of emanations from the numinous realm, of the ultimate reality that presents the psychic reality of the patient in the here and now of the session. In other words, the focus is again on the value of minus as a counterpoint or a step in the mind's processes to apprehend reality.

The issue is presented around the sexual instinct and its presentations: *"The sexual instinct is an integral part of the psycho-analytic theory, but the element of sex in the sense of something for which I need to look is not sex but that from which the presence of sex may be deduced"*. Bion proposes to look for elements that betray the presence of *"some more fundamental thing"*, out of the unknown. The element is a

"precursor" (of sex, for example) and must be intuited in the realm
of its physical or material lack—the realm of minus (all quotations,
EP, 74). All of this is the embryo of the later formulations around
"transformations in O"; it interests us now as the first forays into
the formulations and practical use of the realm of "minus", the
numinous realm.

Its importance is seminal: it can avoid a concretization and
literal understanding by analysts. As a model, one may see that
pornographic movies that advertise themselves as possessing
scenes of "explicit sex" are not sexual at all; and many among the
so called "art films" can be deeply sexual with no actual sex being
visually portrayed.

The issue is clearly stated with the re-introduction of the idea of
"negative growth"—presented the year before as -Y. The quasi-mathematical symbol is abandoned but the 'geometrical' model of a
spectrum of senses or directions is not. A more polished and clear
version of the concept is given, in a way one may notice that marks
Bion's work. The following quotation contains the technical hint to
be used in the session and is closely related to Schiller's view of the
artist's outlook (which was attributed to Verdi by Sir Isaiah Berlin),
that of naivety; and Goethe's observations on achieving something
by one's own means rather than by inheritance. Naivety is that
which enables the analytic observer to make forays into the realm
of minus. Freud and Bion called it the unknown:

> I introduce the idea of negative growth as a method of approach-
> ing the aspect of learning from experience; I do *not* mean denuda-
> tion which I associate with hostile and destructive impulses such as
> envy. Denudation implies impoverishment of the personality . . . A
> capacity for negative growth is needed partly to revivify a formu-
> lation that has lost meaning, partly to establish a link in making
> private knowledge public, but perhaps most important of all to
> achieve naivety of outlook when a problem is so overlaid by expe-
> rience that its outlines have become blurred and its possible solu-
> tions obscure. One of the advantages of the grid is that its use in
> thinking about material that emerges in psycho-analytic practice
> stimulates reconsideration of familiar phenomena such as dreams
> or Oedipal material and their corresponding psycho-analytical
> theoretical formulations. The ability of an analyst to retain the

substance of his training and experience and yet achieve a naïf view of his work allows him to discover for himself and in his own way the knowledge gained from his predecessors. [EP, 85–6]

It would still take twelve years for Bion to give a clearer formulation of this attempt:

It is commonly understood that an analysand talks to keep the analyst correctly informed and the psycho-analyst has a similar aim. It is easily demonstrated that such a supposition is erroneous: so would be the case with the opposite supposition. Questionnaires are drawn up and they are supposed to formulate searching questions to which revealing completions would be provided and the result would be—"revealing". In psycho-analysis it is supposed that no questions are formulated and replies to the *No-Question* would be more revealing. I propose an extension of this procedure—the invention of the *No-Questionnaire*. [AMF, I, 89]

MYSELF Perhaps I can illustrate by an example from something you *do* know. Imagine a piece of sculpture which is easier to comprehend if the structure is intended to act as a trap for light. The meaning is revealed by the pattern formed by the light thus trapped—not by the structure, the carved work itself. I suggest that if I could learn how to talk to you in such a way that my words "trapped" the meaning which they neither do nor could express, I *could* communicate to you in a way that is not at present possible . . .

A musician would certainly not deny the importance of those parts of a composition in which no notes were sounding, but more has to be done than can be achieved in existent art and its well-established procedure of silences, pauses, blank spaces, rests. The "art" of conversation, as carried on as part of the conversational intercourse of psycho-analysis, requires and demands an extension in the realm of non-conversation . . .

I have suggested a "trick" by which one could manipulate things which have no meaning—the use of sounds like "α" and "β". These are sounds analogous, as Kant said, to "thoughts without concepts", but the principle, and a reality approximating to it, is also extensible to words in common use. The realizations which approximate to words such as "memory" and "desire" are opaque. The "thing-in-itself", impregnated with the opacity, itself becomes opaque: the O, of which "memory" or "desire" is the verbal counterpart, is opaque.

I suggest this quality of opacity inheres in many O's and their verbal counterparts, and the phenomena which it is usually supposed to express. If, by experiment, we discovered the verbal forms, we could also discover the thoughts to which the observation applied specifically. Thus we achieve a situation in which these could be used deliberately to obscure specific thoughts.

BION Is there anything new in this? You must often have heard, as I have, people say they don't know what you are talking about and that you are being deliberately obscure.

MYSELF They are flattering me. I am suggesting an aim, an ambition, which, if I could achieve, would enable me to be deliberately and *precisely* obscure: in which I could use certain words which could activate precisely and instantaneously, in the mind of the listener, a thought or train of thought that came between him and the thoughts and ideas already accessible and available to him. [AMF, I, 189–191]

The negative Grid and column 2

The tool "Grid" is explained in its own entry in this dictionary. What interests us now is its allowance for "minus". It can be found both in the categories of column 2—lies—and in the idea of a "negative grid". Column 2 is expanded in the entries "Grid" and "Transformation in hallucinosis".

The "negative grid" must be explained now. It is important to the extent that it fills a gap about the function of minus. It bridges the two seemingly different functions of it, namely, that of a counterpoint and that of a destructive force directed towards that which is. The negative grid is also a manifestation of Bion's scientific honesty, in trying to improve a tool he regarded as defective:

I am aware that the grid not only can be but requires to be improved. I have felt that col. 2 might be replaced by a negative sense to the horizontal axis. It is plausible and would conform to a pleasing similarity with the systems of Cartesian co-ordinates as used in the development of algebraic geometry. Furthermore, it would simplify some difficulties if, instead of the present arrangement, the horizontal axis read
$-(n), -(n-1)\ldots -5, -4, -3, -2, -1, 1, 2, 3, 4, 5, \ldots (n-1), (n)$ with the column 2 standing for what is, in the present grid, column 3.

Then one might say that all the "uses" $1 \Leftrightarrow n$ can be used negatively, as a barrier against the unknown or known but disliked. [EP, 99]

That is, when the no-breast is flatly rejected, under the guidance of pleasure, a negative grid and growth ensues; its aftermath is a destructive stance and outlook. The minus realm, formerly a fertile ground for the evolving unknown, gives rise to an "already known" perennial negation of whatever it is. It would be just this sense of "minus", that is, the evolutions and involutions of these barriers *"to the unknown and the known disliked"* that Bion explores in his next book, *Transformations*.

The lies-generator function of column 2 and negative Grid are duly formulated: *"As a column 2 element all felt emotion is a 'no-emotion'. In this respect it is analogous to 'past' or 'future' as representing the 'place where the present used to be' before all time was annihilated.*

The 'place' where time was (or a feeling was, or a 'no-thing' of any kind was) is then similarly annihilated. There is thus created a domain of the non-existent" (AI, 20).

Final delimitation of the realm of minus: Geometry, Naming and Hallucinosis

A finer formulation appears, relative to the experience of the no-breast, with the renewed aid of another mathematical model. The idea of minus stems from the idea of negative numbers, that is, from the arithmetical branch of mathematics; now the geometric branch is called to help, with the idea of point.

There is another contribution, drawn from clinical experience, that enters into the attempt to explore the realm of minus: the act of naming. The psychotic's difficulties—or better, the psychotic difficulty—with verbal thought and thought in general, as part of the human attempt to apprehend reality, were the sources of this contribution. It summarizes the bulk of Bion's so-called earliest phase from the fifties:

The name, in its function of binding a constant conjunction, partakes of the nature of a definition; it commences by being significant, but meaningless, till experience gives it accumulation of meaning; it derives negative force both by virtue of its genesis as part of thought and by the necessary logic of its coming into existence precisely because the constant conjunction it binds is *not* any of the previous and already named constant conjunctions. Dislike of it is therefore derived from its genesis and from fear of the implications of its "use" (Cf. Aristotle and definition. Topics, VI, 4, 141b, 21). [T, 63]

In short, the word "breast" is not recognized as a word representing a breast, but is thought to be the outward manifestation of a "no-breast", one of the characteristic qualities, so to speak, of the "no-breast" itself. It is in this way that a certain class of patient "concludes" that a thought is a thing, albeit a "thing" in a sense that a rational being does not ordinarily understand. Such a view contrasts with that which enables a mathematician to use a point, however represented, to elaborate a geometric system.

Similarly, it contrasts with the ordinary view of the word "breast" or "point" that enables it to be used to elaborate anatomical or physiological or artistic or aesthetic (in the philosophical sense) systems. [T, 76–7]

I have previously given my reasons for supporting the definition of a definition as something negative *in essence*; a definition should implicitly or explicitly be a statement that the statement itself is not any *past* statement (if not, where would be the need for the statement?) and has no meaning (if it had there would be no need for a definition) to bind the constantly conjoined elements; for they are to be bound so that their meaning can be determined. It is therefore quite appropriate that we should arrive by way of discussion of the no-thing at characteristics which are impregnated with a quality regarded by the scientist (proceeding in thought to H1?) as undesirable. [T, 88]

[The symbol H1? refers to the Grid. It means, the development of thought from more primitive stages towards the most sophisticated hitherto available, mathematical calculus.]

Naming can be regarded as the psychological origin both of the realm of minus as well as the nest of the difficulties that encircle its realization, which belongs to that which is immaterial and ultimately ineffable.

Naming and definitory hypotheses

That which Bion calls "definitory hypothesis" is such a "negative". It is a contrasting counterpoint to be confronted with the realizations that will "saturate" it. Please see "Pre-conception", "Conception" and "Saturation. The definition of the concept can be seen in the entry "Grid" but some reminders are cogent now. It interests us to use this category—the earliest attempt to think hitherto known—as a way to enhance our grasp of the definition of the minus field both in its contrapuntal, epistemological function in the processes of knowing and its function as a negative force at the service of not-knowing:

> ... the definitory hypothesis is to mark a constant conjunction and the exclusion of all previously recorded constant conjunctions (the "negative" quality of definition) ...

> The negative aspect of the definitory hypothesis is strengthened so that the exclusive function of the hypothesis is not a barrier against irrelevance but a denial of the domain to which the hypothesis belongs. For example, the term "cat" would not bind a constant conjunction that excludes "dogginess", but binds a constant conjunction so restrictively that it excludes all animal characteristics. Carried to extremes, the term "cat" is merely a sign analogous to the "point" as the "place where the breast used to be" and should mean the "no-cat". Further denudation leads ultimately to the point which is merely a position without any trace of what used to occupy that position. [T, 98 and 99]

Armed with geometry and the vicissitudes of naming, Bion is able to formulate an integrative view of the two functions he had established of the realm of "minus", as depicted at the beginning of this entry. The result is a new definition that does not replace but extends the definitions of this realm hitherto available:

> Implicit in the name as that which signifies constant conjunction, and inseparable from this significance, is the quality of negation. A constant conjunction, thus bound by a name, is *not* whatever the personality has observed as existing previously, but may be similar to it. This has been a cause of difficulty as far back as Aristotle (Topics, VI.6, 143 b 11). In practice it presents difficulty to the patient who cannot tolerate frustration, and in whom envy, greed and cruelty are dominant.

> In the illustration the problem centres on the fact that the absent breast, the "no-breast", differs from the breast. If this is accepted the

"no-breast" can be represented by the visual image of the point. But if this is a column 2 phenomenon the point lacks the quality of a definitory statement and approximates to an object with column 3 characteristics. It therefore has the meaning that it is a breast that has been reduced to a mere position—the place where the breast was. This state appears to the patient to be a consequence either of greed that has exhausted the breast, or of splitting that has destroyed the breast leaving only the position. [T, 54]

Therefore the realm of minus will be seen as the realm of something that existed but is no more. This "no more" is not tolerated initially because of desire and evasion of pain; later it cannot be tolerated because of the guilt of having been destroyed by hate and greed. This is an important distinction and determines perennially mounting abhorrence towards the no-breast; the lack, the absence, the realm of minus:

The point and the line . . . are used by certain patients, who believe others do the same, as if they or their signs in painting, music, words, etc., were things. That is to say, such a patient hearing me say "point", or seeing a dot, behaves as if the point, however it is signified or represented, marks the place where the breast (or penis) was. Now this "place" seems to be invested by the patient with characteristics that less disturbed people might attribute to an object they would call a ghost. The point (.) and the term "point" are taken as sensible manifestations of the "no-breast". In so far as I can express it in ordinary terms, the patient seems to think that the fact that the word "point" is used, is a sign of the presence of a non-existent breast, "the place where the breast was" having many of the characteristics of a breast that is hostile because it no longer exists. [T, 76]

Meaninglessness and the experiencing of minus in the session

The denudation of the object produces a state that can be described as "meaninglessness". Due to transformations in hallucinosis (q.v.) and concretization, this state is disguised by rational discourse and acting-out. Their appearance is a sign that one is in fact immersed in the realm of minus but is not aware of it. As a matter of consequence one deals with it in the same way one would deal with actually existent things, facts and persons.

Its clinical significance lies in the possibility of accomplishing real psycho-analysis or not; the following quotation provides a summary of the issues adumbrated in *Learning from Experience* to the extent that they are necessary to realize what is at stake when a person acquires a capacity to mimic talking, but with the intention of evading pain, obtaining reassurance and abhorring the unknown. In other words, the avoidance of minus as a counterpoint leads to the prevalence of the destructive minus.

The no-breast, if tolerated, allows a jump into the unknown. This is not always the case. The pre-conception can be seen as the "already known"; the realization is the unknown and the experience of it provides the experiencing of the jump into the unknown. The "negative force" destroys, in hallucination, the real breast and the person "populates" a real unknown with falsely known "things" (usually bizarre objects). *"The ability of 0 [meaning, zero] to increase thus by parthenogenesis corresponds to the characteristics of greed which is also able to grow and flourish exceedingly by supplying itself with unrestricted supplies of nothing"* (T, 134). The final result seems to be, *"a raging inferno of greedy non-existence"*.

The following quotation depicts a session of analysis that risks degenerating into such an activity.

> The infant's experience of the breast as the source of emotional experiences (later represented by terms such as love, understanding, meaning) means that disturbances in relationship with the breast involve disturbance over a wide range of adult relationships. The function of the breast in supplying meaning is important for the development of a capacity to learn. In an extreme instance, namely the fear of the total destruction of the breast, not only does this involve fears that he has ceased to exist (since without the breast he is not viable) but fears that meaning itself, as if it were matter, had ceased to exist. In some contingencies the breast is not regarded as the source of meaning so much as meaning itself. This anxiety is often screened by the fact that the analyst gives interpretations and thus seems to provide evidence that meaning exists. If this is not observed the patient's intolerance of meaninglessness is not interpreted: he will pour out a flood of words so that he can evoke a response indicating that meaning exists either in his own behaviour or in that of the analyst. Since the first requisite for the discovery of the meaning of any conjunction depends on the ability

to admit that the phenomena may have no meaning, an inability to admit that they have no meaning stifles the possibility of curiosity at the outset. The same is true of love and hate. The need to manipulate the session to evoke evidence of the existence of meaning extends to a need to evoke evidence of the existence of love and hate. Anyone with experience of the psychotic personality will be familiar with the probing, incessantly active, designed to tap sources of counter-transference. The patient's associations are directed to obtaining evidence of meaning and emotion (here broadly divided into two all-embracing categories of love and hate). Since the patient's attention is directed to finding evidence of meaning, but not to finding what the meaning is, interpretations have little effect in producing change until the patient sees that he is tapping a source of reassurance to provide an *antidote* to his problem and not a *solution* of it.

The thought, represented by a word or other sign, may, when it is significant as a no-thing, be represented by a point (.). The point may then represent the position where the breast was, or may even *be* the no-breast. [T, 81–2]

The intolerance of the realm of minus producing the state of hallucinosis can be stated thus:

Suppose now that the personality cannot tolerate frustration. This is associated with "that state in which ideas may be supposed to assume the force of sensations through the confusion of thought with the objects of thought, and the excess of passion animating the creations of imagination". *(I use Shelley's formulation of his poetic intuition to provide the background realization for the statement "hallucinosis".) Memory of the satisfaction is used to deny the absence of satisfaction. Denial of time is used to deny that the breast is the place where the breast used to be and to maintain that it is where the breast now is. [T, 133–4]

*Shelley, P.B.: Hellas. His sixth note on the poem.

Final encirclement of the unconscious, abstinence and the realm of minus

The first (night of the soul) has to do with the point from which the soul goes forth, for it has gradually to deprive itself of desire for all the worldly things which it possessed, by denying them to itself; the which denial and deprivation are, as it were, night to all the senses of man. The second reason has to do with the mean, or the road along which the soul must travel to this union—that is, faith, which is likewise as dark as night to the understanding. The third has to do with the point to which it travels, namely, God. Who, equally, is dark night to the soul in this life.*

I use these formulations to express, in exaggerated form, the pain which is involved in achieving the state of naivety inseparable from binding or definition (col.1). Any naming of a constant conjunction involves admission of the negative dimension and is opposed by the fear of ignorance. Therefore at the outset there is a tendency to precocious advance, that is, to a formulation which is a col. 2 formulation to deny ignorance—the dark night of the senses. The relevance of this to psychological phenomena springs from the fact that they are not amenable to apprehension by the senses . . . Similarly the intuitive approach is obstructed because the 'faith' involved is associated with absence of inquiry, or "dark night" to K. [T, 158–9]

* The Ascent of Mount Carmel, 1, 1, and 2.

Then Bion abandoned the theological model and resorted to colloquial language to depict the issue:

WATSON Shall I shut him up?

SHERLOCK HOLMES My *dear* Watson!

BION (outraged) What the devil do you mean by butting into my serious discussion? Are you not aware that I am raising serious issues?

MYCROFT (in no way impressed) Go on, Sherlock. This is more your line than mine. *You* tell him.

WATSON (before Sherlock intervenes which he appears unlikely to do) My dear sir, Mister Holmes and his brother really must not be interrupted: it's a private and important matter.

BION But, my good man, are you not aware that you are entirely fictitious characters? I am a qualified doctor!

WATSON So am I; and an M.D.

BION Nonsense! Purely imaginary and not very bright even in the estimation of your fellow spooks. I am a past President of the British Psycho-Analytical Society and past Director of the London Clinic of . . .

MYCROFT & SHERLOCK (together burst into a gale of laughter)

WATSON (contains his mirth with difficulty, but manages to be civil.) Excuse me sir, but I must admit that I have never heard of your existence. I do not want to hurt your feelings or to appear to boast, but although Mycroft has always been of a retiring disposition, Sherlock, and to a lesser extent myself, has a world-wide following. You yourself were admitting that there are imaginary characters who are infinitely better known than countless generations of nonentities. Now excuse me. I am a very busy man—allow me to suggest that you get on that couch there and sleep it off quietly.

BION (with a gesture of despair, abandons his office to the three intruders and goes to sleep)

SHERLOCK I hope you weren't too rough with him, Watson.

WATSON Real people have to be treated roughly if the universe is to be made safe for imaginary people. If you remember, this problem cropped up before with real numbers. Quite impossible for the simplest mathematical problem even to be formulated till negative numbers destroyed the tyranny of being confined in the restricted space of addition—just more real numbers.

MYCROFT What was the problem, Sherlock? I had the impression it was something simple.

SHERLOCK The simple part of it has been dealt with by Watson. You heard that fellow Bion? Nobody has ever heard of him or of Psycho-analysis. He thinks it is real, but that his colleagues are engaged in an activity which is only a more or less ingenious manipulation of symbols. There is something in what he says. There is a failure to understand that any definition must deny a previous truth as well as carry an unsaturated component. [AMF, I, 91–2]

Recommended cross-references: Emotional Turbulence, (−K), O, Transformation in hallucinosis.
Suggested cross-references: Conception, Grid, Growth, Preconception, Psycho-analytic Object, Saturation.

&; This author has proposed a practical term that defines the analytical posture as an offshoot of Bion's formulation of the realm of minus and the negative force: tolerance of paradoxes (Sandler, 1997, 2001, 2003).

Models: Bion, as did Freud, used models in the scientific (Kantian) sense of the term. See especially *The Interpretation of Dreams* (Chapter VII, especially items A and F); "The unconscious"; "Constructions in analysis". They are initial tools for tackling a real issue or problem or unknown facts. Freud called them scaffoldings. He disposed of them as soon as new empirical data made this necessary. These data were made visible just due to the use of the soon-to-be-superseded model—as it occurs in science. Bion was fully aware of Freud's use of models and exactly followed his line as depicted in *The Interpretation of Dreams* and in the *Project for a Scientific Psychology*. His references to Freud are copious and clear (LE, 56, 57, 61).

Bion defines models as "*a construction in which concrete images are combined with each other; the link between concrete images often gives the effect of a narrative implying that some elements in the narrative are the causes of others. It is constructed with elements from the individual's past . . .*" (LE, 64).

Experiences are models for future experiences; "*the value of a model is that its familiar data are available to meet urgent inner or outer need . . .*

Model making during the experience relates to the model needed for that experience . . . The personality abstracts from . . . elements the model that will preserve something of the original experience but with enough flexibility to permit adaptation to new but supposedly similar experiences . . . I shall use the term model where the construct is forged to meet an 'urgent need' for concreteness" (LE, 74–5).

Models are used both by patients and analysts. Patients use them to represent their states of mind; they range from the manifest content of dreams to statements such as "I hate you" (EP, 76–7) They are tools for research into the unknown of the unfolding fresh emotional experiences that make up an actual analytic session.

Did Bion use models from other fields? "*Mathematics, science as known hitherto, can provide no model*" (AMF, I, 61). Medicine and biology offer a contrast. They are used throughout Bion's work.

Following Freud's own path, Bion used those branches of human knowledge to furnish models that allow clinically fruitful approaches to mental functioning. More specifically, he uses the digestive and reproductive systems as models for his theory of thinking. Also like Freud, he used myths as models to get near human mental functioning. Myths also serve as models.

Two paradoxes mark model-making, and in his characteristic non-absolute way, Bion depicts both:

(i) Models serve both concretization and abstraction. Concretization is here understood as the lower level, or empirical data—the point from where we start in science. Abstraction is here understood as the basic process of thinking, that is, to think in the absence of the concrete object. Prototypically, according to Bion's theory of thinking, the breast.

(ii) Models bring in themselves the seeds of their replacement, in a living sense that is akin to human life itself as well as revolutionary movements:

> The use of a model has a value in restoring a sense of the concrete to an investigation which may have lost contact with its background through abstraction and the theoretical deductive systems associated with it . . .

> A model has also qualities which enable it to fulfil some of the functions of an abstraction. It enables the investigator to use an emotional experience by applying it as a totality, to a subsequent experience, or to some aspect of it. These merits carry in themselves the elements that finally make the model outdated. No experience exactly matches a past experience . . . models can only be an approximation to the realization and vice-versa. [LE, 64]

🕐 Bion did not change his use of and ideas on models throughout the whole of his work:

1962:

> The model may be regarded as an abstraction from an emotional experience or as a concretization of an abstraction . . . In the group the myth has some claim to be regarded as filling the same role in the society as the model has in scientific work of the individual . . .

> Models are ephemeral and differ from theories in this respect; I have no compunction in discarding a model as soon as it has served

or failed to serve my purpose. If a model proves useful on a number of different occasions the time has come to consider its transformation into a theory. [LE, 79]

1973:

Models are expendable; theories are not. [BLI, 31]

Models and abstractions

Abstraction is defined as an idea that emerges from the tolerance of the absence of a material object. Abstractions are almost impossible for the psychotic. They are more flexible and more widely applicable due to the fact that they have lost an anchor in particular concrete images.

Models and abstractions originate from an emotional experience and their application is in a fresh emotional experience. If models are *"constructed with elements from the individual's past . . . the abstraction is . . . impregnated with preconceptions of the individual's future"* (LE, 64).

Compared with models, the elements of an abstraction *"are not combined by narrative but by a method intended to reveal the relationship rather that the objects related"*—the models stress the actual elements. The abstraction stresses the relationships between the actual elements (LE, 65).

Bion used models that aided him to communicate psychoanalytically relevant issues. We may divide them and offer just a few examples:

(i)   His clinical expositions: for example, that of clouds (T, 117), that of surgical shock (AI, 12).
(ii)   His theories: Alpha-function, to present the way sensuous data are transformed into data useful for thinking.
(iii) Real analysis. Mainly in *A Memoir of the Future*:
       ● Maid-mistress—to present sadistic pleasure and the fallacy of absolute values and the danger of relying on appearances.
       ● The English Farm—to present that which is a transcendence, in the guise of England and violence.
       ● War—to present human inhumanity to man.

- Priest and P.A.—to present seemingly different approaches to reality that are paradoxically identical in their inner ways.
- Somites—to present primitive states of mind
- Ultra and Infra-sensuous—to present immaterial facts of psychic reality
- Devil—to present the establishment: schooling, hypocrisy.
- Mycroft/Sherlock/Watson—to present the actionless pure thought/the ability to interpose thinking between impulse and action/and pure action.

Freud's models of primary and secondary processes, id, ego and super-ego seemed to have been taken concretely by many in the psycho-analytic movement.

Models and the in-session, here and now experience

> Those excluded from the psycho-analysis cannot gain from the psycho-analyst's formulations because they are formulations dependent on the presence of the experiences being formulated. They are thus in the position analogous to one whose mathematical ability has not reached a point where it can deal with the problem of objects when the objects are not there. His position vis-à-vis the problem is similar to that of the man who has to experiment with the original object without the aid of an intervening model which he can manipulate . . . The lack of a counterpart to the model, the direct manipulation of the original, denies the psycho-analyst one of the tools required for his job and contributes to the state of perpetual acting-out. This last is evidence that the psycho-analyst is not, and cannot behave as if he were, dealing with models (verbal or otherwise) of his problem but with the original itself. [ST, 146–7]

Any analysis that continues the research into deeper psychotic "strata" or personality will have to tackle the situation that, in contrast with the analysis of the non-psychotic, *"the relationship with external reality undergoes a transformation parallel to the relationship with psychic reality which lacks an intervening (or 'interceding') model. There is no 'personality' intervening between the psycho-analyst and the 'unconscious'"* (ST, 147). This corresponds to the idea that psychotics have no resistances and their unconscious emerges directly and unhampered and cannot be interpreted. It is quite normal that a patient with a prevailing psychotic personality utters, unknowingly and deaf to his own words, "I want to have sex with Mom".

Models are brokers. They have in analogy one of their outstanding media.

Suggested cross-references: Alpha-function, Analogy, Beta-elements, Binocular view, Emotional Experience, K-link, Links, Medicine, Myths, Selected Fact.

Multiplicity of theories:

> Patients and analysts are constantly using different terms to describe situations that appear to have the same configuration . . . What is needed is a solution that will dispose finally of diversity of terms, at present required to describe the experience . . . and the far more serious defect associated with it, namely, the elaboration of as many theories as there are sufferers, matched by almost as many theories as there are therapists, when it is acknowledged that the configurations are probably the same . . .

> I wish to introduce as a step towards formulations that are precise, communicable without distortion, and more nearly adequate to cover all situations that are basically the same. [T, 124]

During Bion's lifetime many of the alternative theories were "anti-Freud". Their authors intended to display Freud's inadequacies on the basis of non-empirical findings that could refute his theories. There was a sense of rivalry, such as the ideas of Stekel, Jung, Adler and Rank. They produced brainy "logicalities" devoid of an empirical basis. Others advertised themselves as "beyond Freud": Moreno's "psychodrama", Szondi, Binswanger's "existential analysis", Reich's "orgonetherapy". Their names are legion. Others still, such as Carl Rogers' "psychotherapy focused on the person" could not claim much more than depicting the same facts in different words.

The tendency began to be felt within the analytical movement: Heimann's claim that Freud was wrong in his concept of counter-transference; Kohut's diatribes with metapsychology and narcissism; the ideas on "borderlines" and "enactment" follow the trend of fashionable non-sense that are as evanescent as they seemed to be all-pervasive during a kind of "extraordinary popular delusions and madness of the masses".

A repetition compulsion seems to exist that denies that any novelty is but oblivion; ideas of concrete causes periodically return and go without leaving trace. From the biochemistry of mental illness to neuroscience, it seems that a cycle of a mere thirty years buries the perception of the waste of misguided psycho-analysis, abhorring "luminous ideas".

> The defect of the existing psycho-analytic theory is not unlike that of the ideogram as compared with a word formed alphabetically; the ideogram represents one word only but relatively few letters are required for the formation of many thousands of words. Similarly the elements I seek are to be such that relatively few are required to express, by changes in combination, nearly all the theories essential to the working psycho-analyst. [Bion's footnote: Compared with the tendency to produce ad hoc theories to meet a situation when an existing theory, stated with sufficient generality, would have done. Compare Proclus, quoted by Sir T. L. Heath, on Euclid's Elements (Heath, T. L: *The Thirteen Books of Euclid's Elements*, chapter 9, CUP, 1956)]. [EP, 2]

Religions have a multiplicity of saints; more primitive religions, a multiplicity of gods. The multiplicity of theories displays a kind of eternal chaotic chasing of facts without ever touching them; it marks the non-existence of, or ignorance about, the possible existence of a generalizing theory that encompasses individual facts.

There is a peculiarity of psycho-analysis that adds to it:

> Because psycho-analytic theories are a compound of observed material and abstraction from it, they have been criticized as unscientific. They are at once too theoretical, that is to say too much a representation of an observation, to be acceptable as an observation and too concrete to have the flexibility that allows an abstraction to be matched with a realization. Consequently a theory, which could be seen to be widely applicable if it were stated abstractly enough, is liable to be condemned because its very concreteness makes it difficult to recognize a realization that it might represent ... The defect ... is twofold: on the one hand description of empirical data is unsatisfactory as it is manifestly what is described in conversational English as a "theory" about what took place rather than a factual account of it and on the other hand the theory of what took

place cannot satisfy the criteria applied to a theory as that term is employed to describe the systems used in rigorous scientific investigation. [EP, 1]

One of the factors in creating many theories is the longing for explanation and a hasty collecting of sensuously apprehensible data without waiting for the emergence of constant conjunctions, selected facts and invariances that could illuminate an underlying connective fact. The enunciation of this fact leads to the scientific theory. An example of the multiplicity of theories is that of the discussion about an excess or lack of narcissism as the cause of mental illness.

> If the individual analyst built up for himself an anthology of working psycho-analytic theory on a foundation of a few good basic theories well understood and capable, individually and in combination, of covering a great many of the situations he might expect to meet, it might help the creation of [a system of] notation. [LE, 42]

Mathematicians had to deal with the same issue and from them stemmed the first successful attempts at generalizing theories—that were later extended to other scientific fields. *"The mathematical problem resembles a psycho-analytic problem in that it is necessary that the solution should have a wide degree of applicability and acceptance and so avoid the need to apply different arguments to different cases when the different cases appear to have essentially the same configuration. Any analyst will recognize the confusion that is caused, or at best the sense of dissatisfaction that prevails, when a discussion by members makes it quite clear that the configuration of the case is apprehended by all, but the arguments formulated in its elucidation vary from member to member and from case to case. It is essential that such a state of affairs should be made unnecessary if progress is to take place, The search must be for formulations that represent the essential similarity of the configurations, recognized by all who deal with them, and thus to make unnecessary the ad hoc nature of so many psycho-analytic theories"* (T, 83–4).

Or, in brief, one must search for underlying invariances: "It will be noted that in writing of 'similar configurations' I am pre-supposing the presence of invariants which are consciously or unconsciously recognized as such" (T, 84).

Freud was able to intuit a basic configuration or invariance of mankind, a fact apprehended by Bion: *"The advantage of using the Oedipus myth . . . is economy and avoidance of a whole series of* **ad hoc** *models and theories for different problems that have the same configurations"* (T, 96).

Suggested cross-reference: Manipulations of symbols.

Mystic:

> ALICE You say you have never had direct experience of a mysterious event; do you mean by that that you have not been in a room at the time when someone, not you, was under the influence of a mystical force?

> P.A. I have had no evidence that either I or the other was passing through such an experience. I only remember two or three occasions when an analysand of mine actually claimed a mystical origin for the event. I have been more impressed when the individual was *not* consciously making such a claim. [AMF, III, 525]

In resorting to verbal formulations originally found in Plato's theory of forms, in Kant's unearthing of them, in the Jewish and Christian Cabbala and in Buber's extensions of them, Bion used a most misunderstood analogy to describe the psycho-analytic negative realm of the id and of the unconscious. (See the entries Atonement; "O".) A discussion of the common misunderstanding related to the use of metaphors is to be found in the entry, Models.

There is a strong similarity between Bion, Freud and Freud's forerunners in the German Romantic movement: all of them were also accused of being "mystics" in their time; even Hume was accused of this.

Bion regards religion as relevant as a school of thought; he nourishes some objections that nevertheless do not preclude his appreciation of the achievements of this *"school of thought"*. In one of the many passages where he resorts to a confrontation between the imaginary character "Psycho-analyst" ("P.A.") and the imaginary character, "Priest", Bion states:

> P.A. One of my objections to your school of thought is that it appears to encourage a belief in unlimited times such as life after death.

PRIEST Unfortunately we are debited with the views—usually mistaken—that people have about what we teach.

P.A. You yourself appear to debit me with views about psycho-analysis which I do not hold; it would be a part of my task if you were an analysand to elucidate your assumptions so that you could contrast and compare them with any other ideas you might enter-tain. In this respect I think that our activity is different from yours. *You* aspire to tell others how and what to think. *We* aspire only to show what people think—the rest is their choice. [AMF, II, 388]

The term has serious practical usage and links with the coun-terparts in reality hinted at by the term "intuition", in the here and now of the decisive moment of the analytic interpretation.

Let us resort to Bion in order to try to illuminate the issue in psycho-analytical terms:

The intuitive psycho-analytic background is that which I have "bound" by terms such as pre-conception, definition, notation, attention . . . [Note by this dictionary's author: the reader must have firmly in his or her mind that last and last-but-one terms are Freud's functions of the ego. See Freud, "Formulations on the two principles of mental functioning", 1910.] I shall borrow freely any material that is likely to simplify my task, starting from Plato's theories of Forms. As I understand the term, various phenomena, such as the appearance of a beautiful object, are significant not because they are beautiful or good but because they serve to "remind" the beholder of the beauty or the good which was once, but no longer is, known. This object, of which the phenomenon serves as a reminder, is a Form. I claim Plato as a supporter for the pre-conception, the Kleinian internal object, the inborn anticipation . . . Phenomena, the term being used as Kant might use it, are trans-formed into representations. [T, 138]

Bion states that the final products of transformations (q.v.) may be regarded as representations of the individual's experience of the numinous realm, reality, O, the id. Nevertheless, he also states that the significance of O is not that of an "O-in-itself" which corre-sponds, in experience, to the idea of owning absolute truth—but rather, this significance *"derives from and inheres in the Platonic Form"* (T, 138).

Lest any doubts remain about Bion's ideas on religion, one may read one of his last formulations:

> BION . . . I wonder how many plausible theories have been used and bewildered the human race. I would like to know. I am not sure of the ease with which "plausible" theories are produced. In this context of "plausible theories" about which we are talking, the plausible theory or "convincing interpretation" may be hard to come by. It can be plausible and false. Witness the idea that "the sun rises"—what trouble that has caused! We do not know the cost in suffering associated with the belief in a Christian God, or the god of Abraham's Ur, or Hitler's Germany, or peyotism—or god of any kind. [AMF, I, 172]

In discussing his last books, which try to be *"a description of psycho-analysis"* (AMF, I, 86) Bion makes clear his kind of relationship with religious manifestations: *"I have to employ an extremely inadequate apparatus to discuss it. I have to manufacture the apparatus as I proceed. I claim that it is artistic though the art has not yet been created; it is religious though the religion has not been and never can (without ceasing to be a religion) be made to conform to any of the dogmata and institutions hitherto regarded as characteristic of religion"* (AMF, I, 88).

Suggested cross-references: Atonement, Correct Analysis, O, Philosophy, Science versus Religion, Truth, Ultra-sensuous, Thoughts without a thinker.

Myth, private myth: Bion's rescuing of the **function** of myths in depicting mind's functioning may be regarded as an outstanding contribution to psycho-analysis. This rescue harks back to the attempts of the Renaissance and Romantic authors, such as von Herder and Nietzsche—even though there is no evidence that he consciously based himself on their works. Anyway, it illuminated the function they had for Freud. Freud's use of myths is debased into a transplant of mythology to psycho-analysis.

Otherwise they could remain obscure and mysterious, giving rise on one hand, to concretized repetitive uses and on the other, to explanatory uses. They were and still are sizable parts of the psycho-analytic movement that do not care too much about the experience of psycho-analysis according to Freud's attempts. This has resulted in its replacement by intellectual, rationalized, and concretized understanding. Or many use myths according to their historical, philosophical, or literary functions. Freud's use of myths is debased into a transplant of mythology to psycho-analysis.

The myth's function in apprehending, working through and preserving transcendent insights about mankind's nature and psychology are denied or even despised by western civilization's so-called "modern" and "post-modern" thinking. Its hallmark is memory and understanding. Experiencing, transcendent truth and mind are not taken into consideration.

This illuminates why members of the psycho-analytic movement look for mythologists. They hope to get help in grasping the meaning of myths, as if this study could lead them to finding out psycho-analytic matter. One may fail to see that myths were early attempts to study human mind and nature. It is the same object that interests analysts, but with two seminal differences. The two differences constitute the medical vertex, applied to analysis:

(i)   the myth makers were not interested in individual people,
(ii)   much less, in alleviating or taking care of individual people's suffering.

The private myth

The medical vertex understood in this way is contrasted with the pseudo-medical idea of cure (q.v.). Actually this kind of idea is a chimera in real life and in medicine, as a rule. This vertex is clearly seen in Bion's novel concept of "private myth". It conserves the myth's scientific quality, that of simultaneous generalizing/particularizing powers:

> The private myth has this important role in the individual's attempt to learn from experience analogous to that played by public myths as systems of notation and record in the development of groups . . . The myth must be expected to appear in a private version. [EP, 67]

This vertex—Freud's vertex—according to the research of the author, is furnished by the Enlightenment and improved by the Romantic movement. It came to be known as "Medicine" (q.v.), or in Bion's parlance, the medical vertex. This interest in the individual also gave rise to social movements seen as "revolutionary". If one loses sight of this vertex, one's fate is to be a mythologist, a historian, a literary critic rather than an analyst. *"The erudite can see that a description is by Freud or Melanie Klein, but remains blind to the thing described"* (AMF, I, 5).

🜨 Bion's observation, or the rescuing of Freud's ethos, first appeared in *Elements of Psycho-analysis,* 1963. It seems to be yet more explicit in the preparatory study that was to remain unpublished until 1992, "Tower of Babel: possibility of using a racial myth":

> This brings me to the application of our myth to the problem that it is to interpret. The scientist must know enough mathematics to understand the nature and use of various mathematical discoveries and formulations, such as the differential calculus or the binomial theorem: the psycho-analyst must know his myth. The scientist must also know enough to have an idea when he is confronting a problem to which a particular mathematical procedure would apply: the psycho-analyst must know when he is facing a problem to which a myth would provide the psycho-analytic counterpart of the algebraic calculus. *This, one might say, is precisely what Freud did: he recognized, as a scientist, that he was confronted by a problem to the solution of which he would have to apply the Oedipus myth. The result was the discovery, not of the Oedipus complex, but of psycho-analysis. (Or is it man, or man's psyche, that is discovered when these elements are constantly conjoined?)* It is in this sense that I believe that the myth of Babel, or Oedipus, or Sphinx must be used as a tool comparable to that of the mathematical formulation. [C, 228; my italics]

The same idea would resurface in a compacted form in *Elements of Psycho-analysis*: *"The Oedipus myth may be regarded as an instrument that served Freud in his discovery of psycho-analysis and psycho-analysis as an instrument that enabled Freud to discover the Oedipus complex"* (EP, 92). As often happens, Bion's "repetitions", as they are regarded by many, a fact he recorded in his introduction to *Seven Servants*, are evolutions and growing insight about an invariance. These fresh formulations have the same function as the athlete and the music performer's exercises—prior to the show.

Myths and the practical decisive moment: the here and now of the analytic session

> The interpretation can be . . . a theory used to investigate the unknown. The most obvious example of this is the Oedipus myth

as Freud has abstracted it to form the psycho-analytic theory. The function of the theoretical formulations in this category are interpretations being used with an intention to illuminate material, that would otherwise remain obscure, in order to help the patient to release still further material. The primary object is to obtain material for satisfaction of the impulses of inquiry in patient and analyst. Note that the probing quality of such interpretations may help to account for differences of reaction in the patient from those he would display to interpretations in category 1 or 4 [definitory hypothesis and notation, that is attentive initializations]; this component can be distinguished from those derived from the content of the interpretation. [EP, 19]

A fact finding tool

The helping hand provided by the myth during the session as research into the unknown of each individual's specific mental structuring and creative ways on the spur of the moment, or non-creative ways, displays *"the value of the myth as a fact-finding tool"* (EP, 66). The conscious rescuing of the seriously endangered ethos of Freud's discoveries and psycho-analysis itself was pursued by Bion. It is clearly stated and seemed to be a feasible task through this specific use of myth and the concept of private myth: *"I wish to restore it to its place in our methods so that it can play the vitalizing part there that it has played in history (and in Freud's discovery of psycho-analysis). . . It is also an object of investigation in an analysis as part of the primitive apparatus of the individual's armoury of learning"* (EP, 66).

Myths and dreaming

Myths are seen as a kind of dreaming with social expressions and utilities; the kinship of dreaming and myths could be elicited after Freud brought dreams to scientific consideration as self-epistemological tools of the self. In making unconscious that which was originally sensuously apprehended, dreaming serves as a working through function: the working through of emotional experiences. The back and forth movement from conscious sensuous apprehension to the unconscious introjection and back to consciousness as the sensuous organ for apprehension of psychic reality and quality (see "Contact Barrier") allowed a continuous evolution and maturation of feelings, emotions and affects. Myths and dreams, as sensible or sensuously apprehensible forms themselves, perform the function of manifest content. They demand an experienced listener or reader who does not take them at their face value and thus is enabled to elicit their latent content, to use Freud's words as used by Bion. In their outward appearance, myths and dreams, a *bricoleur's* work made out of debris from the day or the human tragedy actually experienced, are always queer and not-understandable. This is their power and weakness.

Myths seem to serve functions, socially speaking, in the transmission and conservation of pre-conceptions, biologically founded, of the human species. Myths did not allow comprehension but allowed learning, as evolutions of postulates or definitory hypotheses. This is exactly what Bion does in devising the C-categories of the Grid (q.v.): they come from α-elements, raw sensuous stimuli, things-in-themselves; they may evolve to β-elements and then to myths and dreams. This is a "genetic", or, using Bion's question, "*is man's psyche that is discovered when these elements are constantly conjoined?*", ontogenetic development. This furnishes a "durable" or transcendent quality both to dreams—to the individual, and to myth—and to mankind. Myths and dreams are seen as belonging to the same category, which means they share the same nature or invariance. They have an invariance under knowledge. This implies apprehension of facts, transformation of its materiality into psychic immateriality, storing that confers durability and public-action that confers a communicative power to it. The following phrase must be read while keeping in mind the definition of α-function, that is, it is a "de-sense-fying" function of the mind (q.v.).

> The dream of the individual must be taken to mean that certain α-elements are constantly conjoined . . . The α-function has then served the purpose of making storable, communicable and publishable an emotional experience that is constantly conjoined and has made it possible to record the latter fact . . . If myth and manifest content of a dream are to be regarded as the group and individual versions of the same thing—and that thing is an assertion that certain α-elements are constantly conjoined—to what use are we to put this statement? If we regard it as analogous to $(a+b)^2 = a^2 + b^2 + 2ab$, then presumably we need to know how the statement has

been constructed and what the rules are that have to be obeyed if we are to use the statement correctly.

> ... all dreams have one interpretation and only one—namely, that α-elements are constantly conjoined ... every dream has a corresponding realization, which it therefore represents ... its resemblance to the dream that represents it is so nearly conscious that the dreamer has an illusion that he expresses by saying he had a dream that came true ... *certain factual experiences will never be understood by the patient, and therefore will never be experiences from which he can learn, unless he can interpret them in the light of his dream or the myth in which the group has enshrined both the dream and the belief in the dream's validity for all members of the group.* [C, 229–31; my italics]

The "rules" in psycho-analysis can only be learnt through the actual experience of psycho-analysis itself. Mankind's commonsensical experiences are birth, death, love and hate, narcissism, envy and greed, a capacity for bestiality and sublimity. They furnish generalizations that encompass their individual variations or transformations. The rules belong to the unconscious numinous realm of truth "O". They cannot be apprehended and much less learnt by rational procedures such as readings of texts.

Dreams: private myths

The dream itself is seen as a private myth (EP, 92). The dream, the myth and the private myth are something that belongs—perhaps philogenetically—to that part of each individual apparatus that caters for contact with reality. Summing up: they are part of the ego. In this sense, there is a precursor of Oedipus in a sense that differs from that observed by Klein (please refer to the entry, Pre-conception): "*I postulate an α-element version of a private Oedipus myth which is the means, the pre-conception, by virtue of which the infant is able to establish contact with the parents as they exist in the world of reality. The mating of this α-element Oedipal pre-conception with the realization of the actual parents gives rise to the conception of parents*" (EP, 93).

There is more than the singularity of a given parental couple; what is at stake is the very conception of parents and parenthood. In other words, "relativity", meaning, one is not alone; one was not a parthenogenetic production, but is "related to". (The use of Einstein's verbal formulation is intentional.)

The private myth has certain primitive characteristics that further illuminate the nature of the pre-conception as a kind of generator—both of private myths and of expressions of the peculiar structuring of the personality. They guide the specific and wholly personal ways of structuring it. This view allowed Bion to observe and to formulate the hypothesis of an Oedipal pre-conception.

Thus the human being would have at least two pre-conceptions: that of the breast and Oedipus. In practice, it allows one to grasp the function of seemingly incoherent material. They are expressions of the destruction of this pre-conception and the consequent loss of the *"apparatus essential for gaining a conception of the parental relation-ship and consequently for resolution of Oedipal problems: it does not fail to solve those problems—it never reaches them"* (EP, 93) (see entries, "Pre-conception", and "Disaster").

Myths are a way of exercising alpha-function (q.v.) to the extent that they provide a narrative form that binds the component of a history. Their time-related components are sensuously apprehensible data that belie the timeless quality of the unconscious. This quality must be elicited in the listener's mind. The time-components give ideas of "Causes" and "Effects" in the narrative; they are characteristics of the narrative but not of the reality. The concrete appearance of characters, space demand to be "de-sense-fied" too, in order to attain a narration that displays how things and facts and immaterial emotional facts really are, quite independent of time and space. This furnishes the transcendent quality of the invariance that the myth strives to convey. In this sense, Babel and the expulsion from Paradise display an invariance: "prohibition to knowledge and truth". The Ajax myth displays an invariance, "hubris" or "omnipotent fame".

Mythologies: bad science?

"Thoughts without a thinker" is a concept (q.v.) that profits from that which Descartes thought of as being absurd. The trend of profiting from that which was seen as waste to other disciplines was set by Freud who profited from dreams. Positivism dismissed dreams as senseless waste. Science is set forth in this faction: do not be fooled by apparent lack of importance or a single immediately given sense. Sir Alexander Fleming's intuition about penicillin displayed that mould was not waste. Bion's rescuing of the myth's function in the wake of Freud relies on this attention to obvious detail of reality as it is. More often than not the detail passes unnoticed.

In suggesting the detection of "elements of psycho-analysis" (q.v.) Bion states that they must have an extension in the *"domain of myth"* (EP, 11), besides extensions in the domains of sense and passion. *"It is . . . difficult to give a satisfactory explanation of what I mean by extension in the domain of myth. I cannot conceive the possibility without it of model making as part of the equipment available to the psycho-analyst. Suppose that a patient is angry. More meaning is given to a statement to that effect if it is added that his anger is like that of a 'child that wanted to hit his nanny because he has been told he is naughty.' The statement in quotation marks is not an expression of a theory in a genetic exposition. It must not be supposed to express a theory that small boys hit their nannies if they are called naughty. It is a statement akin to the type of statement that philosophers contemptuously dismiss as mythologies when they use the term pejoratively to describe bad theories. I require as part of analytical scientific procedure and equipment, statements of this kind. They are not statements of observed fact, or formulations of a theory intended to represent a realization: they are statements of a personal myth . . . I shall refer to this dimension as the myth or 'as if' component"* (EP, 12).

One of the scientific functions of the myth is that of notation (in Freud's terms) or record (EP, 48). Is it possible to imagine a Science devoid of a system of notation or recording?

This is an issue that displays how Bion was not subject to the Establishment, represented by authors such as Karl Popper during his time, and Thomas Kuhn in later times.

Myths and growth See entry, "Growth".

Origins

There is evidence that Bion's grasp of the function of myths is linked to his acquaintance with R. B. Onians' *Origins of European Thought* (for example, pages 55 and 59, CUP, 2000 reprint) and Giambattista Vico's revolutionary dealing with myths. Onians is quoted in *Elements of Psycho-Analysis*, page 40; and Vico, in *A Memoir of the Future*, volume I, p. 98.

&; On the functions of the myth: there is the now forgotten fundamental push given by Georg Hamann, Kant's teacher and von

Herder, Goethe's teacher. They were similar to Vico's historic approach but in certain senses more profound in grasping transcendences. They furnished, more than anyone else before or after, a way out of the blind authoritarian dogmata that encircled the Bible and Greek works. For the first time they were not regarded as texts to be mechanistically repeated and adored or as pagan works. They began to be examined as myths—therefore, outside the religious view. Nietzsche and Schopenhauer developed this stream of thought. Vico is quoted in Volume I, A Memoir of the Future. The former is quoted by Bion in Brazilian Lectures I. The author found no evidence of Bion's acquaintance with the work of Hamann and von Herder. It is possible that the intellectual environment they founded and that was developed by Goethe, Hegel, Schopenhauer and Nietzsche had some kind of unconscious influence on Freud's discoveries—including profiting from Greek mythology's wisdom on human nature (Sandler, 1997–2003).

During Bion's centennial, a group of Brazilian analysts extended the suggestion of Bion around the myth of Ajax; another author, around the myth of Satan (Sandler, E. H. et al, 1997; Chuster, 1997).

Suggested cross-references: Alpha-function, Cause, Conception, Oedipus, Pre-conception.

N

Nameless dread: A concept seen as a most primitive experience or perhaps a human endowment. At first it was seen as an experience from the earliest phases of life. The little infant tries to project her feelings of annihilation into the mother, according to Klein's discoveries about projective identification. If the mother is unable to exercise reverie, the fear of annihilation is returned with doubled force, as a "nameless dread". This is depicted in *Learning from Experience*.

In later times, the concept was seen as a natural endowment of the human species. It was remarkably linked to the ultimate reality of life itself—"O". It is related to the human capacity for cruelty. One of its depictions is:

> ROLAND There is a remarkable durability about the human capac-
> ity to believe in God. Religion affords a continuing source of study.
> The persistence of the belief is used by some people as an argument
> in favour of the existence of God—as if one could not believe, still
> less that the race could not believe, in the existence and even
> worship of a reality which somehow approximates to the reality
> of the human and animal impulse to worship. The mouse or rat

sometimes looks as if it were imploring, in a positively worship-ping posture, the mercy of the cat who is licking its whiskers preparatory to making a meal of its prey. The human animal, which has achieved a degree of articulate speech, certainly seems to be aware of its equipment of cruelty and the need to glut it, or at least feed it with the appropriate diet for its cruel impulses. "But not on us", the oysters said, "turning a little blue", is a formulation of the material which is to nourish and sustain cruelty in vigorous health. You remember there is a well-known history—it is even attributed, amongst others, to Jesus the eponymous hero of the Christian reli-gion. "My God, my God", he is reputed to have said, "why hast thou forsaken me?" If he had thought of his Father as greedy and cruel he would have more rationally complained about being remembered—in time to satisfy his hunger for the satisfaction of his cruelty. But usually the cornered rat seems to feel, in extremis, the advisability of adoration and worship, "morituri te salutemus" is a succinct formulation of the principle.

In the civilized world it is more comfortable to believe in its civi-lized qualities, to obscure the cruel laughter . . . which might evoke, through memory and desire, the configuration evocative of dread. It seems clear that the attempt is inherent to ward off, or to ward off awareness of, something which is dread or terror and behind that the object that is nameless. There are many formulations of dread, unformulated and ineffable—what I denote O. [AMF, 76, 77]

📕 Isaac Bashevis Singer's *The Moskat Family* and *Satan in Goray*.
Suggested cross-references: Alpha-function, Controversy, Growth, Real Psycho-analysis, Reverie, O.

Narcissism and social-ism:

. . . narcissism, apparently primary narcissism [Freud, "Instincts and their vicissitudes", 1915c, SE14], is related to the fact that common sense is a function of the patient's relationship to his group, and in his relationship with the group the individual's welfare is secondary to the survival of the group. Darwin's theory of the survival of the fittest needs to be replaced by a theory of the survival of the fittest to survive in a group—as far as the survival of the individual is concerned. [C, 29]

Bion grasps Freud's psychodynamic with no simplification expressed by ideas of pathology, cure, causes and rationalized discussions about its excess or lack. Bion's starting point is Freud's "Instincts and their vicissitudes"

Narcissism is defined in conjunction with social-ism. The two concepts are inseparable. The model can be that of an old type mechanical scale that functioned with two plates in tandem, with counter-weights.

The grasping of the concept has a pre-condition, namely, to grasp the concept of life and death instincts as also operating in tandem. Narcissism and social-ism refer to the conjoint operation of four variables: narcissism, social-ism, life instincts and death instincts. It can be said that it demands a thinker capable of working in four realms to use the concept.

The concept was created by Freud, albeit not stressing the word "socialism". He was schooled by Ehrlich's biology, a doctrine that is still valid today. The essential point here is that of "passivity-activity", in which some tendencies of many living beings seem to challenge individual interests in favour of the group. To Freud this was biologically determined and perhaps because of this fact he did not explicitly stress the word socialism (Freud, 1915, 125, 133, 140). More attention is given to the biologically-determined, non-understandable instinctual fusion and defusion of instincts and to the non-rational social-istic tendency where individuals perish. In the present day we have the "Muslim" expression of it; sixty years ago, called "kamikaze".

It seems that Bion resorted to this graphic resource of hyphenation in order to avoid the already-existing penumbra of associations to that word. He stressed the joint operation and their relative balance and/or imbalance, with a close intertwining that implies the tandem between love and hate described by Freud in the paper that served as inspiration to Bion.

Definition. Narcissism and social-ism are seen as two **tendencies** of man. If narcissism prevails, the underlying constellation is that life instincts are directed towards the ego; simultaneously the death instincts are directed to the group. Conversely, if and when social-ism has the upper hand, it means that death instincts are directed to the ego and life instincts to the group (C, 122).

They form a continuum, a range, a spectrum. Each one may fall off in intensity. The other one will increase correspondingly (T, 80). Besides Ps⇔D, narcissism⇔social-ism would be the only other definition where the double arrow ⇔ would be used by Bion.

🕐 This concept is one of the few that were more presented than defined when first introduced publicly, that is, in 1965. It is explained and dissected in some preparatory papers that were written before—but were published only in 1992, thanks to Francesca Bion's efforts. Its latest version, which corresponds to the first publication, does not include the definition.

In 1959 he defines them without hyphenation in the word socialism. He was at odds with the division between ego instincts and sexual instincts, as expressed by Freud up to 1915. One may consider that Freud himself was at odds with it too, for he changed it five years later. Bion proposes to replace Freud's division by "*one between narcissism on the one hand, and what I shall call socialism on the other*" (C, 105).

He offers a clear-cut definition then: "**By these two terms I wish to indicate the two poles of all instincts** . . . *The exclusive mention of sexuality ignores the striking fact that the individual has an even more dangerous problem to solve in the operation of his aggressive impulses, which, thanks to this bi-polarity, may impose on him the need to fight for his group with the essential possibility of his death, while it also imposes on him the need for action in the interests of his survival . . .*

This struggle contributes to the forces that lead, in certain circumstances, to the splitting—and in extreme cases the weakening and finally the destruction—of the ego ... There is, therefore, in extreme cases a weakening or even destruction of the ego through splitting attacks that derive from the primitive instinctual drives which seek satisfaction for both poles of their nature and turn against the psychic organ that appears to frustrate both alike. Hence the appearance, noted by Freud, of hatred of reality— now hatred of the ego which links with reality—characteristic of the severely disturbed patient seen in the psychoses" (C, 106; my bold).

In 1960 he defines that the terms "*might be employed to describe tendencies, one ego-centric, the other socio-centric, which may at any moment be seen to inform groups of impulsive drives in the personality. They are equal in amount and opposite in sign. Thus, if the love impulses are narcissistic at any time, then the hate impulses are social-istic, i.e., directed towards the group, and vice-versa . . . if one group of impulses is dominated by narcissistic trends, then the remaining impulses will be dominated by social-istic trends*" (C, 122).

Characteristically, the concept is in evolution. Bion applies his continuing questioning ability: "*Love of self need not be narcissistic;*

*love of the group need not be social-istic. At one pole is one object; at the
other pole an infinitude of objects"*. Or, in other words, one may dedi-
cate narcissistic love for one person and social-istic love (split in
groups of emotions or groups of objects) for another (C, 122).
Perhaps it was this further questioning that made him leave aside,
in the final definition, the specific matter of the poles. They could
not be made only of instincts, but they can also be made of split
objects.

In 1962 he mentions the concept again, related to the psycho-
analytic object and its possibilities of growth and decay:

> Growth may be regarded as positive or negative. I shall represent
> it by ($\pm$ Y). The plus and minus signs are employed to give sense or
> direction to the element they precede in a manner analogous to
> their mode of employment in co-ordinate geometry ... Whether (Y)
> is preceded by plus or minus sign will be determined only by
> contact with a realization. Abstraction from the psycho-analytic
> object will be related to the resolution of the conflicting claims of
> narcissism and social-ism. If the trend is social (+Y) abstraction will
> be related to the isolation of primary qualities. If the trend is narcis-
> sistic ($-$Y) abstraction will be replaced by activity appropriate to
> $-$K ... [LE, 70]

In 1965 he suppresses the comments about the matter that the
poles are made from: *"Narcissism and Social-ism may be regarded as at
opposite poles; I shall not consider what they are poles of ..."* (T, 80).

The parts of the definition that would remain would be the
"poles", the notion of the spectrum and the tandem mode of functioning; the stress would be in the splitting of the poles with the
resulting prevalence of one of them.

Origins

Probably Bion's experiences of war as well as the loss of his first
wife aided him to accept more smoothly than his contemporaries
Freud's review of a division between ego and sexual instincts. The
clue may lie in Freud's observation, which many years later would
be clearer to Bion too, namely, that hate is the most primitive form
of love. Hate against one's own self expresses itself as love towards
the group. The final integration of love and hate made him conjec-

ture, many years later, on the utility of serving one's contemporaries. Or, in other words, the medical profession as well as the conscious intentions of the social reformers or many among the soldiers of warring nations. He made it clear in *The Long Week-End* and *War Memoirs* that, in his own view, his narcissism prevailed.

> ROBIN Yet the boy . . . did not surrender when the alternative was clearly death. Perhaps you think it was not clear—that he chose it under some misapprehension.

> P.A. Such devotion was, and still is, beyond my capacity. In situations of great danger I always had a belief that I would probably survive. Had I realized—been compelled by some dreadful wound to realize—that such a belief was nonsense, I would have dodged the danger. Nobody told me—nor would I have understood them if they had—that war service would change utterly my capacity to enjoy life. Are we, even today, prepared to tell our children, or children's children, what price they would have to pay if they served their fellows? [AMF, III, 508]

The implication of narcissism ⇔ social-ism of the analyst is emphasized:

> The fiction can be so rhetorical as to be incomprehensible; or so realistic that the dialogue becomes audible to others. There is thus a double fear: that of the conversation being so theoretical that the thoughts might be taken for meaningless jargon; and that of the seeming reality. Having two sets of feelings about the same facts is felt as madness and disliked accordingly. This is one reason why it is felt necessary to have an analyst; another reason is the wish for me to be available to be regarded as mad and used to being regarded as mad. There is a fear that you might be called an analys- and, or reciprocally, that you may be accused of insanity. Should I then be tough and resilient enough to be regarded and treated as insane while being sane? If so, it is not surprising that psycho-analysts are, almost as a function of being analysts, supposed to qualify for being insane and called such. It is part of the price they have to pay to being psycho-analysts. [AMF, I, 113]

&, The origins of these concepts are related to femininity and aspects of PS⇔D. They are part of an attempt to examine early roots of Bion's contributions to psycho-analysis as they seem to appear in *War Memoirs* and *A Memoir of the Future* (Sandler, 2003).

Negative: See entry, "Minus". This realm was first described by Kant. He delimited, in the *Critique of Pure Reason*, the numinous realm as a *"limit concept"*, as a *"mere negative"*. Later, Hegel developed this concept, in the *Philosophy of Mind*, in order to research into the *"absolute"*.

Even though the term "Negative" can be regarded as philosophically more cogent, the realm that it refers to in the work of Bion was called by himself "Minus".

Neurotic part of the personality: A term used interchangeably with the term "Non-Psychotic Personalities". See entry, "Psychotic and Non-Psychotic Personalities (or Psychotic Part of the personality and Neurotic Part of the personality)".

No-breast: It is **the** condition for the inception of thinking processes. When the infant has a frustrating experience of realizing that the breast it wants, needs and pre-conceives is not the actual breast, it "thinks" the breast. The wished for, needed and pre-conceived breast is never the real breast. The real breast is both the actual external breast that is offered and the final non-attuned tuning that marks the introjected breast.

The no-breast is the mark of symbolizing processes to the extent that one may think in the absence of the concrete object.

> Suppose the infant is fed; the taking in of milk, warmth, love, may be felt as taking in a good breast. Under dominance of the, at first unopposed, bad breast, "taking in" food may be felt as indistinguishable from evacuating a bad breast. Both good and bad breasts are felt as possessing the same degree of concreteness and reality as milk. Sooner or later the "wanted" breast is felt as an "idea of a breast missing" and not as a bad breast present. We can see that the bad, that is to say wanted but absent, breast is much more likely to become recognized as an idea than the good breast which is associated with what a philosopher would call a thing-in-itself or a thing-in-actuality, in that the sense of a good breast depends on the existence of milk the infant in fact has taken. The good breast and the bad breast, the one being associated with the actual milk that satisfies hunger and the other with the non-existence of that milk, must have a difference in psychical quality. [LE, 34]

Suggested cross-references: Atonement, Breast, Conception, Mathematization, Pre-conception, Real psycho-analysis, Thinking, Transformations in hallucinosis.

Non-psychotic personality: A term used interchangeably with the term "neurotic part of the personality". See entry, "Psychotic and Non-Psychotic Personalities (or Psychotic Part of the personality and Neurotic Part of the personality)".

Non-sensuous: A term that corresponds to the term "non-sensible" in philosophy. It refers to the phenomena that cannot be apprehended by the sensuous apparatus. A non-sensuous realm was described by Plato and unearthed by Kant; namely, the numinous realm. Its practical application was given by Freud and a few years later by Planck and Einstein in physics.

Misuses and misunderstandings: Strictly speaking, to avoid confusion, the term non-sensuous that was used by Bion in a clear way may perhaps be replaced by a more precise formulation, namely, non-sensuously apprehensible. A problem emerged among Bion's readers due to a reification of the term; many people who advertise themselves as Bion's followers came to use the term as if there was a counterpart in reality of the "non-sensuous", that is, a "non-sensuous reality", which would represent a contradiction in terms and a lack of philosophical grasp and psycho-analytical practice. Nothing can be sensuous, except the sensory organs themselves. This attitude degenerated into a bashing of the sensuous experience and a transformation of psycho-analysis into an esoteric, disincarnate practice; a solipsism and idealism clothed by quasi-analytical terms. Bion himself seems to have been aware of such a distortion. His attempts to correct it can be seen in the term, "Reality sensuous and psychic" used to name a chapter in the book *Attention and Interpretation,* and in the terms ultra-sensuous, infra-sensuous (see this specific entry).

No-thing: Corresponds to the experience of the no-breast whose tolerance leads to:

(i)   the inception of thinking,
(ii) the possibility to symbolize,

(iii) the search for saturated meanings and verbal processes,
(iv) the looking for a mate.

"*Every word represents what is not—a 'no-thing', to be distinguished from 'nothing'*" (T, 79). The capacity to use words can be seen as a possibility of tolerating the no-breast. Intolerance of the no-thing equals psychosis; it means that the person seeks an ever and wholly-fulfilling object, fact or situation. Intolerance of the no-thing is expressed by hallucination—a perception devoid of object—and delusion.

Suggested cross-references: Atonement, Circle, Point and Line, Mathematization of psycho-analysis, Principles of mental functioning, Transformations in hallucinosis.

O

"**O**": A quasi-mathematical symbol created to denote the numinous realm of the unconscious, where the human and individual truth resides—ultimate reality, absolute truth.

Bion introduces it for the first time in *Transformations*, page 12. It is a built-in part of the applications of the theory of transformations and invariances to psycho-analysis. He takes the example from a landscape and a painter who sees it and afterwards paints it, and makes an analogy of this simple model with the analyst's task both with his patients and with his colleagues. The task is basically that of "*public-action*": to make available to himself and others his and his patient's "fight-for-an-insight". The insight is a product of a "language of achievement" (q.v.): to glimpse transiently aspects of the emanations that present immaterial, psychic reality, "O".

> A sign to represent the realization would denote . . . the landscape as a thing-in-itself, and therefore distinguish it from both $T_2\alpha$ [the painter's processes of transformation of that which he saw] and $T_2\beta$ [the readied painting]. The sign would denote something that is not a mental phenomenon and therefore, like Kant's thing-in-itself, can never be known. I introduce the idea of the thing-in-itself in order

to make clear the status of $T_2\alpha$ and $T_2\beta$ as signs for mental phenomena.

The use of these signs may be clarified by an illustration: The patient enters and, following a convention established in the analysis, shake hands. This is an external fact, what I have called a "realization". In so far as it is useful to regard it as a thing-in-itself and unknowable (in Kant's sense) it is denoted by the sign O. The phenomenon, corresponding to the external fact, as it exists in the mind of the patient, is represented by the sign T(patient)α . . .

The experience (thing-in-itself) I denote by the sign O (T, 12–13) . . .

I shall therefore assume that the material provided by the analytic session is significant for its being the patient's view (representation) of certain facts which are the origin (O) of his reaction. [T, 15]

This quasi-mathematical notation, to the extent that it symbolizes the numinous realm (after Kant, 1781) of the non-sensuous experience, the thing-in-itself, corresponds to Plato's Ideal Forms. It is ultimately unknowable and corresponds to psychic facts as they are, appertaining to the realm of the unconscious and of the id.

"O" corresponds to "origin". This is explicitly stated: *"I shall therefore assume that the material provided by the analytic session is significant for its being the patient's view (representation) of certain facts which are the origin (O) of his reaction"* (T, 15). At least once Bion had referred to it as "zero" (AMF, I, 44).

One may evolve from it or to it. One should not be identified with it, one cannot describe it verbally, one cannot know it. One can, through *becoming* (T, 140–1ff.; AI, 26), be O. *"O does not fall in the domain of knowledge or learning save incidentally; it can 'become', but it cannot be 'known'"* (AI, 26).

A Theory?

It is not, as it would seem, a theoretical formulation *per se*, but rather a practical one. Bion states it in many parts of his work, stressing its utility during an analytic session, as something to be pursued. He adjoins it to descriptions of the analyst's task as established by Freud:

The psycho-analyst tries to help the patient to transform that part of an emotional experience of which he is unconscious into an emotional experience of which he is conscious. If he does this he helps the patient to achieve private knowledge. But since scientific work demands communication of discovery to other workers the psycho-analyst must transform *his* private experience of psycho-analysis so that it becomes a public experience. The artist is used here as a model intended to indicate that the criteria for a psycho-analytic paper are that it should stimulate in the reader the emotional experience that the writer intends, that its power to stimulate should be durable, and that the emotional experience thus stimulated should be an accurate representation of the psycho-analytic experience ("Oa") that stimulated the writer in the first place. [T, 32–3]

The obstacles to intuit it are sometimes seemingly insurmountable. It depends on the activity of feeble beings—we, human beings—using a new tool, psycho-analysis. What slowly emerges in *Transformations* is that the very inaccessibility of O is its betrayal, not to the senses, but to our fleeting apprehension. To deal with resistances, lies (or column 2 categories of the Grid) and hallucinations are ways of glimpsing "O" transiently, exactly in the sense depicted by Freud in *The Interpretation of Dreams* and his grasping of the paths to the formations of symptoms (*New Introductory Lectures*).

Bion puts this into terms of an observational theory. It seems to furnish a fresh new perspective about facts that were—and still are—being buried by the psycho-analytical establishment. "*. . . The most profound method known to us of investigation—psycho-analysis—is unlikely to do more that scratch the surface*" (BLI, 52).

"*P.A. The practical point is—no further investigation of psycho-analysis, but the psyche it betrays.* **That** *needs to be investigated through the medium of* **mental** *patterns;* **that** *which is indicated is* **not** *a symptom;* **that** *is not a cause of the symptom;* **that** *is not a disease or* **anything** *subordinate. Psycho-analysis itself is just a stripe on the coat of the tiger. Ultimately it may meet the Tiger—The Thing Itself—O*" (AMF, I, 112).

The analyst must focus his attention on O, the unknown and unknowable. The success of psycho-analysis depends on the maintenance of a psycho-analytic point of view; the point of view is the psycho-analytic vertex: the psycho-analytic vertex is O. With this the analyst cannot be identified: he must *be* it.

Every object known or knowable by man, including himself, must be an evolution of O. It is O when it has evolved sufficiently to be met by K capacities in the psycho-analyst . . . In so far as the analyst becomes O he is able to know the events that are *evolutions* of O". [AI, 27]

In practice this means that I shall regard only those aspects of the patient's behaviour which are significant as representing his view of O; I shall understand what he says or does as if it were an artist's painting . . . From the analytic treatment as a whole I hope to discover from the invariants in this material what O is, what he *does* to transform O . . . [T, 15]

The postulate is that . . . designated by O. To qualify O . . . I list the following negatives: Its existence as indwelling has no significance whether it is supposed to dwell in an individual person or in God or Devil; it is not good or evil; it cannot be known, loved or hated. It can be represented by terms such as ultimate reality or truth. The most, and the least that the individual can do is to be with it. Being identified with it is a measure of distance from it. The beauty of a rose is a phenomenon betraying the ugliness of O just as ugliness betrays or reveals the existence of O . . . The rose *is* itself whatever it may be *said* to be. [T, 139–40]

O, representing the unknowable ultimate reality can be represented by any formulation of a transformation—such as "unknowable ultimate reality" which I have just formulated. It may therefore seem unnecessary to multiply representations of it; indeed, from the psycho-analytic vertex that is true. But I wish to make it clear that my reason for saying that O is unknowable is not that I consider human capacity unequal to the task but because K, L, or H are inappropriate to O. They are appropriate to transformations of O but not to O. [T, 140]

My theory would seem to imply a gap between phenomena and the thing-in-itself and all that I have said is not incompatible with Plato, Kant, Berkeley, Freud and Klein, to name a few, who show the extent to which they believe that a curtain of illusion separates us from reality. Some consciously believe the curtain of illusion to be a protection against truth which is essential to the survival of humanity; the remainder of us believe it unconsciously but no less tenaciously for that. Even those who consider such a view mistaken and truth essential consider that the gap cannot be bridged because the nature of the human being precludes knowledge of anything beyond phenomena save conjecture. From this conviction of the inaccessibility of absolute reality the mystics must be exempted . . . We must therefore consider further the gap between O and knowledge of phenomena and transformations of O.

The gap between reality and the personality, or, as I prefer to call it, the inaccessibility of O, is an aspect of life with which analysts are familiar under the guise of resistance. Resistance is only manifest when the threat is contact with what is believed to be real. There is no resistance to anything because it is believed to be false. Resistance operates because it is feared that the reality of the object is imminent. *O represents this dimension of anything whatever—its reality.*

It is not knowledge of reality that is at stake, nor yet the human equipment for knowing. The belief that reality is or could be known is mistaken because reality is not something which lends itself to being known. It is impossible to know reality for the same reason that makes it impossible to sing potatoes; they may be grown, or pulled, or eaten, but not sung. Reality has to be "been"; there should be a transitive verb "to be" expressly for use with the term "reality". [T, 147–8].

. . . I propose to extend the significance of O to cover the domain of reality. [T, 156, my italics]

Further dwellings on the realm of O

Earlier suggestions on elements of psycho-analysis are expanded: dread, pain, birth, death, hate and love: *"There are many formulations of dread, unformulated and ineffable—what I denote O. Plato named it 'forms', of which sensuous objects are the unreal but sensible counterpart"* (AMF, I, 77).

O is by definition indestructible and not subject to, circumscribed by, beginnings and ends, rules, laws of nature or any construct of the human mind. In the domain of human comprehension Melanie Klein could not reconcile herself to the fact that whenever she had made herself understood, the fact rendered what she understood no longer "alive". [AMF, I, 88–9]

"Passionate love" is the nearest I can get to a verbal transformation which "represents" the thing-in-itself, the ultimate reality, the "O", as I have called it, approximating to it. [AMF, I, 183]

ROSEMARY Alice, I think it's time we left. I feel I am not in a sufficiently serious state of mind to keep in touch with these two

BION I should have thought both of you might know very well what I am talking about—the thing-in-itself as contrasted with the language about it. You may find yourselves as inadequate as I am talking *about* it, that is, in trying to tell someone else—lateral communication. I cannot feel optimistic of my chances of making it clear even to myself.

MYSELF I see your point.

BION Then it can't be the point.

MYSELF You mean I am wrong?

BION No, I don't; but you are now.

ALICE Rosemary, do you think we shall ever understand this?

ROSEMARY . . . I feel I am "becoming" it even if I do not, and never shall, "understand" what I am "becoming" or "being".

BION In short, "being" something is different from "understanding" it. Love is the ultimate which is "become", not understood.

ALICE (looking at Rosemary) I have "become" something and this, if I could say it, would depend on my saying, "I love". [AMF, I, 182–3]

The difference between apprehension of transient, if truthful aspects of O and feelings of owning "absolute truth"

There is a profound difference between "being" O and rivalry with O. The latter is characterized by envy, hate, love, megalomania and the state known to analysts as acting out, which must be sharply differentiated from acting; which is characteristic of "being" O. [T, 141]

This illuminates the damaging situation of idolization.

Formulations of O in psycho-analysis

Bion considers the existence of *"intersections"* of the *"human being with the evolving O"* (AI, 85). They have been depicted since 1963 as "elements of psycho-analysis". In his opinion, they are presented by Oedipus, the interplay between PS and D and container contained, as well as the formulations of the two principles of mental functioning and the theory of instincts.

Recommended cross-references: Minus, Oedipus.

Suggested cross-references: Absolute truth, Analytic view, Atonement, Becoming, Disturbed personality, Facts, Jargon, Nothing, Real analysis, Reality Sensuous and Psychic, Thoughts without a thinker, Transformations in Hallucinosis and Transformations in O, Truth, Unknowable, Unknown.

&; Attempts at explorations into the realm of O can be seen, in a comparative way with other disciplines, in the series "*A Apreensão da Realidade Psíquica*" (1997–2003), by the author.

Objectives of psycho-analysis: See Analytic view, Atonement, Real Psycho-analysis.

Observational theory: Bion distinguished a system of Psycho-Analytical Theory from a system of Theories of Observation. He did this in order to enhance the scientific status of psycho-analysis (T, 160). After many warnings about *ad hoc* theorizing (see this specific entry, as well as the entry, "Manipulations of symbols") and of different descriptions applying to the same basic configurations that lost sight of these underlying configurations, he tried to develop observational methods that could ensure the "pursuit of truth-O" (AI, 9, see entries, "Real psycho-analysis", "O").

More than this, he tried to get descriptions that, if put into analytical terms could lack the necessary precision demanded by scientific communication among peers. "*Most analysts have had the experience of feeling that the description given of characteristics of one particular clinical entity might well fit with the description of some quite different clinical entity*" (EP, 2).

One is not erring if one states that most of Bion's contributions to psycho-analysis are of observational theories. His theory of thinking, the theory of container/contained (q.v.) and the adjoining of the theory of pre-conception of the Breast and of Oedipus to man's innate capacities, are the main exceptions to this rule. Even the theory of alpha-function which is in many quarters held as a new theory of psycho-analysis, cannot be regarded as such: "*The theory of functions and alpha-function are not a part of psycho-analytic theory. They are working tools for the practising psycho-analyst to ease problems of thinking about something that is unknown"* (LE, 89). They do *"not diminish or increase existing psycho-analytic theories"* (LE, 89).

He would try his hand again in a paper named "Metatheory". Nevertheless, this was a posthumously published work and was not expanded. Many of its hypotheses—mainly that of violent emotions—contributed to his other contributions.

Bion made theoretical contributions mainly in the form of extensions of the existing body of psycho-analytic knowledge, which he used extensively. His contributions were never replacements, but rather non-rival improvements:

(i)   Of Freud's theory of dreams, to include a closer scrutiny of waking life dream work.

(ii) Of Freud's theory of a time succession between conscious and unconscious, that demanded to be added with the idea of a simultaneous occurrence of both in the psychotic personality.

(iii) Extensions of the study of Oedipus, which came to reach the non-formation of Oedipus.

(iv) Developments on the genesis and vicissitudes of thought processes, an extension of Freud's two principles of mental functioning in terms of functions of the ego and the genetics of thought processes.

(v)   Klein's theory of projective identification, to include its function as a method of communication.

(vi) Klein's theory of symbolization, to include the more extensive forms of communication and primitive symbolization performed by acts or apprehensions of psychotics.

He added to the analyst's capacity for observation and assessment of analytical situations and verbal statements. Both the Grid and the application of the theory of transformations are part of this. Perhaps they are the most powerful tools hitherto available to this task, with the possible exception of the analyst's personal analysis. It cannot be a comparison with this, on Bion's own terms. On many occasions he recommended analysts to look for the best analysis they could. He believed his books were inaccessible to non-analysts.

Bion would state a number of times that his were theories of observation:

In 1965: *"The theory of transformations and its development does not relate to the main body of psycho-analytic theory, but to the practice of psycho-analytic* **observation**" (T, 34).

In 1970: *"The theory formulates a recurrent pattern of emotional experience . . . It does not replace any existing psycho-analytical theory, but is intended to display relationships which have not been remarked"* (AI, 87).

It is easy to see that the theory of alpha-function is a theory that observes the "behaviour" of the sense stimulus in its path in becoming immaterial psychic facts. Also, that the theory of objects of psycho-analysis tries to encompass the processes of thinking in terms of observing the mother–baby relationship in the first place—and how it affects the patient's capacity to observe facts in life. The Grid is an observational theory to gauge the truth-value of the analyst and patient's verbal statements.

Oedipus:

> We are accustomed, thanks to Freud's discoveries, to attribute great significance and importance to the Oedipus complex, and consequently it has come to be regarded as if it were the starting point of a dynamic process. [C, 200]

> If the Oedipus story is the weapon that reveals homo, it is also the story that conceals, but does not reveal, that by which it will destroy itself. [AMF, I, 61]

> I shall consider in what respect it is meaningful to regard the Oedipus myth as an important component of the content of the human mind . . .

> Features that can serve as symbols for the mechanics of thinking contribute to my suspicion that it is inadequate to regard the Oedipus situation as a part of the *content* of the mind. [EP, 47 and 49]

Freud opened many broad avenues to research. Few analysts ventured to push this research beyond the limits established by the end of Freud's physical life. Bion tackles the task of trying to do this in at least four aspects of Freud's theories: dreams, the two principles of mental functioning, Oedipus and the nature of free associations.

Bion introduces the suggestion of the existence of a "private myth", that must be seen as a particular presentation and realization of a universal myth. *"The private myth, corresponding to the Oedipus myth, enables the patient to understand his relationship with the parents"* (EP, 66). With this suggestion he invites analysts to give up two tendencies: (i) that of using Oedipus as a pre-patterned moulding which could justify an artificial fitting of the patient's material into it; (ii) the tendency to reify and concretize the content of Oedipus. This posture is made at the expense of an assessment of the function of Oedipus in each individual. How it is conceived by each individual is not examined. The content is dealt with as an end-in-itself. Bion shows that it is a conveyor, a vehicle of the function. From prejudice to pre-conception would be a synthetic manner to put the issue of the gradual loss of sight of Oedipus. Did it cause decadence of the psycho-analytical movement? Bion sees Oedipus as a pre-conception that seeks a realization, namely the *"realization of the actual parents gives rise to the conception of parents"* (EP, 93).

More specifically, he invited the analyst actively to seek *"Oedipal components and the events of the consulting room"* (EP, 68). In doing this, he tried to circumvent the failure to see that there is a tendency to devalue myths as *"fact-finding tools"* (EP, 66). *"I wish to restore it [the myth] to its place in our methods so that it can play the vitalizing part there that it has played in history (and in Freud's discovery of psychoanalysis)... It is also an object for investigation in an analysis as part of the primitive apparatus of the individual's armoury of learning"* (EP, 66).

If used in this way, which differs from that of the theologian, anthropologist, mythologist or historian, myth emerges as a scientific tool to the extent that it is a generalization flexible enough to be applied to particular cases as observed in the here and now of the session.

Myth of Oedipus and theory of Oedipus

The Oedipus theory and its various formulations belong to the areas encompassed by the functions of the ego, namely, attention and inquiry; moreover, concepts derived from attention and inquiry and scientific approaches obtained by such attention and inquiry. The myth, in contrast, belongs to the areas encompassed by dreaming activity (EP, 58).

Bion deals with the Oedipus situation in a way that resembles, at least to the author, that offered by Giambatistta Vico (one of his intellectual forebears; AMF, I, 88 and 119) as regards the history of mankind and religion, and that of von Herder when he focused on the so called sacred scriptures, namely, as chronicles and apprehensions of human nature and life (Sandler, 2001a, 2002, 2003b). This posture has at least two consequences: in its use in the session and in the way one deals with Freud's legacy. Bion views Freud's study in an un-sanctified way; not as a taboo, as a postulate unearthed from nothing, or an issue above discussion because it was uttered by Freud. Also, Bion applies Vico, von Herder and Freud's sense of "historicity" and consideration about historical conditions, in terms of each individual's history.

His earliest statement seems to date from circa 1960: *"The scientist must know enough mathematics to understand the nature and use of various mathematical discoveries and formulations, such as the differential calculus or the binomial theorem: the psycho-analyst must know his myth. The scientist must also know enough to have an idea when he is confronting a problem to which a particular mathematical procedure would apply: the psycho-analyst must know when he is facing a problem to which a myth would provide the psycho-analytic counterpart of the algebraic calculus. This, one might say, is precisely what Freud did; he recognized, as a scientist, that he was confronted by a problem to the solution of which he would have to apply the Oedipus myth. The result was his discovery, not of the Oedipus complex, but of psycho-analysis. (Or is it man, or man's psyche, that is discovered when these elements are constantly conjoined?)"* (C, 228).

Bion used this thinking (published in 1992, in *Cogitations*) later, in his typical way. Namely, in a condensed form, in 1963: *"The Oedipus myth may be regarded as an instrument that served Freud in his discovery of psycho-analysis and psycho-analysis as an instrument that enabled Freud to discover the Oedipus complex"* (EP, 92).

His last theorization about Oedipus was:

The oedipal situation, or its even more primitive roots, would have a different configuration according to whether the vertex of the group was psycho-analytic, religious, financial, legal, or some other. This itself increases the variety of experiences opened up within the limits of even rigid psycho-analysis. The messianic expectation, formulated and institutionalized in the Christian religion, may represent the evolved aspect of an element which is represented also at its evolved stage by the Oedipus myth.

Similarities in the configurations suggest a common origin and common disorders associated with the problem of containing the mystic and institutionalizing his work. The emotional impact of $\male\female$ will be proportionately greater the more closely it is related to the forces represented by the messianic hope, the Oedipus myth, the Babel myth, and the Eden myth; the greater the emotional impulse the greater the problem. These myths are evolved states of O and *represent* the evolution of O. They represent the state of mind achieved by the human being at his intersection with the evolving O. [AI, 84–5]

The ferocity with which children sometimes play games is evidence that the players are not feeling that they are playing, or the observer witnessing, "just a game". The idea of "game" is an inadequate description for what is being witnessed. It is being wrongly categorized by the name of "game". I think of a mathematical analogy. If the "universe of discourse" does not facilitate the solution of 3 minus 5, then real numbers are no good, but must be enlarged by "negative numbers". If the mathematical "field of play" is not suitable for the manipulation of "negative numbers" it has to be extended to provide conditions for "games" with negative numbers. If the world of conscious thought is not suitable for playing "Oedipus Rex" the "universe of discourse" must be enlarged to include such plays. [AMF, I, 175–6]

Being a kind of tool for apprehending reality, myths are related to mathematics. Bion left some attempts to display the possible analogies and links. They are just preliminary papers, later published in *Cogitations*. They relate Oedipus, Pythagoras' triangle, Euclid's Pons Asinorum and Lewis Carroll's mathematics (see entry, Mathematization of Psycho-Analysis).

Bion's integration of Freud and Klein: extensions of the Oedipus myth

The model of container and contained (q.v.) and its fundamental basis, the double arrow ⇔ can be seen as an outgrowth that integrates Freud's use of the Oedipal situation and Melanie Klein's theory of the positions—as lived by an analytic couple during an actual session, when thinking and a vivid intercourse takes place between two people. *"It will be observed that PS is capable of functioning as if it were a form of ?"* (EP, 43) in the sense that PS *"may be regarded as a cloud of particles capable of coming together"* (EP, 42). A mystery of life, that is, the prodigality of a male ejaculation when it encounters an ovum may be used as an approximate realization of it (incurring the risk of being too concrete to some readers). Conversely, D is regarded as *"an object capable of being fragmented and dispersed, PS"*, as a *"field of fragmentation"* (EP, 42–3)—due to the very fact that it can *"be regarded variously as an integrated object, as an agglomeration produced by the convergence of elementary particles . . . or as an especial instance of integrated object, namely, either ? or ?"* (EP, 42–3). One must keep firmly in mind that this refers to the human being's bi-sexuality as first described by Freud. The thinking process is *"used as a term to describe the processes by which thoughts are produced and the processes by which they are subsequently dealt with"*. Therefore an analytic session is a kind of creative production of thoughts about the psychic reality of the patient, striving to elicit truthful features of it.

The process shares a creative quality with Oedipus: *"Although I shall speak of the Oedipal situation as if it were the content of thoughts it will be apparent that thoughts and thinking may be regarded as part of the content of the Oedipal situation"* (EP, 44), lived in every minute of life and in every minute of the life of an analytic couple. The possibility of making creative couples or destructive couples is always at stake and can be glimpsed in a session. Oedipus is a kind of "compact" that presents this mystery of the evolving human life itself. *"The term 'Oedipal situation' may be applied to the (1) realization of relationships between Father, Mother and child, (2) emotional preconception, using the term 'preconception' as I have used it here as that which mates with awareness of a realization to give rise to a conception, (3) a psychological reaction stimulated in an individual by (1) above. . .*

Freud's use of the Oedipus myth illuminated more than the nature of the sexual facets of the human personality. Thanks to his discoveries it is possible by reviewing the myth to see that it contains elements that were not overshadowed by the sexual component in the drama" (EP, 44–5).

Re-examination of Oedipus and sex in terms of immaterial (psychic) reality

Bion considers that not too much weight can be attributed to any of the discrete possible contents and elements of the myth: "*The developments of psycho-analysis make it possible to give more weight to other features . . . No element, such as the sexual element, can be comprehended save in its relationship with other elements; for example, with the determination with which Oedipus pursues his inquiry into the crime despite the warnings of Tiresias. It is consequently not possible to isolate the sexual component, or any other, without distortion. Sex, in the Oedipal situation, has a quality* that can only be described by the implications conferred on it by its inclusion in the story. If it is removed from the story it loses its quality unless its meaning is preserved by an express reservation that 'sex' is a term used to represent sex as it is experienced in the context of the myth. The same is true of all other elements that lend themselves to abstraction from the myth***".

This point becomes more clear when I discuss the use of ideational content of a statement as a method of expressing feeling.

** *Particularly curiosity—the K link (EP, 45–6).*

Bion observes other elements that are combined in myth (all quotations, EP, 46–7): curiosity, self-curiosity—that correspond to sexual development, to the extent that sexual curiosity, according to Klein, already a manifestation of self-curiosity towards one's own body, evolves to a curiosity about mind. Self-curiosity is in fact self-consciousness, "*or curiosity in the personality about the personality*". Not without a serious sense of humour, Bion states that "*psycho-analytic investigation thus has origins of respectable antiquity*"; the pronouncement of the Delphic Oracle; the warning of Tiresias, who had already paid the price—blindness—for having witnessed sexual intercourse; the riddle of the sphinx; Oedipus' hubris; disaster (the plague, suicides and homicides—Laius, Jocasta, the Sphinx, Oedipus' blinding).

> I . . . wish to show that the problems involved in the interplay between the Positions have also prompted attempts at resolution analogous to those to which I point as associated with the matrix or matrices of the Oedipus myth. [C, 200–1]

Oedipus as an inborn pre-conception of the human mind

Bion explores the possibilities opened up by a "*suspicion*", namely, *"that it is inadequate to regard the Oedipus situation as a part of the* **content** *of the mind"*. One may use the term "content" here as evoking the meaning of the term "essence" in philosophy. He deals with Oedipus as a multiple and complex compact of many functions of the mind.

In one of his explorations, he uses the horizontal categories of the Grid (if the reader is not acquainted with the definitions of this tool, refer to the specific entry in this dictionary). They include Freud's functions of the ego. He shows that the pronouncement of the oracle can be seen as functioning as a definitory hypothesis; Tiresias corresponds to a falsity (column 2) maintained to act as a barrier against anxiety (see especially EP, 80); the myth as a whole is a kind of notation; the Sphinx corresponds to the functions that Freud attributed to attention.

Another function of the myth, already existent in Freud's description, can be stated as follows: *"The classical psycho-analytical employment of the myth sheds light on the nature of L and H links; it is equally illuminating for the K link"* (EP, 49). In this sense, if the functions of the mind may be seen not as contents, but as constitutive factors, one may see the coherence of Bion's statement, that *"it is inadequate to regard the Oedipus situation as a part of the* **content** *of the mind"*. It is coherent with his earlier contributions on stress functions of the mind. It has a practical consequence that can be healthy for the analytic movements, analysts and patients alike. The content of the myth can be seen as a conveyor, a presenter, and as a manifestation of the myth. This view avoids its usage as a symbol to be manipulated.

A patient seemed to be friendly and co-operative. In fact he tried to hide from himself the intense pain he experienced. He always said that the analyst was *"right"*, but at the same time furnished baffling, *"stupefied silence"* as well as *"apathetic acquiescence"* followed by more disjointed, if rational verbal material, as a response to Bion's interpretations. This situation turned a dynamic situation into a static one, a condition that Bion named "reversion of perspective" (q.v.). The practical—not pre-patterned—use of Oedipus illuminated the situation. *"There was ample evidence, after interpretations had established the reality of the patient's inability to comprehend, of the severity of his pain.*

In each instance, the perspective that enabled me, but not the patient, to grasp the meaning of the associations, was afforded by the Oedipus theory. In every instance, that which appeared to cause the patient to reverse the perspective, was the Oedipus myth" (EP, 58).

In *Cogitations*, one is bound to find many more seemingly incoherent manifestations of patients or at least manifestations that seemingly do not cohere with Oedipus, such as *"hallucinations associated with intense deprivation . . . blockading effect of . . . envy . . . destruction of all links . . . murderous super-ego . . . dreams, speech . . . stammer . . . painting and drawing, and reports of difficulty with musical execution . . . no information in terms of ordinary conversation . . . attacks on positions"* but an ability to *"create an impression . . . As I attempted to show in my paper on the attacks on linking, this means that the two main routes by which the patient can maintain communication with the sources essential for healthy development are both obstructed with degrees of thoroughness dependent on the severity and duration of the attacks on the links . . . for the present . . . consider what these vitalizing sources are from which the patient is isolated. . . . I believe they are sources that betray their presence and activity in the Oedipus myth . . . I wish now to regard the Oedipus myth . . . and Freud's own discoveries as all being attempts at the resolution of a developmental crux. I hope to show that these attempts at resolution are far more widespread in time and far more various in the form and method of resolution adopted, than has hitherto been realized or even suspected"* (C, 198–200).

Bion writes "myth", not "theory"—and considers that *"the distinction is important"* because of the fact that the Oedipus theory affords situations that belong to the realm of attention and notation of concepts and of scientific theories; the Oedipus myth affords situations that belong to the realm of dream activities.

These expansions on the functions of Oedipus led Bion to postulate *"a precursor of the Oedipal situation"*; Oedipus would not only be a fact-finding tool for the practising analyst during a session. More than that, it would be a fact-finding tool for any human being. In this sense he differs from Klein's usage of the term in her classical paper, "Early phases of the Oedipus complex" (EP, 93)—*"but as something that belongs to the ego as a part of its apparatus for contact with reality . . . a private Oedipus myth which is the means, the pre-conception, by virtue of which the infant is able to establish contact with the parents as they exist in the world of reality. The mating of this . . . Oedipal preconception with the realization of the actual parents gives rise to the conception of parents"* (EP, 93).

This difference with Klein is not couched in rival terms; it is an amendment. Bion makes full use of Klein's observations to reach a point that was not available before: a kind of non-Oedipus in certain patients, or, using his later terminology, "the place where Oedipus might be". The Oedipal situation cannot be found in many cases but not due to a defect of psycho-analysis—provided the analyst has dealt with his Oedipus in his analysis or otherwise:

> If, through envy, greed, sadism or other cause, the infant cannot tolerate the parental relationship and attacks it destructively, according to Melanie Klein the attacking personality is itself fragmented through the violence of the splitting attacks. Restating this theory in terms of the Oedipal pre-conception: the emotional load carried by the private α-element Oedipal pre-conception is such that the Oedipal pre-conception is itself destroyed. As a result the infant loses the apparatus essential for gaining a conception of the parental relationship and consequently for resolution of Oedipal problems: it does not fail to solve those problems—it never reaches them.

> The significance of this for practice is that scraps of what appear to be Oedipal material must be treated with reserve ... The investigation must be directed to distinguishing amongst the elements of Oedipal material those that are fragments of Oedipal pre-conception from those that are fragments of the fragmented Oedipal situation. Since the experience of learning from which the patient is thus debarred is that of the parental relationship, the importance for the patient's development and for a successful outcome of analysis, depending on the resolution of the Oedipus complex, are gravely prejudiced. [EP, 93–4]

Intuitive psycho-analysis

Bion always coupled this term with Oedipus. In Kant's terms, it is a typical "sensible intuition", learned by experience:

> ... the analyst must have a view of the psycho-analytic theory of the Oedipus situation. His understanding of that theory can be regarded as a transformation of that theory and in that case all his interpretations, verbalized or not, of what is going on in a session may be seen as transformations of an O that is bi-polar. One pole of O is trained intuitive capacity transformed to effect its juxtaposition

with what is going on in the analysis and the other is in the facts of the analytic experience that must be transformed to show what approximation the realization has to the analyst's preconceptions—the preconception here being identical with Taβ as the end-product of Taα operating on the analyst's psycho-analytic theories.

Freud stated as one of the criteria by which a psycho-analyst was to be judged was the degree of understanding allegiance he paid to the theory of the Oedipus complex. He thus showed the importance he attached to this theory and time has done nothing to suggest that he erred by overestimation; evidence of the Oedipus complex is never absent though it can be unobserved.

Melanie Klein, in her paper on 'Early phases of the Oedipus complex', made observations of Oedipal elements where their presence was previously undetected. [T, 49–50]

Misuses and misunderstandings: The quotations in this entry try to furnish empirical data about Bion's profound respect and allegiance to Freud's work and the enlightening continuity and expansion of Freud's work that he was able to deliver to any practising psycho-analyst. Remarkably, it is just around the issue of Oedipus that there is a tendency to compare Bion's work with that of Freud, with a sense of superiority of the former over the latter. The other issues in Bion's work that were seen in this same sense by these readers are the theory of consciousness and the theory of transformations.

His attempts to improve the theory and its application scientifically were read by some readers as if they were a statement of rivalry and obsolescence. Perhaps they misunderstood some texts such as the following one (all quotations, LE, 76–78):

1. Suppose that the patient has produced a number of associations and other material. The analyst has available:

(1)   Observations of the patient's material;

(2)   Various emotional experiences of his own;

(3)   A knowledge of one or more versions of the myth of Oedipus;

(4)   One or more versions of the psycho-analytical theory of the Oedipus complex;

(5)   Other fundamental psycho-analytic theories.

Some aspects of the session will appear familiar; they will remind him of past experiences analytical and otherwise. Others will seem to bear a resemblance to the oedipal situation. From these sources the analyst can form a model; the problem is to decide whether the analyst is confronted by a realization of Freud's theory of the Oedipus complex.

Then comes a seminal phrase:

The Oedipus theory does not correspond closely to what a physicist would call a scientific deductive system but can be formulated to qualify for inclusion in such a category. Its weakness as a member of this class is likely to be its lack of abstraction and the peculiar structure by which its elements are related to each other. In part this is due to the fact that the more concrete the elements the less they lend themselves to variation of combination.

The fact that the myth was buried and perhaps made more sense to the ancient Greeks than it made intuitive sense to modern audiences until the advent of Freud illustrates this weakness. The word "weakness" is important here; perhaps some readers think that it refers to Freud's theory and not to the power of myths to serve as scientific theories. Were they the most primitive scientific theories available? Does this mark some of their limitations for that purpose?

2. In addition two factors (1) the actual nature of the network of relationships in which the elements are held, and (2) the derivation of the elements from a myth contrast with the elements in a scientific deductive system as used by a physicist. The latter purports to derive from one realization and to be able to represent another, whereas the psycho-analytic formulation is derived from and expressed by the emotional experience of a folk narrative and is said to represent a realization encountered in psycho-analysis.

The situation is stated with a difference from the kind of realization of the scientist. Bion needed three years more—to adopt Heisenberg's contributions—to question the kind of evidence claimed by the so-called hard sciences, concerning their materiality and objectivity. Let us follow him:

Freud derived his theory from the emotional experience of psycho-analytic inquiry, but his description could not be comparable with the formulations usually supposed to represent scientific discovery.

The difficulty here lies in the criteria of reproducibility and falsifiability as defended by people such as Popper. In due course Bion would see that these criteria are highly questionable. Reading his notes in his copies of Popper's book and the chapters in *Cogitations* shows this—as did his proposals that began in *Transformations*. There he finally adopted with less timidity Freud's view, stemming from his own analytic practice with psychotics, of the interference of the observer in the observed object. Anyway, his attempt was to furnish a sound scientific basis to analysis, rather than to criticize Freud:

I wish to discuss only two methodological weaknesses in the Oedipus theory and these are:

(1)   The theory as it stands is so concrete that it cannot be matched with its realization; that is to say no realization can be found to approximate to a theory whose elements, concrete in themselves, are combined in a narrative network of relationships that is intrinsic and essential. Without the narrative the elements lose their value.

Conversely:

(2)   If the elements are generalized the theory becomes an ingenious manipulation of elements according to arbitrary rules—the commonest formulation of this suspicion of the theory is the criticism that analyst and analysand indulge in a taste for jargon.

3. A theoretical formulation that appears to be too concrete and yet too abstract requires to be generalized in such a way that its realizations are more easily detected, without the attendant weakness, most often seen in mathematics, appearing to be an arbitrary manipulation of symbols. Can it retain its concrete elements without losing flexibility so essential in psycho-analytic application?

4. I am convinced of the strength of the scientific position of psycho-analytic practice. I believe that the practice of psycho-analysts in making psycho-analysis an essential training experience deals with the fundamental difficulties for the time being because it makes conscious and unconscious available for correlation; but I do not

consider the need less pressing to investigate the weaknesses that
spring from faulty theory construction, lack of notation and failure
of methodical care and maintenance of psycho-analytic equipment.
("Care", "maintenance", "equipment",—again the implicit model).

The last phrase could preclude the confusion of Bion's work
with the structuralist, textualist tendency as well as the post-
modernist tendency.

The text compacts the issue of scientific deductive systems that
was dealt with in many preparatory papers that appeared in *Cogitations* (chiefly, pages 2, 8, 76, 147, 151, 154). The basic problem was
stated first by Bacon and consists in the ability to transpose raw
empirical data into generalizations that can be regarded as scientific, to the extent that they would encompass particular cases.

The text clearly depicts:

(1)   The starting point, with no criticism or disagreement about
      Oedipus.
(2)   The abysmal gap between Freud's scientific outlook *vis-à-vis*
      that which was considered to be science in those days, which
      continued with Bion, namely, the positivist view of science.
      Bion courted neo-positivist views, which differ considerably
      from the positivist ideas; he abandoned this as he increasingly
      leaned towards forms of science that proved to be more
      adequate to the kind of phenomena that involved no distinc-
      tion between matter and energy (or mind), namely, psycho-
      analysis itself and post-Planck and post-Einstein physics.
      Nevertheless, when the text quoted above was written, the
      prevailing view of science was still the positivist one, as well
      as the neo-positivist attempts. Bion tried to adapt analysis to
      the latter. He recognized that some criticism levelled against
      the use of Freud's concepts by so-called followers of Freud
      had some basis. The whole issue is expanded in the entry,
      "Manipulations of symbols".

The "jewel" was to be polished in his next book, and the same
statement, a defence of the scientific approach in psycho-analysis as
well as a warning to the psycho-analytic establishment can be seen
again:

Psycho-analytic theories suffer from the defect that, in so far as they are clearly stated and comprehensible, their comprehensibility depends on the fact that the elements of which they are composed become invested with fixed value, as constants, through their association with other elements in the theory. This phenomenon is analogous to the phenomenon of alphabetic script where meaningless letters can be combined to form a meaningful word. The elements in Freud's theory of the Oedipus situation, for example, are combined, by their association to form the narrative of the Oedipus myth, and so achieve a contextual meaning that gives them a constant value. As elements in a description of a realization that has been already discovered this is essential to their usefulness: as components of a theory that is to be used in the illumination of realizations yet to be discovered it is a defect because the constant value impairs the flexibility needed. [EP, 5]

Then Bion recommends some measures for using the elements of the theory during an actual session; it is clear that he is referring to *the usage* of the theory by many, and not to the theory itself. This is a preparation for the instrument of the Grid as well as for his next book, *Transformations*. There he proposes a theory of observation in psycho-analysis. It is implicitly a critique of the psycho-analytic movement, which was transforming itself into a psycho-analytic establishment. It is also an implicit critique so typical of the British Renaissance and Enlightenment. Thomas Browne, Dr Johnson and Alexander Pope were Bion's forebears, as he makes clear in *Learning from Experience, Attention and Interpretation* and mainly in *A Memoir of the Future*. This means that a tradition of a refusal to submit to dogmas; lack of erudition is present in this text. In the same way that a theory may be used in an "immobilized" way, it can be bandied about in a repetitive, pre-patterned way that causes *ad hoc* theorizing.

In the same text, he deals with Oedipus using a quasi-mathematical formula: $♀♂ \geq 2$, which conveys a sense of mother, father and their possible offspring—Oedipus. Why should it be necessary to do this? It may have the same sense as the letters in the alphabet forming words or the quotations of pages in standardized editions in writing a paper that he proposed in the text of 1962, reproduced above. He seems to strive to keep open the investigative ethos of an analytical session itself, as practised by Freud. It was being extinguished by authoritarian, ossified repetitions and manipulations of symbols. There is no departure from or attack on Oedipus; quite the contrary, Bion strives to unearth it.

In the end, he contributed to the analytic movement in the sense that clinical work must discover particular configurations of Oedipus. These may be variable as fingerprints and are always unknown. They are unknown—unconscious—to the patient and are unknown to the analyst. The work of analysis is an attempt to glimpse aspects of it.

Bion states it clearly, in one of the, at the same time, rare and outstanding illuminations we may have both of Oedipus and free associations:

> . . . The interpretation can be verbally identical in each case—but it is a theory used to investigate the unknown. The most obvious example of this is the Oedipus myth as Freud has abstracted it to form the psycho-analytic theory. The function of the theoretical formulations in this category are interpretations being used with an intention to illuminate material, that would otherwise remain obscure, in order to help the patient to release still further material. [EP, 19]

It is in this sense that Bion made an affirmation that is at the base of many serious objections to his contributions, stemming from people whose grasp of psycho-analysis itself and views about the nature of life differ in an unbridgeable way:

> Freud's use of the Oedipus myth illuminated more than the nature of the sexual facets of the human personality. Thanks to his discoveries it is possible by reviewing the myth to see that it contains elements that were not stressed in the early investigations because they were overshadowed by the sexual component in the drama. The developments of psycho-analysis make it possible to give more weight to other features. First, the myth by virtue of its narrative form binds the various components of the story in a manner analogous to the fixation of the elements of a scientific deductive system by their inclusion in the system: it is similar to the fixation of the elements in the corresponding algebraic calculus where that exists. No element, such as the sexual element, can be comprehended save in its relationship with other elements; for example, with the determination with which Oedipus pursues his inquiry into the crime

> despite the warnings of Tiresias. It is consequently not possible
> to isolate the sexual component, or any other, without distortion.
> [EP, 45]

This is linked to some misunderstandings about the mathematical model that is used here, as an analogy: that of relationships
between objects. Psycho-analysis, mathematics and music share a
common invariance, namely, the three disciplines are able to study
relationships among objects.

Recommended cross-references: *Ad-hoc* theorizing, Container–
Contained, Dream, Grid, Manipulations of Symbols, Mathematization of Psycho-analysis, Myth and Private Myth.

Opinion (of the analyst): This entry is intended to clarify a frequent
misreading of Bion's work, in the view of the author. And it is quite
a dangerous one for the patient, for the psycho-analyst and for the
idea that the encircling social milieu has and will have about analytical practice.

It seems that the authoritarian-minded or idealistic reader is
prone to excise some single phrase from its whole context and use
it to legalize an analyst's belief, view, opinion or idea. This kind of
reading runs against the whole ethos of Bion's work and tries to
make it an affiliate of a philosophical trend born from unresolved
paranoid nuclei. It was variously called subjectivism, idealism (in
Kant's time), solipsism (in Freud's time) and nowadays, relativism.

It constitutes a serious denial of the existence of truth itself.
According to it there would be only personal views of the universe,
world and facts; in its extreme forms, reality itself would always be
a creation of an individual mind. There is no possibility to apprehend reality as it is; reality and truth are not issues to bother with,
except to naïves and simpletons unaware of social or ideological
determinants. Reality and truth are confused with absolute truth.
The ultimate unknowability of ultimate reality is mistaken for its
alleged non-existence; truth is reduced to a matter of individual
opinions, thus enthroning the emitter of the opinion, who becomes
indistinguishable from an opinionated being. There are already
some attempts to mix Bion's work with the post-modernist fashion.
Its accepted fashionable form appears under the guise of "individual readings", which would be the maximum one can attain.

Heisenberg's uncertainty principle was transformed, or better, debased into a principle of ignorance.

The relativist reader can dismiss this entry from the start, levelling against it the accusation that is his customary shield. What follows is just this author's "reading" of Bion, rather than a writing of Bion. Or that I—or anyone—is forbidden to follow Ruskin's advice, that one should try not to put one's own meanings into a text, but should try to see the author's meaning. This being the case, let Bion's writings speak for themselves.

Cogitations brought us Bion's reflections that were to be expanded later. The issue of truth and the analyst's opinion—that would resurface in *Transformations*—was first stated there. In the attempt to test a theory (dream-work-α) with empirical data, the issue of the truth value of the analyst's interpretations is emphasized.

> It is very important that the analyst knows not what **is** happening, but that he *thinks* it is happening. That is the only certitude to which he lays claim. If he does not know that he thinks such-and-such is happening, he has no grounds for making the interpretation . . . The theory that is being subjected to empirical test must be related to its power to enable the analyst to feel certain that he *thinks* that x is the case—not to its power to make certain that x is the case. The fact susceptible of empirical test is the certainty, or the degree of certainty, that the analyst can achieve about what he thinks is going on. He could say, "I quite realize that my view may be entirely wrong, but I do know that I am certain at any rate that *this* is my view". [C, 70]

The idealistic reader who is also prone to jump irritably and hastily to conclusions (because one cannot be sure that all idealists do this) would benefit from observing that Bion does not state that what *is* happening cannot be approached; he states that no approach to what is happening is possible if the analyst is not sincere with him(her) self. He sharply differentiates and establishes a priority, namely, that the "*power to enable the analyst to feel certain that he **thinks** that x is the case*" differs from the "*power to make certain that x is the case*"; and that the "*power to enable the analyst to feel certain that he **thinks** that x is the case*" is more important in a session than "*its power to make certain that x is the case*". There is no statement, at any time, that the analyst would have *"power to make certain that x is the case"*.

Years later he would throw more light on the issue: *"O, representing the unknowable ultimate reality can be represented by any formulation of a transformation—such as 'unknowable ultimate reality' which I have just formulated. It may therefore seem unnecessary to multiply representations of it; indeed from the psycho-analytic vertex that is true. But I wish to make it clear that my reason for saying that O is unknowable is not that I consider human capacity unequal to the task but because K, L, or H are inappropriate to O., They are appropriate to transformations of O but not to O"* (T, 140) (see entries K, L, H, O and Transformations). Or: *"reality is not something which lends itself to being known. It is impossible to know reality for the same reason that makes it impossible to sing potatoes; they may be grown, or pulled, or eaten, but not sung. Reality has to be 'been': there should be a transitive verb 'to be' expressly for use with the term 'reality'"* (T, 148).

In *Learning from Experience* Bion stressed the importance that truth has to the mind, comparable to that of water and nourishment to the physical body. And there appears a plea to analysts, to their sincerity. Perhaps this kind of statement may sound to relativistic ears to be a statement of contingency of truth or of its non-existence. But an unprejudiced ear can catch another gist:

> The aim in making the choice L, H or K [a choice that determines what kind of link, love, hate or knowledge, will dictate the nature of an interpretation] is to make one statement that is to the best of the analyst's belief true. It need not be a statement that accurately represents a realization of which it is the counterpart; the statement must seem to the analyst to be a true reflection of his feelings and one on which he can rely for a particularly important purpose, namely to act as a standard to which he can refer all the other statements that he proposes to make. [LE, 45]

In other words, echoing Thomas Paine, Bion elicits the faithfulness one must keep before oneself. It is not the belief in itself that matters. This being so, the analyst would be the most important person in the room. What matters is how faithful the analyst is to his belief, whatever it may be.

The first time that Bion inserts some matters of convenience for the analyst can be seen in the third chapter of *Transformations*. He is trying to classify the material that comes as the final views construed by the patient after receiving any stimulus. He names the original stimulus or experience "O", ultimate reality (q.v.) and the "material" (which also comprises an immaterial dimension), the final products of the transformations effected by the patient in "O", as Tpβ (q.v.):

> The problem of classifying the material is complicated because it contains elements of all three: TP, Tpα and Tpβ. It is a matter of consequence because the decision depends on what is most convenient for the analyst ... The problem is to reformulate Tpβ in conversational, but precise, English. [T, 26]

The *convenience* is restricted to a necessary direction that enables the communication to achieve the maximum possible effectiveness. That is, the convenience is patient-oriented rather than analyst-oriented, even though paradoxically it has to take into account each analyst's limitations. To know those limitations, albeit partially, ensures using them profitably (to make the best of a bad job), or avoiding them, etc. The paradox is often abhorred and in its "resolution", the professional tends to exaggerate the analyst's prerogatives, tastes, conveniences. A theory devised to discipline desire is used to enforce the analyst's desire.

The "opinion of the analyst" is in Chapter IV of the same book. The often-used phrase is *"Verbal expression must be limited so that it expresses truth without any implication other than the implication that it is true in the* **analyst's opinion***"*. Let us return it to the original text instead of splitting it off; it was adumbrated in the text of 1959 quoted above:

> Theory leaves us free to give Taβ (q.v.—the final products of the analyst's transformations on a given reality that is not created by the analyst) the value of the analyst's verbalization of his experience in the session, or the emotional state induced in his patient. That the analyst works on his patient's emotions as a painter might work on his canvas would be repugnant to psycho-analytic theory and practice. The painter who works on his public's emotions with an end in view is a propagandist with the outlook of the poster artist. He does not intend his public to be free in its choice of the use to which it puts the communication he makes. The analyst's

position is akin to that of the painter who by his art adds to his public's experience. Since psycho-analysts do not aim to run the patient's life but to enable him to run it according to his lights and therefore to know what his lights are, Taβ either in the form of interpretation or scientific paper should represent the psycho-analyst's verbal representation of an emotional experience. An attempt to exclude by restriction to verbal expression any element from Ta that would make it pass from the domain of communication of knowledge to propaganda would be inadequate. Verbal expression must be limited so that it expresses truth without any implication other than the implication that it is true in the *analyst's opinion*. How this is to be attempted lies outside the scope of this discussion, but for certain implications which I shall now consider. The first concerns the route by which we have arrived at this conclusion. It is sometimes assumed that the motive for scientific work is an abstract love for truth. The argument I have followed implies that the grounds for limiting the values that may be substituted for Taβ to true statements lies in the nature of values *not* so limited and their relationship to other components in the T theory. If truth is not essential to all values of Taβ, Taβ must be regarded as expressed in and by manipulation of the emotions of patient or public and not in or by the interpretation; truth is essential for any value of Taβ in art or science. How is truth to be a criterion for a value proposed to Taβ? To what has it to be true and how shall we decide whether it is or not? Almost any answer appears to make truth contingent on some circumstance or idea that is itself contingent. Falling back on analytic experience for a clue, I am reminded that healthy mental growth seems to depend on truth as the living organism depends on food. If it is lacking or deficient the personality deteriorates. I cannot support this conviction by evidence regarded as scientific. It may by be that the formulation belongs to the domain of Aesthetic. [T, 37–8]

That is, the text is almost an ode to the necessity for the analyst to be sincere with himself; to discipline his desire. But if it is taken out of context it can be used to enthrone the analyst's opinion or legalize the issuing of mere belief. Bion's passionate stress is on a necessity, namely, the analyst's active avoidance of delinquency, self-interest or vested-interests. Relativistic reading risks inducing the opposite of this, for an analyst indulging in his or her beliefs, conveniences or opinions is just imposing himself at the expense of anything else, including an attempt at useful practice. The restrictive posture would seem to put any other desires into abeyance and the analyst would just give personal opinions, thus sparing the patient undue influences, as, for example, of transference phantasies that turn analysis into counselling. But if it is enforced in a manner that diminishes the analyst's responsibility—he or she would be just giving "personal opinions", after all—it will have the opposite effect; the Olympian analyst thus created would speak with no responsibility other than to give personal ideas. It pleases the paranoid individual, who values his personal opinions so much, to the point of phantasizing that they would be a matter of importance to anyone other than him. The "analytic view" expressed by Bion would be a matter of no consequence. The freedom of the patient to use the analyst's communication as he can or prefers is taken at face value and will have no importance whatsoever to continuing investigating, and what the consequences are for the patient who uses them. If suicide or homicide ensues, the "opinionated analyst" has no reasons to bother; if the use is usefully used or not is the same; again, there is an open door for the "opinionated analyst" to act out unchecked.

Also, just the attitude that Bion explicitly recommends avoiding will be unchecked, namely, the seductive appeal that a free-for-all posture implicit in the libertine voicing of personal opinions that have no obligation other than to be personal opinions, allows. The solipsistic legalization of the individual opinion had, has and will have a broad appeal to mankind and prove to be popular: it is desire-fulfilling, pleasure-satisfying, omnipotence-serving. It has the appeal of drugs, *"substitutes employed by those who cannot wait"* (C, 299).

Giving personal opinions, in its extreme form, precludes scientific research, proof, refutation, evidence, counterparts in reality and is sheltered by a kind of pseudo-spontaneity: a seductive appeal, which turns the professional into a propagandist. Some patients, who are prone to aloofness, indifference, ideas of superiority, human insensitivity, will be especially attracted by this offer. They will collude and invite collusion: the very areas that would demand analysis will remain untouched, even though the analysand will display a syntonic and sympathetic attitude towards this kind of analyst. The professional who openly states "it is just a personal opinion" can also convince the patient of his profound awareness of his limitations, and humble attitudes may be seductive propaganda. Disguised as humbleness, paranoia is free to be rampant.

The best the "opinionated analyst" can aspire to is to be ineffectual and to waste his own and his patient's time. To take it lightly has serious consequences; not because according to some, "time is money", an optimistic and concretized outlook, but because time is life and there is no return of the time lost. There would be no room, for the "opinionated analyst", to consider phrases—to quote just one that was written in the preceding paragraphs: *"Since psychoanalysts do not aim to run the patient's life but to enable him to run it according to his lights and therefore to know what his lights are, Taβ either in the form of interpretation or scientific paper should represent the psycho-analyst's verbal representation of an emotional experience"* (T, 37).

Other goals of an analysis are stated in the entries **Analytic view, Atonement**

Let us examine in more detail the opinionated analyst's favourite catch-phrase extracted from Bion's text: *"An attempt to exclude by restriction to verbal expression any element from Ta that would make it pass from the domain of communication of knowledge to propaganda would be inadequate. Verbal expression must be limited so that it expresses truth without any implication other than the implication that it is true in the analyst's opinion"* (T, 37)

The emphasis is on an avoidance of a manipulation of the analysand's mind through omission and insincerity—Bion's passionate warning on refraining from giving a sincere opinion is followed by a recommendation of sincerity, rather than aloofly giving of personal opinions. The analyst's opinion is uncompromising with regard to truth but it is compromised with the patient's emotional experiences and views. It is external (patient's) reality-dependent, rather than exclusively inner (analyst's) reality dependent. The influence of the analyst's inner reality is a fact to be taken into account in order to be disciplined, rather than to get the upper hand. The analyst's personal formation, previous analysis, counter-transference, use of the Grid, are dealt with elsewhere in Bion's texts. They are real and taken for granted, and an awareness of them, albeit incomplete, is mandatory.

The opinionist falls short from perceiving that there is a fine paradox to be dealt with; truth obtrudes as a contrapuntal insight into the negative realm: *"The argument I have followed implies that the grounds for limiting the values that may be substituted for Taβ to true statements lies in the nature of values **not** so limited and their relationship to other components in the T theory"* (T, 37).

There is strong evidence of Bion's awareness of this danger. In discussing the immaterialness of the analytic endeavour, he makes a comparison with the mathematicians' task, who also works in the absence of objects: *"A theory of transformations must . . . constitute a system capable of the greatest number of uses . . . if it is to extend the analyst's capacity for working on a problem with or without the material components of the problem present.*

*This may seem to introduce a dangerous doctrine opening the way for the analyst who theorizes unhampered by the facts of practice, but the theory of transformations is inapplicable to any situation in which observation is not an essential. Observation is to be made and recorded in a form suitable for working **with** but inimical to wayward and undisciplined fabrications"* (T, 39–40).

The analyst who really thinks he is involved in an activity devoid of responsibility, and that his job is well done when he has just issued his opinions, could compare his catch-phrase and other mention of belief with: *"In general it may be said that the cultural background against which analytic work must be done is hardly a matter with which the individual analyst can concern himself; yet the culture may concern him . . . it is a matter of importance to analysts that the public image of our work is not distorted to produce a climate of opinion in which difficulties, already great, are enhanced"* (T, 11).

Suggested cross-references: At-one-ment, Becoming; O, Transformations in O, Transformations in K, K.

📖 *The Sense of Reality,* by I. Berlin; *Fashionable Non-Sense* by A. Sokol and J. Brickmont; *Against Relativism,* by I. Norris.

P

Pain: Pain was regarded by Bion as one of the elements of psycho-analysis (q.v.). This means that pain qualifies as something basic, fundamental, endowed with a structuring function in the human mind. As a matter of consequence, pain is a function in an analytic session.

> The case for acceptance of pain as an element of psycho-analysis is reinforced by the position it occupies in Freud's theories of the plea-sure–pain principle. It is evident that the dominance of the reality principle, and indeed its establishment, is imperilled if the patient swings over to the evasion of pain rather than to its modification; yet modification is jeopardized if the patient's capacity for pain is impaired. [EP, 62]

The relationship between pain and growth is discussed in the specific entry Growth. There is some evidence that Bion learnt from his varied life experiences, namely, war, the physical loss of a wife, and the psychic loss of his first wife and to a certain extent, of a daughter. All these experiences added to his doubts about his capacities for love and hate. His view of pain and fear does not deal with them as things-in-themselves. His focus is invariably directed to the difficulties of tolerating and enduring pain and fear. Specifically, the difficulties in making the quantum leap from—to quote his own terms—*"feeling pain"* to *"suffering it"* (AI, 9).

This is in stark contrast to the popular view, endorsed by the vast majority of professionals in the field of so-called mental illness, that one must unquestionably extinguish any pain, with no attention to its quality or quantity and much less to each individual's way of dealing with it. Freud had a view similar to Bion but he was not heard.

In one of his earliest papers Bion quotes John Donne in a telling way. It deals with pain, avoiding being prey either of the easy allegiance to attempts to extinguish it or attempts to co-opt it through sadism: *"Donne said that 'affliction is a treasure and scarce any man hath enough of it. No man hath affliction enough that is not matured and ripened by it.' No one to-day is likely to complain that there is any shortage in this commodity, but it is possible that our elaborate machinery, social as well as individual, for the denial of the existence of everyday troubles and difficulties has led to a revolt that has taken the form of an artificial production of calamity on a vast scale?"* (C, 346).

Bion's Huguenot (non-conformist offshoot of the Reformation) Christian formation as well as his grasp of the Christian and Jewish mystics probably exerted a great influence on his views. They were constantly conjoined with Freud's ideas on the need for abstinence in analytical work.

> Pain cannot be absent from the personality. An analysis must be painful, not because there is necessarily any value in pain, but because an analysis in which pain in not observed and discussed cannot be regarded as dealing with one of the central reasons for the patient's presence. The importance of pain can be dismissed as a secondary quality, something that is to disappear when conflicts are resolved; indeed most patients would take this view. Furthermore it can be supported by the fact that successful analysis does lead to diminution of suffering: nevertheless it obscures the need, more obvious in some cases than in others for the analytic experience to increase the patient's *capacity* for suffering even though patient and analyst may hope to decrease pain itself. The analogy with physical medicine is exact; to destroy a capacity for physical pain would be a disaster in any situation other than one in which an even greater disaster—namely death itself—is certain.
> [EP, 61–2]

The technical hint in dealing with pain relies on the concept of reversible perspective and it is seminal in clinical practice. Reversible perspective is a special use of projective identification in order to render a dynamic situation static.

> The work of the analyst is to restore dynamic to a static situation and so make development possible . . . the patient manoeuvres so that the analyst's interpretations are agreed; they thus become the outward sign of a static situation . . . In reversible perspective acceptance by the analyst of the possibility of a capacity for pain can help avoidance of errors that might lead to disaster. If the problem is not dealt with the patient's capacity to maintain the static situation may give way to an experience of pain so intense that a psychotic breakdown is the result. [EP, 60 and 62]

The word "static" can be seen as a verbal formulation of a manifestation of the death instincts; conversely, "dynamic" is the hallmark of life itself. There is an added complication, linked to the "economic problem of masochism": sadism is a way of establishing and inflicting pain in order to achieve pleasurable sensations.

The psychotic creation of pseudo-pain is akin to sadistic relationships; together with incapacity to suffer pain it runs parallel to, and disguises the capacity to feel pain. They are highlighted in Bion's work in many ways. Most useful is dependence on one's capacity to keep in touch with one's mind:

> There are patients whose contact with reality presents most difficulty when that reality is their own mental state. For example, a baby discovers its hand; it might as well have discovered its stomach-ache, or its feeling of dread or anxiety, or mental pain. In most ordinary personalities this is true, but people exist who are so intolerant of pain or frustration (or in whom pain or frustration is so intolerable) that they feel the pain but will not suffer it and so cannot be said to discover it. [AI, 9]

The analyst's state of mind is under scrutiny in that which puts analysis at stake:

> Developments of memory that are inevitable to the psycho-analyst are . . . the primacy of pleasure–pain (in contrast with reality or truth), and "possession" with its reciprocal, fear of loss; all have been acquired in close association with the senses.

The impulse to be rid of painful stimuli gives the "content" of the memory ... an unsatisfactory quality when one is engaged in the pursuit of truth O ... An analyst with such a mind is one who is incapable of learning because he is satisfied. [AI, 29]

If these excerpts lead some readers to conclude that there is an enshrining of pain (despite the quotation from EP, 62, above) they must be duly weighed:

The emotion to which attention is drawn should be obvious to the analyst, but unobserved by the patient; an emotion that is obvious to the patient is usually *painfully* obvious and avoidance of unnecessary pain must be one aim in the exercise of analytic intuition. Since the analyst's capacity for intuition should enable him to demonstrate an emotion before it has become *painfully* obvious it would help if our search for the elements of emotions was directed to making intuitive deductions easier. [EP, 74]

There was movement at the other end of the hall. Two or three men and a woman came in with a jug of water and what might have been surgical instruments. The water was cold. They talked amongst themselves, but otherwise paid no attention to the two girls except to wash them and clean their bodies thoroughly, with no more concern for them than if they had been inanimate ... A little later Rosemary, exasperated by an unusually painful scrape between her fingers—they were usually too expert to inflict pain unless with intent ...

the team withdrew and were replaced by medical assessors. The room which had been allowed to become dark, was flooded with bright light. This time there was no conversation and when Alice asked one man if they were to be given food and facilities of a sanitary kind, she was so alarmed by his ferocious gaze that she fell silent.

The medical examination was minute and thorough. The wishes of the two girls were of no consequence. There could have been no more convincing evidence that they were irrelevant than the way the examination was carried out on this and subsequent occasions. It was a daily routine expeditiously carried out. [AMF, I, 27–8]

📖 Pain and avoidance of it, as well as its linking with projective identification, are fully realised in Bion's autobiographical cycle, *A Memoir of the Future*, *The Long Week End* and *War Memoirs*.

Paramnesias: Bion asked if all psycho-analytic theory should be regarded as a vast paramnesia intended unconsciously to fill the void of our ignorance (*Bion's Brazilian Lectures*, I, 1973; "Evidence", 1976; "Emotional turbulence", 1977; *A Memoir of the Future*). An earlier approach to the issue was made through warnings about *ad hoc* theorizing (in *Transformations*).

> ROLAND Yes; but is there any evidence for a mind at all? It has no colour, smell, or any other sensuous component. Why should not the whole of psycho-analysis be just a vast, towering Babel of paramnesias to fill the gap where our ignorance ought to be? [AMF, III, 540]

Please refer to the entries, "Analytic view" and "Manipulations of symbols", where the issue is further expanded.

Parasitic: From biology, Bion suggests a model of a link, to be amended to the model of container and its possible relations with the contained. This model entails three possibilities of relationship between a host and its guest: the commensal, the parasitic and the symbiotic. Bion uses this model in order to illuminate (i) the real link between mother and child; (ii) the parental relationship; (iii) the relationship of analysand with the analyst during the session; (iv) and the process of thinking.

See entry, "Link". The parasitic link is further expanded under the heading, "second model of links".

Penis: Bion dedicated himself more to the development of observational theories for the psycho-analyst's use, rather than creating new theories of psycho-analysis. The latter, after all, usually simply add to the huge apparatus of plausible theories already available—quite independent of their practical value.

One of the few exceptions—that would remain unpublished during his lifetime—was a paper entitled "Metatheory". It was an attempt to describe *scientifically* some elementary basics of psycho-analysis. One of its items is entitled, "Penis"; like "breast" it was devised to function as a practical guideline that served to discern a "*class of interpretations*" (C, 253).

Bion's attempt was to formulate a stopgap during an epoch when a fully scientific theory and method were not available in psycho-analysis: *"I propose to improvise temporary solutions of our problems by these short interjections of metatheory between the discussions of successive elements of theory"* (C, 254). The *"interpretation penis"* is made in conjunction with the *"interpretation breast"* (please refer to the entry, Breast). All that Bion says about the Breast applies to the Penis (C, 253). It is *"in its visual aspect ... more elongated than the breast . . . These two interpretations, breast and penis, are plastic; that is to say that in the mind their visual image can alter enormously and yet retain its identifiability without loss or diminution"* (C, 254).

Suggested cross-reference: Breast.

Penumbra of associations: A quest for precision in psycho-analytical communication marks all of Bion's work. He took many measures to be as unambiguous as possible when using verbal formulations. At the same time he tried to illuminate the possible penumbra of associations that some terms already had, or could be invested with. With this illumination he could use the term with the meaning he wished to convey.

In this sense his writings echo Freud's; both seemed to be constantly "talking" with imaginary readers—who could be quite critical! In Bion's case the criticisms appear not always to be imaginary. Some came from himself, constituting self-criticisms. Some were the result of the previous reading of the manuscripts by some of his friends or colleagues.

The first time one spots a mention of a penumbra of associations is in the Introduction to *Learning from Experience*. Those who read the paper "A theory of thinking" (q.v.) had already noticed a sudden and quite unexpected use of the philosophy of mathematics (see entry Circle, Point, Line). There Bion puts the question of the number three, referring to Oedipus, and two, referring to the me and not-me (the breast). Or, in more precise terms, the senses of "two-ness" and "three-ness". The reader informed in mathematics would instantly recognize Gottlob Frege's theories of numbers. Nevertheless Bion would make the origin of this sense of quality explicit only nine years later, in 1970, after also resorting more heavily to other achievements in the philosophy of mathematics, that of the concept of transformations and invariances (q.v.).

One may consider the paper "A theory of thinking" as a kind of first chapter of *Learning from Experience*. But he chose as the

Introduction to this book a rather different text (from which we have at least one other version that was published in *Cogitations*, thirty years later).

This text is crystal clear concerning his use and borrowing (the term to borrow is Bion's) of concepts and verbal formulations stemming from philosophy and mathematics. Perhaps it would be useful to keep in mind what he writes there when reading any of his texts:

> It may seem that I am mis-using words with an established meaning, as in my use of the terms function and factors. A critic has pointed out to me that the terms are used ambiguously and the sophisticated reader may be misled by the associations of both words with mathematics and philosophy. I have deliberately used them because of the association, and I wish the ambiguity to remain. I want the reader to be reminded of mathematics, philosophy and common usage, because a characteristic of the human mind I am discussing may develop in such a way that it is seen at a later stage as classifiable under those headings—and others. [LE, second page of the Introduction]

In this case, Bion was specifically concerned with the terms factor and function, but the situation applies throughout his writings. The reader who takes the term "ambiguity" too literally will split it off from the context, and will be misled. He will lose sight of the fact that ambiguity means having two meanings. This is the basis of the analytic approach: the manifest discourse has underlying meanings that can be elicited. Any practising psycho-analyst is accustomed to the fact that patients often accuse him of mis-using their words. The issue at stake is the fact that the analyst searches for underlying meanings—a quest often stressed by Bion (see entry "Analytic View").

Bion's quest for precision in communication can be seen, for example, when eliciting the concretization involved in the psychotic's intolerance of the breast. He classifies it as an extraordinary view and compares that view with an ordinary view of the no-breast, which tolerates it:

> I can differentiate the views by regarding the extra-ordinary view as backward-looking and relating to what has been lost, and the

ordinary view as forward-looking and relating to what can be found. Such a differentiation is not convenient because it implies a penumbra of associations, and therefore has implications, that limit my freedom of discussion. I shall therefore denote the extra-ordinary view by the sign −K and the ordinary view by the sign K. [T, 77]

Once he used it in order to display the usefulness of colloquial language: *"If the psycho-analytical situation is accurately intuited—I prefer this term to 'observed' or 'heard' or 'seen' as it does not carry the penumbra of sensuous association—the psycho-analyst finds that ordinary conversational English is surprisingly adequate for the formulation of his interpretation"* (ST, 134).

Therefore one may conclude that he avoided penumbras when they meant cloudy confusions.

Personal equation: Freud observed the "personal equation" (Freud, 1926, 1938)—the fact that the analyst's personality influences his perceptions. With this he showed that the observer interferes in the object observed. He did this years before the quantum physicists finally discovered it.

The issue was revived by Ferenczi alone. To know at least part of this interference and how to deal with it is decisive in analysis. It is decisive because the object of study and the method of studying it are the same—the human mind. How can we gauge if the analyst's views about his patient are not attributable to himself?

Freud's method of minimizing the personal factor was the analyst's personal analysis. Bion equates the personal equation described by Freud to countertransference, as did Freud:

I shall ignore disturbance produced by the analyst's personality or aspects of it. The existence of such disturbance is well known and its recognition is the basis for analytic acceptance of the need for analysts to be analysed and the many studies of counter-transference. While other scientific disciplines recognize the personal equation, or the factor of personal error, no science other than psycho-analysis has insisted on such a profound and prolonged investigation of its nature and ramifications. [T, 48]

Earlier Bion had emphasized the need not to pass judgement when analysing or observing, resorting to a quotation from Darwin [LE, 86]

Phenomena: Bion uses this term exactly in the sense that Kant used it—phenomena are the ways that emanations and presentations of real reality (or numinous realm), or the secondary qualities of objects can be apprehended by the human sensuous apparatus.

It is used in "A theory of thinking", in *Learning from Experience*, and in *Elements of Psycho-analysis* in order to present the first and final versions of the theory of alpha-function (q.v.) (ST, 115, LE, 67; EP, 6–9). This function depicts a process of depuration where the sensuous and concrete component of the phenomena is extracted. It was further expanded when dealing with transformations (T, 12).

The non-sensuous immaterial counterpart of phenomena, that is, the noumenon, is symbolized by "O". See entry "O".

Philosophy:

> Abandonment of memories and models derived from physical medicine involves experience of problems which the psycho-analyst may regard as outside his province or capacity; often they appear to belong to disciplines to which his training is not extended. The psycho-analyst's experience of philosophical issues is so real that he often has a clearer grasp of the necessity for a philosophical background than the professional philosopher. The academic philosophic background and the realistic foreground of psycho-analytical experience approach each other; but recognition of the one by the other does not occur as often or as fruitfully as one might expect. [ST, 151–2]

Bion uses past achievements of philosophers but he makes sharp distinctions between the analyst and the philosopher; as a matter of consequence, between psychoanalysis and philosophy. Psycho-analysis since the time of Freud is part of scientific endeavour to the extent that it deals with truth, reality and mind. Before there was a Freud to think psycho-analysis, the task of investigating or at least nourishing interest in truth, reality and mind fell to philosophers. It is no wonder that Bion draws from their experience.

> . . . I am primarily concerned to present a theoretical system. Its resemblance to a philosophical theory depends on the fact that philosophers have concerned themselves with the same subject matter; it differs from philosophical theory in that it is intended, like all psycho-analytical theories, for use. [ST, 110]

... one advantage that the psycho-analyst possesses over the philosopher; his statements can be related to realization and realizations to a psycho-analytic theory. [T,44]

Five years later he would reaffirm the same: *"... the psycho-analyst is concerned **practically** with a problem that the philosopher approaches **theoretically**"* (AI, 97).

When, as psycho-analysts, we are concerned with the reality of the personality there is more at stake than an exhortation to "know thyself, accept thyself, be thyself", because implicit in psycho-analytic procedure is the idea that this exhortation cannot be put into practice without the psycho-analytic experience. The point at issue is how to pass from "knowing phenomena" to "being" that which is "real". [T, 148]

The use that Bion makes of Kant and of some mathematical theories is often seen as "wrong" by narrow-minded academics (please see the entry, "University"):

It may seem that I am mis-using words with an established mean-ing, as in my use of the terms functions and factors. A critic has pointed to me that the terms are used ambiguously and the sophis-ticated reader may be misled by the association of both words with mathematics and philosophy. I have deliberately used them because of the association, and I wish the ambiguity to remain. I want the reader to be reminded of mathematics, philosophy and common usage, because a characteristic of the human mind I am discussing may develop in such a way that it is seen at a later stage to be classifiable under those headings—and others. [LE, Introduction, 2]

Therefore, due to Freud, an issue that hitherto was the concern of philosophers and religious people is now the object of science. The following phrase echoes Freud's posture:

Psycho-analytic procedure pre-supposes that the welfare of the patient demands a constant supply of truth as inevitably as his physical survival demands food. It further presupposes that discov-ery of the truth about himself is a precondition of an ability to learn the truth, or at least to seek it in his relationship with himself and others. It is supposed at first that he cannot discover the truth about himself without assistance from the analyst and others. [C, 99]

The limitations of the philosophers to deal with the issues the analyst deals with are emphasized; this emphasis alone should help to discriminate Bion's use of some philosophical contributions: ". . . *the philosopher . . . falls back defeated when the factor of emotional impulses obtrude. This will, I am sure, be very ably denied. That is my point: it is the function of philosophy to deny it"* (C, 341).

Bion's philosophical sources

The following table is an attempt to summarize some of Bion's philosophical sources. Many of them were made apparent in *A Memoir of the Future*
  1)   Confirmed (see Table 2a)
  2)   Inferred, to be confirmed (see Table 2b)

Point: Many readers of Bion still wonder, what has the point to do with psychoanalysis?
  This mathematical achievement, point, is regarded by Bion as the graphic representative of the tolerance of the no-breast. It depends on the tolerance of frustration in mankind. It is an early attempt to deal with psychosis. The point is both a representative and a representation. Later it may represent the thought whose inception was marked by the tolerance of the no-breast. *"The thought, represented by a word or other sign, may, when it is significant as a no-thing, be represented by a point (.). The point may then represent the position where the breast was, or may even be the no-breast"* (T, 82)
  Taking into account that this dictionary already has an entry named "Circle, Point, Line", why are we including an entry exclusive to the point? It is because of its basic nature: the point is the barest, irreducible, ultimate and most resilient bastion of reality itself. If it is a device that gauges everyone's ability to tolerate frustration and therefore reality as it is—in its simplest terms—it is refractory to hallucination and imagination.
  The point is indestructible because it is not sensible to mind's attempts at evasion and subservience to the principle of pleasure/ displeasure. It is indestructible to the same extent that reality itself is

Table 2a   Confirmed philosophical sources (writings of Bion and the personal library of Wilfred and Francesca Bion)

Category	Period/group	Name	Inspiration and use	Where to find the reference	Where is it in Bion's work?
Philosophers	Antiquity	Plato	Ideal forms Nous–mind which thinks about itself	*Republic, Phaedro*	T; AMF I, II, III LE; EP. T; AI
		Aristotle	Mathematical objects–psychoanalytical objects	*Metaphysics*	
	Judaeo-Christian tradition	Isaac Luria	He established a system of interpretative construction through the "sepiroth" that extracts from the "holy" scriptures some implicit, deeper and truthful meaning that is not given directly by words, but is already there. Therefore the text reveals itself but means things other than itself	*On the Kabbalah and its Symbolism* (George Scholem, Martin Buber)	AI; AMF I, II, III
		Meister Eckhart	Human truth and divinity		T; AMF I, II, III
		St John of the Cross	The domain of "minus", intuiting the truth on the basis of experiencing the negative, sensory dispossession, abstinence and pain		T; AMF I, II, III
		William Blake	On cruelty, on woman, and on the truth	Blake's engravings to his books and novels *The Book of Urizen* and *The Book of Job*	AMF I, II, III; C, e.g. p. 125

(continued)

Table 2a Confirmed philosophical sources (*continued*)

Category	Period/group	Name	Inspiration and use	Where to find the reference	Where is it in Bion's work?
Philosophers	Middle Ages and Renaissance	Thomas Browne	Non-subordination to dogmatic authority		EG
		Francis Bacon Giambattista Vico	Facts as they are Historicity	*Essays*	T; AMF I, II, III AMF I, II, III
		René Descartes	Bion criticizes Descartes for having advocated philosophical doubt without practising it. The concept of "thought without a thinker" was an original formulation of Descartes, but he argues that such an idea is absurd. There is a similarity with Freud, who distinguished a scientific validity in facts which are spurned by positivist science, like dreams. Bion employs Descartes's idea without being under the sway of the "great philosopher"—he shows how it is useful to take into account the fact that thoughts are epistemologically prior to the thinker	*Discourse on Method*	ST (*A Theory of Thinking*); LE; EP; T; AI; AMF I, II, III

(*continued*)

Table 2a Confirmed philosophical sources (*continued*)

Category	Period/group	Name	Inspiration and use	Where to find the reference	Where is it in Bion's work?
Philosophers	Philosophers of the Enlightenment and the Romantic period	John Locke	"Common sense" (it is different from trivialization, "commonplace" and "good sense")	*Essay on Human Understanding*	LE; EP; C
		David Hume	Constant conjunction	*An Enquiry Concerning Human Understanding*	ST (*A Theory of Thinking*); EP; T
		Samuel Johnson	The truth of facts as they are	*Life of Samuel Johnson* (Boswell)	ST (*A Theory of Thinking*); EP; T; AMF I, II, III
		Alexander Pope	Warnings against false science; trivialization, "the English spirit"	Alexander Pope *Epistle to Dr. Arbuthnot* *Essay on Criticism* (quoted in Bion AMF I, p. 42)	AMF I, II, III
		Immanuel Kant	Primary and secondary qualities; noumena and phenomena; the concepts and sensible intuition	*The Critique of Pure Reason* (Kant, 1990) *History of Philosophy* (Copleston)	EP; T;, AMF I, II, III
		Johann Goethe	Errors of value-judgement; method of dialogical writing, Woman	*Faust*	AMF I, II, III

(*continued*)

Table 2a   Confirmed philosophical sources (*continued*)

Category	Period/group	Name	Inspiration and use	Where to find the reference	Where is it in Bion's work?
Philosophers	Philosophers of the Enlightenment and the Romantic	W. F. Hegel	Perception of the truth, limits of idealism, religion, rational processes and the acquisition of human consciousness, the infinite and the absolute	*Nature and Destiny of Man* (Niebuhr, 1941–43) *History of Philosophy* (Copleston); *Scientific Explanation* (Bradley and Prichard, quoted by Bion, C, pp. 3, 14, 27, 32, 84, 151, 157	ST (*A Theory of Thinking*); EP; T; AI; AMF I, II, III; C
		F. Nietzsche		*History of Philosophy* (Copleston)	AMF I, II, III
Philosophers of Mathematics		Blaise Pascal	Intuition, limits and possibilites of the search for truth	*Penséea*	ST (*A Theory of Thinking*); EP; T; AMF I, II, III
		Sylvester and Cayley	The concept of T and invariants	Eric Temple Bell	
		Jules Henri Poincaré	Selected fact, intuition	Poincaré's *Science and Method* (quoted by Bion, C, pp. 2, 284)	ST (*A Theory of Thinking*); EP; T; AMF I, II, III
		Brouwer	Intuitionism, non-Euclidean geometry, non-Euclidean logic	*Intuitionism—An Introduction* (Heyting, 1971)	AMF I, II, III

(*continued*)

Table 2a   Confirmed philosophical sources (*continued*)

Category	Period/group	Name	Inspiration and use	Where to find the reference	Where is it in Bion's work?
Philosophers of Mathematics		A. N. Whitehead / B. Russell	Theory of numbers	*History of Mathematics* (Whitehead, 1911)	
Philosophers of Physics		Max Planck	Quantum theory, resistance to new ideas	Scientific autobiography	T
		Albert Einstein	Relativity		AMF I, II, III
		Werner Heisenberg	Uncertainty principle		T; AMF I, II, III;
					C
Philosophers of Science	Historians of scientific ideas	Prichard	The idea that intuition allows for the direct perception of concrete objects and permits knowledge of universals and their relations	*Knowledge and Perception* (Prichard)	C
		Braithwaite	Ideas and reality, Kant and Hegel	*Scientific Explanation* (Braithwaite)	C
	Neo-positivists	Bradley	Humean induction, probability, causality	*The Principles of Logic* (Bradley)	C
		Karl Popper	Bion profited from Popper's opinion on *ad hoc* theories. He refutes Popper's criteria of scientificity for psycho-analysis (Popper, 1959)	*The Logic of Scientific Discovery* (Popper)	LE; T; AMF I, II, III
		P. Tarski	Value–truth of assertions	*History of Philosophy* (Copleston), *Introduction to Metamathematics* (Kleene)	T
		Rudolph Carnap	Rules for making assertions	*Introduction to Meta-mathematics* (Kleene)	T

Table 2b   Inferred philosophical sources (personal library of Wilfred and Francesca Bion)

Category	Period/group	Name	Inspiration and use	Where to find reference	Where is it in Bion's work?
Philosophers	Enlightenment and Romantic Period	Voltaire	Critique of discourse, the outside as a source of scorn	*Candide*	AMF I, II, III
		Denis Diderot	Formulation of human truth in the form of dialogues		AMF I, II, III
Philosophers of Mathematics		Bertrand Russell	Russell's paradoxes, theory of numbers personal authority	*History of Western Philosophy* (Russell)	T
Philosophers of Science	Historians of scientific ideas	Isaiah Berlin	Sense of reality	*The Sense of Reality* (Berlin)	ST (*A Theory of Thinking*); EP; T; AI; AMF I, II, III

indestructible. The perception of it can be obliterated, damaged and even extinguished during a human being's lifetime. Nevertheless, reality itself is not destroyed if the perception of it is. "*Truth is robust*" and will prevail (for example, AMF, III, 499).

The point may be the most irreducible representation of truth hitherto available, the truth of frustration: "*The fragmentation of point and line cannot go beyond the point; though the line may be annihilated, having been transformed into a series of points, to a single point, to the place where the point was, this last is still a point. The point is thus indestructible*" (T, 95).

Suggested cross-references: Circle, Point, Line, Mathematization of Psycho-analysis, Real psycho-analysis.

Pre-conception, preconception, premonition:

> This term represents a state of expectation. The term is the counterpart of a variable in mathematical logic or an unknown in mathematics. It has the quality that Kant ascribes to an empty thought in that it can be thought but cannot be known. [LE, 91]

Bion suggests that human beings have two innate pre-conceptions. The concept of pre-conception is used in the sense first formulated by Kant. It corresponds to Freud's protophantasies (Freud, 1920). Bion isolated two basic pre-conceptions to start with: that of the Breast (in "A theory of thinking") and that of Oedipus (In *Elements of Psycho-analysis*).

Fresh pre-conceptions are continuously formed during any period of learning. Depending on the epistemophilic, life, and death instincts, the process may span a given individual's whole period of life. They add to a growing arsenal of knowledge. There is a difference between the two initial or start-up pre-conceptions and those that mark an evolution in maturation and its opposite (see below).

Bion tackled the vicissitudes of apprehension of reality, internal and external. In order to do this he makes a conjunction of Plato, Kant, Freud and Klein. Many regarded Bion's as a novel approach. A detailed scrutiny of the history of western civilization's ideas shows that Klein and Freud were not only inheritors of the Platonic approach—they gave a practical application to it. Bion made this fact explicit; the novelty concerns the integrative form of the approach but not the approach in itself.

In order to deal with the inception of thought processes—thus inserting himself in the field of the researchers of the ontology of human thinking—Bion looks for elementary elements. He adds an earlier stage to the functions of ego as described by Freud in 1910/11 ("Formulations on the two principles of mental functioning"). This stage is so primitive that it precedes the infant's obstetric birth; therefore it precedes the phase of notation described by Freud.

Through living experience with people (the so-called psychotics) who could not form concepts, Bion created a practical application of philosophical problems. *"I am anxious to establish the elements of psycho-analysis on a foundation of experience"* (EP, 8).

The Kantian concept that Bion uses is that of "pre-conceptions". They correspond to a priori knowledge, which is quite independent of pure reason or dogma. It refers to inborn notions with which humans seem to be endowed. In Kant's work there are two "a prioris": time and space. As we have seen, Bion hypothesizes that there are two inborn pre-conceptions: that of the breast and that of Oedipus.

First he tackles the breast: *"The pre-conception may be regarded as the analogue in psycho-analysis of Kant's concept of 'empty thoughts'. Psycho-analytically the theory that the infant has an inborn disposition corresponding to an expectation of a breast may be used to supply a model"* (ST, 111).

Bion makes an attempt to display the evolution of thought processes. At first he adumbrates a theory of thinking. In 1961, he proposes that pre-conceptions mate with realizations and thus form conceptions. This mating is always incomplete. It is just its incompleteness that allows the inception of thought processes. The experience of a negative realization, the para 100 quanta of no-breast, allows for an abstraction of the "breastness". It is abstracted from the breast. The abstraction is immaterial; it shapes psychic reality; it is the psychic realization (or symbolization) of the Breast. A breast (concrete, sensuously apprehensible) turns into Breast.

"If intolerance of frustration is not so great as to activate the mechanisms of evasion and yet is too great to bear dominance of the reality principle, the personality develops omnipotence as a substitute for the mating

of the pre-conception, or conception, with the negative realization" (ST, 114). This is the first moment in Bion's work that he refers to the Hegelian realm of the negative, which is also the realm of Platonic Ideas, the realm of the unconscious. Bion does not quote Hegel.

Two years later (1963), in *Elements of Psycho-Analysis*, the concept of pre-conception was further developed in two directions. (i) One of them was as a part of the theory of thinking, now more expanded to fit into Freud's functions of the ego in thinking processes; (ii) the other was an embryonic attempt to depict the analyst's mental states, to be further developed in his next book, *Transformations*.

The first direction materializes in the Grid (for a more detailed description please refer to this entry). It is an epistemological tool to evaluate the truth-value of verbal statements and the relative value of these statements in terms of emotional growth. In this first direction we must distinguish two situations: (i) the term was placed as a step in genetic development of thoughts (corresponding to the Grid's vertical axis, or lines); (ii) the term refers to counterparts in reality that it (the term) strives to approximate; the Grid provides still another category which Bion named "Definitory hypothesis".

The second direction is linked to the analyst's mental state. It was named "preconception", non-hyphenated, by Bion. We shall see this later.

Pre-conception

Definitory hypothesis is also a Kant-inspired concept and would correspond to a primitive state of a proto-mind. It is an inchoate; in terms of the Grid it performs the function of the ego and it is at the same time a genetic concept. It is a kind of origin of thoughts. With reference to its function, it shares with pre-conceptions the status of an expectant state. It carries within it the ethos of a pre-conception but it differs from it to the extent that it is more primitive. Being inborn, it is previous to sensory stimulation and previous to the influx of beta-elements. It waits for them.

Now Bion assigns a new function to the 3-year-old concept of pre-conception which depends on the fate of definitory hypothesis. This new function slightly alters the earlier definition. Pre-conception is now much more a turning point, albeit a fundamental one, rather than a starting point of thoughts as it was hitherto. It admits even more primitive precursors—definitory hypotheses, beta-elements, alpha-elements.

The new function of pre-conceptions fits it more clearly into Freud's theory of functions of the ego. Genetically speaking, when beta-elements, so to say, are "thrown over" an individual (external or internal stimuli) they may "strike" with definitory hypotheses.

The model shows that from there on alpha-elements may ensue through the action of alpha-function. They are the building blocks of myths, dreams, dream thoughts. From there the pre-conceptions, heirs of a phylogenetic and ontogenetic development, will happen.

Bion defines pre-conceptions in a more precise way compared with his definition of 1961 through assigning line 4 of the Grid to them: "*this corresponds to a state of expectation. It is a state of mind adapted to receive a restricted range of phenomena. An early occurrence might be an infant's expectation of the breast. The mating of pre-conception and realization brings into being the conception*" (EP, 23 [Phenomena are always understood in the Kantian sense; EP, 9]). The preconception has a quasi-mathematical notation: the formula of a constant (ψ) together with an unsaturated element (ξ).

Instead of assigning the value of naming to concepts and instead of seeing them as fixed, Bion now assigns the activity of naming to the formation of pre-conceptions. But now they are at once, paradoxically, "fixed"—thus the constant (ψ) element, and the unsaturated (ξ) element. Both the constant or fixed and the mobile or not-fixed function together. The constant is needed to encircle a field and prevent infinite fragmentation: "*It will be observed that this theory of the name as that which prevents scattering of phenomena so that they can function as a pre-conception . . .*" (EP, 88). This development occurred together with the development of the concept of container/contained (q.v.) This notion would linger on in invariances and transformations (q.v.) two years later. For now, Bion makes explicit that, "*The term 'pre-conception' is ambiguous because it denotes a tool, the function for which exists and the use to which it may be put . . .*" (EP, 89).

Definitory hypotheses and pre-conceptions both share the qualities of being precursors.

Preconception

Let us now turn to the second direction. It is related to the analyst's state of mind and was named "preconception", non-hyphenated. Preconception is defined as belonging to *"the domain of emotion"*. Bion adumbrates it as *"something that is reminiscent of the relationship of pre-conception to conception"* (EP, 75).

The original edition of *Elements of Psycho-Analysis* contains a misprint: the word pre-conception in this phrase omitted the hyphen. Preconceptions (non-hyphenated) are now defined as *"the analyst's theoretical preconceptions"*, which refers *"to the use of a theory"*.

While pre-conceptions appertain to **line** 4 of the Grid, preconception means states of ego, or stages of ego functions (in Freud's sense), namely, notation and attention—**columns** 3 and 4. This is a sharp difference between pre-conceptions and preconceptions: the former is the verbal formulation of a **genetic** phase in the evolution of thoughts and the latter is the verbal formulation of an **emotional** state concerning the **analyst's use** of analytic theories.

Those theories are used as ancillary frameworks that may help the analyst's expectant state when he may detect precursors of emotions. This is fundamental to detecting the elements of a psycho-analytic session and of a patient's psychic reality. It is a way to diminish the pain involved in the patient's specific plight and in analytic intuition (EP, 74).

The search is for precursors; it allows the exercising of **premonition**. The analyst does not look for properties only; the analyst does not stop at appearances. At that time, Bion did not have available the concept of invariances. The concept of selected fact seemed to have some limitations when emotions were involved and it seems that he was trying to find more effective means to find out what really happens during an analytic session—a question that brings to the fore the goals of psycho-analysis. At that time, it seemed that to look for fundamentals—elements—was one of those goals. It seemed to endow the analytic theory with scientific soundness. The search for the underlying unconscious fact was the task: *". . . for my purpose the term 'element' cannot be properly seen to denote something that would appear to be a property of some more fundamental thing whose presence it betrays . . . if the hate that a patient is experiencing* *is a precursor of love its virtue as an element resides in its quality as a precursor of love and not in its being hate"* (EP, 74) (see also entry Minus).

Premonition

To detect precursors, Bion resorts to still another definition: *"The counterpart of the preconception is the **premonition**. Directly observed emotional states are significant only as premonitions"* (EP, 75). Or, "O" is unknowable, and when an analyst and a patient are in the session, they tend to deal with emotions as if they were ultimate realities. In fact they are pointers that both indicate and hide something. This concept is examined under its specific entry in this dictionary.

☮ Twelve years later, the question of theories, pre-conceptions, preconceptions and premonitions were presented in novel forms in some good-humoured ways. This writing is from his later phase; he was free to draw analogies from mystics and from music and poetry. One notices that "precursors", "pre-conceptions" and so on are replaced by terms such as "prelude":

> PAUL . . . St. John of the Cross even said that reading his own works could be a stumbling block if they were revered to the detriment of direct experience. Teachings, dogma, hymns, congregational worship, are supposed to be preludes to religion proper—not final ends in themselves.
>
> P.A. This sounds not unlike a difficulty which we experience when psycho-analytic jargon—"father figures" and so forth—
>
> ROBIN Touché!
>
> P.A. —are substituted for looking into the patient's mind itself to intuit that to which the psycho-analyst is striving to point: like a dog that looks at its master's pointing hand rather than at the object the hand is trying to point out. [AMF, II, 267]

In 1965 he made clear those origins of his work. They could be seen by the attentive, or philosophically and psycho-analytically informed reader. He makes clear that Melanie Klein was not in agreement with him about the pre-conception of the breast. Perhaps it was his scientific honesty that made him make public this private talk with Klein. It is recorded in *Transformations*, page 138.

> I claim Plato as a supporter for the pre-conception, the Kleinian internal object, the inborn anticipation. Melanie Klein objected in conversation with me to the idea that the infant had an inborn pre-conception of the breast, but though it may be difficult to produce evidence for the existence of a realization that approximates to this theory, the theory itself seems to me to be useful as a contribution to a vertex I want to establish. Phenomena, the term being used as Kant might use it, are transformed into representations, Tβ. Tβ may then be regarded as a representation of the individual's experience O, but the significance of O derives from and inheres in the Platonic Form. [T, 138]

As pointed out above, aside from the breast, Oedipus was seen as one of the pre-conceptions. A reminder may be not outside the scope of this dictionary: the Kantian concept was extensively demonstrated by Darwin and Mendel; Freud used it and Bion unearthed it—now more explicitly. Pre-conceptions are used by Bion as a step in the genesis and evolution of thought processes, but the pre-conceptions he described bridge material with psychic reality. Perhaps in the future other researchers will be able to describe other pre-conceptions, if they exist at all.

The ethos of the concept of pre-conception as well as that of the psycho-analytical object (q.v.) would survive as the ontogenetic model of the process of thinking.

With regard to a finer view of those processes in the analytic session, as a part of a theory of observation, the theory of Transformations and Invariances would supersede it. The unsaturated component would be seen as a question of cycles of transformations, where the final products of a given cycle serve as a starting point for a new process of transformations. The Invariances correspond to the constants.

Bion and Klein

The pre-conceptions proved to be expansions of Freud and Klein. As we stated above, Bion makes clear that Melanie Klein put forward, in a private communication with him, her disagreement about the existence of a pre-conception of the breast. Also, his suggestion of a precursor of the Oedipal situation is not made, according to him, in *"the sense that such a term might have in Melanie Klein's discussion of 'Early Phases of the Oedipus Complex', but as something that belongs to the ego as part of its apparatus for contact with reality"* (EP, 93). This is a private myth, and is dealt with in its corresponding entry of this dictionary.

Suggested cross-references: Concept, Conception, Myth, Premonition.

Premonition: Bion uses this term in *Elements of Psycho-analysis* in order to represent some emotional states as compared with ideational contents. In this sense, they are precursors of more developed mental states. The latter are called "pre-conceptions".

The emotions that pervade a premonition define it. They are *"a sense of warning and anxiety. The feeling of anxiety is of value in guiding the analyst to recognize the premonition in the material ... Analysis must be conducted so that the conditions for observing pre-monitions exist, a conclusion compatible with Freud's definition of the analytic situation as one in which an atmosphere of deprivation is dominant. If premonitions cannot be experienced correct interpretation becomes difficult for the analyst to give and difficult for the analysand to grasp; unnecessary pain ... becomes more likely"* (EP, 76).

Suggested cross-references: Pre-conception, Real Analysis.

Principle of pleasure/pain: A verbal formulation equivalent to Freud's formulation of the principle of pleasure/displeasure. The modification was not explicitly explained; it was simply presented in many parts of his work.

⏚ Perhaps the first time it was formulated is in *Elements of Psycho-analysis*, p. 62; it was repeated in *Transformations*, p. 73 and in *Attention and Interpretation*.

See entry, Principles of Mental Functioning.

Principle of reality: See entry, Principles of Mental Functioning.

Principle of uncertainty: Heisenberg's uncertainty principle is used by Bion in *Transformations* and in *A Memoir of the Future*—as well as in some preparatory papers included by Francesca Bion in *Cogitations*.

His first mention is a warning on not splitting parts from a whole. To focus on the relationships between them is of paramount importance (T, 2). Thereafter he uses the principle as a warning on the access one may have to facts, at least in physics, *"because the facts to be observed are distorted by the very act of observation"* (T, 45).

Later he would use Heisenberg's warning on the fallacy of the sense of having discovered a theory which is as false as the one it was intended to replace—in the case of multiple causation as a "face saving" device to replace the causation theories (T, 57).

Contrary to appearances, Bion "dialogued" with the texts: Heisenberg writes: "What will be the outcome of this impact of a special branch of modern science on different powerful old traditions?" Bion completes: *"What will be the impact of powerful old traditions on this special branch of modern science?"* (C, 60).

The re-arrangement is typically psycho-analytical. It offers a new perspective in examining a patient's material. Without adding, falsifying or changing the basic idea, it elicits a hitherto unseen but existent meaning. He offers an example of two different constant conjunctions based on the same elements. Through unearthing a previously unseen view, under a new vertex, analysts elicit paradoxes that are growth promoting.

Bion's main use of Heisenberg is his backing of a criticism of positivistic views of science, namely, rationality and pretensions to objectivity. His basis is Freud:

> In the natural sciences the quantum mechanical theories have disturbed the classical concept of an objective world of facts which is studied objectively. And the work of Freud has at the same time excited criticism that it is unscientific because it does not conform to the standards associated with classical physics and chemistry; it constitutes an attack on the pretensions of the human being to possess a capacity for objective observation and judgement by showing how often the manifestations of human beliefs and attitudes are remarkable for their efficiency as a disguise for unconscious impulses rather than for their contribution to knowledge of the subjects they purport to discuss. [(C, 84–85]

The personal factor

This may be stated in terms of the "personal equation" (q.v.). It approximates quantum physics to psycho-analysis; we can know to a certain extent some features of the stimulus we make on the object observed. In the physicist's laboratory it is known as the beam of light or another source of energy that is bombarded on unknown material. In the analytic room the analysis of the analyst, his knowledge of himself, of his theories, of his customary vocabulary, and the simplified setting provide a situation similar to the physicist. Under given parameters, one observes something that is real.

How can the paradox contained in Heisenberg's uncertainty principle be tolerated? It allows real knowledge and at the same time, that this knowledge is transient. It may or may not be furthered: "... *the 'uncertainty principle' (borrowed from Heisenberg) used by me both formulates and destroys the formulation* ..." (AMF, I, 88).

> ROLAND You said, if "thinking" turned put to be a by-product of glandular activity it would be a mare's nest. Why should one deny the reality of thinking; or refrain from turning *that* to good account even if glands originated ideas?
>
> P.A. I did not mean to suggest it was a "mere" product of glandular activity. It does not surprise me if I betrayed such hostility to thought or its lowly glandular origin. I am too familiar with that kind of intolerance to suppose that I am free of it. I, like my fellow brothers and sisters, aspire to a messianic superiority to my fallible origins. Hatred of our origins seems to be inseparable from any advance.
>
> ALICE Perhaps especially when we owe a debt to the origins from which we rise to "higher things". How beastly we are!
>
> ROLAND And were. But how admirable we shall shortly become! It would seem to be an advantage if we could find out the conditions propitious to real progress.
>
> P.A. Or if we knew the direction in which we were progressing. I sometimes doubt it.
>
> ROBIN I thought you psycho-analysts had no doubt about it. You talk as if you were certain at least about your own "progress" because you have been analysed.
>
> P.A. "Certainty" is a part of life as is "uncertainty". We cannot avoid either; they are opposite poles of the same feeling. I do not know what name to give the "same feeling"—that is, the feeling of

which they are opposite poles. Perhaps if I were a poet or philosopher I could. It does not help that I am thought to be a psychoanalyst because that is my profession. [AMF, III, 513]

Misuses and misunderstandings: The idealistic professional who believes that the universe is a product of the mind mistakes Heisenberg's uncertainty principle and Bion's resorting to it with a "principle of ignorance". They deny that Heisenberg observed that it is impossible to determine precisely the position of a quantum particle in space and simultaneously to determine its spin or orbital velocity precisely. It is possible to determine both probabilistically. This does not mean, as Erwin Schrodinger showed, that it is impossible to determine each one in isolation precisely. The gain in precision of a measure implies a proportional loss of precision of the other measure.

Suggested cross-references: Analytic View, Atonement, O, Transformations in O, Truth.

Principles of mental functioning: It would not be an exaggeration to state that the whole of Bion's work stems from four of Freud's broad ideas that can be subsumed by the following formulations:

(i)   The two principles of mental functioning
(ii) Dream-work (including free associations and day dreaming)
(iii) Epistemophilic, life and death instincts
(iv) Oedipus.

His dwelling on thinking processes comes from an integration of all four. Even his furthering of Klein's furthering of Freud's observations on the existence of death instincts is linked to them.

There is, nevertheless, an important difference between Freud's possibilities and Bion's expansion of them. This difference enriches Freud's observations within Freud's own frame of reference. It uses Freud's observations about the timelessness of the unconscious and brings them to a higher pitch. Bion also profited from expanded clinical work with psychotics, made possible by Klein's observations.

In brief, he takes Freud's idea that at first thinking was unconscious; he integrates it with Klein's early roots of Oedipus and the presence of a rudimentary ego and super-ego at birth. Then he proceeds, from clinical observation, with the idea that projective identification is an early form of thinking. If thinking was designed (after Freud) to disburden the psyche of accretions of stimuli and if projective identification does exactly this, it follows that projective identification is a primitive form of thinking. In 1961, Bion hypothesizes that it is *the* primitive form of thinking

The modification Bion proposes demands a firm grasp of the timelessness of the unconscious in a field—thinking—that Freud opened but perhaps did not have time to explore fully:

> The link between intolerance of frustration and the development of thought is central to an understanding of thought and its disturbances. Freud's statement suggests that the reality principle is sequent to the pleasure principle; it needs modification to make both principles co-exist. [LE, 29]

> To make theory correspond to these clinical findings I have suggested an emended version of Freud's pleasure principle theory so that the reality principle should be considered to operate co-existentially with the pleasure principle. [LE, 31]

Pain

The pleasure–displeasure principle is written in the work of Bion in a manner that differs from that of Freud. Instead of writing it as the pleasure–displeasure principle (*lust–unlust*) he writes "pleasure/pain principle". There is a case to be argued whether it is a lack of precision or faithfulness to the original or an implicit proposal of change. The proposal was not made explicitly in any of his works.

The phrase appears as such in many parts of his work, as for example in *Elements of Psycho-analysis, Transformations* and *Cogitations*. In stating that pain qualifies to be regarded as an element (a basic foundation) both of psycho-analysis and of psycho-analytic work, Bion writes that the "*case for acceptance of pain as an element of psycho-analysis is reinforced by the position it occupies in Freud's theories of the pleasure-pain principle*" (EP, 62).

If it seemed convenient to change the verbal form of the principle of pleasure/unpleasure the same is not true to the principle of reality. The long march towards tackling it occupies the bulk of Bion's contributions to psycho-analysis.

Projective identification: Bion uses Klein's definition of projective identification in the same sense that Klein established in 1946 except for the fact that he extends it. Initially this extension was not dissimilar to Herbert Rosenfeld's. He observed its communicative use by babies with their mothers, and use by patients who suffer from severe disturbances of thinking processes.

Babies resort to projective identification in order to attain a sense of protection against annihilation. Good enough mothers (to borrow a term from Donald Winnicott, who also observed the phenomena, albeit using different terminology) are able to "contain" their own anxiety and therefore, through reverie (q.v.), they "return" a detoxified experience.

This summarizes Bion's formulation of projective identification as a method of communication up to 1963. In 1961 this special use of projective identification was named "realistic projective identification". In the end it is neither just a form of communication nor just a special use of projective identification. Bion suggests that the mechanism is both more universal and original: "*In its origin communication is effected by realistic projective identification*" (ST, 118).

"*If mother and child are adjusted to each other projective identification plays a role in the management through the operation of a rudimentary and fragile reality sense; usually an omnipotent phantasy, it operates realistically ... As a realistic activity it shows itself as behaviour reasonably calculated to arouse in the mother feelings of which the infant wishes to be rid*" (ST, 114). "*Normal development follows if the relationship between infant and breast permits the infant to project a feeling, say, that it is dying into the mother and to reintroject it after its sojourn in the breast has made it tolerable to the infant psyche*" (ST, 116). Later he would suggest that reverie makes reintrojection possible.

Bion suggests that the failure of the mother leads to the perpetuation of projective identification that loses its realistic meaning and purpose. It acquires a repetitive nature:

"*A well-balanced mother can accept these and respond therapeutically; that is to say in a manner that makes the infant feel it is receiving its frightened personality back again but in a form that it can tolerate— the fears are manageable by the infant personality. If the mother cannot*

tolerate these projections the infant is reduced to continued projective iden-
tification carried out with increasing force and frequency. The increased
force seems to denude the projection of its penumbra of meaning" (ST,
115). *"If the projection is not accepted by the mother the infant feels that*
its feeling that it is dying is stripped of such meaning as it has. It there-
fore reintrojects, not a fear of dying made tolerable, but a nameless dread"
(ST, 116).

In adulthood, *"The internal object starves its host of all understand-*
ing that is made available. In analysis such a patient seems unable to gain
from his environment and therefore from his analyst" (ST, 115). The
analysis continues with denigration of the analyst, who through
projective identification is provoked to feel he or she is useless,
unworthy, suicidal.

One may say that this is a dream-like state entertained by babies
and children. To quote an example drawn from this author's experience: an illiterate, lower-class mother brought her almost dying,
2-week-old child to a large public hospital famed for the excellence
of its services—against the will of her family, who judged the case
as needing spiritual help. The child would not accept nourishment
and vomited as soon as she suckled it. There was an innate steno-
sis of the oesophagus; this mother's reverie was active to intuit the
child's need for a surgeon. It being a shared phantasy, she could not
in fact save the child. But she could take steps in this direction.

All Bion's so-called "clinical papers" describe in a way not available anywhere, before or after, the minute following of projective
identification and its phantastic nature, expressed by hallucination.
His last expansion of projective identification as a method of
communication was made through the exaggeration expressed by
Hyperbole (q.v.)

Projective identification is also used by Bion as an integrative effort between Freud and Klein's contributions to psycho-
analysis. When he elicits that which was implicit, namely, its use to
unburden the psyche of excessive accretions of stimuli, projective
identification is the mechanism used to achieve it. Therefore it lies
in the very origin of thinking itself (LE, 31).

Suggested cross-references: Arrogance, Curiosity, Schizophrenia, Hyperbole, Transformation in Hallucinosis.

📖 On Arrogance, Notes on the Theory of Schizophrenia,
Development of Schizophrenic Thought, Differentiation of the

Psychotic from the Non-Psychotic Personalities, On Hallucination, Attacks on Linking.

Projective transformations: A name suggested by Bion to classify projective identifications (after Klein). It forms part of a unifying observational theory in analysis, that of transformations and invariances.

    Suggested cross-references: Transformations, types of.

Proto-resistance: This seems to be a term that did not gain widespread usage. It is a development of a term, "premonition" (q.v.) that was defined earlier.

    It is a depiction of the analyst's state of mind favourable to the issuing of an interpretation. Its origins are the finding that an interpretation must be born from the tolerance of PS and of lies as a way to get to the truth. It can also be stated as the tolerance to perceive the evolution of an element that belongs to column 2 of the Grid (statements known to be false).

    Its importance cannot be overstated. It is one of the many attempts to furnish a psycho-analytic posture, with regard to not being deceived by outward appearances as well as perceiving a continuous dynamic situation that characterizes the living act we call "psycho-analysis".

> The emergence of the column 2 dimension may be observed in the contingency of the analysis as a step in the evolution of the statement and from it the analyst can judge that the conditions for interpretation have arrived; but it does not mean that an interpretation must be made; for the analyst's thought also must reach maturation. When he can see the column 2 element in his thoughts the conditions for interpretation are complete: an interpretation should be made. In terms of analytic theory it is approximately correct, but only approximately, to say that the conditions for an interpretation have arrived when the patient's statements provide evidence that resistance is operating: the conditions are complete when the analyst feels aware of resistance in himself—not counter-transference which must be dealt with by analysis of the analyst, but resistance to the reaction he anticipates from the analysand if he gives the interpretation. Note the similarity of the analyst's resistance to the response he anticipates from the patient to his interpretation and the patient's resistance to the analyst's interpretation . . .

So far the "distance" between the analysand's statement (association) and the analysand's statement (interpretation) has been stated in terms of time required for the emergence of the column 2 element in the statement of the analysand and "proto-resistance", to coin a phrase, in the analyst to a response that has not yet been made. The analyst's proto-resistance must be a projection of his own resistance to one dimension of his proposed interpretation. The interpretation he does give is a theory, known to be false, vis-à-vis an unknown contingent circumstance, but maintained as a barrier against turbulence expected to occur were it not so maintained. [T, 168–69]

Suggested cross-references: Emotional Turbulence, Premonition.

PS: Sometimes this is also written as Ps. A quasi-mathematical, shorthand symbol for the paranoid–schizoid position, first proposed in *Elements of Psycho-Analysis*, p.4 (see entry PS⇔D).

PS⇔D:

... the individual's capacity for learning depends throughout life on his ability to tolerate the paranoid–schizoid position, the depressive position, and the dynamic and continuing interaction between the two. [C, 199]

A quasi-mathematical notation created by Bion around 1960 and first published in 1963 to symbolize the second element of psycho-analysis. *"It may be considered as representing approximately (a) the reaction between what Melanie Klein described as the paranoid–schizoid and depressive positions and (b) the reaction precipitated by what Poincaré described as the discovery of the selected fact"* (EP, 3).

It was sometimes written as Ps⇔D. It represents a dynamic, living tandem movement, back and forth, existing as long as life subsists. It was first mentioned in a short note written circa 1960. It highlights dynamic interaction rather than a static goal; it brings home the existence of a primitive mechanism throughout life:

The Positions are not to be regarded simply as features of infancy, and the transition from paranoid–schizoid to depressive position as something that is achieved once for all during infancy, but as a continuously active process once its mechanisms have been successfully established in the early months. If, therefore, this is not established at the outset, then its operation remains defective throughout life (in varying degrees of intensity . . . [C, 199–200]

Suggested cross-reference: Elements of Psycho-analysis.

Psycho-analytical object: One of Aristotle's fundamental contributions to mathematical knowledge is the concept of mathematical **object**. This metaphysical concept allows manipulation and dealing with mathematical problems without the concrete presence of that which is objectified; that is, the problem itself, which constitutes an abstraction, and the tools used to deal with it, which are also abstracted from the nature of the problem.

Bion, inspired by those objects, and tackling an equally immaterial object, mind itself, proposes the creation and use of "psycho-analytical objects". Through an analogic and metaphorical model he presents the internalization of the parental object "father". The child learns to utter the word, "Dad", when the Mother nourishes love towards both; the naming is simultaneous to and conditional of knowing who his (her) father is and what a father is all about:

> The use of the term hypothesis as a name for the object that would more often be described as a concept is an expression of the problem presented by (3) [Note: point (3) describes the name given to a selection of feelings, impressions, etc., which are felt, by virtue of the selected fact, to be related and coherent] as it emerges when investigated psycho-analytically. The problem presented by the psycho-analytic experience is the lack of any adequate terminology to describe it and in this respect it resembles the problem that Aristotle solved by supposing that mathematics dealt with mathematical objects. It is convenient to suppose that psycho-analysis deals with psycho-analytical objects and that it is with the detection and observation of these objects that the psycho-analyst must concern himself in the conduct of an analysis. (3) describes an aspect of these objects. [LE, 67–8]

The concept of psycho-analytical object superimposes itself on the term "object" in Freud and Klein's work, and at the same time it is an attempt to enhance its scientific scope through a more specific approach to its functioning in the mental processes and its function in the personality.

This enhanced scientific scope includes something that is basic in science: communication (between analysts and their patients as well as among analysts). Psycho-analytical objects, at the beginning of life, are the internal objects or imagos, but development makes those prototypes function as patterns of learning—and non-learning, or idiosyncratically restrictive learning—that defines modes of thinking and the objects with which the mind (that specific mind) deals.

A model

Psycho-analytical objects cannot be observed directly. They are models; abstractions (EP, 7).The psycho-analytical object is a model of something that occurs in the numinous realm of the unconscious. It becomes; therefore, some manifestations of the psycho-analytical object may be observed by the mother; it can be "used" by its beholder, the child itself through its emotional development; its state can be intuited by an analyst.

Bion proposed a quasi-mathematical notation for a "psycho-analytical object": ψ (ξ)(M). The definition of this quasi-mathematical notation is on page 69 of *Learning from Experience*. This notation compacts the whole of the observational theory described in "A theory of thinking". This is one of the moments where Bion incurred the risk of being regarded as obscure and difficult just when he made efforts to be clear. The use of symbols is felt as alien to the analytic field. Let us describe them:

(ψ) = a constant
(ξ) = an unsaturated element which determines the value of the constant y as soon as it is identified.

One may remember that in mathematical formulae, ax may be put to use. For example, in a linear function that can be represented by ax + b. x corresponds to that which Bion denotes as the symbol (ψ) and a corresponds to that which Bion denotes as the symbol (ξ).

Psycho-analytically speaking:

(ψ) = innate pre-conceptions
(ξ) = realization

In the realm of real facts we have the following realizations of (ψ) and (ξ).

(ψ) = innate pre-conceptions. Bion describes two innate pre-conceptions that are not contents of mind, but functions:
- {(ψ) Breast }(Bion, 1962a, b e 1963).
- {(ψ) Oedipus }(Bion, 1963, p. 49).

(ξ) = a realization that meets the incomplete nature of the pre-conception.

(ψ) = Breast, Fathers, Mothers, Possible marriage mates, abilities that can be sublimated into professions, activities.

This means that: (ψ) (ξ) = conception (experience).

Now we have a mental function. The secondary qualities determine the value of the unsaturated element (ξ) and therefore the value of (ψ)(ξ). The previously unsaturated element (ξ) together with the unknown constant (ψ)(ξ) *"share a component, that is the inborn character of the personality"* (LE, 69), represented by M.

Bion states that the value of (ψ), as well as of (ξ), are determined by the *"emotional experience stimulated by the realization, that is . . . the contact with the breast"*. Therefore the psycho-analytic object (ψ)(ξ)(M) possesses a precise and definite value determined by two experiences: an identification of the emotional experience of a contact with the breast and the value of the unsaturated element.

The psycho-analytical objects are amenable to undergoing a process of **development**, which Bion denotes with the letter **Y**; they are also amenable to be subject of **K** (knowledge). To know involves making abstractions of psycho-analytical objects. Both development and growth can be negative (debasing and falsity).

We can try our hand at exercising this kind of notational system: we may think of the psychic–biological function "parental couple"

Formation of conception: {(ψ) Oedipus}{(ξ) creative parental couple} = Conception parental couple.

Formation of its correspondent "psycho-analytical object" that may be introjected and projected: {(ψ) *Oedipus*}{(ξ)*creative parental couple*}{(M) *emotional experience-breast*} = Conception *parental couple*.

This psycho-analytical object may develop (Y, in Bion's notation), decay (−Y), be known (K), or not (−K). To the extent that one of those outcomes occurs, or a combination of them, a given person's possibility of forming a couple when grown-up will be determined. To be known it will need as the experience of forming a couple, to divest itself from transference, meaning a repetitive attachment to the original object of cathexis—which is often imaginary. And thereafter, it can make elective affinities through "tropisms" (q.v.).

> If the trend is social, (+Y) abstraction will be related to the isolation of primary qualities. If the trend is narcissistic ($-Y$) abstraction will be replaced by activity appropriate to $-K$. [LE, 70]

Those trends should be understood as occurring at the beginning of life. The social trend leads to the apprehension of the breast-as-it-is; the narcissistic trend leads to contempt of it and creates an imaginary breast-as-it-should-be.

The concept of psycho-analytical object as well as that of pre-conception (q.v.) would survive as ontogenetic models of the process of thinking. With regard to a finer view of those processes in the analytic session, as part of a theory of observation, they would be superseded by that of "Transformations and Invariances" (q.v.). There, the unsaturated component would be seen as a question of cycles of transformations, where the final products of a given cycle serve as a starting point for a new process of transformations. The Invariances correspond to the constants.

> Psycho-analytical objects are associations and interpretations with extensions in the domain of sense, myth and passion ... requiring three grid categories for their representation. [EP, 103–4]

Suggested cross-references: Elements of psycho-analysis, Grid, Growth, Tropisms, Saturation.

"Psycho-analytic" paramnesias: See entry, "manipulations of symbols".

Psychological turbulence: See entry "Emotional turbulence".

Psychotic part of the personality: A denomination often used interchangeably with Psychotic Personality. See entry, "Psychotic and Non-Psychotic Personalities (or Psychotic Part of personality and Neurotic Part of the personality)".

Psychotic and non-psychotic personalities (or psychotic part of personality and neurotic part of the personality): Melanie Klein expanded Sigmund Freud's discovery of the universality of neuroses. She stated more explicitly that psychotic nuclei were also a primitive endowment of all human beings. One may argue that Freud was aware of this, inasmuch as observing primary narcissism and the powerfully violent instinctual endowment meant that destructive drives were a hallmark of human beings. Freud's earlier studies had already suggested that seemingly neurotic phenomena, such as transference phenomena, had a hallucinatory—that is, psychotic—basis.

If Klein illuminated more fully the nature of these universal psychotic features of the human mind—the occupying of the paranoid–schizoid position—and displayed them brilliantly in the analysis of children, one may state that one of the seminal contributions that Bion made to the practising analyst was to make Klein's expansion operative in adult analysis.

It was a fact that occurred from pure experience; at first it came from the idea of pathology, for it was discovered through the analysis of the so-called schizophrenics. As with all revolutions that implode the milieu that generated them, the discovery of a way to deal with the universality of psychosis outdated the idea of psychosis as a pathological condition.

The verbal formulation seemed from the beginning to have some limits. In 1956 it was first described as *"psychotic and non-psychotic parts of the personality"* (in "Development of schizophrenic thought", ST, 39). Bion seemingly needed to change the term to "Psychotic and non-psychotic personalities" in 1957 but at the same time it added to, rather than replaced the terms, "Psychotic part of the personality" and "Neurotic part of the personality", which are used in the conclusion of the paper.

As with any verbal formulation, both suffer from some built-in drawbacks, to the extent that they try to encompass or subsume their counterparts in reality but fall short of fulfilling such a task.

One of these counterparts is the monistic nature of the issue, which includes a pair and a paradox. The definition included an antithetical pair: the Psychotic and Non-Psychotic lingered on together. In this sense, the adjoining wording, "Psychotic Part of the Personality" and "Neurotic Part of the Personality" makes this point more clear. That is, it is clear right from the start that the "Personality" is a discrete one. Due to splitting, in phantasy, it *functions as if* it were two separate entities or personalities. One must remember that the one and only real effect of projective identification is that of the splitting of thinking processes (Klein, 1946).

This aspect of the definition is fundamental. Without a firm grasp of it the whole concept is doomed to remain out of the reader's reach. The monistic paradox of the existence of two modes of functioning, that function in tandem, calls for experience of the user, rather than rational understanding. This feature is shared by all basic concepts of workable or real psycho-analysis.

The differentiation proposed by Bion deals with *"awareness of internal or external reality"*. The psychotic personality has disturbances of this awareness. There occurs *"a minute splitting of all that part of the personality that is concerned with awareness of internal and external reality, and the expulsion of these fragments so that they enter into or engulf their objects"* (ST, 43).

The personality functions as if there were two; one uses the other. This concept of mutual use needs to be firmly grasped; it is a paradox of one entity functioning as two and at the same time as one. The psychotic cannot grasp that "monistic nature" of a whole personality and therefore cannot apprehend this "mutual use": *"there is an ever-widening divergence between the psychotic and non-psychotic parts of the personality until at last the gulf is felt to be unbridgeable"* (ST, 39).

We may use Bion's definition in order to make this mutual use more apprehensible to the reader—leaving aside for the moment that real apprehension perhaps may be achieved only during an actual analysis. The phrase, *"all that part of the personality that is concerned with awareness of internal and external reality"* refers to the non-psychotic personality, or neurotic part. When it is split, it uses and was used by the psychotic personality, which performs the splitting. The splitting itself gives form to the psychotic personality, which now has the upper hand and becomes prevalent. The expulsion of the fragments that enter or engulf objects is psychotic functioning; each fragment is a kind of "mini-neurotic-personality".

It is used to clothe the object of a neurotic presentation—meaning, rational, plausible, and seemingly sane. Each fragment becomes a "whole mini-personality", complete with ego, super-ego, etc. The neurotic part used the psychotic part to "externalize" itself; the psychotic part used the neurotic part to achieve, so to say, in hallucination, a life of its own.

In practice, it demonstrated that the psychotic is able to form a transference relationship. Nevertheless, transference presents itself differently if compared with that presentation more typical of that which appears when neurosis is prevalent. For this reason it passed unnoticed by earlier researchers: it is *"tenuous and tenacious"* (ST, 37); the relationship is *"premature, precipitated and intensely dependent"* (ST, 44).

The experienced analyst who profited from Freud and Klein's contributions soon perceived that this description fitted the experiences he (she) had with his (her) patients who were not certified psychotics. If analysis is deep enough, psychosis emerges in its use of the neurotic "layer". It was exactly this that happened with Bion—as one may vouch for in his second thoughts about cure, and later, about pathology. Indeed, one of the two main bases of this now classic paper is Freud's differentiation between neurosis and psychosis (Freud, 1924). Neurotics try to suppress *"part of the id (the life of instinct) whereas in the psychosis the same ego in the service of the id, withdraws itself from a part of reality"* (Freud, 1924, quoted in ST, 45). That is, both outdistance reality. Freud was aware of the use that both (neurosis and psychosis) made of each other (*"in the service of . . ."*). In the consulting room, a rule-of-thumb can be formulated: if one deals with neurotic behaviour, one must look for the underlying psychotic personality that is making use of a neurotic presentation; and if one deals with a psychotic presentation, one must look for the underlying neurotic mechanism which puts psychosis at its service.

Bion makes two modifications of Freud's descriptions, which acquire more precision. They stem from Bion's more extensive experience with patients labelled as psychotics. He observes that *"contact with reality is never entirely lost"* (ST, 46), meaning that both psychosis and neurosis are present as a sub-layer; one always underlies the other. They co-exist, albeit each one may remain unseen. In this phrase, it is neurosis that makes the sub-layer. And that *"withdrawal from reality is an illusion"* (ST, 46), means that in neuroses a psychotic sub-layer is at work. The psychotic withdrawal would not be real and would not be due to delusional processes, but surprisingly enough, to illusion, that is, neurosis. *"As a result of these modifications we reach the conclusion that patients ill enough, say, to be certified as psychotic, contain in their psyche part of the personality, a prey to the various neurotic mechanisms with which psycho-analysis has made us familiar, and a psychotic part of the personality, which is so far dominant that the non-psychotic part of the personality, with which it exists in negative juxtaposition, is obscured"* (ST, 47).

What is psychosis under the analytic vertex?

The psychotic aspect was manifested through minute splitting and projective identification; in this Bion integrates Freud and Klein. *"One concomitant of the hatred of reality that Freud remarked is the psychotic infant's phantasies of sadistic attacks on the breast . . . the psychotic splits his objects, and contemporaneously all that part of his personality, which would make him aware of the reality he hates, into exceedingly minute fragments, for it is this that contributes materially to the psychotic's feelings that he cannot restore his objects or his ego. As a result of these splitting attacks, all those features of the personality which should one day provide the foundation for intuitive understanding of himself and others are jeopardized at the outset. All the functions which Freud described as being, at a later stage, a developmental response to the reality principle . . . have brought against them, in such inchoate forms as they may possess at the outset of life, the sadistic splitting eviscerating attacks that lead to their being minutely fragmented and then expelled from the personality to penetrate, or encyst, the objects. In the patient's phantasy the expelled particles of ego lead an independent and uncon-trolled existence, either contained by or containing the external objects . . . In consequence the patient feels himself to be surrounded by bizarre objects . . . Each particle is felt to consist of a real object which is encap-sulated in a piece of personality that has engulfed it"* (ST, 47).

The successful operation of the hallucinosis of *"having . . . rid him-self of the apparatus of conscious awareness of internal and external reality"* enables the patient under the sway of the psychotic personality to present himself to himself and others—especially the analyst—in *"a state which is felt to be neither alive nor dead"* (ST, 38).

> P.A. I agree it does make them seem full, but I think these formu-lations have content. I am talking about "something" and I think it

would be worth having respect for "seeming". I doubt the equivocation of the fiend that lies like truth. [AMF, II, 363–4]

The shape of things to come in Bion's work appears in the form
of events as they happen in the consulting room, as hinted at in the
last phrase of the paper's conclusion:

> . . . I do not think real progress with psychotic patients is likely to
> take place until due weight is given to the nature of the divergence
> between the psychotic and non-psychotic personality, and in partic-
> ular the role of projective identification in the psychotic part of the
> personality as a substitute for regression in the neurotic part of the
> personality. The patient's destructive attacks on his ego and the
> substitution of projective identification for repression and introjec-
> tion must be worked through. Further, I consider that this holds
> true for the severe neurotic, in whom I believe there is a psychotic
> personality concealed by neurosis as the neurotic personality is
> screened by psychosis in the psychotic, that has to be laid bare and
> dealt with. [ST, 63]

⊕ The use that the psychotic personality makes of the neurotic
personality, a socially palatable, rational cover-up may well be
named the psychosis of everyday life. This was dealt with in a more
explicit way twelve years later, with the eliciting of the transformations in hallucinosis (q.v.).

& Many analysts who accustomed themselves to work through
powerful instinctual manifestations, came to realize a corollary of
Bion's paper. Namely—to paraphrase him—that patients certified
as neurotic contain in their psyche part of the personality, a prey to
the various *psychotic* mechanisms with which psycho-analysis has
made us familiar. They are dumb, so to speak, in common social
settings.

If and when the person tries to develop more intimate relationships with him (her) self and with others, then some more propi-
tious conditions for the emergence of these psychotic parts are
created—usually implying turbulence. Marriage, paternity and
psycho-analysis may provide such conditions of intimacy. This is
perhaps one of the main implications of Bion's paper.

Public view: This entry must be read together with at least one of
the following entries: Catastrophic Change, Transformations in

hallucinosis, K and O. The issue is presented in the opening and closing chapters of *Transformations* (I and XXII) and developed in *Attention and Interpretation* and *A Memoir of the Future*. Please refer to the entry, "Establishment", to scrutinize these expansions.

Definition. It refers to the individual's view, *vis-à-vis* the view of the group. In the analytic situation the group is the analytic couple.

Public view and hallucinosis

The situation of hallucinosis depends on the analyst's view. This includes his premonitions. Please refer to this term as well as its expansion (mainly in *Attention and Interpretation*, p. 51); it refers to an intra or extra-session examination of his own state of mind when he is evoking *"the resistance-proliferating elements"* with the due aid of the patient's provoking thrusts.

There is a resistance *"based on hatred and fear"* of the movement of growth (T, 163). Namely, from a state of **knowing about** "something" to a state of becoming that which **is** that "something". The something was formerly the object or goal of knowledge. *"Any interpretation may be accepted"* when it is taken for granted that it is an interpretation intended to achieve knowledge (or, using Bion's quasi-mathematical notation, "in K") but it is rejected when it propitiates being and becoming ("in O") (T, 164). *". . . acceptance in O means that acceptance of an interpretation enabling the patient to know that part of himself to which attention has been drawn is felt to involve 'being' or 'becoming' that person. For many interpretations this price is paid. But some are felt to involve too high a price, notably those which the patient regards as involving him in 'going mad' or committing murder of himself or someone else, or becoming 'responsible' and therefore guilty. There is one class of interpretations, which seems to illuminate good qualities, to which the objection is not so easy to understand. The extreme example, interpretations which involve 'becoming' O are dreaded as inseparable from megalomania, or what the psychiatrists or public might name delusions of grandeur or other diagnosis implying grave pathological disorder. The public or psychiatric view is more important than might appear as it introduces the social or group component in mental disorder and its treatment . . .*

A patient will manipulate his analysis and his environment in a manner which is consistent, determined, bearing the impress of a plan which is set but of which the pattern remains obscure. With most patients it is easy to understand that his disabilities are a trial to himself and his associates but with a few his pain, obvious enough, seems to matter far less to him than it does to everyone else, including the analyst. Relatives and associates are frightened by his irresponsibility into accepting, however powerless they may be, the responsibility he will not accept himself; he who has the power won't exercise it, they, who have not, are forced to do so. His company, so painful to himself, is nurtured and developed so that it will be even more painful to others" (T, 164).

This situation is felt by the public in three ways (T, 165). The public here can be the analyst; or it can be the relatives and associates:

(i)   Ambivalent feelings that entrap the onlooker are aroused: a choice between hating the patient, or feeling guilty of inexperience of the world as it is; that *"the analyst is unaware of the feelings that all men of common sense would be bound to entertain about his conduct of the case"*; (T, 165).

(ii)   Feelings of superiority, either displayed by the patient towards the analyst (*"The total experience, typical of many, demonstrates the crudity of expression and of the ideas expressed by the analyst as contrasted with the subtlety and evocative potency* [fn: Learning from Experience—beta-screen] *of the analysand's ideas and methods of expression"* or the public or the other way round. In the end, the patient displays the *"superiority of the aim to exacerbate pain over the aim to alleviate it"* (T, 166).

(iii) Forebodings and forebodings about the forebodings—outstanding among them, *"that a grave threat to analyst and analysis is impending"* (T, 165).

Bion sums up the situation in general terms:

... the analysis has been changed into a contest between (a) thought against action, (b) therapeutic use of insight against insight used to exacerbate, (c) pairing and dependent group against flight fight group, (d) individual against group.

The patient's dilemma, in so far as he too is trying to be co-operative, reparative and creative, lies in his having to choose between "sanity" which is powerful, destructive and devoted to exacerbation, on the one hand, and creativeness which is impotent and "insane" on the other. If he wishes to be destructive his choice is between sanity which is creative and destructiveness which is insane. [T, 166]

Taking into account that the assumption underlying *"loyalty to the K link"* (T, 129) and *a fortiori*, to the transformations in O, that is, concern for truth and life, is *"that the personality of analyst and analysand can survive the loss of its protective coat of lies, subterfuge, evasion and hallucination and may even be fortified and enriched by the loss. It is an assumption strongly disputed by the psychotic and a fortiori by the group, which relies on psychotic mechanisms for its coherence and sense of well-being"* (T, 129), it is no wonder that the psychotic ideas of superiority, and superiority of a sanity that is destructive, proves to be popular.

This public view determines that it is a matter of increased difficulty *"for the analyst to conduct himself in such a manner that his association with the analysand is beneficial to the analysand. The exercise, in the patient's view, is the establishment of the superiority of rivalry, envy and hate over compassion, complementation and generosity"* (T, 143).

Since Freud, the public view is not favourable to analysis. Ideas of cure by the analyst ensures his smooth membership of the group. The relationship of groups with truth proves to be turbulent.

Suggested cross-references: Atonement, Catastrophic Change, Real psycho-analysis, Transformations.

R

Real psycho-analysis/correct analysis/correct interpretation:

> The remainder of the session, after appropriate interpretation, took on an entirely different stamp . . . [C, 199]

> P.A. . . . We do not aspire to be leaders or shepherds; we hope to introduce the person to his "real" self. Although we do not claim to be successful, the experience shows how powerful is the urge of the individual to be led—to believe in some god or good shepherd). [AMF, II, 266]

> P.A. I am concerned with what he says and what it is about. My interpretation is my attempt to formulate *what* he says so that he can compare it with his other ideas. [AMF, II, 269]

Around 1960 Bion was looking for sounder, more reliable methods of communication that could endow psycho-analysis with scientific credibility (albeit not endorsing the positivistic "science"): "... *what in fact does happen in correct analysis? What is correct analysis, and what is the essential germ without which we have recorded virtually nothing?*" (C, 175).

A quarter of a century later he would state, coining the expression, "real analysis": "*P.A. Mystery is real life; real life is the concern of real analysis. Jargon passes for psycho-analysis, as sound is substituted for music, verbal facility for literature and poetry, trompe l'oeil representations for painting*" (AMF, II, 307).

Real analysis and growth

> The central postulate is that atonement with ultimate reality, or O, as I have called it to avoid involvement with an existing association, is essential to harmonious mental growth. [ST, 145]

> It is believed and intended that the analyst's theories, if correct in content and expression, exert a therapeutic effect. [EP, 17]

> In psycho-analytic methodology the criterion cannot be whether a particular usage is right or wrong, meaningful or verifiable, but whether it does, or does not, promote development. [LE, Introduction, 3]

> ROBIN So you admit that psycho-analysis can do harm?

> P.A. It does neither harm nor good; but the person may use the experience for whatever purpose he will. After all, if a surgeon heals a thief or murderer he makes them more efficient, but not more moral.

> ROLAND Nobody expects him to do so.

> P.A. Believe me they do! The analyst is often held responsible for the behaviour of a man or woman who has at some time been to a psycho-analyst. [AMF, II, 322]

⊕ The term "real analysis" seems to have been coined during 1973–4. It was uttered for the first time in a public situation in Bion's Brazilian lectures (1974). It was not only mentioned but used extensively in *A Memoir of the Future*, vols. II and III (written from 1976–78).

It had to do with Bion's perceptions of the deleterious effects of formalism, *ad hoc* theorizing, pre-patterned rules and erudition, and with his defence of exercising observation and intuition, leading to insight:

In the practice of psycho-analysis it is difficult to stick to the rules. For one thing, I do not know what the rules of psycho-analysis are. There are plenty of people who will say "Don't you know the theories of psycho-analysis?" and I could say, "No I don't, although I have read them over and over again. I now feel that I only have the time to read the very, very best psycho-analytic theories—if only I knew what they were". However, that is what I would try to limit myself to. The practice of *real* psycho-analysis is a very thorough job indeed. It is not the kind of thing which should be chosen as a nice, easy comfortable way of life. Theories are easily read and talked about; practice of psycho-analysis is another matter. [BLII, p. 114]

The real life that Bion talks about is both the patient's external life and the intra-session life, lived during the here and now: *"Any O not common to both* [analyst and patient] *is incapable of psycho-analytic investigation; any appearance to the contrary depends on a failure to understand the nature of psycho-analytic interpretation"* (T, 49).

Real life, psychosis and psycho-analysis

ROBIN I thought psycho-analysis was all sex.

P.A. .... As psycho-analytic theories are about, or purport to be about, human beings, you would feel they should resemble real life, real people ... [AMF, II, 303]

Real analysis is indivisible from real life—the realness of an analysis is given by real life as it is. The problems associated with both real life and real analysis have their roots in the origin of psychosis. The latter may be regarded as a basic denial of reality itself. Psychosis is a manifestation of a blind allegiance to the principle of pleasure/unpleasure constantly conjoined with fear and pain. These in their turn are in a vast majority of cases phantasized, stemming from inner aggression and violence of emotions.

P.A. .... But just as it would be impossible to explain to anyone who had not been in action what it would be like to be a combatant soldier or a regimental stretcher bearer, so is it impossible to describe to anyone who has not been a practising psycho-analyst what it is to experience real psycho-analysis.

ROBIN Surely you do not seriously mean that an analytic session is comparable with going into action?

P.A. Comparable, yes. Imminent death is not expected, although there is that possibility. That does not weigh the anxiety—fear in a low key. One shrinks from giving the unwelcome interpretation.

ROBIN Is it not just fear that the patient is going to be angry at being criticized?

P.A. I don't think so; the patient may be angry at a critical comment, perhaps even murderously angry, but I do not think that possibility consciously deters.

ROBIN Is it some unconscious fear—the counter-transference of which you spoke?

P. A. It is. Though one is not "conscious" of it—to obviate that is one reason why we think analysts must themselves be analysed—there is an inherent fear of giving an interpretation. If a psycho-analyst is doing proper analysis then he is engaged on an activity that is indistinguishable from that of an animal that investigates what it is afraid of—it smells danger. An analyst is not doing his job if he investigates something because it is pleasurable or profitable. Patients do not come because they anticipate some agreeable imminent event; they come because they are ill at ease. The analyst must share the danger and has, therefore, to share the 'smell' of danger. If the hair at the back of your neck becomes erect, your primitive, archaic senses indicate the presence of the danger. It is our job to be curious about that danger—not cowardly, not irresponsible.

ROLAND You must think highly of yourself if you are such a paragon.

P.A. I am trying to describe the job—not my fitness or otherwise for it. I have enough respect for the psycho-analyst's task to tell the difference between this social chat about psycho-analysis—or even a technical discussion of it—and the practice of psycho-analysis. Anyone who is not afraid when he is engaged on psycho-analysis is either not doing his job or is unfitted for it.

ROBIN An airman or seaman who is not afraid of the elements, afraid of the sea and the skies, is unfit to navigate. The line between fear and cowardice is faint.

P.A. Quite so. I would add, the line between daring and stupidity is similarly faint.

ROLAND How would you define it?

P.A. I would not. In practice, where to draw the line depends on the facts, including the facts of one's personality, with which one judges—the total capacity. Definition is only a matter of theory— useful for discussion and communication of ideas. In practice one does not rely on anything so ambiguous as verbal formulation. [AMF, III, 516–17]

Real analysis must be both jargon- and desire-free. It presents Bion's final formulation to improve the scientific status of psychoanalysis, achieved after twenty five years of continuous development. It replaced earlier terms such as "correct analysis" and "correct interpretation".

The phrase "real analysis", if compared with those terms, seems to present some advantages. One of them is the fact that it has no taints of judgmental values in the possible associations (or penumbra of associations as Bion called them) that can be evoked by the listener.

Bion seems to have achieved the formulation as soon as he replaced the desire for cure by attempts to help growth: *"The psychoanalytic problem is the problem of growth and its harmonious resolution in the relationship between the container and contained, repeated in individual, pair, and finally group (intra and extra psychically)"* (AI, 15–16).

The term "harmonious" is detectable up to his latest work. It has aesthetic, rather than judgmental, implications. It provides an opportunity to think about a persistent (mis)reading of Bion's works linked to attempts to debase it into a kind of "opinionism". "Harmony" belongs to a transcendent and commonsensical appreciation, **outside** and **beyond** personal opinions.

The "opinionism" is an idealistic manifestation that tries to disguise opinionated authoritarianism. It is an expression of difficulties in working through paranoid aspects of the paranoid–schizoid position. The professional tends to enthrone his own opinion as the one and only possibility that is left to him. Harmony in art is an existent, underlying fact, rather than a creation of the artist or an opinion of the onlooker. Both can apprehend it and convey it in an individual form. The conveyance is many times mistaken by the thing conveyed.

The "opinionist" tendency presents itself as modesty. It advertises a self-acknowledged limitation of the analyst. The outward appearance is deceptive. Its unobserved underlying factor is the restriction of possibilities so typical of dictatorships. This posture states that the analyst may just issue personal opinions to the patient he is seeing. The opinions would not be weighed according to their truth-value. For truth, says the opinionist, does not exist outside one's own views. This was known in earlier times as the idealistic, subjectivist, or solipsistic *Weltanschauung*.

The self-advertised modesty of the "opinionist" is that he is not able to "own the truth"—as if such a pretension would demand conscious advertisement, as if this would be a possible alternative for someone. The heightened and unchecked ownership of truth and an extreme lack of responsibility constitute a disguise. If no correct interpretation is possible at all why would one bother oneself with an attempt at improving one's intuition and observational skills?

This posture mistakes Heisenberg's uncertainty principle as a "principle of ignorance". This takes a single phrase of one of the writings of Bion, splits it from the whole of his work—"opinion of the analyst" (q.v.) and subsumes that transformations can exist with no reference to invariances (see also Transformations and Invariances). As the famed industrialist, Henry Ford once said, "You may acquire a Ford painted any colour, provided it is black". Ford was an admirer of Hitler, up to 1941. Also, Sir Francis Bacon observed (in his essay "On the Unit of Religion") that "All colours agree in the dark".

This posture in reading of Bion's work was present right from the beginning; it 'legalizes' everyone's views, with no attempt at truthful interpretations. It is observable now in other places of the world where his work took more time to catch on. It is easy to see why. Subjectivism, idealism, and solipsism were, are, and probably will continue to be popular, for they are hooked on human allegiance to pleasure and intolerance of frustration and pain. It also pleases the unscientific outlook. It is easier to be performed intra-session for many reasons: it facilitates collusion in the sense that the patient and the professional hallucinate that the patient is an authority (the transference of a father figure in the classical sense); it facilitates evasion of pain (see below).

In the view of the author, this view challenges the scientific attempt that Bion made. This entry is partially devoted to displaying some counterbalancing references to the parts of his work that are necessarily denied or ignored by the "opinionists". They may be useful in order to get a view that can be entitled to be seen as comprehensive and therefore faithful to his writings.

The "opinionist" appeared in the wake of the popular "countertransference" bandwagon. This denies the existence of the analyst's unconscious. If unconscious personal limitations—in this case, to other approximations to reality as it is—could be consciously known, it could be possible to look for, and perhaps find, alternatives to them. This fact would discard a person's unconsciously maintained limitations, up to a point.

Desire and real life

Confusion seems to exist between desire, pleasure and freedom. Desire sets that which must be; it produces morals. In contrast, freedom is to be free to become that which each one **is**. Real analysis does not provide light to a patient—it reveals the patient's light. It does not tell the patient what he must do; it illuminates what he is doing.

Correct interpretation, K, L, H and O

Let us examine Bion's statements as they are worded (or as they are). Even though "invariances in literacy" (T, 3) cannot guarantee that one will be able to find the text's meaning, it may well be worth a try, if one attempts to leave aside, even momentarily, one's prejudices.

There is an evolution in Bion's concept of a correct interpretation. At first, he seemed more prone to try his hand at psychoanalytic postures that resemble those of the neo-positivists (notably Schlick, the young Wittgenstein, Carnap, via Prichard and Braithwaite). During this period, which lasts from 1956–65, he stressed the necessity to interpret through the K-link:

> The peculiarity of a psycho-analytic session, that aspect of it which establishes that it is a psycho-analysis and could be nothing else, lies in the use by the analyst of all material to illuminate a K relationship . . . The patient communicates information that has significance by virtue of criteria of his own: the analyst is restricted to

interpretations that are an expression of a K relationship with the patient. They must not be expressions of L or H. [EP, 69–70]

Bion looked for some practical indications that could help the analyst. They were in-built features of the emotional experiences one had during an analytic session. The main hints were derived from the scientific search for truth, and obstacles to performing such a task. They can be subsumed as belonging to the following categories:

(i)   Presence of judgmental values—Bion dwells on them in "A theory of thinking" and in *Elements of Psycho-analysis*. Judgemental values preclude the discrimination between truth and falsity. Under the sway of judgement, the former is replaced by "right" and the latter by "wrong". Moreover, the link between true and false—represented graphically by the preposition "and"—is replaced by "or". Summing up: the situation "true or false" remains unseen; it is replaced in the mind of the onlooker by "right or wrong". Bion quotes Darwin (*"judgement obstructs observation"*; LE, 86). The ability to misunderstand (minus K) is linked to those judgements. They reflect a sense of superiority.

(ii) Pain

(iii) Anxiety.

(iv) Fear; (ii), (iii) and (iv) are expanded in *Elements of Psycho-analysis* in many guises. The developments from pain, anxiety and fear during a session lead to the description of premonitions. There are two built-in feelings that characterize a premonition: *"warning and anxiety"*. They are to be regarded as a kind of compass. *"The feeling of anxiety is of value in guiding the analyst to recognize the premonition in the material . . .*
Analysis must be conducted so that the conditions for observing premonitions exist, a conclusion compatible with Freud's definition of the analytic situation as one in which an atmosphere of deprivation is dominant. If premonitions cannot be experienced correct interpretation becomes difficult for the analyst to give and difficult for the analysand to grasp; unnecessary pain . . . becomes more likely" (EP, 76).

The latest development of those obstacles appears in *Transformations* and in *Attention and Interpretation*. They are put into terms of resistance and lies; in other words, resistance to the obtrusion of truth. The possibility to make an interpretation is succinctly formulated: "*... if I am attempting to establish a K link, which is after all the case with any interpretation, there must be no emotion belonging to the H or L group. This may seem a commonplace of counter-transference theory, but it is not*" (T, 61).

As late as the seventh chapter of *Transformations* Bion continued using this tone, even though some winds of change could be felt. In discussing the theory of causation, which he recognizes as false, he regards it as an example of the use of theories known to be false that could be usefully employed as a provisional step. This imposes a demand on the listener. He or she must be able to transform that which is said in order to get some meaning from it.

A psychotic seems to be "*unable or unwilling to make for himself the adjustment of a conversational phrase which would make the phrase meaningful to him*". With this kind of patient or with this kind of experience with any patient, a further exactitude is needed. It seems not to be obtained with interpretations that establish a K link. The K link is a necessary measure to take care of the emotional tone accompanying the interpretation—but something more is needed. This does not mean that Bion denied his ideas on the analyst issuing interpretations that must not be expressions of L and H. It does mean that K does not suffice. To meet an arising necessity Bion pays attention to "O" and truth. This attempt occupies the last parts of *Transformations* and would fill his writings to the end of his life with the concepts of Transformations in O and Atonement (q.v.).

Bion states that all psycho-analysts would agree that 'correct analysis' demands that the analyst's verbal formulations obey a need, namely, to "*formulate what the patient's behaviour reveals*" (T, 35). A correct interpretation presumes that "*the analyst's judgement should be embodied in an interpretation and not in an emotional discharge (e.g. counter-transference or acting-out)*" (T, 35).

Analysis is many times called "*treatment*"—at least as late as 1970. "O" seemed to further the strength of it. For example, "*From the analytic treatment as a whole I hope to discover from the invariants in this material what O is*" (T, 15). The idea of a therapeutic application—as different from cure (q.v.)—linked to development persists in his later works: "*Formulations of the events of analysis made in the course of analysis must possess value different from that of formulations made extra-sessionally. Their value therapeutically is greater if they are conducive to transformations in O; less if conducive to transformations in K"* (AI, 26).

Oedipus and real analysis

Correct or real analysis may be stated in the following terms: "If analysis has been successful in restoring the personality of the patient he will approximate to being the person he was when his development became compromised" (T, 143).

Perhaps the nearest that psycho-analysis came to the presentations of "O" is the Oedipal theory. Bion states explicitly that *"a successful outcome of analysis"* depends on *"resolution of the Oedipus complex"* (EP, 94). This is plainly stated in *Elements of Psycho-analysis*. Oedipus, qualifying as an element, is fully integrated in Klein's theory, especially concerning splitting, which leads to the practical significance of looking for Oedipal material in unexpected places. This view synthesizes all the issues earlier in this entry: truth-O, ultimate reality unknowable but intuitable, the deceptive seduction of appearances and others:

> Since the experience of learning from which the patient is thus debarred is that of the parental relationship, the importance for the patient's development and for a successful outcome of analysis, depending on resolution of the Oedipus complex, are gravely prejudiced. [EP, 94]

Imitations of analysis

Many fields would not admit an imitative device as a replacement for the real thing; forgery may function for a dishonest art dealer who finds a greedy collector, but who would prefer an imitative surgeon, engineer or aircraft pilot? The immaterial nature of analysis seems to facilitate the infiltration of idealistic relativism. A dangerous offshoot is the imitation commonly expressed by erudite learning of jargon (please refer to the entries, "Opinion of the Analyst" and "Jargon"):

> ... considering any psycho-analytical session as an emotional experience, what elements in it must be selected to make it clear

that the experience had been a psycho-analysis and could have been nothing else?

Many features of a psycho-analysis may be regarded as typical but they are not exclusively so. Departures from the common rule of meetings between two people may seem insignificant, but the number of such apparently insignificant departures taken together ultimately amounts to a difference that decides the need for a special term. A catalogue of such difference is likely to establish what constitutes an *imitation* of psycho-analysis rather that what is genuine, unless the difference can be stated in elements. [EP, 14]

One may see a practical application of it in the then popular pre-patterned mould of the imagined effects of the week-end, "*like a barber's chair, that fits all buttocks*" (Shakespeare, *All's Well that Ends Well*). This idea of week-end breaks is popular in some scholastically-oriented environments in the psycho-analytic movement.

. . . I have assumed that a week-end break, O, exists, and that the phenomena associated with O by the patient is something I denote by T(patient). In some circumstances it may be adequate to say that the patient was talking about the week-end break. It may be adequate to say this in an analysis. But, as analysts know, such a statement will not provide an answer that is adequate to all breaks in analysis. [T, 17]

This phrase hints at the danger represented by fashion inter-twined with authoritarian ways. The underlying paranoid phan-tasy is that one is entitled to state what is right or wrong. The person deals with these statements as if they were absolute truths rather than relative to an arbitrary set of individually- or socially-established rules. At the time when Bion wrote that piece it was already customary to state that almost everything that the patient did or said had some connection with the week-end break.

This attitude tried to replace the participant observation of the analyst with a pre-patterned, a priori mould where one "fits" the material through rational manipulations. It seemed to provide an easy, at-hand interpretive panacea. One cannot guarantee that this situation is not prevalent today, despite warnings such as this from Bion. In this case, a kind of "a priori formalism" tries to furnish one, and only one, correct interpretation quite disentangled from the context in which it is given. The correctness stems from the idolized or scholastic superiority of a chosen school of thinking, duly administered by a supervisor or the like. No observation is necessary; just a mechanical repetition of establishment-backed and accepted clichés will suffice. In group situations, when there is prevalence of the basic assumptions of a messianic leader, fight/flight or pairing, if this issue is not assessed, correct interpretation is always authority-bound, rather than truth-bound.

> ... I was able to narrow choice of interpretations to two or three. But even two or three interpretations can be an embarrassment when one only is wanted and that one correct in the context in which it is given. [T, 16]

The context is seminal here; given the context and the point(s) of view or vertex(es), one is not obliged to be restricted to the opinion of the analyst. The correct interpretation cannot be achieved through pre-patterned theorization; it cannot be attained in the superficiality of appearances. An underlying factor is to be looked for:

> The practical point is—no further investigations of psycho-analysis, but the psyche it betrays. *That* needs to be investigated through the medium of *mental* patterns; *that* which is indicated is *not* a symptom; *that* is not a cause of the symptom; *that* is not a disease or *anything* subordinate. Psycho-analysis itself is just a stripe on the coat of the Tiger. Ultimately it may reach the Tiger—The Thing Itself—O. [AMF, I, 112]

Or, in an earlier formulation:

> Superficially an analytic session may appear boring, or featureless, alarming, or devoid of interest, good or bad. The analyst, seeing beyond the superficial, is aware that he is in the presence of intense emotion; there should be no occasion on which this is not apparent to him.

> The intense experience is ineffable but once known cannot be mistaken; this chapter must be understood to relate to and be in preparation for participation in it for if such a contact is maintained the analyst can devote himself to evaluating and interpreting the central experience and, if he sees fit, the superficialities in which it is embedded.

One such group of superficialities pertains to the circumstances in which analysis is conducted. These are usually physically comfortable and bear the stamp of unadventurous civilized existence. They therefore conspire against awareness that analysand and analyst are engaged on a venture which is as hazardous as activities in which the perils are more obvious and dramatic. In what the danger consists will depend on circumstances, but danger and awareness of danger are features of the situation with which the analyst should be in contact. The approach to it, to be effective, is "binocular"; the analyst must be aware, while attending to the patient's material, of the dangers of his association with that particular patient: he should also be able to see what the danger is that the patient is inviting him by his presence to share. [T, 74]

The problem here, taking into account that *"The patient's activity most in evidence in an analysis is thinking"* and that *"The analyst can see the use he makes of the analytic situation"* (EP, 91), is that of apparent coherence or logical linking. We are used, because of our formation heavily based on Euclidean–Cartesian deductive and inductive logic, or classical logic, not to consider the irrational forces underlying rational thinking. This prevents the experiencing of PS$\Leftrightarrow$D during the analytic session and makes for prevalence of understanding, memory and desire. Many analysts are prone to ask many questions of their patients in order to "understand". "Why did you do this and that", "what do you feel" and so on are characteristic doubts. This is a resistance of the analyst to experiencing uncertainty, the PS$\Leftrightarrow$D movement. If the patient is entitled to answer correctly, he or she does not need analysis. If not, some analysts use the rational argument of "exploring" the analysand's reactions. This would be incompatible with the analytic posture, hampering the flow of free associations.

The patient may be describing a dream, followed by a memory of an incident that occurred on the previous day, followed by an account of some difficulty in his parents' family. The recital may take three or four minutes or longer. The coherence that these facts have in the patient's mind is not relevant to the analyst's problem. His problem—I describe it in stages—is to ignore that coherence so that he is confronted by the incoherence and experiences incomprehension of what is presented to him. His own analysis should have made it possible for him to tolerate this emotional experience though it involves feelings of doubt and perhaps even persecution. This state must endure, possibly for a short period but probably longer; until a new coherence emerges; at this point he has reached PS⇔D, the stage analogous to nomination or "binding" as I have described it. From this point his own processes can be represented by $Q\,\male$—the development of meaning. [EP, 102]

Binding does not demonstrate any "real" aetiological link or cause; binding is—during this phase of Bion's work—a signal that a constant conjunction, or better, a selected fact, has been achieved. A psycho-analytic object (q.v.) is thus established. We are marching here towards a correct interpretation, the establishment of selected facts, of a psycho-analytic object out of emotionally lived experiences. At this point Bion makes a definite use of myths as the model for this: "... *the importance of the myth lies in the fact that it represents a feeling and as such its place in a grid category denotes a psycho-analytic element. Taken with other similar psycho-analytic elements it and the other elements together form the field of incoherent elements in which it is hoped that the selected fact, that gives coherence and relatedness to the hitherto incoherent and unrelated, will emerge. Thus 'nominated', 'bound', the psycho-analytic object has emerged. It remains to discern its meaning. This verbally same myth may then be a psycho-analytic object which is instrumental in giving meaning to the totality of elements, one of which was the feeling represented by the myth in its grid category. Correct interpretation therefore will depend on the analyst's being able, by virtue of the grid, to observe that two statements verbally identical are psycho-analytically different*" (EP 103).

PS⇔D and the analyst

In *Elements of Psycho-analysis* as well as in papers such as "Reverence and awe", from 1963 and 1967 respectively, Bion furnishes technical hints to try to achieve a correct interpretation according to its context. One of them is the seminal necessity that the analyst experiences both PS, D, and back to PS and D. The former marks an evolution from Melanie Klein's explicit emphasis on the study of PS and D in the patient: one may couple it to the study of this living movement in the analyst too.

Bion emphasizes that the analyst must endure the movement. In order to endure the patient's PS⇔D, the back and forth movement, the analyst must experience it *during the session*. Many facts exist but cannot be experienced: the blood flowing through one's arteries or microwave magnetic radiation such as those emitted by radio and cell phones. To be attentive to one's own PS⇔D depends on one's own analysis. The analyst is enabled to take advantage of this, to make the best of that which may seem to be a bad job, namely, human frailty. This may be denied by those who think that to be an analyst entitles one to be free from PS.

Models

Model making is essential to achieve correct interpretations. The model corresponds to Kant's schemes, on theoretical grounds. In the session, it can be observed that *"The failure of the patient to solve his problems may in some cases depend on the fact that he employs models wrongly. In making his own model the analyst needs in such cases to be aware of and to lay bare the model used by the patient. The analyst's model must be such that it enables him to arrive at an interpretation of the facts that present themselves for scrutiny"* (LE, 82). In 1976 ("Evidence") he would state that an analyst must know his vocabulary in order to compare the use that the patient makes of it and of his and the analyst's words.

The situation of the analyst is not simplistic even though it is simple. It is laborious; it goes beyond appearances, it demands continuous and long observation. There are no shortcuts, shorthands, a priori thinking, patterned rationales.

In 1967:

> I suggest that for a correct interpretation it is necessary for the analyst to go through the phase of "persecution" even if, as we hope, it is in a modified form, without giving an interpretation . . . Again, he should not give an interpretation while experiencing depression; the change from paranoid–schizoid to depressive position must be complete before he gives his interpretation. [C, 291]

The situation may be felt by many as complicated or more difficult due to the analyst's necessity to have at his or her disposal an *"analytically trained intuition"* (T, 18). It seems that this statement enraged many in the analytical movement. *"The analyst conducting a session must decide instinctively the nature of the communication that the patient is making"* (T, 35).

This brings us to a most useful category of the Grid concerning the analyst's search for a correct interpretation, namely, the column 2. This column refers to statements known to be false. The analyst must avoid by all means making formulations belonging to column 2:

> The generally accepted view amongst psycho-analysts is that interpretations are expressed verbally, that they should be terse and to the point, namely to make the patient aware of his unconscious motivations. The orthodox view can be expressed in my terms thus: the medium of transformation is conversational English. The analyst's statements should belong to the categories F1, 3 and 4. The link with analysand should be K, not H or L. He should not express himself in any terms other than those used by an adult; theoretically this excludes certain categories (notably column 2) but, as I have shown, it is possible to regard the patient's statement in different ways, so that sometimes one dimension is thrown into relief, at other times another, and it is equally open to the patient to do just that. It is because he does so that his response to an interpretation may appear anomalous. Therefore although the analyst is under an obligation to speak with as little ambiguity as possible, in fact his aims are limited by the analysand who is free to receive interpretations in whatever way he chooses. In a sense it can seem that the analyst is hoist with his own petard: he is free to decide how to interpret the statements of the analysand how he will; the analysand retorts in kind. The analyst is not free except in the sense that when the patient comes to him for analysis he is obliged to speak in a way which would not be tolerable in any other frame of reference and then only from a particular vertex.
>
> The patient's response would also be intolerable if there were no psycho-analytic indulgence to excuse it, or, if it were not for a psycho-analytic vertex. [T, 144–5]

Thus the correct interpretation must be free of lies. A correct interpretation, being an approximation to the patient's truth-O, a pursuit of truth-O, depends on the evolution of the unknown and does not have official speakers. It stems from the non-spoken, the negative or numinous realm. This has a seminal significance for the work of the analyst concerning what he will or will not say of his choice of issues, of the rationality and lack of it that are involved:

"Nobody need think the true thought: it awaits the advent of the thinker who achieves significance through the true thought. The lie and its thinker are inseparable . . . The only thoughts to which a thinker is absolutely essential are lies . . .

Whether the thoughts are entertained or not is of significance to the thinker but not to the truth. If entertained, they are conducive to mental health; if not, they initiate disturbance . . .

Since the analyst's concern is with the evolved elements of O and their formulation, formulations can be judged by considering how necessary his existence is to the thoughts he expresses. The more his interpretation can be judged as showing how necessary **his** *knowledge,* **his** *experience,* **his** *character are to the thought as formulated, the more reason there is to suppose that the interpretation is psycho-analytically worthless, that is, alien to the domain O"* (AI, 103 and 105).

The correct interpretation belongs to the immaterial realm of the evolving O. It must be divested of any impulse to attach some concreteness to it. This attitude often seems to be reassuring in vouching that it is correct. It was already adumbrated in the turbulently anxious situation that is implied in the uncertainty involved in tolerating PS and the movement between PS and D.

Real analysis and psychological turbulence

Bion uses the term psychological turbulence in a specific way:

My term "psychological turbulence" needs elucidation. By it I mean a state of mind the painful quality of which may be expressed in terms borrowed from St John of the Cross. I quote:

"The first (night of the soul) has to do with the point from which the soul goes forth, for it has gradually to deprive itself of desire for all the worldly things which it possessed, by denying them to itself; the which denial and deprivation are, as it were, night to all the senses of man. The second reason has to do with the mean, or the road along which the soul must travel to this union—that is, faith, which is likewise as dark as night to the understanding. The third has to do with the point to which it travels— namely, God, Who, equally, is dark night to the soul in this life" [The Ascent of Mount Carmel, 1, 1 and 2].

I use these formulations to express, in exaggerated form, the pain which is involved in achieving the state of naivety inseparable from binding or definition (col. 1). Any naming of a constant conjunction involves admission of the negative dimension and is opposed by the fear of ignorance. Therefore at the outset there is a tendency to precocious advance, that is, to a formulation that is a col. 2 formulation intended to deny ignorance—the dark side of the senses. The relevance of this to psychological phenomena springs from the fact that they are not amenable to apprehension by the senses. [T, 158–9]

In examining the analyst's state of mind Bion deals with counter-transference in a sharply different way from the Heimannian change from Klein. He firmly puts this fact into the realm of the analyst's analysis. He looks for situations outside this realm that can interfere with the analyst's work. His focus is on the patient's attitude; the patient has an inability to face that some facts have no meaning (in the wake of the patient's inability to tolerate the no-breast). This intolerance stifles curiosity, love and hate at their outset:

Since the first requisite for the discovery of the meaning of any conjunction depends on the ability to admit that the phenomena may have no meaning, an inability to admit that they have no meaning stifles the possibility of curiosity at the outset. The need to manipulate the session to evoke evidence of the existence of meaning extends to a need to evoke evidence of the existence of love and hate ... Since the patient's attention is directed to finding existence of meaning, but not to finding what the meaning is, interpretations have little effect in producing change until the patient sees that he is tapping a source of reassurance to provide an *antidote* to his problem and not a *solution* of it. [T,81–2]

This leads us to *incorrect interpretations*. Rationality, plausibility, causes and explanations are almost invariably manifestations of manipulations of symbols and the habit of theorizing *ad hoc*, which makes the whole of psycho-analysis a candidate to be *"a vast paramnesia to fill the void of our ignorance"*:

SHERLOCK The simple part of it has been dealt with by Watson. You heard that fellow Bion? Nobody has ever heard of him or of Psycho-analysis. He thinks it is real, but that his colleagues are engaged in an activity which is only a more or less ingenious manipulation of symbols. There is something in what he says. There is a failure to understand that any definition must deny a previous truth as well as carry an unsaturated component. [AMF, 92]

BION Is it not just there that the danger lies? One more plausible theory is created to swell the enormous supply of plausible theories.

MAN Of course. But fear of what might happen is a bad master.

BION So is plausibility. I wonder how many plausible theories have been used and bewildered the human race. I would like to know. I am not sure of the ease with which "plausible" theories are produced. In this context of "plausible theories" about which we are talking, the plausible theory or "convincing interpretation" may be hard to come by. It can be plausible and false. Witness the idea that "the sun rises"—what trouble that has caused! We do not know the cost in suffering associated with the belief in a Christian God, or the god of Abraham's Ur, or Hitler's Germany, or peyotism—or god of any kind. [AMF, I, 172]

The unsaturated component corresponds to the negative realm of the noumena; in the intuitive *"pursuit of truth-O"*, pain and frustration are unknown. The first attempts at formulating technical hints were made through the borrowing of the model of the "dark night of the senses" from St. John of the Cross. That is, they were warnings about the deleterious effects of memory, desire and understanding: "illuminations" that definitely blinded those who could not tolerate Freud's transient "artificial blinding". Also, it amplifies and rescues Freud's recommendation that the patient comes to tell what he does not know; and we tell him, equally, that which he does not know either:

The domain of personality is so extensive that it cannot be investigated with thoroughness. The power of psycho-analysis demonstrates to any practising psycho-analyst that adjectives like "complete" or "full" have no place in qualifying "analysis". The more nearly thorough the investigation, the clearer it becomes that however prolonged a psycho-analysis may be it represents only the start of an investigation. It stimulates growth of the domain it investigates. This difficulty I mean to exploit in this way: if it is true that the proportion of the known to the unknown is so small at the *end* of analysis, it must be even smaller *during* analysis. Therefore to spend time on what has been discovered is to concentrate on an irrelevance. What matters is the unknown and on this the psychoanalyst must focus his attention. Therefore "memory" is a dwelling on the unimportant to the exclusion of the important. Similarly, "desire" is an intrusion into the analyst's state of mind which covers up, disguises, and blinds him to, the point at issue: that aspect of O that is currently presenting the unknown and the unknowable though it is manifested to the two people present in its evolved character. This is the "dark" spot that must be illuminated by "blindness". Memory and desire are 'illuminations' that destroy the value of the analyst's capacity for observation as a leakage of light into a camera might destroy the value of the film being exposed. [AI, 69]

These warnings were hints in a negative sense, telling what-not-to-do in order to keep analysis fit. His latest hints were more in the positive sense, an attempt to exemplify the exercising—intrasession—of a "language of achievement" (q.v.):

MYSELF Perhaps I can illustrate by an example from something you *do* know. Imagine a piece of sculpture which is easier to comprehend if the structure is intended to act as a trap for light. The meaning is revealed by the pattern formed by the light thus trapped—not the structure, the carved work itself. I suggest that if I could learn how to talk to you in such a way that my words "trapped" the meaning which they neither do nor could express, I *could* communicate to you in a way that is not at present possible .

BION Like the "rests" in a musical composition?

MYSELF A musician would certainly not deny the importance of those parts of a composition in which no notes were sounding, but more has to be done than can be achieved in existent art and its well-established procedure of silences, pauses, blank spaces, rests. The "art" of conversation, as carried on as part of the conversational intercourse of psycho-analysis, requires and demands an extension in the realm of non-conversation . . .

I have suggested a "trick" by which one could manipulate things which have no meaning—the use of sounds like α and β. These are sounds analogous, as Kant said, to "thoughts without concepts", but the principle, and the reality approximating to it, is also extensible to words in common use. The realizations which approximate to words such as "memory" or "desire" are opaque. The "thing-in-itself", impregnated with the opacity, itself becomes opaque; the O, of which "memory" or "desire" is the verbal counterpart, is opaque. I suggest this quality of opacity inheres in many O's and their verbal counterparts, and the phenomena which it is usually supposed to express. If, by experiment, we discovered the verbal forms, we could also discover the thoughts to which the observation applied specifically. Thus we achieve a situation in which these could be used deliberately to obscure specific thoughts.

BION Is there anything new in this? You must often have heard, as I have, people say they don't know what you are talking about and that you are being deliberately obscure.

MYSELF They are flattering me. I am suggesting an aim, an ambition, which, if I could achieve, would enable me to be deliberately and *precisely* obscure; in which I could use certain words which could activate precisely and instantaneously, in the mind of the listener, a thought or train of thought that came between him and the thoughts and ideas already accessible and available to him.

ROSEMARY Oh, my God! [AMF, I, 189–191]

Pain

The issue of pain has merited passing references until now. It is seminal in order to achieve a *"successful analysis"*, *"correct interpretations"* and *"correct analysis"* and above all, in its more precise, more scientific and less pedagogical formulation, *"real analysis"*:

Pain cannot be absent from the personality. An analysis must be painful, not because there is necessarily any value in pain, but because an analysis in which pain is not observed and discussed cannot be regarded as dealing with one of the central reasons for the patient's presence. The importance of pain can be dismissed as a secondary quality, something that is to disappear when conflicts are resolved; indeed most patients would take this view. Furthermore it can be supported by the fact that successful analysis does lead to diminution of suffering: nevertheless it obscures the need, more obvious in some cases than in others, for the analytic experience to increase the patient's *capacity* for suffering even though patient and analyst may hope to decrease pain itself. The analogy with physical medicine is exact; to destroy a capacity for physical pain would be a disaster in any situation other than one in which an even greater disaster—namely death itself—is certain. [EP, 61–2]

To deal with pain in analysis requires the notion of reversible perspective (q.v.). It is a special use of projective identification in order to render a dynamic situation static.

"The work of the analyst is to restore dynamic to a static situation and so make development possible....the patient manoeuvres so that the analyst's interpretations are agreed; they thus become the outward sign of a static situation . . . In reversible perspective acceptance by the analyst of the possibility of an impairment of a capacity for pain can help avoidance of errors that might lead to disaster. If the problem is not dealt with the patient's capacity to maintain a static situation may give way to an experience of pain so intense that a psychotic breakdown is the result" (EP, 60 and 62). Therefore real analysis cannot be achieved in an environment where abstinence of desire is not achieved, at least in the greatest possible degree one can achieve.

Circular argument

Correct interpretation is couched in the following terms: *"The interpretation should be such that the transition from* **knowing about** *reality to* **becoming real** *is furthered"* (T, 155). Bion develops a concept that had not been pursued further. It tries to describe the construction of an analytic session in terms of a verbal intercourse between analyst and patient: the **circular argument**. It is a concept destined to gauge the effectiveness of an interpretation given by an analyst *vis-à-vis* the patient's statements. As quoted above, a "correct interpretation" must be such that one avoids being restricted to "knowing about" but reaches "becoming" (q.v.). Please refer to the specific entry, circular argument.

Compassion

Finally, Bion includes in the possibility of making correct interpretations, in the *"result of analytic cure"* (T, 143) the possibility of exercising a *"mature compassion"* (T, 143). With certain patients this may present a kind of catch-22 situation. The patient in question is one who resorts to hallucination and phantasies of superiority. The phenomenal manifestation in the session is rivalry and envy. They almost invariably are successful in turning a correct interpretation into an incorrect one quite independently of the interpretation itself. As far as it is more analytically correct it will be received as the *"analyst's fault"*. The only way out is to return the issue to its origins, or to use an analytical vertex. That is, to undo a relationship that is locked into the view that analyst and analysand are rivals and to turn it into an intrapsychic conflict of rival methods within the analysand. If the analyst is compassionate, the "superior" patient turns this compassion into the analyst's superiority (please refer to the entry "Compassion").

Misuses and misconceptions: Many who usually dismiss Bion's work after 1961 off-hand are used to writing that it is in D that a cure is reached; that it is in D that a patient thinks; that PS equals no-thinking at all. Let us quote Bion in one of the many parts of his work that suggest that this kind of misapprehension is a deep-rooted problem of personality: *"The patient feels that the association between the depressive position and verbal thought is one of cause and effect"* (ST, 26).

It seems to constitute a backward step to a psychiatric-authoritarian view of cure. This idea denies or perhaps ignores that Bion wrote, as we reproduced above, that *"The analyst can see the use he makes of the analytic situation"* (EP, 91). *The coherence that these facts have in the patient's mind is not relevant to the analyst's problem. His problem—I describe it in stages—is to ignore that coherence so that he is confronted by the incoherence and experiences incomprehension of what is presented to him. His own analysis should have made it possible for him to tolerate this emotional experience though it involves feelings of doubts and perhaps even persecution"* (EP, 102).

Those readers would profit from a more attentive reading of "Reverence and awe", especially pages 287–292, quoted above.

A correct analysis assumes a state of atonement; to be at one with oneself, as one really is. This state is feared; it involves depression because of truthful recognition of one's envy, delinquency, greed and violence, which is unjustifiable for the needs of survival. Also, for some people this means facing one's own impoverished self and mindlessness. For many among those people atonement may be indistinguishable from suicide or homicide:

> The psycho-analyst accepts the reality of reverence and awe, the possibility of a disturbance in the individual which makes atonement and therefore, an expression of reverence and awe impossible.

The central postulate is that atonement with ultimate reality, or O, as I have called it to avoid involvement with an existing association, is essential to harmonious mental growth. It follows that interpretation involves elucidation of evidence touching atonement, and not evidence only of the continuing operation of immature relationship with a father . . . Disturbance in capacity for atonement is associated with megalomanic attitudes. [ST, 145]

The revision of the concept of cure seemed to bewilder some of Bion's readers. They came to deprecate the medical model. Are they trying to be more royalist than the king? This reading appeals to idealistic readers, to those who are not willing to take on human responsibilities. To them, analysis would be an activity for its own sake, a circularity whose effect is indistinguishable from one who devotes himself to making his bank account fatter; or from academic or religious musings that lead to an endless supply of more musings. They deny the existence of a correct interpretation stating that there is no such thing. They make a split reading of parts of Bion's texts—especially of *Transformations*, in which they deny the "invariance" part of it. They insist that the analyst should just issue "opinions" (q.v.). In maintaining that truth is *always and ever contingent* and therefore non-existent, they deny any attempt to help people in their suffering. Those people like to deny the medical nature of analysis and try to stress that a poetic or literary or any other nature should replace it. How can one reconcile this reading with, for example:

Psycho-analytic procedure pre-supposes that the welfare of the patient demands a constant supply of truth as inevitably as his physical survival demands food. It further presupposes that discovery of the truth about himself is a pre-condition of an ability to learn the truth, or at least to seek it in his relationship with himself and others. It is supposed at first that he cannot discover the truth about himself without assistance from the analyst and others. [C, 99]

I assume that the permanently therapeutic effect of a psycho-analysis, if any, depends on the extent to which the analysand has been able to use the experience to see one aspect of his life, namely himself as he is. It is the function of the psycho-analyst to use the experience of such facilities for contact as the patient is able to extend to him, to elucidate the truth about the patient's personality and mental characteristics, and to exhibit them to the patient in a way that makes it possible for him to entertain a reasonable conviction that the statements (propositions) made about himself represent facts.

It follows that a psycho-analysis is a joint activity of analyst and analysand to determine the truth; that being so, the two are engaged—no matter how imperfectly—on what is in intention a scientific activity. [C, 114]

If analysis has been successful in restoring the personality of the patient he will approximate to being the person he was when his development became compromised. [T, 143]

This would serve people who think that Bion was just interested in observing for its own sake, and not in being helpful, interested or who cared little for people. This is one of the prevailing views in some parts of the world. The same befell Freud, who was seen as hard and dispassionate by the medical establishment of Vienna. That attitude proved to be excessively prone to blindness to transference hallucinations and seduction; the same accusation was levelled against Klein, years later.

Poetic and religious expressions have made possible a degree of "public-action" in that formulations exist which have achieved durability and extensibility . . . the psycho-analyst's attention is arrested by a particular experience to which he would draw the attention of the analysand . . . he must employ methods which have the counterpart of durability or extension . . .

it is certainly my impression that the experience of psycho-analysis is supposed or intended to have an enduring effect. [AI, Introduction, page 2]

The idea of a correct analysis, real analysis and interpretations, would be enriched with the expansions of the theory of container/ contained, $\varphi \, \sigma$ (q.v.). The "life" feature of a real analysis is at stake:

The patient will be at a loss to convey his meaning, or the meaning he wishes to convey will be too intense for him to express properly, or the formulation will be so rigid that he feels that the meaning conveyed is devoid of any interest or validity. Similarly, the interpretations given by the analyst, ϑ, will meet with the appar-ently co-operative response of being repeated for confirmation, which deprives ϑ of meaning either by compression or by denuda-tion. Failure to observe or demonstrate the point may produce an outwardly progressive but factually sterile analysis. The clue lies in the observation of the fluctuations which make the analyst at one moment φ and the analysand ϑ and at the next reverses the roles. When this pattern is observed the links (commensal, symbiotic, or parasitic) within the pattern must also be observed.

The more familiar the analyst becomes with the configuration φ and ϑ, and with events in the session that approximate to these two representations, the better. The essential experience is not the read-ing of this volume but the matching of the real event in the psycho-analysis that approximates to these formulations. [AI, 108–9]

Perhaps the most touted part of Bion's recommendations about a "correct analysis" is linked to his recommendations on eschewing memory, desire and understanding. The analyst must develop a discipline, far from an easy-going posture; see especially "Notes on memory and desire", 1967. A sharp differentiation between "remembering" and "memory" is made three years later.

The analyst who comes to a session with an active memory is there-fore in no position to make "observations" of unknown mental phenomena because these are not sensuously apprehended. There is something that has often been called "remembering" and that is essential to psycho-analytic work; this must be sharply distin-guished from what I have been calling memory. I want to make a distinction between (1) remembering a dream or having a memory of a dream and (2) the experience of the dream which seems to cohere as if it were a whole, at one moment absent, at the next present. This experience, which I consider to be essential to evolu-tion of the emotional reality of the session, is often called a memory, but it is to be distinguished from the experience of remembering. In memory, time is of the essence. Time has often been regarded as being of the essence of psycho-analysis; in the growth process it has no part. Mental evolution or growth is catastrophic and timeless . . .

In every session the psycho-analyst should be able . . . to be aware of the aspects of the material that, however familiar they may seem to be, relate to what is unknown both to him and to the analysand. Any attempt to cling to what he knows must be resisted for the sake of achieving a state of mind analogous to the paranoid–schizoid position. For this state I coined the term "patience" to distinguish it from "paranoid–schizoid position", which should be left to describe the pathological state for which Melanie Klein used it. I mean the term to retain its association with suffering and tolerance of frustration . . .

"Patience" should be retained without "irritable reaching after fact and reason" until a pattern "evolves" . . .

For this state I use the term "security" . . . I consider that no analyst is entitled to believe that he has done the work required to give an interpretation unless he has passed through both phases— "patience" and "security" . . . Few, if any, psycho-analysts should believe that they are likely to escape the feelings of persecution and depression commonly associated with the pathological states known as the paranoid–schizoid and depressive positions. In short, a sense of achievement of a correct interpretation will be commonly found to be followed almost immediately by a sense of depression. I consider the experience of oscillation between "patience" and "security" to be an indication that a valuable work is being achieved. [AI, 107–8; 124]

His last attempt to stress the *"evolution of the emotional reality of the session"* and the *"Mental evolution or growth"* that *"is catastrophic and timeless"*—partaking of the features of the unconscious—would be made through a hitherto untried form, which seems to be more life-like than the earlier attempts.

In the dialogic *A Memoir of the Future*, the term "correct" would be definitely and definitively replaced by the more precise "real".

Judgemental values

The expression was used by some readers, as if passing judgement. The paranoid or delinquent reader tends to use it with rivalling purposes, trying to compare it with "classical analysis" as if "classical" meant obsolete, inferior. This was enhanced due to errors in translation to some Latin languages, which mistook "real" for "true". Hence the term "true analysis" among readers who tried to express themselves in those languages. Those readings served to fuel "wars among analysts" but they are unwarranted distortions of the original writings. How can we continue with a superior approach after scrutinizing, for example, text such as:

> P.A. The hope is that psycho-analysis brings into view thoughts and actions and feelings of which the individual may not be aware and so cannot control. If he can be aware of them he may, or may not, decide—albeit unconsciously—to change them.

> ALICE I don't see how this differs from what has been done by parents, teachers, saints, philosophers, for countless generations of prophets of one kind or another.

> P.A. What I said—and I cannot say it any better—is a description, which could apply to many time-honoured procedures. You would be right to assume from my description that there is no particular reason to attribute any primacy to a psycho-analytic approach. That is why most people do not put themselves to the expense in time and money to go to a psycho-analyst. The "real psycho-analysis" to which we aspire is at best only a reaching out towards that "real psycho-analysis". But it is real enough to make people aware that there is "something" beyond the feeble efforts of psycho-analyst and analysand. I think it optimistic to suppose that we do more than scratch the surface in our struggles to achieve it. [AMF, III, 509–10]

Dangers implied in real analysis

The practice of real analysis is linked to the hatred of truth. Social groups being masses whose sense of well-being is derived from questioning the value of truth, the analyst risks hate stemming from the group. A successful analysis usually leads people to take action in situations that do not subject the interests of the individual to the interests of the Herd. Conversely, a successful analysis may temporarily enhance the appeal to psychotic mechanisms of defence and manipulations of the patient's environment—by the patient himself—to destroy analysis. Many times the analyst can be seen as the messenger of bad news. For news that is felt as unpleasant—the realization of one's meanness, envy and unjustified hate—is usually felt as meriting extinction, and its messenger suffers the same fate. Primary envy and primary narcissism are associated with an inability to face truth. Bion deals with public opinion in chapter I of *Transformations*. The issue is reviewed in this dictionary under the entries, Truth, Lies, Psychotic Personality.

> P. A. People frequently assume that I am devoid either of culture or of technical equipment—or both.
>
> ROLAND You sound hardly used.
>
> P.A. No; it is part of the analyst's profession to be familiar with the real world, whereas laymen think they can afford to be deaf and blind to these unpleasing components of real life. [AMF, III, 528]

> The fiction can be so rhetorical as to be incomprehensible; or so realistic that the dialogue becomes audible to others. There is thus a double fear; that of the conversation being so theoretical that the thoughts might be taken for meaningless jargon; and that of the seeming reality. Having two sets of feelings about the same facts is felt as madness and disliked accordingly. This is one reason why it is felt necessary to have an analyst; another reason is the wish for me to be available to be regarded as mad and used to being regarded as mad. There is a fear that you might be called an analysand, or reciprocally, that you may be accused of insanity. Should I then be tough and resilient enough to be regarded and treated as insane while being sane? If so, it is not surprising that psycho-analysts are, almost as a function of being analysts, supposed to qualify for being insane and called such. It is part of the price they have to pay for being psycho-analysts. [AMF, I, 112–13]

Suggested cross-references: Analytic View, Atonement, Circular Argument, Compassion, Cure, Disaster, Judgmental values, Lies, Reverence and awe, Sense of Truth, Truth and Transformations in O.

Reality sensuous and psychic: This verbal formulation heads chapter III of *Attention and Interpretation*. With it Bion rescues the ultimate monistic nature of the human being. One may say, after Hegel, the "holistic" nature of human nature (Sandler, 2003b). It was intuited as such for the first time in the history of western civilization by Freud. From time to time the apprehension of this nature was rescued by the work of some individual's from the darkness of denial and splitting. Some were subjected to cooptation and debasement such as Plato, Spinoza, Kant, Shakespeare, Goethe, Nietzsche, Freud and Einstein; some are damned into oblivion, such as Hamann, Maimon and possibly Bion. The positivistic-minded pseudo-scientific establishment never grasped psychic reality; the idealistic minded anti-scientific hermeneutics abhor material reality. Philosophy lost itself in this splitting, today being a shadow of its former self. The psycho-analytic establishment soon tried to deny the truth presented by Freud's expressions, "psychic reality" and "material reality" and their offshoots, such as the death and life instincts.

Freud, and Bion after him, realized that the two forms in which reality presents itself are in fact one and only one. One cannot name ultimate reality; therefore Freud or Bion's denominations are unavoidably clumsy. One can only intuit its existence, and use it, and be at one with it. Its transient nature means that it can be lived as it becomes, but it cannot be understood, named, owned. It is ineffable. But one can describe two of its forms of presentation, and this is what Plato, Kant, Freud, Einstein and Bion did.

In coining the phrase "reality sensuous and psychic", Bion rescues both Freud's insightful original verbal formulation, and Freud's ethos of psycho-analysis. It was expressed in chapter VII of *The Interpretation of Dreams*. There Freud identifies two forms of existence, namely, material reality and psychic reality. The term "material" replaced the term "factual", which had been used for a few years.

There is a kind of catch that seems to have proved elusive for the psycho-analytic movement. The issue can more easily be seen with the aid of a clinical example. There are patients who mistake sex with sexuality. They split sex from sexuality; in this sense, they cannot realize the monistic character of two forms of the same existence. They imagine that there are two existences.

Reality sensuous and psychic is a verbal formulation that emphasizes the concrete, factual, material presentation of that which is not concrete, is not necessarily factual and is immaterial. It may be named "reality sensuous and psychic" to the extent that the factual, the material, the concrete are in most cases amenable to being apprehended by the human sensuous apparatus. Or, in Bion's words, to be sensuously apprehensible. Is there any "psychic" equivalent of this apparatus? Freud attributed this condition to consciousness.

The newness in Bion's verbal formulation *vis-à-vis* Freud's is the explicit insertion of the conjunction "and". "And" displays that

R   635

there is tolerance of a paradox, namely, the existence of two forms
of discrete reality. It stresses the indissoluble link—the monism.
Terms such as psyche and soma, for example, are superfluous when
one realizes that those terms reflect only our (human) difficulties in
grasping the whole or in apprehending that which demands to be
apprehended, rather than understood. An analogy may be made
with a coin: the two faces of the coin are two forms of presentation
of the same discrete reality, the coin itself. They cannot be seen
simultaneously. The same analogy can be made with a human
hand. These concrete analogies are easier to grasp, but reality
sensuous and psychic or reality material and psychic may be more
difficult to realize for the concretizing mind.

Misuses and misunderstandings The term was written like
this: "reality sensuous and psychic". It seems to be advisable not to
split it. Some readers did split it and talked about an alleged "reality sensuous" or "sensuous reality". Bion did not write this and it
has no counterpart in reality. There is no sensuous reality. Kant
showed that this kind of reliance on the sensuous organs leads the
human being to conclude that reality is restricted to that which the
sensuous apparatus can apprehend. He showed that the product of
this idea is not reality at all. He called those who believe in this
"naïve realists". Reality can be, to an extent, sensuously apprehensible. It is due to the fact that we human beings were provided with
a sensuous apparatus whose perceptual powers encompass a
comparatively narrow spectrum of absorption.

In the same way, great care should be taken in using the term
psychic reality. Its disembodied use repeats an error. It has been
variously named as the idealist, subjectivist or solipsistic error. This
was an error that Kant tried to warn about. Freud was never prey
to it. "Sometimes a cigar is just a cigar", he was forced to claim once
when faced with the wild hermeneutics of his own time. The solip-
sist relativism denies the nature of the unconscious to the extent
that it "immaterializes" it. It denies that the instinctual drives are
born from that which we call "body". The idealistic error is gradually prevailing in the psycho-analytic movement as medically
trained practitioners are being replaced by professionals who have
trained in other areas. The hermeneutic and post-modernist trends
are the forms that express this mistake.

🕐 May reality present itself under forms of presentation other than material (sensuously apprehensible) and psychic? Is there a reality "out there", external to us, which partakes of the monistic nature that has been adumbrated as existing in the innermost "internal milieu", as represented by instincts? Usually those infinite spaces offer an opportunity to jump to conclusions such as "God". The first part of the following quotations includes psychic reality but something more seems to be hinted at too:

> Recently, by mechanical means, it has been possible in the biological range (human sub-category) to detect disturbances of great violence which have completely escaped detection by animals dependent on sight, even when sight is augmented by instruments such as telescopes, spectrographs, cameras and preparations of film collated with fine grains receptors—all macroscopic. Yet, these perturbations are matters of the greatest crudity and violence!

> Though extremely rare and scattered over a huge range of temporal space, they only appear to be extremely rare because of the crudity and triviality of recorded time as an instrument of measure. Time as a concept is as inadequate as topological space to provide a domain for the play of such enormous thoughts as those liberated by freedom from dependence on a thinker. The breakdown is trivial, though made to appear vast by the inadequacy of the framework as, to take a very gross but simple analogy, that which occurs if a simple operation such as the subtraction of five from three is attempted with sensuous objects or even a relatively sophisticated mathematics best limited by being exclusive of negative numbers though well stocked with real numbers. [AMF, 70]

At the end of his life Bion seemed to be open to this possibility. He hinted at it in his lectures all around the world (mainly in São Paulo and New York) and in *A Memoir of the Future*. He suggested that some other facts, possibly of a material nature albeit not apprehensible by the human sensuous apparatus, may be at stake when a patient affects the analyst—something that is not covered by the theories of transference and projective identification. Those hints are dealt with in other entries of this dictionary.

Suggested cross-references: Analytic view, Atonement, O, Real psycho-analysis, Ultra-sensuous and Infra-sensuous.

&c This author's theory of Tolerance of Paradoxes as necessary to the analytic posture (Sandler, 1997, 200b, 2001b).

Reason: Bion's critique of pure reason stems from Freud's insights into the realm of the unconscious. His distrust of classical logic and reason stems not only from his Humean and Kantian origins but also from his experiences of life—notably, his experiences of war and of reactions from the establishment (school, officialdom, societies of psycho-analysis). Medical and war experiences provide opportunities to divest oneself of illusions of reason.

There are at least two passages in Bion's work that make clear the following point: pretensions to reason—later called "rationalization" by Freud, are at the service of the principle of pleasure. *"Reason, as the slave of the passions, transforms psycho-logically necessary meaning into logically necessary meaning"* (T, 73), writes Bion, fully profiting from his integration of Hume and Freud.

Rationalization occupies a curious place in the history of psycho-analytic ideas. It has never received the status of a mechanism of defence and stems from Freud's insights about Judge Schreber's memories. Ernest Jones tried to highlight the problem, which was tackled more effectively on its deepest level by Bion. It is a psychotic mechanism—a fact usually denied.

> When thoughts have to be used under the exigencies of reality . . . the primitive mechanisms have to be endowed with capacities for precision demanded by the need for survival. We have therefore to consider the part played by the life and death instincts as well as reason, which in its embryonic form under the dominance of the pleasure principle is designed to serve as the slave of the passions, has forced it to assume a function resembling that of a master of the passions and the parent of logic. For the search, for satisfaction of incompatible desires, would lead to frustration. Successful surmounting of the problem of frustration involves being reasonable and a phrase such as the "dictates of reason" may enshrine the expression of primitive emotional reaction to a function intended to satisfy not frustrate. The axioms of logic therefore have their roots in the experience of a reason that fails in its primary function to satisfy the passions just as the existence of a powerful reason may reflect a capacity in that function to resist the assaults of its frustrated and outraged masters. [EP, 35–36]

In allowing the existence of two kinds of reason one may see that a reasonless reason, the "powerful reason", is sometimes required. In the words of the bard, *"I must be cruel, only to be kind"*

(Hamlet). This "powerful reason" emerges due to the fact that *"These matters will have to be considered in so far as dominance of the reality principle stimulates the development of thought and thinking, reason, and awareness of psychic and environmental reality"* (EP, 36).

Bion deepens the idea in a re-examination of the Humean constant conjunction and suggests the existence of a "psycho-logic": *"A constant conjunction is a function of consciousness in the observer. The observer feels that it is a necessity **for him** that the conjunction should have a meaning **for him**. Meaning is a function of self-love, self-hate or self-knowledge. It is not logically, but psycho-logically necessary. The constant conjunction, once named, must then be found, as a matter of psychic necessity, to have a meaning. Once psycho-logically necessary meaning has been achieved, reason, as the slave of the passions, transforms psycho-logically necessary meaning into logically necessary meaning"* (T, 73).

That is, reason is an artefact devoted to alleviate the mind of frustration and fear of the unknown. There seem to be two kinds of meaning: a real one and a fabricated one, the real one being that which is linked to reality itself:

> Inadequacy of hallucinatory gratification to promote mental growth impels activity designed to provide "true" meaning; it is felt that the meaning attributed to the constant conjunction must have a counterpart in the realization of the conjunction. Therefore the activity of the reason as the slave of the passions is inadequate. In terms of the theory of the pleasure/pain principle there is a conflict between pleasure principle and reality principle to obtain control of the reason. [T, 73]

The issue of reason is serious to the extent that it concerns primary or non-primary narcissism. The narcissistic personality is able to find reason for everything and becomes an advocate of pleasure and desire. Lack of answers is felt as abominable and outrageous, potentially annihilating. Scientific outlook becomes impossible and is replaced by the religious outlook.

> The objection to a meaningless universe (however big or small it may be thought to be) derives from fear that the lack of meaning is a sign that meaning has been destroyed and the threat this holds for essential narcissism. If any given universe cannot yield a meaning

for the individual, his narcissism demands the existence of a god, or some ultimate object, for which it has a meaning from which meaning he is supposed to benefit. In some instances meaninglessness is attacked by splitting and projected into an object. Meaning or its lack, in analysis, is a function of self-love, self-hate, self-knowledge.

If narcissistic love is unsatisfied the development of love is disturbed and cannot extend to love of objects.

Disturbed self-love is accompanied by intolerance of meaning or its lack. The one contributes to the other. [T, 73]

In other words, explanations, general meanings and external laws are expressions of this. In fact, the Stalinist and Nazi regimes were wholly logical, in terms of their internal logic.

Misuses and misunderstandings: to mistake a critique of pure reason for irrationality is to be oblivious to the very meaning of the terms "rational" and "irrational".

Suggested cross-references: Analytic view, Atonement, Catastrophic Change, Transformations in Hallucinosis.

Relationship: Bion stressed that "relationship" or "link" is a basic necessity of the human being and especially of mental functioning. Starting from the fact that the mind functions through pairs of opposites (dialectical opposites) as Freud and Klein had shown, Bion made more explicit how those opposites are always functioning in tandem—through a link.

The two principles of mental functioning, the instincts of death and life, sadism and masochism, love and hate, paranoid–schizoid and depressive positions, container and contained, are examples of this. This also happens in the sphere of thinking, reality and hallucination. An emotional experience is indissoluble from a relationship (LE, 42).

The links in tandem admit growing and sophisticated improvements when a creative dialectical pair is present. It leads to syntheses. The link, formerly made between pairs, comes to be a triad: Oedipus furnishes a classical example of it.

Bion's use of the mathematical theory of functions and of mathematical analogies is founded on the idea of relationships among objects. The concept is valid biologically—life emerged when relationships between elements were made. It is also valid under any vertex one considers: anthropological, musical. Living systems (Miller, 1965) are possible because of relationships.

> Relativity is relationship, transference, the psycho-analytic term and its corresponding approximate realization. [AMF, I, 61]

Relationship and paradox

> The failure to grasp the trivial range of the biological spectrum, even when the field of the living is extended by the dead, the animate by the inanimate, has been matched with the vastness of the extent of the relatively minute. This is due, in part, to the failure to grasp the nature of relativity, in particular the fact that it includes paradox. The restriction imposed by the limitation of thought to thoughts with thinkers implies the polarization "truth" and "falsehood", complicated further by morals: uninvestigated "moral" systems, and extensions of Plato's thoughts to moral views of the functions of poets and artists. A similar seepage from the domain of religion may likewise be traced to the inability to respect the "thought without a thinker", and, by extension the "relationship without related objects". How this has affected even the so-called practical thinking is seen in the difficulty of the "public" to grasp that an analogy is an attempt to vulgarize a relationship and not the objects related. The psycho-analytical approach, though valuable in having extended the conscious by the unconscious, has been vitiated by the failure to understand the practical application of doubt by the failure to understand the function of "breast", "mouth", "penis", "vagina", "container", "contained", as analogies. Even if I write it, the sensuous dominance of penis, vagina, mouth, anus, obscures the element signified by the analogy . . . [AMF, I, 70–71]

> Mathematical terms could be used to formulate a problem and demonstrate relationships between invariants and constants with such accuracy that the configuration presented by the newly disposed elements was familiar and unwelcome. [AMF, I, 183]

In trying to display the utility of the theory of transformations as applied by him to psycho-analysis, Bion states that the psycho-analytical theories, the analyst's and patient's statements are representations of an emotional experience. He suggests an ability, namely, to apprehend the "process of representation" that could help us to understand both the representations and that which is being represented—be it a person, a fact, even a dream, a concept, an idea or an object. The theory of transformations is intended to illuminate a network, chain, cluster or string of phenomena in which the apprehension of a link, or even only an aspect of this link, can illuminate or guide the apprehension of other links and related objects. Obviously, Bion's emphasis is in the "analytic session". This statement can be found in Transformations, page 34.

Relationship and caesura

Please refer to the entry, Caesura.

Misuses and misunderstandings: "relationship" or "link" as a basic necessity of the human being and especially of mental functioning does not mean, as many understand, either that Bion was a member of the school of object relations, or a forerunner of the intersubjectivists or "enactists". When he stresses the functions of the related objects, he does not partake of these tendencies. He stays within the limits of science. Functions are amenable to be studied and to a certain extent, known or at least intuited and used.

There are seminal differences between Bion's work and the "relationist" school of the psycho-analytic movement that became popular in the nineties.

(i)   That school disparages Freud's metapsychology.
(ii) That school puts Freud as a positivist.
(iii) That school is a school.
(iv) That school denies that which is intra-psychic.
(v)   That school believes in cure and explanatory ideas, including those of cause and effect.

Resistance: Bion uses the term resistance in exactly the same way as Freud. He puts an explicit emphasis on an implicit aspect. It has basically to do with truth: the human mind seems to nourish hate towards truth. There is no resistance to lies.

Bion makes a minute application of the concept through its embodiment in a theory of observation of the decisive moments of the analysis. In order to get a proper reading of the following quotation one must keep in mind the following lexicon:

Column 2: the second vertical category of the tool "grid"; the vertical categories represent the uses under which the thinking processes can be put in; column 2 is made up of statements known to be false.

K: processes of knowledge, and the link of knowledge.

O: quasi-mathematical symbol for the numinous realm, the thing-in-itself.

Transformations in K: e(/in)volutions in the processes of knowledge.

Transformations in O: e(/in)volutions in the processes of apprehension of reality; also called, "becoming".

(If this brief lexicon proves not to be enough for a reader, he or she may consult the specific entries in this dictionary.)

> When he can see the column 2 element in his thoughts the conditions for interpretation should be made. In terms of analytic theory it is approximately correct, but only approximately, to say that the conditions for an interpretation have arrived when the patient's statements provide evidence that resistance is operating; the conditions are complete when the analyst feels aware of resistance in himself—not countertransference which must be dealt with by analysis of the analyst, but resistance to the reaction he anticipates from the analysand if he gives the interpretation. Note the similarity of the analyst's resistance to the response he anticipates from the patient to his interpretation and the patient's resistance to the analyst's interpretation . . . [T, 168]

> Interpretations are part of K. The anxiety lest transformation in K leads to transformations in O is responsible for the form of resistance in which interpretations appear to be acceptance but in fact the acceptance is with the intention of "knowing about" rather than "becoming". In other terms, it is an acceptance to preserve the K link as a col. 2 element against transformations in O. By agreeing with the interpretation it is hoped that the analyst will be inveigled into a collusive relationship to preserve K without being aware that he is doing so . . . [T, 159–60]

Bion states that if the manoeuvre is successful, transformations in K fulfil a role of false concepts. They prevent the inception of a process of transformation that evolves into a final product; this product is equated with a transformation from knowing to becoming.

The same issue is more developed in *Attention and Interpretation*, including the concept of cure and its reassuring use.

Suggested cross-references: Analytic view, Cure, Lie, Transformations in O.

Reverie: The term has both poetical and musical penumbras of previous associations. Bion warned about a penumbra of previously existent meanings of verbal formulations, be it either in theoretical constructs or during the analytical sessions. In some cases he felt it was useful to avoid the penumbra, and in other cases he felt it was useful to incorporate it.

This seems to be the case with the term reverie. One is safely authorized to use the sense conveyed by timeless musical masterpieces such as *Traumerei* by Robert Schumann in order to evoke that which Bion means with this word in the psycho-analytical context. It is an integral part of his theory of thinking and its links with the capacity to tolerate frustration, the need for love and the processes of knowledge.

Why specifically Schumann's *Traumerei*, taking into account that other authors also composed pieces with this title? Because *War Memoirs*, probably the last work of Bion ever to be published, seems to indicate the seed of this, as the author has tried to show elsewhere (Sandler, 2003).

The issue touches on the question of alpha-function (q.v.) to the extent that alpha function "de-sense-fies" or turns into immaterial that which was material in its origin. Reverie also has to do with this transformation from material into immaterial.

⏾ The first time Bion mentions reverie with an analytic purpose was in 1959: "*in the psychotic we find no capacity to reverie*".

This was written in connection with his expansion of Freud's theory of dreams (please refer to the entry "Dreaming the patient's material"). There is an unequivocal link of the term with a capacity to dream, or a special usage of dreaming: "*Intolerance of frustration makes for intolerance of reality and . . . hatred of reality. This leads to reinforcement of projective identification as a method of evacuation. This in turn leads to dreams that are evacuations, not introjectory operations*" (C, 53). Which equals saying that in this usage dreams cannot perform the function of tools for self-knowledge.

I have pointed out that it is essential to mental efficiency to be able to "dream" a current emotional experience, whether it is taking place while the person is awake, or while asleep. By this I mean that the facts, as they are represented by the person's sense impressions, have to be converted into elements such as visual images commonly met in dreams as they are ordinarily reported. Such an idea will not seem strange if the reader consider what happens in reverie—the word itself, chosen to name the experience, is significant of the widespread nature of the experience. [C, 216]

One or two years later, the term is actively used to form a theory for the first time. In "A theory of thinking", page 116 of the version published in *Second Thoughts,* the sense of a dreamy, maternal state of loving care that allows for solace, warmth and serene sleep is implied: *"Suppose the infant is fed; the taking in of milk, warmth, love, may be felt as taking in a good breast"* (LE, 34).

This has a seminal importance in his theory because from now on Bion gives a more precise picture of his theory of thinking. It can be synthesized by the statement that a thought requires an absence. If one is left with satisfaction, one is left with beta-elements (q.v.) *"Both good and bad breasts are felt as possessing the same degree of concreteness and reality as milk. Sooner or later the 'wanted' breast is felt as an 'idea of a breast missing' and not as a bad breast present"* (LE, 34).

This is a kind of turning point for the human mind. It performs for the inception of thought processes the same role that the history of the "Cape of Good Hope" (later, Cape Town) had for the Portuguese explorers who discovered an alternative route from Europe to India by sea. The cape, first discovered by Bartolomeu Dias in 1487, was initially named "Cape of Torment" due to its inclement weather. Because he was sailing uncharted and inhospitable waters, Dias was afraid of a mutiny and did not go very far beyond the cape. Upon returning to Europe, the cape was renamed "Cape of Good Hope", perhaps as an attempt to draw attention away from the relative failure of Dias's aborted voyage, and instead underscore the optimistic hope of one day securing the route to India. Ten years later, the Portuguese explorer Vasco da Gama finally managed to circumnavigate the cape and, with it, the southern tip of Africa, sailing all the way through to India and securing the coveted alternative route. *"We can see that the bad, that is to say wanted but absent breast is much more likely to become recognized as an idea than the good breast which is associated with what a philosopher would call a thing-in-itself... in that the sense of a good breast depends on the existence of milk the infant has in fact taken"* (LE, 34).

The importance of this cannot be overstressed; in science, it created positivism, the abhorrence towards that which is "negative"; Kant called it "naïve realism". *"The good breast and the bad breast, the one being associated with actual milk that satisfies hunger and the other with the non-existence of that milk, must have a difference in psychical quality"* (LE, 34). The difference is just the inception of thinking that the experience of frustration allows. He had expanded this point in chapters V-VI of the same book (see forced splitting). But now, at this point, Bion supposes *"an infant to have been fed but to be feeling unloved"*.

In this case he had a problem to solve. He needed to expand Freud's theory of consciousness, but at first he was sceptical about it. After musing for some months about a "dream work alpha", which was fated to be left aside, he finally accepted the way Freud puts it: consciousness is the sense organ for the perception of psychical quality. Once accepting this, the problem was to know how *"consciousness comes into existence"* (LE, 35). Given his theory of alpha-function—which states that *"the existence of consciousness and unconsciousness depends on the prior production of alpha-elements by alpha-function"*, and therefore accords *"chronological priority to beta-elements over alpha-elements"*—is to be coherent with the whole idea in the formation of thinking processes: tolerance of frustration will define the outcome.

"Intolerance of frustration could be so pronounced that alpha-function would be forestalled by immediate evacuation of the beta-elements". The baby cannot think the breast in absence of it. *"The mental component, love, security, anxiety, as distinct from the somatic* [digestion of milk] *requires a process analogous to digestion"* (LE, 35).

Now Bion brings the mother to the fore and defines reverie: *"What this* [the mental digestion] *might be is concealed by use of the concept of alpha-function but a value may be found for this by psychoanalytic investigation. For example, when the mother loves the infant what does she do it with? Leaving aside the physical channels of communication my impression is that her love is expressed by reverie"* (LE, 35). Why does he bring the mother to the fore? Because this is the way real life is; the mother is in the forefront of whatever happens and in the fact that anything will happen.

Therefore one must necessarily assume that the issue is to get a capacity for thinking; this capacity cannot be obtained autistically or with satisfaction (invariably hallucinated). It demands a relationship. The mother comes to the fore in the sense that love is necessarily related to thinking and knowledge. Alpha-function alone, being intrapsychic to the infant, cannot cope with more than food for thinking (alpha-elements) but cannot provide thinking itself. Reverie can provide the means for that.

Reverie is not love; reverie is a way to express love. *". . . reverie is that state of mind which is open to the reception of any "objects" from the loved object and is therefore capable of reception of the infant's projective identifications whether they are felt by the infant to be good or bad.* [LE, 36]

Misuses and misconceptions: Many debase the concept into a soft-humanism or a corny commonplace.

Suggested cross-references: Concepts, Conceptions, Preconceptions, Projective identification, Psycho-analytical objects, Transformations.

Reversal of alpha-function: In chapter 10 of *Learning from Experience*. Bion describes a destruction of the contact-barrier (q.v.). This concept describes a kind of filter that both divides and unites unconscious and conscious.

There is *"a replacement of alpha-function by what may be described as a reversal of direction of the function"* (LE, 25). The concept of reversal of alpha-function is intertwined with the concept of contact barrier and its destruction.

"The reversal of direction is compatible with the treatment of thoughts by evacuation; that is to say that if the personality lacks the apparatus that would enable it to 'think' thoughts but is capable of attempting to rid the psyche of thoughts in much the same way as it rids itself of accretions of stimuli, then the reversal of alpha-function may be the method employed" (LE, 101). *"Instead of sense impressions being changed into alpha-elements for use in dream thoughts and unconscious waking thinking, the development of the contact-barrier is replaced by its destruction. This is effected by the reversal of alpha-function . . ."* that *"means the dispersal of the contact barrier and is quite compatible with the establishment of . . . bizarre objects"* (LE, 25).

Bion explains that the contact-barrier is a function and the ego is a structure. For this reason the *"reversal of alpha-function . . . affects the ego"*. This is important to the extent that it *"does not produce a simple return to beta-elements, but objects which differ in important respects from the original beta-elements which had no tincture of the personality adhering to them. The beta-element differs from the bizarre object in that the bizarre object is beta-element plus ego and superego traces. The reversal of alpha-function does violence to the structure associated with alpha-function"* [that is, the ego] (LE, 25).

Bion would never return to this theme.

&? The author made an attempt to extend clinically Bion's concept of the reversal of alpha-function. Profiting from Bion's own revision of his earlier ideas of pathology and cure (1967 and 1970) as well as from later expansions into the realm of minus, there emerges a suggestion about the existence of a model of an anti alpha-function. Therefore, it is not just a reversal of the alpha-function nor a pathological case, but it is a counterpoint to alpha-function. Anti alpha-function "takes" psychic data to start with and turns them into concrete and sensuous things. The emphasis on pathology is nil. This function would be necessary for certain purposes such as communication as it is found in art, early life and in any public-action that demands action in the material outside world, concrete survival (Sandler, 1990, 1997a).

Suggested cross-references: Alpha-function, Contact barrier.

Reversible perspective: A model that depicts the use of projective identification to make a dynamic situation static. It is drawn from academic psychology—the figure that can be seen as representing either a face or two vases, brought in to deal with a serious clinical problem.

From (psycho)dynamics to (psycho)static

The clinical origin is the observation of a false agreement. The silent denial of an interpretation is accompanied by an overt acceptance of the interpretation. The force of the interpretation is drained and sucked out. *"The patient reverses perspective to make a dynamic situation, static"* (EP, 54, 55, 61).

It differs from common forms of resistance due to its travestied presentation. The patient is keen to detect some ambiguities in the analyst's expressions, wording and so on, and gives to the *"interpretation a slant that the analyst does not intend"* (EP, 56).

For example: a patient detects a note of satisfaction in the analyst's voice and responds in a tone conveying dejection; a patient detects a moral supposition in an interpretation and his response is a silent rejection of that which he feels as a moral supposition. The silent denial is the outstanding clinical feature.

Reversible perspective differs from the attacks that the personality makes on its objects that has as its aftermath the minute fragmentation of both personality and objects; the component of dynamic splitting is lacking (EP, 58). It is a situation that favours the observation of the psychotic and non-psychotic personalities.

Reversible perspective is evidence of pain and is linked to extinguishing its sources as they are felt by the patient. Conflict, debate, disagreement are unspoken; the pseudo-agreement itself is lifeless, through making it insignificant. Its insignificance is achieved through a denial of the analyst's assumptions and vertexes. The disagreement is clothed by agree-able rational devices inserted in the discourse and pleases both parties.

The detection is subtle: *"the disagreement between analyst and analysand is apparent only when the analysand appears to have been taken unawares"*. There is a pause, and **this** pause is useful as a tool to detect that the perspective is being reversed. *"The pause is not being employed to absorb fully the implications of the interpretation, but rather to establish a point of view, not expressed to the analyst, from which the analyst's interpretation, though verbally unchanged and unchallenged, has a meaning other than the one the analyst intended to convey"* (EP, 55). If the patient is successful in avoiding the pain this way and the analyst likewise is successful in avoiding the pain, the result is that *"after many months of apparently successful analysis the patient has gained an extensive knowledge of the analyst's theories but no insight"* (EP, 55). There is a display of the denied disagreement.

The perspective, so to say, "un-reversed" that allowed Bion to *"grasp the meaning of the associations, was that afforded by the Oedipus theory. In every instance, that which appeared to cause the patient to reverse the perspective, was the Oedipus myth"* (EP, 58).

The situation must be "un-reversed" in order to *"restore dynamic to a static situation and so make development possible"* (EP, 60). Please refer to the entry, "Growth".

Bion emphasizes a distinction between myth and theory. The Oedipus theory and its various formulations belong to the areas encompassed by the functions of the ego, namely, attention and inquiry. Concepts derived from attention and inquiry are scientific approaches. The myth, in contrast, belongs to the areas encompassed by the dreaming activity (EP, 58).

The building of a delusion

The patient takes subtle but violent measures to ensure that his analyst's interpretations are agreed; "*they thus become the outward sign of a static situation*". But the analyst's interpretations do not permit this as far they can be alive, real, and evocative. The patient may feel them provocative and is "*unlikely always to command sufficient nimbleness of mind to match the interpretation with a shift that reverses the perspective in which the interpretation is viewed*". To ensure success "*the patient employs an armoury that is reinforced by delusion and hallucination. If he cannot reverse the perspective at once he can adjust his perception of the facts by mis-hearing and mis-understanding so that they give substance to the static view: a delusion is in being.*

If this is not sufficient to keep the situation static the patient resorts to hallucination . . . in order to preserve, temporarily, an ability to reverse perspective; and reversed perspective in order to preserve a static hallucination" (EP, 60).

The hallucinations and delusions appear through the covert-subtleties pattern. They are static, evanescent and clothed by the non-psychotic appearance. Agreements determine that "*. . . the true significance of the patient's behaviour as a sign of delusion or hallucination is not apparent unless the analyst is alert to this possibility . . .*

The lesson to be drawn from this discussion is the need to deduce the presence of intense pain and the threat that it represents to mental integration" (EP, 61).

The issue is not to avoid pain—the issue is ongoing undetected pain. It is doubly serious in the so-called "training analysis", where collusion is a feature often found (please refer to the entry, "Pain").

Synonyms: Reversed perspective, reversion of perspective.

Suggested cross-references: Growth, Pain, Real psycho-analysis.

S

Satisfaction: Freud regarded satisfaction—often understood as happiness—as an impossible achievement. The development of the concept of a principle of reality in his paper of 1920 considers something "beyond" satisfaction. It equates Nirvana with death. The "interminability" of an analysis as well as the tribulations of the scientist compared to the consolation provided by religion (described in his paper about *Weltanschauung*) display his observations.

This word is often linked to mistakes due to the prevalence of the principle of pleasure/displeasure in the mind of the reader. Satisfaction of instinctual needs (or objectives, as described in *"Instincts and their vicissitudes"*) cannot be confused with satisfaction of desire. Freud himself needed almost 20 years to discern them fully.

Bion's use of the term appears in "A theory of thinking" and in *Learning from Experience*. It is put into the terms that a pre-conception finds a realization. It satisfies the "need for a realization". It does not say that the realization fully satisfies the pre-conception. For an ever-fulfilling goal, the object is never possible; or it is a hallucinated situation.

There is a mathematical sense of this word as used by Bion. In discussing the term "factor", he writes that *"It may be represented by the unsaturated element(ξ) in $\psi(\xi)$ and there must be a realization approximating to it. What the realization is that satisfies it, in the mathematical sense of satisfying the terms of an equation, is a matter to be determined by the psycho-analytical investigation itself"* (LE, 89).

☺ The issue is developed in terms of science: Bion states that there are no problems that can be resolved; the resolution of a problem leads to the formulation of unexpected new problems.

The disciplinary recommendation of being careful with manifestations of desire is the clearest indication of his ideas on satisfaction. From 1969 onwards Bion was fond of quoting a phrase from Maurice Blanchot which André Green had told him: *"La réponse est le malheur de la question"*.

He invariably refused to answer his audience's questions in the traditional manner. And a few days before dying, he was quoted by a close friend as uttering: *"Life is full of surprises—most of them unpleasant"*.

Misuses and misunderstandings: There lingers the same difficulty that encircled Freud's writings. Many readers mistake the attempt of instincts at their instinctual-satisfaction for the so-called satisfaction of pleasure. Similarly, people suppose that the preconception is satisfied by a realization. What is satisfied is the need for a realization. The satisfaction of the pre-conception's goal does not imply that the satisfaction of the "pre-conception-in-itself" was achieved. The real breast furnishes the satisfaction of the goal, but not the satisfaction of the pre-conceived breast. The former allows, due to its "non-satisfaction" quota, the inception of thinking and symbolization; the latter originates the hallucinatory processes.

The misuse of the term, which tries to attribute to it a sense that is the opposite of the original, displays how resilient is the prohibition to knowledge. This fate usually falls on outstanding psycho-analytic achievements. It is in itself a proof of Freud and Bion's views. To regard them as "pessimists" is an expression of cravings for satisfaction.

Saturation:

> Since I wish to find a system of representation that would serve for all these systems, and some of whose existence I am unaware, I seek

a system of representation that is unsaturated ($\psi(\xi)$) and will permit of saturation. [T, 118]

Definition. This concept refers to a **system of representation** that tackles the saturation of meaning in thinking processes. An analogy may be drawn from chemistry: some elements or materials may be diluted in (or by) others, up to a point and in variable degrees of saturation of the medium (the dilutent).

This entry can be read more easily after the reader has obtained a firm grasp of the contents of the entries, Elements of Psycho-Analysis, Grid, O, Psycho-analytical objects.

☺ The concept was initially developed to describe the matching of pre-conceptions with realizations (q.v.). The prototype is the breast and the baby's pre-conception of the breast. In this case it was already stated that the saturation of the pre-conception was an idealized chimera. There is always a non-saturation—meaning, the no-breast was seen as the condition for the inception of thinking processes. The concept was then used in the description of the formation of psycho-analytic objects and elements of psycho-analysis (see the specific entries).

The final use of the concept (1965) is in the framework of the theory of transformations and invariances (q.v.). It seems to have had a function in the adoption of the theory. It involves verbal communications which have seminal consequences in the analytic endeavour. In brief: the various evolving cycles of transformations that encircle the invariances are cycles of increased saturation and ensuing de-saturation. The movement towards more sophisticated levels of saturation and their accompanying fresh "de-saturation" corresponds to the successive experience of the paranoid–schizoid and depressive positions. The path corresponds to entering into the darkness of the unknown and from there, becoming that which the person is. It can be viewed through the continuing experience of a container looking to contain a contained which looks for a container. To state the last phrase in practical terms: the container is the verbal formulation (either the analyst's or the patient's). The contained is that which strives to be communicated and/or not communicated (feelings, emotions, emotional experiences, interpretations, etc.).

It would not be an exaggeration to state that the concept of saturation, as a movement of the mind, as the basis of thought processes, integrates all of Bion's contributions to psycho-analysis as a cohesive whole.

The saturation would be seen as the very formation—in genetic terms—of thought. The model of the Grid (q.v.) is wholly constructed on the basis of successive saturation. Definitory hypotheses "searched for" saturation. All Grid categories of the vertical axis may be seen as steps in the direction of increased saturation and non-saturated conditions "looking for" saturation. The process, desaturation–saturation, expresses the development (growth) of thinking.

> Evidently the impulse to achieve saturation is unlikely to be fulfilled because in addition to the limitations of human capacity there is the factor of "the void and formless infinite", which, whether thought of as in the mind of man or outside it, cannot be known but must be "become", that is, saturated in a particular way. [T, 155]

His last formulation on saturation was made in 1975. The kernel is maintained—an idealized breast, and its dissatisfaction as the *sine qua non* condition for the inception of thought processes and maturation. The form tries to integrate all the earlier contributions. Saturation, O, the drama of communication; the limitation of all sensuously based media, the implications for the analyst, the scientific attitude—they are all there.

The reader may keep in mind that the appeal to symbols invites a de-saturation. Colloquial words such as "man" are overloaded with that which is already known. They are saturated with shared prejudiced views that prevent further investigation. In the session, one should say, beware of the already known, including known words:

> Suppose I drew λ and claimed it was, or was a picture of, a man. You who are looking at this could, if the conditions existed in which we could converse, agree that I looked "just like that" and that it was a meritorious and continuing example of my artistic genius. This book could be hailed as bearing, in itself, resemblance to its paternity—that it could not be mistaken for someone else's "brain child". But I may have a different aim; say, that of writing a description of psycho-analysis. To me, that the book bore witness to its

mental origins might be an unwelcome irrelevance, a feature additional to the main component of my wish to communicate and your wish to receive. It is this double quality of the communication and the fact that significance might be attached in varying degrees, now to one, now to the other component, that I wish to discuss. I want to stress that the components are not "bi-valent" but multi- or poly-valent even if at first I denote it by a "bi-valent" symbol—this, $\lambda\xi$. The signs I am choosing are the Chinese λ and the Greek ξ. If I write it as λ (ξ) I wish λ to represent a constant, (ξ) an unknown variable. But what is this? Why have symbols appeared? The experience of my existence stimulates curiosity about me and my objects—of people or things like me.

Since I do not know for sure what these objects are, but want in fact to discuss them, I need to have some way of referring to them . . . I want to discuss man, but as soon I say that, I realize the word "man" has a definite, perhaps misleading and frustratingly definite, meaning . . .

The places in the following few sentences marked by _ are places representing "some thing" I want to talk about. "Some thing" is not adequate; it is too impregnated with pre-existing meaning—too saturated (λ) and at the same time not saturated (ξ) enough. I am now as wide awake, conscious, rational, sane as I am ever likely to be between the moment of writing and the day of my _. I pick upon the _ for although I do not know when that is, I imagine that the empty _ will at some time be, like an algebraic variable in the course of mathematical calculations or a legal register of births, marriages and deaths, completed . . .

λ (ξ) denotes a domain without beginning, end, or other dimension. I have to employ an extremely inadequate apparatus to discuss it. I have to manufacture the apparatus as I proceed. I claim that it is artistic though the art has not yet been created; it is religious though the religion has not been and never can (without ceasing to be a religion) be made to conform to any of the dogmata and institutions hitherto regarded as characteristic of religion. I do not expect the art to be analogous to music, painting, literary expression, sculpture or quantum mechanics; the "uncertainty principle" (borrowed from Heisenberg) used by me both formulates and destroys the formulation together with λ (ξ). O is by definition indestructible and not subject to, circumscribed by, beginnings and ends, rules, laws of nature or any construct of the human mind. In the domain of human comprehension Melanie Klein could not reconcile herself to the fact that whenever she had made herself understood, the fact rendered what she understood no longer "alive". [AMF, I, 86–9]

Saturation and absence of object

Thinking depends on the interaction of the no-thing with the realization—that is felt as approximating that very same no-thing. In this context, Bion means by thought (the term, "*I mean*", is Bion's), that which enables the person to solve problems "*in the absence of the object*" (T, 107). "*Indeed, unless the object is absent there is no problem*" (T, 107).

In the definition of the psycho-analytic object. Bion proposed a quasi-mathematical notation for it: $(\psi)(\xi)(M)$. (ξ) stands for the unsaturated component of the object.

Both the search and discovery of elements perceived in space are part of the procedure by which definitory hypotheses begin to acquire meaning. The definitory hypothesis has a negative quality. It is discarded or replaced by new elements "*that saturate the elements (ξ) of $\psi(\xi)$*" (T, 106).

Saturation is therefore a **necessary step** in the march into the unknown.

The following quotation summarizes the issue. The quasi-mathematical formulations mean, if translated into verbal formulations:

(i)   T (ξ) means the transformation of an unsaturated element;

(ii) C2 means that a verbal formulation is amenable to be seen as a false myth or dream;

(iii) A1 means that a verbal formulation is amenable to be classified as a definitory hypothesis. Therefore the quasi-mathematical formulation that is used in the quotation below—T (ξ) = C2 → A1—which is in the form of an equation, means that a saturated hallucination, from a real unsaturated object (for example, a breast) is amenable to be transformed into a hypothesis that potentially can be used by furthering the search into reality. "Is the ideal breast I crave, real?" could be another verbal formulation of it. The question T (ξ) = C2 → A1, replacing the absolute truth C2 allows further research, further saturation:

By analogy, we, having bound the constantly conjoined elements of the analytic experience by the formulation T (ξ) = C2 → A1, may now resort to further analytical experience for evidence which will provide us with meaning; in other terms, to saturate the unsaturated element (ξ); or, again, to put it in another way, we hope to find evidence from analysis for a more precise understanding of this particular patient's transformation. [T, 14]

In Bion's example, the clinical situations were a handshake and the emotional experience provided by the sight of a dog.

Saturation as a Need and Saturation as a Wish (Desire)

All realizations just approximate the pre-conception. They always fall short of fulfilling it. The problem of the absent object—breast, father, etc.—is associated to the "non-approximation factor" of the realization (para 100). "*With the psychotic personality the approximation has to be extremely close*". Consequently (ξ) often remains unsaturated. The problem, when associated with forced splitting and excessive concretization, is that the "*active no-thing, without a corresponding thing, is associated with the dis-satisfaction in the domain of alimentation when hunger exists, but there is no food*" (all quotations, T, 107).

Saturation and verbal communication

Statements from the analysand are either unsaturated or saturated. The former are free associations and daytime dreaming activity; the latter call to be de-saturated. For example: if one hears a dream's manifest content and the accompanying free associations, they are to be constantly conjoined with the analyst's trained intuition and previous experience with the patient. This leads to unsaturated latent contents. These are offered to the analysand for further saturation in the following "cycle of transformation".

It follows that the "*verbal communication is therefore one that cannot represent O by virtue of the accepted meaning of the sign employed nor can it represent O by access of meaning through saturation*" (T, 118). [O is a quasi-mathematical notation for ultimate reality; please refer to this specific entry.]

Saturation in verbal communication brings with it some intrinsic limitations. The de-saturation may prove to be difficult. In chapter 9 of *Transformations*, Bion furnishes a dream-like account of his contact with a patient:

Two people are present: myself and a patient. I am detached and so is he, though for both of us the experience is important. As he lies on the couch and I sit I imagine that a cloud begins to form rather in the way that clouds can sometimes be seen to form above a hot-point on a summer's day. It seems to be above him. A similar cloud may be visible to him, but he will see it arising from me. These are probability clouds. [T, 117]

Bion goes on and intuits that the "*hot points*" and "*clouds*", visual and tactile imagery, are "de-sense-fied", and conjoined with "*pressure*" and "*probability*" turn into immaterial "*tension*"; further evolutions display clouds of "*certainty*", and also "*clouds of depression, guilt, hope, and fear likewise*". There is a "total situation" going on:

I associate pressure with both tension and clouds. The total situation I have tried to describe pictorially I would like to be able to describe odoriferously—as a dog might smell it, and, if he were sufficiently gifted might delineate it odoriferously. And similarly with all other sensuous media available. Since I wish to find a system of representation that would serve for all these systems, and some of whose existence I am unaware, I seek a system of representation that is unsaturated (ψ (ξ)) and will permit of saturation . . .

I must replace the C1 elements, visual images of clouds, analyst, analysand, etc., and replace them by elements approximating to ψ (ξ). It is clear that the C1 elements must not be denuded because were that to occur they would be replaced by β-elements.

I can do this by using the point (.) to represent the "place where" a some-thing (as contrasted with no-thing) could be and the line (———) as the locus of a point or the place where the point is going. The analogy is defective because it is saturated by a meaning of movement . . .

The changes I have had to make throughout this book *from analogy to more precise formulation, and from more precise formulation to analogy, illustrate some of the difficulties with which I am attempting to deal. All these changes are examples of transformation* . . .

the model (represented by verbal signs of C category) of analyst and patient served to communicate by virtue of the rigidity (invariant quality) of the images. This same rigidity meant the model was saturated and therefore unsuitable for use as a pre-conception (column 4 element). [T-118–9 and 121; my italics]

Saturation and Becoming

The transition from "knowing about" to "becoming" O can be seen as a particular instance of the development of the conception from the pre-conception (row E from row D). I have described that process as one of saturation of an unsaturated element $\psi\,(\xi)$, to become $\psi\,(\psi)$ (ξ). That is to say, a pre-conception becomes a conception and retains its dimension of "usability" as a pre-conception. [T, 153]

An example of saturation: Oedipus

The pronouncement of the oracle defines the theme of the story and can be regarded as a definition, or definitory hypothesis. It resembles a pre-conception, or an algebraic calculus, in that it is an "unsaturated element" that is "saturated" by the unfolding of the story; or an "unknown", in the mathematical sense, that is "satisfied" by the story. It is the statement of the theme of the story that is to unfold: the description of the criminal who is wanted. [EP, 48]

Misuses and misunderstandings: In some parts of the world the concept is taken as a judgmental rule. It dictates that interpretations and thinking should never be "saturated". The saturation is seen as an enemy to be fought. The dynamic process of saturation/de-saturation is lost in favour of an established, ossified, and judgmental theory—far from Bion's writings.

Schizophrenia, theory of: Note on terminology In 1967 Bion had already developed his observations on the inadequacies of the curative model to the psycho-analytic endeavour. Then he had clearer ideas on the limited utility of psychiatric diagnoses to the here and now of the analytic session. For example, his warning appears in the remark, *"for the practising psycho-analyst, the terms used in 34[1] are almost useless and I would now use them with circumspection"'* (ST, 139).

Those were the times of his quasi-didactic recommendations on the analyst's need to discipline him(her) self on memory, desire and explanatory understanding in order to be able to attain the psychoanalytic vertex. They appear in the Commentary to *Second Thoughts* as well as in the now classical paper "Notes on memory and desire". Both can be regarded as preparatory papers to *Attention and Interpretation* (which would be published in 1970).

Therefore he jumps from the psychiatric diagnosis to a truly psycho-analytic appreciation stemming from Melanie Klein's observations: "*The patients in whom the difficulties described occur are important for the degree to which destructive ambitions are active*'" (ST, 139).

The modern reader should take into account the development that Bion enjoyed and the second thoughts that he entertained as a matter of consequence, before using the definitions and postures.

Theory of Schizophrenia: Bion states that Melanie Klein's work occupies a central position in his views about the theory of schizophrenia. His approach to this issue was rather uncommon in his time and continues to be so: he sets out to scrutinize verbal thought. That is, both the processes through which thought is formed and a noticeably complex form of it that Bion names "verbal thought". There are non-verbal thoughts—dream thoughts, for example. The latter kind of thought is largely based on the human capacity to *formulate* perceptions in a sensuous form (pictograms and visual imagery).

This is not as original an approach as it might seem. Bion has psychiatric ancestors such as Von Domarus' research that illuminated the non-syllogistic thinking so typical of "schizophrenics". One may look for his epistemological motives. As did Freud and Klein, Bion tackled schizophrenia using the accurate clinical observations provided by psychiatry. Also, one may see that many epistemologists, the very founders of all theories of knowledge—Locke, Hume, Voltaire, Hamann, von Herder, and more recently Wittgenstein, had an acute awareness of the links between reality, thinking, and language. Wittgenstein built a whole theory in which reality is figured by language itself—not as a representation, but as "propositions" (*Tractatus Logico-Philosophicus*).

Bion uses Locke's ideas on common sense, Hume's ideas on constant conjunctions. He was acquainted with Bertrand Russell, whose influence is felt in many parts of his work, as for example in issues of personal authority and **responsibility** (q.v.). Russell tutored Wittgenstein. The contemporary and intellectual climate may have influenced Bion's interest in verbal thought. This was not an issue much developed in Freud and Klein's work. It was just hinted at in "Two principles of mental functioning" and in Klein's forays into symbol formation and the language of infants.

Bion paid more than lip service to language—psycho-analysis being the "talking cure", wholly practised via verbal thought and language. If Shakespeare and Goethe can be seen as Freud's great sources in his research into the realm of human nature, one may well respect Bion's concern for verbal thought and its disturbances.

Bion seems to have been conscious of resistance to his seemingly novel approach. One cannot know now if he suffered from the criticisms or if he was able to forecast criticisms due to some kind of personal intuition or due to his long experience with human beings, in terms of groups' **basic assumptions** (q.v.). One must remember that those times (the fifties) were ridden with quasi-wars of serious accusations of deviations from psychoanalytic theory and technique; accusations of "dissidence" were quite common and had adversely affected the work of Melanie Klein a few years earlier: *"By approaching the subject through consideration of verbal thought I run the risk of appearing to neglect the nature of the schizophrenic's object relations"* (ST, 23). He emphasizes his view that *"the peculiarity of the schizophrenic's object relations is the outstanding feature of schizophrenia"*. There are reasons to pursue a seemingly novel path: *"the importance of the points that I wish to make lies in their capacity to illuminate the nature of this object relationship of which they are a subordinate function"* (ST, 23).

Bion hints at a possible collaboration that psycho-analysis makes with epistemology—the object relations theory and its links with language. This was Bion's second purely psycho-analytical published study, the earlier papers having a strong sociological bent.

The paper hints at two scientific tools he will use in order to apprehend psychic reality (mental life):

i.   Research into the "nature" of the phenomena of psychic reality.
ii. Research into the functions that those phenomena perform in psychic reality.

The first tool (i) derives from a conjunction of Freud's papers on the two principles of mental functioning (1911 and 1920) with some epistemological achievements by Plato and Kant. The second tool (ii) embodies mathematical modes of thought. Bion was not interested in mathematics *per se* but rather in the history and philosophy of mathematics.

Thus armed, he endeavoured to elicit *factors, functions and their correlates* in order to make approximations to Truth or Reality ("**Truth-O**", q.v.), the thing-in-itself (adopting Kant's parlance), the Platonic Forms, or "**O**" (adopting Bion's quasi-mathematical symbol to denote the numinous realm). In psycho-analytic terms, Bion attempts explorations into the unknown, the realm of the unconscious, the Id. Those are not explorations to make final, teleological discoveries but allow flashing, transient insights of a "**becoming**" (q.v.), in the way of forays into the unknown using unknown tools that are forged in the spur of the moment. They are intuitively made to the extent that "mother necessity" demands them, just as the practising psycho-analyst does in the here and now of the session.

Later Bion would explore differently some paths he opened here. He equates the attitude one has towards one's verbal thought to one's attitude *"to his potency and his equipment for work and love"* (ST, 27). In this sense, the capacity for verbal thought and hate and ambivalence against this capacity may express themselves as hate towards analysis. The patient may feel like a *"prisoner of psycho-analysis"* (ST, 27). In more colloquial terms it means that the hate and ambivalence towards verbal thought means hate towards the very existence of psychic reality. Psycho-analysis, after all, is a mode of getting in touch with psychic reality (mental life).

With the advancements made by Bion concerning the universality of psychosis, one may see that those clinical manifestations make their appearance in so-called neurotic patients. Many of them act out rather than think; many communicate through provoking emotional rather than verbal responses; some use their discourse to disguise their feelings.

The loss of verbal capacity entails the loss of an ability to build in a rational way the systems of evasion from contact with inner truth. In analysis it expresses itself, as far as Bion's experience goes, through manifestations such as, *"I have lost my words"*, meaning, *"as further analysis disclosed, that the instrument with which he had effected his escape had been lost in the process. Words, the capacity for verbal thought, the one essential for further progress, have gone"* (ST, 27). Bion observes a paradox: both the gain and the loss of verbal capacity are feared. The individual falls back willingly on using the improvements in his or her verbal capacity as a *"mode of action"*. *"From the patient's point of view, the achievement of verbal thought has been a most unhappy event. Verbal thought is so interwoven with catastrophe and the painful emotion of depression that the patient, resorting to projective identification, splits it off and pushes it into the analyst. The results are again unhappy for the patient; lack of this capacity is now felt by him to be the same thing as being insane. On the other hand, reassumption of this capacity seems to him to be inseparable from depression and awareness, on a reality level this time, that he is 'insane'. . ."*

The analyst's problem is the patient's dread, now quite manifest, of attempting a psycho-analytic understanding of what they meant for him, partly because the patient now understands that psycho-analysis demands from him that very verbal thought which he dreads" (ST, 32).

In 1967 Bion modifies some of his apprehensions of schizophrenia and verbal thought. He expands it not only with concern to the ever present psychotic under-layer but also in something that seems to be a human necessity: religious thinking—idolization and capacity for **reverence and awe** (q.v.) (ST, 145; C, 284). For the extensive exploring of science, religion and psycho-analysis, see the talks between the characters P.A. and Priest in volumes II and III of *A Memoir of the Future*—and the entry "Science versus Religion" in this dictionary.

Not dissimilar to Wittgenstein's work, Bion would develop the psycho-analytical clinical exploration of the links between words, verbal thought, reality and truth.

The psychotic clinical feature is linked not to psychiatric diagnoses but to aspects of the paranoid–schizoid position such as self-interest, arrogance, contempt for the object, persecution, and hatred of truth. One of his statements in 1973 may illustrate the issue: *"I can see that this is compatible with a culture in which it is assumed as a matter of course that you do not believe what you are told by anybody. It is difficult to see how they ever manage to get anything done in which you would have to know the truth ... you simply assume that the person who is speaking is speaking an untruth, or at any rate is being dishonest in the sense of making a communication that is primarily for its own purposes, not for the communication of a true statement to some other person. It throws an entirely new light on the problems of psycho-analysis and the fact that nobody is likely to believe that one is trying to tell them something that it is worth their while to hear"* (C, 357).

In 1965, Bion observes that a problem involved in analysing the psychotic patient seems to be his impossibility of working without the presence of the objects which, and about which, the work must be done. This produces, as a matter of consequence, a *"tendency to produce problem situations instead of solving problems"*. He follows by putting the issue primarily in the realm of perception: *"If we could suppose that there was a failure to develop a system of notation and record which could also be used for manipulation in the absence of the object; it might explain a number of features associated with the psychotic's behaviour"* (T, 40).

His clinical observations hark back to his papers on schizophrenia. He noticed that the psychotic sometimes behaves as if *"in order to 'think' something he had to wait for that thing to appear in the world of external reality. Similarly he seems unable to think or imagine a situation but has to act it out"*. Bion states the situation in terms of the theory of transformations. In this theory, there is a system of signs. T is the sign that Bion uses to represent the phenomenal counterpoint of O; O is the sign that Bion uses to represent the ultimate reality, or that which belongs to the realm of noumena; $Tp\beta$ is the sign to represent the final products of the patient's transformations. In this case, it seems that the patient cannot transform T (the phenomenal counterpart of O). It seems that the patient has a direct contact with the ultimate reality ("O") and cannot transform O into T.

The situation must be examined from two perspectives: the person can never know the thing-in- itself, he can just know the primary and secondary qualities, which are amenable to be apprehensible by the human sensuous apparatus. But the psychotic seems to be unable to know anything other than the thing-in-itself. *"This apparent attitude has similarities with another apparent attitude, namely, that postulated by the theory of projective identification. He behaves as if parts of his personality had physical properties and could be split off and projected into others as physical objects which the other object could modify or use. Since a psychotic patient can express words and sentences it seems reasonable to suppose that he can think. But thinking, in the sense of manipulating words and thoughts to do work in the absence of the object, seems to be just what the patient cannot do. I have said* [Learning from Experience] *that such patients do not have memories but only undigested facts. The breakdown appears to occur in the necessity for an object into which the patient feels he is able to project parts of his personality for their development and manipulation. If he feels there is no such object, and no such possibility as 'splitting off parts of his personality' disturbance is set up"* (T, 40–1).

This posture develops that which was earlier suggested in the paper "On arrogance": the triad arrogance-stupidity-curiosity emerges when the patient feels impeded to exert projective identification. It shows that PS is not an enemy or synonymous with illness.

Recommended cross-references: Intuition (especially the last part, on "Gist"), Transformations.

Suggested cross-reference: Mathematization of Psycho-analysis.

"Science versus religion": Have science, and as a matter of consequence, psycho-analysis, anything to do with religious activity? Or with theology?

Appearances are deceptive. The psycho-analytic movement may have misjudged Freud's writings about religion, thus creating a religious counter-religion, whose fanaticism may pass unnoticed. The general disapproving tone attributed to a so-called "psycho-analytic view of religion" has been hampering a real appreciation of Freud's views. Passing judgement precludes appreciation (see the entries, Judgmental Values and Sense of Truth). *"Psycho-analysis tells you nothing; it is an instrument, like the blind man's stick, that extends the power to gather information"* (C, 361). The claim that an analyst is entitled by his condition of being an analyst to have a say in any issue is not scrutinized. It is not scrutinized even by analytic standards that could, for example, reveal omnipotence. This belief in an "analytic view on . . ." anything precluded appreciating Freud's respect towards approaches that differed from his own. The reading of his paper, "On the question of a *Weltanschauung*" (the last of the *"New Introductory Lectures"*) may dispel this commonly found misunderstanding.

Bion also seemed to be free from these two prejudices (of attributing to the analytic view an overpowering reach, and deprecating religion) both of which may be credited to hubris, haughtiness and self-righteousness and other aspects of the paranoid–schizoid position:

P.A. Psycho-analysts are trained to do psycho-analysis only—a considerable undertaking. I would not feel qualified by my training to do more than that although like surgeons, engineers and other citizens, I am expected to carry my civil obligations as well as my professional ones. But I deprecate the idea that my expertise extends beyond that of psycho-analyst; it is hard enough trying to be an "expert" in one's own profession. Yet we are constantly expected to be expert far beyond our professional domain and are regarded with contempt if we fail to live up to expectations which we strive not to arouse. [AMF, III, 507]

Bion's integration of psycho-analysis with the philosophy of mathematics and philosophy itself cannot be seen as belonging either to cross-disciplinarity or interdisciplinarity or even trans-disciplinarity. The integration is genetic; the irradiating kernel of these branches is the same right from the start. Under that vertex, philosophy, theology, and science are different ways of the same underlying attempt: the apprehension of reality itself. He regards philosophers and theologians as primeval psycho-analysts.

P.A. The hope is that psycho-analysis brings into view thoughts and actions and feelings of which the individual may not be aware and so cannot control. If he can be aware of them he may, or may not, decide—albeit unconsciously—to change them.

ALICE I don't see how that differs from what has been done by parents, teachers, saints, philosophers, for countless generations of prophets of one kind and another. [AMF, III, 509–10]

Some kinships between analysts and religious people are: the healing pretensions, secularization, mystic tradition, as well as pretensions to deal with immaterial facts such as distress, mind and reality. Also, that which is commonly regarded as the distortion of analysis, medicine and religion: a tendency to self-idealization, a sense of mission, authoritarianism and messianic ideas of owner-ship of absolute truth, and denial of hate and self-hate.

Is the sensuous concrete debasing of theology into seculariza-tion as pointed out by countless individuals and groups such as St. Francis of Assisi, the Jansenists, and the Reformists akin to the debasement of psycho-analysis into the mindlessness that charac-terizes much of the psycho-analytic movement?

Bion calls the religious establishment an "organization", in the social sense of the term.

🕒 Bion's first suggestion that helped him to encircle the analytic endeavour with the help of a theological analogy resorted to the metaphor of the mystic which is part of *Transformations* and *Attention and Interpretation*.

This attempt reaches maturity in the novel form of a quasi-Socratic dialogue between part-objects embodied in *A Memoir of the Future*.

Possible analogies

Bion elicits some striking, unexpected similarities between the theological posture and psycho-analysis, and the religious and psycho-analytic establishments. He stresses the differences and above all, the paradoxical psycho-analytic view entertained by religion *vis-à-vis* the religious view entertained by the imitative psycho-analysts. They depend on real human limitations, as for example, the movement in tandem of PS to D and back to PS. There is a tendency to worship when helplessness prevails.

This entry can be read separately but it is potentially enriched by the reading of the entries, Atonement, Mystic, Facts and Real Analysis.

> ROSEMARY . . . You two (addressing Priest and P.A.) have arrived at an agreement. I am glad—
>
> PRIEST It is more apparent than real.
>
> P.A. We have arrived at the same fence at the same time and that gives an illusion of agreement liable to obscure the fact that we are on different sides of the fence.
>
> ROSEMARY Fence? What fence?
>
> PRIEST Alas! It is invisible, impalpable, insensible . . .
>
> P.A. Nearly inexpressible but for our borrowings from disciplines not our own.
>
> ROSEMARY Then you are in agreement in "acquisition".
>
> P.A. No. He steals or borrows from me: I do the same from him. We both resent each other and even ourselves as we have to collude with each other. Collusion, robbery, theft—what do we not owe to them!

PRIEST Bigotry, ignorance, intolerance—how much science owes to them!

P.A. How firm the foundations on which the Church must build!

PRIEST How persistently the scientists rob us of faith! How unsleeping must be our resistance to their attacks!

ALICE A plague on both your houses and may they soon perish. [AMF, II, 384–5]

P.A. The Intuitionists would say that logical and intuitionist mathematics can exist happily with one another provided the logicians admit the reality of another approach. Quantum mechanicists do not deny the existence of wave motion. [AMF, III, 554]

The earliest attempts to find knowledge were—and still are—linked to helplessness, bewilderment and fear. These seem to be among the most basic feelings and emotional experiences that encircle and permeate human life from birth to death. The encircling environment is both hostile and facilitating to life. The universe, external and internal, is an immeasurable amount of inexplicable and non-understandable facts and ways.

More often than not the human capacity to construe and even to fathom scales of measurement, the facts we must deal with, whatever they may be, occur in such a domain that the scales of measurement are at their best caricatures of that which demands to be measured. The scales suffer the same limitations of the apprehension of the facts itself. The phenomena occur in scales infinitely small or large, in comparison to the scale we may imagine. This is valid quite independently of the invented unit of measurement one chooses to rely on, such as macroscopically defined sizes, range of apprehension of human senses, etc.

In brief, the human being must deal with the unknown, but accustomed himself to denying it. Intolerance of these facts is linked, as Freud showed, to a reaction that generates omnipotent and omniscient ideas. They are usually projected outside in deities or explanations about the origins and ends of the universe.

PRIEST Where do you suppose that reality originates—only from the genes, the chromosomes, DNA, the double helix?

P.A. I don't know.

PRIEST That's the wisest admission you have made.

P.A. I could not aspire to a scientific inquiry without that basic assumption.

PRIEST I could not aspire to God without a similar admission.

P.A. My objection to your people is that they claim an omniscient and omnipotent God.

PRIEST We aspire to a god made in our own image—that is well known; but because we keep company with people that have certain views I don't think we should be debited with those views.

P.A. It is part of my work to point out that all of us are victims of just that experience. Like it or not, of such is the kingdom of men.

PRIEST I don't quarrel with that. [AMF, II, 383–384]

Therefore, in the earliest ways to deal with helplessness and truth as expressed by the religious movement; the final goal is evasion of pain and a simultaneous craving for safety, happiness—even if imaginary. Freud's studies—namely, *The Future of an Illusion, Civilization and its Discontents, Moses and Monotheism,* "On the question of a *Weltanschauung*"—offer a number of hypotheses and conjectures. They also offer theories and hypotheses about these conjectures (C, 378).

This emotional origin hampers the attempts to apprehend reality as it is; sometimes it is really seen or felt as unbearable—an *oeil en trop*, as André Green pointed out (AMF, III, 537). This feeling is linked to the regression of development of thinking to more primitive ways such as moral judgement.

A central point in Bion's work seems to be the replacement of primitive moral judgment by more developed forms of mental functioning. Or to put it in other terms, mindlessness may be replaced or amended by thought.

Moral implications, moral schemata, afflicted him in his personal life to the point of making him take the plunge of joining the British war effort of 1914. These are later seen as conflicting with the scientific outlook (please refer to the entries Lie, Sense of Truth and Truth in this dictionary).

This issue cannot be overemphasized with regard to

(i)   the loss of the psycho-analytical vertex,

(ii)   the possibility or impossibility of achieving real analysis,

(iii   the danger of replacing insight with a given analyst's authority,

(iv)   the persistence of collusive transference hallucination rather than working through of transference. It fuels omnipotence and imitation of analysis—in the here and now of the session.

> The observation of constant conjunction of phenomena whose conjunction or coherence has not been previously observed, and therefore the whole process of Ps⟺D interaction, definition and search for meaning that is to be attached to the conjunction, can be destroyed by the strength of a sense of causation and its moral implications. Patients show that the resolution of a problem appears to present less difficulty if it can be regarded as belonging to a moral domain; causation, responsibility and therefore a controlling force (as opposed to helplessness) provide a framework within which omnipotence reigns. In certain circumstances . . . the scene is thus set for conflict (reflected in controversies such as those on Science and Religion). This situation is portrayed in the Eden and Babel myths. The significance for the individual lies in its part in obstructing the Ps⟺D interaction. [T, 64–5]

The whole issue is dealt with quasi-artistically in *A Memoir of the Future*, through the talks between the characters "Paul" (a priest), "P.A.", "Doctor" (a physician) and "Edmund" (an astronomer) (volume II). The character "Paul" changes name and is called thereafter, "Priest" (in the middle of vol. II and volume III, for example).

The issue is used to raise questions about scientific and analytic behaviour when it is unwittingly distorted in a religious situation. It is a warning about not prejudging religion, at the risk of throwing out the wealth of knowledge about the human mind and human truth that was possible through the religious vertex.

> ROBIN "The Heavens declare the Glory of God". When I was in the RAF I used to think of the verse, "I will take the wings of the morning and fly to the uttermost parts of the Earth". Paul knows it, I'm sure.

> PAUL Of course—we all do.

> TOM I fear I never thought of anything so poetical. I was too filled with petrol fumes.

ROBIN Those were the best years of my life. Although I was scared out of my wits, afraid of death. Afterwards I felt ashamed that I had not been brave enough, like one young boy I knew, to defy the enemy who called him to surrender as he crawled out of his disabled tank.

P.A. What happened?

ROBIN What happened? Why, what could happen? They—

TOM —Shot him of course.

ROBIN Of course; as you say, "Of course" . . .

PAUL You have forgotten that the wings of the morning were to aid flight, ineffectually, from God.

P.A. Perhaps the depths of hell.

ROBIN As Paul said, I had forgotten "the wings of the morning"— a poetical way of escape. I think I must have succeeded—not so effectually as P.A. perhaps, but enough not to go to Church.

P.A. Why do you assume I succeeded?

ROBIN Haven't you? I thought people who were properly analysed, like psycho-analysts, didn't believe in a lot of rubbish like "God's in his heaven, All's right with the world."

ALICE Really, Robin—why don't you read your Browning properly?

ROBIN Why? What have I done wrong now?

ROLAND Pretty well everything I should say—you hadn't read the Bible properly.

TOM You have forgotten your flying regulations.

P.A. I spend a great deal of my time trying to show people which particular god they are currently worshipping. Whether they are right or wrong is for the individual to decide for himself. Robin's god seems, from what he says, to be a solar god, but that would depend on the evidence to which I would try to draw his attention as it became discernible.

ROLAND To him, or to you?

P.A. Both, I should hope. I give my interpretation when I think he and I could both understand it, in the language which I think both could comprehend, and while the evidence is "visible" to two ordinary beings. Just now—

ROLAND Can you give an example?

P.A. —Tom seemed to think that *he* would smell gas, Robin, some visual or religious experience.

ROBIN I certainly said nothing about religion; I gave it up long ago.

P.A. Either you have little respect for what you say, or you say words for which you have no respect. You said "The Heavens declare the Glory of God—"

PAUL —"and the firmament showeth his handiwork" is the text.

ROBIN Good heavens! Can't one talk simple literate English?

P.A. You should hear my psycho-analyst aspirants talking "simple literate" English.

PAUL But you surprise me. Do you really think anyone expects psycho-analysts to talk "simple" English? I thought it was understood that it was a point of honour to talk incomprehensible jargon.

P.A. It is a point of honour when we are playing the game of Who's Top of the Psycho-analytical League Tables, but that is when we are "talking about" psycho-analysis.

ROLAND You have international league championship matches too. I've read some accounts in your journals. The language is ferociously incomprehensible. [AMF, II, 225–278]

In the previous dialogue one may detect a critique of the existence of sharp differences about the religiosity one may find in members of the analytic movement and religiosity found in overtly religious people. This allows a practical illustration of an analyst at work. One may see the peculiar way that the character P.A. deals with the wording attributed to the character "Robin".

The similarities fade when it comes to the use of hymns, jingles and other ways so typical of religion. The differences are blurred again in the closing phrase of the character "Robin". They are fitting enough for both the psycho-analytical movement and the religious establishment and their respective wars. The imaginary dialogue follows on with an observation of a most characteristic feature of religion: bigotry. Those who advertise themselves as "freudians", "kleinians", "bionians", "lacanians" would benefit from the following warning. It is evident that the "flooding of riotous meaning" in the last phrase is directed to the self-entitled "bionians" (q.v.).

> P.A. Psycho-analysts can "in truth" claim, like physicians, to be engaged in a respect-worthy occupation deserving the use of a language which can be employed by people who respect the truth, without having to be ashamed of technical precision on the one hand, and "primitive" precision on the other. Terms which are no longer permitted in socially oriented cultures—
>
> ALICE Such as?
>
> P.A. Shit. If you can indicate the cultural boundary I can guess whether the term would arouse anger. Show me the drawing and the onlookers before whom it is to be exhibited, and I can guess at the outcome. When Freud said infants had a sexual life people were outraged. Today James Joyce is regarded as permissible. An assertion of a religious manifestation will arouse the hostility and suspicion of psycho-analysts who would deny that they were displaying bigotry.
>
> ALICE Really? You surprise me.
>
> P.A. We are all scandalized by bigotry. We are none of us bigot-generators; that is, we none of us admit to being the spring from whom bigotry flows. As a result we do not recognize those of our offspring of whose characters we disapprove. Indeed, Melanie Klein discovered that primitive, infantile omnipotence was characterized by fantasies of splitting off undesired features and then evacuating them . . .
>
> These primitive elements of thought are difficult to represent by any verbal formulation, because we have to rely on language which was elaborated later for other purposes. When I tried to employ meaningless terms—alpha and beta were typical—I found that "concepts without intuition which are empty and intuitions without concepts which are blind" rapidly became "black holes into which turbulence had seeped and empty concepts flooded with riotous meaning". [AMF, II, 228–9]

The following quotation uses the idea of awesome natural occurrences, such as the eruption of volcanoes to compare that which is attributed to analysts and that which is attributed to religious ministers. Many times the functions change and phrases easily attributable to analysts are "uttered" by the "religious" character, who also warns and many times admonishes the "psycho-analyst" that "his" postures are not easily distinguishable from these of a religiously minded person:

> ALICE I understood Mont Pelée killed lots of Ephemera.
>
> P.A. Of course we dislike it, but I do not see why we should get above ourselves and indulge in our megalomaniac sense of our own importance—there could be something between the extremes of religious abasement and religious exaltation.
>
> PAUL Don't call it religious *please*—it may be psycho-analytic abasement and psycho-analytic exaltation, but don't drag in religion. I believe in God and in God's Truth and in God's Wrath and God's Love, but I don't see why anyone has to confuse their undisciplined human thinking with God. Men are always worshipping their own image and calling it God.
>
> P.A. You are not far away from expressing something to which, as a psycho-analyst, I frequently try to draw attention when I interpret an actual human statement as betraying an omnipotent phantasy. You would be surprised how often it is supposed that we are casting doubt on God. All I purport to do is to give the individual a chance of observing his God-like assumption of God-like attributes. It is not surprising that he finds it difficult to be awestruck by God, though not doubtful about his own God-like qualities.
>
> ROBIN They must be a conceited lot, your patients.
>
> P.A. Yet they are humble enough to submit to not-devotional observation by another by another ordinary human animal.
>
> PAUL By "not-devotional observation by another ordinary human animal" you mean a psycho-analyst?
>
> P.A. I mean myself—. [AMF, II, 242]

Ultimate reality

> ROBIN Really—do you blame us if we don't know what you are talking about?
>
> P.A. No, I don't. I am not surprised at your protest; in extenuation I have found that if I say what I mean it is not English; if I write English it does not say what I mean.

PAUL Theologians are blamed for being incapable of being religious—you are a bad as we are!

P.A. Probably for the same reason: Ultimate Truth is ineffable.

ALICE I think you are hard on him. I don't pretend to understand, but I do have an idea.

P.A. After all, ultimate reality must be a whole even if the human animal cannot grasp it. If I kick open an ant's nest it would no doubt appear to an ant to be an act of God, but it is capable of a simple explanation.

PAUL So you think.

P.A. Quite; I do not see why an infinitely small biological particle being whirled round the galactic centre on a speck of dirt—called by us the Earth—should, in the course of an ephemeral life that does not last even a thousand revolutions round a sun, imagine that the Universe of Galaxies conforms to its limitations.

PAUL The laws of nature are only the laws of scientific thought.

ROBIN It is readily assumed, filled with meaning, that these colossal forces "obey" these laws as we obey social conventions. [AMF, II, 229]

Truth, religion, psycho-analysis and issues of communication

ROLAND We follow the lead given by our shepherds.

P.A. You need not be sheep. We do not aspire to be leaders or shepherds; we hope to introduce the person to his "real" self. Although we do not claim to be successful, the experience shows how powerful is the urge of the individual to be led—to believe in some god or good shepherd.

ROBIN A father figure in fact.

P.A. No; a "father figure" is a technical term, but the individual person believes that there is a real person approximating to such a theoretical term. "God the Father" is a familiar term about which Paul can say more than I can.

PAUL We believe in God, not in Father Figures.

P.A. We do not affirm or deny the reality, but we do wish our analysands to recognize that one root of such an *idea* is a reminiscence of an actual human father. That is not the same as saying that because there is a reminiscence there cannot be a "thing" remembered, or that because we try to draw attention to a pre-existent idea, generated perhaps by a common and unworthy reality, there may not be some other source from which such an idea springs.

PAUL I'm glad to hear it. It has always been one of my objections to psycho-analysis and its devotees that they appear to be so dogmatic, so sure in their refutation of religious truth, that—

P.A. I should not like to replace one dogma by another; the erection of any God should be studied.

PAUL Isn't that what the Church has always advocated?

P.A. It appears to me that the unquestioning belief in God is demanded by the Church or its representatives. Perhaps I am misled by the Institutions of Religion which have obscured for me the chance of going beyond the institution's dogmata to a reality beyond.

PAUL: There are certainly plenty of religious teachers who have deplored that and warned against it. St. John of the Cross even said that reading his own works could be a stumbling block if they were revered to the detriment of direct experience. Teachings, dogma, hymns, congregational worship, are supposed to be preludes to religion proper—not final ends in themselves.

P.A. This sounds not unlike a difficulty which we experience when psycho-analytic jargon—"father figures" and so forth—

ROBIN Touché!

P.A. —are substituted for looking into the patient's mind itself to intuit that to which the psycho-analyst is striving to point; like a dog that looks at its master's pointing hand rather than at the object the hand is trying to point out. [AMF, II, 266–7]

P.A. "Talking about" dreams does not cause dreams. They exist— and some of us think, with Freud, that they are worthy of consideration and debate. The night, the dream, is a "roughness" between the smooth polished consciousness of daylight; in that "roughness" an idea might lodge. Even in the flat polished surface there can be a delusion, or an hallucination, or some other flaw in which an idea might lodge and flourish before it can be stamped out and "cured".

PAUL Yes, but you believe that dreams can be *scientifically* studied. That limits your freedom to investigate lies, falsities, "roughnesses", instead of looking for Truth only.

P.A. The search for truth does not limit my capacity; my freedom is limited by my lack of equipment; lack of capacity to *look* for truth. Your assumption that God exists does limit the search by precluding the discovery that there is no God if in fact there is none. Anyhow—how does one discover a negative?

PAUL In practice I don't find this belief limiting. It certainly would limit my researches into Truth if I worshipped Money or a widely admired footballer *as if* he or it were God.

P.A. We find financiers and sportsmen who practise that, in contrast to the religion professed. That is why it is useful to have terms such as "father figure". It is unfortunate if the term is thought to imply that the *reality* is correctly defined as nothing other than a "father figure".

THEA These distinctions seem to me to be subtle and are exercises in semantics rather that adventures in the realm of Truth. [AMF, II, 267–268]

The scientific and the religious vertexes illuminated—without religious wars; sometimes scientists are more religious than certified religious people.

ROBIN . . . an old man whose capacities were decaying would not be properly sexual.

P.A. The decay you talk of is nothing to do with sex: it is "to do with" anatomy or physiology, and should be distinct from decay or development which "originates" in sex. Similarly, development or decay of religious impulses which originate in religious forces should be distinguished from those which originate elsewhere.

PAUL We *do* contend that there is an important distinction to be made between development originating in God and that originating in the individual's impulses. Isaiah wrote as if there were no doubt that the impulse came from direct experience of God.

ROBIN Would P.A. admit the validity of Isaiah's experience, or would he regard it as having hallucinatory force—a phantom of the mind?

P.A. I do not have scientific evidence for discussion of an event of so many centuries ago.

PAUL The religious experience to which we refer is current—*not* hundreds of years ago—even though history suggests that it occurred from remote ages. In recent times Cowper wrote, correctly: "Sometimes a light surprises the Christian while he sings".

P.A. Cowper was manic-depressive and committed suicide.

PAUL The religious experience is universal; it is not closed to the psychotic, the unfortunate.

ROBIN You don't deny, do you, that religion is often apparently the cause?

P.A. I do not deny cause; I know that it is likely that we would think in terms of causes. Has Edmund any ideas about this?

EDMUND I like to think of causes, but I see no reason for believing that the human mind would ever comprehend the vast universes that surround us. The religious people express optimistic statements.

PAUL "The heavens declare the glory of God; and the firmament showeth his handywork".

EDMUND That is one such statement.

P.A. It is an observation and Paul has formulated what *he* observed. His statement seemed to me to be made from the religious vertex. I know that Edmund maintains that he is without religion and I am left to suppose that his observations and formulations are "only" or "just" scientific. Le Conte said that there was one fact we should *never* know—the composition of the stars. I would be interested to know what Edmund would say about that "*never*".

EDMUND Conte was right to say so, but spectrographic investigation leads us to have definite ideas about stellar composition. [AMF, II, 287–88]

Le Conte managed to be more religious than religious people.

Analysis and religion: do they harm or the obverse?

One often hears that religion is poisonous, toxic or harmful—at least since Marx. The same accusation is levelled against psycho-analysis at another point—that analysis and religion seem to intersect, at least in respect to the social reactions to them.

ROBIN So you admit that psycho-analysis can do harm?

P.A. It does neither harm nor good; but the person can use the experience for whatever purpose he will. After all, if a surgeon heals a thief or a murderer he makes them more efficient, but not more moral.

ROLAND Nobody expects him to do so.

P.A. Believe me they do! The analyst is often held responsible for the behaviour of a man or woman who has at some time been to a psycho-analyst.

PRIEST We have the same difficulty with religious people.

P.A. Do you help your believers to see what kind of god they follow? Or do you assure them that they are good people who are supporting the true God?

PRIEST Of course we try to show them what gods they follow. People try to serve both God and Mammon.

P.A. Has it any effect?

PRIEST In the course of the centuries, yes.

P.A. "In the course of centuries"? There may not be centuries available. That is why we regard analytic procedure as essential if people are to understand what beliefs they hold and by which they are held.

PRIEST Do you find they understand—more quickly?

P.A. Sometimes I think they do, but not often. Nevertheless psycho-analysis enables the psycho-analyst to learn something and even to pass it on. There are occasions when a resistance is surmounted with astounding speed; a number of facts display their relationship for the first time. It is almost a revelation.

PRIEST You use a term which is part of our technical equipment.

P.A. I thought you would notice that. I wished that we could make clear both the verbal fact you mention and the psychic reality which corresponds. The concentration of meaning would require the concision which can be achieved in music or painting. Would my analysand undergo the work necessary to understand if I could achieve such precision? Audiences rarely listen to music or look at pictures; still less do they think it worth while listening to what an analyst says.

PRIEST These difficulties have been familiar to the religious for many centuries. Music, painting, poetry, vestments gorgeous and austere—all have been used as auxiliaries.

P.A. I have found that the auxiliary can easily be transferred by the receptor from the periphery to the centre. Messages intended to convey profound truth—*The Iliad, The Aeneid, Paradise Lost, The Divine Comedy*—have all in turn become famous as gorgeous settings for the precious "stone" which is outshone by its attendant splendour. Krishna warned Arjuna that he might not be able to survive the revelation of the godhead which he, Krishna, was prepared to vouchsafe. Dante has only rarely found a reader able to discern the vision to which he points in Canto XXXI of the *Paradiso*. Milton's mind was overshadowed by a doubt whether he could pass beyond the "evil days" on which he had fallen; it was indeed his tragedy.

PRIEST The most profound expression of despair known to us was, "Why has thou forsaken me?"

P.A. This discovery is one which all are afraid to make. A theory that the human animal is not going to call on God do to for him what he must do for himself in loneliness and despair cannot be formulated; any formulation is a substitute for that which cannot be substituted.

ROLAND Do you suggest that *that* psycho-analytic interpretation is the explanation of Christ's call reported on the Cross?

P.A. You show that I have failed to make clear that I attach the utmost importance, in the practice of analysis, to the presence of analyst and analysand at the same time and in the same place and in conditions in which the consciously discernible facts are available to both people. These are the *minimum* conditions, not the maximum. Only *then* does psycho-analysis become an activity open to the two participants. You suggest that I am making a statement about events reported to have taken place almost two thousand years ago; if you believe that to be the gist of my remarks, what might you not say about my opinions when I am not present to defend them? [AMF, II, 332–3]

P.A. "Worship" you say. I would prefer to use some less emotional term.

PRIEST The word is not emotional. It means exactly what I intend it to mean when I am, as at present, talking about God. I avoid using it in contexts such as "worshipping" Man or our mistress here. If I did I would feel guilty of blasphemy or, at the least, flattering speech.

P.A. Who or what were you speaking of when you used it just now?

PRIEST God, as I have said, I would not consider my "queer" dream as just a dream with a qualifying adjective.

P.A. Effusions of the unconscious—

PRIEST Unconscious—what's that?

P.A. "God"—what is that?

PRIEST I realize you think I know as little about God as you do, and perhaps I know even less about the unconscious, but I meant it seriously when I asked you about the unconscious. Do you know more about it than the usual theories of Freud and Melanie Klein and the rest? Do you know the extent to which qualified psycho-analysts are unconscious of reality, even the realities of psycho-analysis? Those I have seen individually and at their congresses appear to me only to be capable of grasping that narrow range of phenomena which fall, so to speak, within the rational band of the spectrum. Unless you can formulate your "discoveries" within the range of rational, articulate speech you are not satisfied that you "know".

P.A. That is probably so; since we try to conform to the conventions commonly accepted by scientists as "scientific", our formulations are vulnerable to the criticism that they are only rational statements—common sense. Even so, they are challenged as being unsupported by evidence. We are criticised both for being platitudinous *and* incomprehensible—"mad" as it is vulgarly called.

PRIEST I wonder if you have considered "scientists" as you call them.

P.A. May I ask if you have considered Christian Scientists?

PRIEST Yes indeed, as I have also considered Christian Philosophers. I do not exclude consideration of any phenomenon, but we must consider how much time is available for "consideration" between birth and death.

P.A. One of my objections to your school of thought is that it appears to encourage a belief in unlimited times such as life after death.

PRIEST Unfortunately we are debited with the views—usually mistaken—that people have about what we teach.

P.A. You yourself appear to debit me with views about psychoanalysis which I do not hold; it would be a part of my task if you were an analysand to elucidate your assumptions so that you could contrast and compare them with any other ideas you might entertain. In this respect I think that our activity is different from yours. *You* aspire to tell others how and what to think. *We* aspire only to show what people think—the rest is their choice.

PRIEST Fair enough; I have no quarrel with that. But I have a quarrel with psycho-analysts who talk as if they are subject to no such weakness.

P.A. Fair enough—I reciprocate. We object to that kind of psychoanalyst. I would hope not to be of their number.

PRIEST It sounds ideal.

P.A. It is, but we are aware of the difference between the real and the ideal. A few people have existed who have done more to help others to discriminate between the real and ideal than we have.

PRIEST I don't wish to deny you the credit for it; religion also has played an important part in fostering that awareness.

P.A. Scandals of the Church and scandalous behaviour of its devotees could, I suppose, be said to have taught people to discriminate, but that is hardly a virtue of religious activity, or an activity of which religions should claim to be proud.

PRIEST Scandals of psycho-analysis are not different . . . [AMF, II, 387–88]

There is a paradoxical situation. An analyst who consciously espouses the scientific outlook may be prey to a kind of blind fanaticism more typical of followers of the so-called "religious" sects than a self-declared Priest. Who, in his turn, may be more open to the unknown, and therefore more scientific than the self-declared scientist:

P.A. It certainly sounds as if I were lacking in mental flexibility. That is what I suspected about being dead. I never anticipated the possibility of experience after death; either I am not dead, or I shall have to revise my views.

PRIEST Let me recommend the less dogmatic approach, not least because you may be unfamiliar with dogma and its uses.

P.A. I have usually considered dogma to be the analogue of the so called "laws of nature".

PRIEST I believe it to be a formulation of the "thing itself".

P.A. You claim, with the mystics, that you have direct experience of God. I should have thought your organization would have considered that heretical: a psychiatrist would suspect megalomania.

PRIEST There are opinions which question the claim of any human animal to aspire to such experience. Dante only claims such direct experience as a mortal being can have. [AMF, II, 420]

The next dialogue begins with the character "Man", a kind of improved Nazi invader. This character just acts-out, conquers and has rational thinking linked to the bare concrete necessities of survival rather than to the mind's necessities that form real life. The character "Moriarty" was created to represent "Sherlock Holmes's" fiercest enemy.

MAN I shot you so you would lie down and stay down—and out. And silent. Your friend Robin too—years ago. I don't want any ghostly voices around. Anyone would think it wasn't bad enough with religious nonsense investing a future life and angel voices to add to the tumult.

ROBIN I can't see that's any worse than P.A. and his crowd inventing minds and characters and psycho-somatic disturbances.

ROLAND Doctors are as bad—new diseases and expensive new cures and specialists to go with them.

MORIARTY As one who has waged war against religious nonsense much longer than—

P.A. Oh, come—you are a creature of fiction yourself!

SHERLOCK HOLMES But *not* religious fiction. Scientific fiction is entirely superior.

DEVIL I am religious, but certainly I do not consider that I am fictitious. I do not of course hold with the ridiculous theatrical costumes in which I am suppose to appear in gardens of Eden and such primitive landscapes. In fact I have always been most punctilious about my dress. I defy anyone to say they have ever seen me in anything but unobtrusive clothes, quietly and beautifully cut, and manners to which no real lady or gentleman could possibly take exception. Excuse me—you were about to say?

P.A. I confess I had supposed you inhabited the unconscious.

ALICE At my school we certainly were taught that the Devil existed, but none of us believed it was true.

DEVIL My dear lady—I hardly know how to apologize for my lack of perspicacity. I remember your school very well. I frequently gave away the yearly prizes and used to address you at the close of the ceremony which I was vain enough to regard as a particularly pleasing annual tribute to my services. Very charming, if I may say so, you all looked. Your Headmistresses—I knew all of them very well—were gratifyingly deferential. I even donated a fund for a prize to the most promising pupil——for the promises which were unlikely to be kept. It carried a scholarship—a university scholarship—for Moral Philosophy. No, no thanks—I never touch sherry. I find it induces a somewhat genuine geniality.

ROLAND Now I understand why your face is so familiar—at our Prize-giving Days! You were responsible for all our sexual troubles I suppose?

DEVIL Certainly not. Sex, like sherry, often produces perfectly genuine feelings of love and affection. I relied on various religious teachers and moralists to inflame moral hatred for those harmless and agreeable practices—

SOMA My department.

DEVIL Quite so; as my friend P.A. was saying—

P.A. Excuse me; *not* your friend. I do not even believe in you.

DEVIL You amaze me. I would have thought that by this time the facts would have compelled you to catch up with Priest—he at least believes in me.

P.A. I do not waste time believing facts or anything I *know*. I save my credulity for what I do *not* know.

DEVIL Like God?

P.A. Certainly. Both you and God I leave to Priest and his religious department.

ROLAND But ... I suppose you would say you do not believe in men and women because they are facts which you know.

P.A. Certainly—I know some men and some women. I know they have minds as well as bodies.

SOMITE THIRTY Somitically speaking I know a lot that I cannot make clear to you but that is factual enough to me. I have to borrow articulate speech from Soma.

SOMA My difficulty exactly. I cannot make anything clear to Psyche unless I borrow a bellyache or headache or respiratory distress from somitic vocabulary for any of these post-natal structures. I believe in mind and personality as there is no evidence whatever for anything but Body. And when I manage to make somebody aware of a bellyache the probability is that they immediately drag in a "cure". As for my message, God knows—

DEVIL God knows! Is Soma also among the religious?

ROSEMARY You know that as well as I do. Some of the healthier and most well-nourished bellies I know are to be found among the religious. The Celibates look particularly pregnant.

ROLAND I know women who look pregnant. Sometimes they are.

P.A. I *know* pregnant silences—I don't have to believe in them. Seventy-five was speaking of all talking at once as a bedlam.

PRIEST Milton spoke of Pandemonium.

DEVIL That was before Reason took the chairmanship.

P.A. And Bedlam—only because Reason was such a bad Chairman. The so-called *laws* of logic were a prescription for Chaos. They left no living space at all for vitality. Even today it would be still-born if it had not found refuge in what Alice would call craziness or—

DOCTOR Manic-depressive psychosis, or hysteria, or schizophrenia, etcetera, etcetera, etcetera—and quite right too.

P.A. Or the Royal College of Physicians, or the Royal College of Surgeons.

DOCTOR Or the International Psycho-Analytic Association, or the Church. [AMF, III, 444–6]

ROLAND If you cannot believe in a religious solution at least I cannot "believe" in *facts*. Facts do not offer an outlet for a religious impulse—only for scientific curiosity.

P.A. Might they not be the same? The religious people I know certainly think they are concerned with the Truth and nothing but the truth. It is often difficult to retain a sense of awe in the face of what we are more likely to think of as humdrum daily trivialities rather than facts that deserve to be treated with respect.

ROLAND "With respect" I could manage, but not "with awe".

ALICE I would have thought that "awe" is more appropriate left to people who are religious.

P.A. I agree that we should respect the language we use and be careful not to debase it.

ROBIN Is there any fact which you know and regard with awe?

P.A. Certainly—I know awe inspired by the light curtains of the Aurora, mountains—. [AMF, III, 514]

ALICE . . . Religious people often think that "though the body dies the soul shall live for ever".

ROBIN It's a nice idea.

ROLAND "Nice" you call it? I think it perfectly horrible—one life is enough. I do my best to maintain my life and that of my family, but that has provided me with enough pain and anxiety to get on with.

ALICE What does P.A. say? Do you believe in religion and a future life?

P.A. I have no doubt of the "fact" of religion as a part, perhaps an unalienable part, of human character. [AMF, III, 521]

The following dialogue was written after a round of Bion's travels in South America and also in some parts of North America. The book ends with this same reference about his "American Experience". His activity was seen by himself as being distorted into a Priesthood, a fact he noticed and objected to. It seems that he took it with good humour and put himself as the character "Priest". His last-but-one chapter of *Cogitations* is also from this date, where he states that people regarded him as a kind of deity (C, 376).

The attempts to idolize Dr Bion in his travels abroad: misplaced religiosity

Bion seems to think that a kind of priestly self is a part-object of his mind, and that the Priest-Bion is full—as is any priest—of judgemental values; there remains the character "P.A." to bear the load of that which Dr Bion seemed to have as his goal. The most elevated goals of psycho-analysis—among them, the universality of neuroses and psychoses and the search for truth without lies and evasion—are stated again and again:

ALICE (to PRIEST) It is very pleasant to welcome you back to our group. I hope your trip was successful.

PRIEST It was; I am glad to be back and to find you all looking so well. How's the debate been progressing?

ROBIN Well, though I don't think we made any discoveries. We were wondering whether you could re-light the flame which seems to have grown dim to near extinction. How was your conference?

PRIEST Much like others I have known—in fact I suspect my experience has not been so different from yours. Your account could be transferred to the religious conference without verbal alterations—insignificant, but not in the eyes of God.

ROBIN Why drag in God? We have no evidence of his existence.

PRIEST True. But the fact that we cannot prove that God exists may be a matter of importance only to our self-admiring selves. "Self-yeast of spirit a dull dough sours", as the poet says. "But, swollen with wind and the rank mist they draw . . .", as an earlier poet said.

ROLAND You do not mention that the two you quote were of opposing sects.

PRIEST Of opposing sects, yes; but at one in agreeing there is a God.

ROLAND Between them there is not *one* god, but two. In fact there seem to be as many gods as there are people to believe in them.

P.A. I agree, but that is only saying that different individuals have different ideas about whom they are addressing and in what manner they should communicate their approach.

PRIEST That does not prove that there is no God.

ALICE I think the discussion is pointless. Some people have an experience which they cannot explain in any way comparable to that in which they describe other experiences. The sense of contact with God is not similar to other contacts.

P.A. You are, here and now, making just that comparison. That could be because when you speak of "contact with God" you are using "contact" metaphorically; when you speak of contact with air or water or Tom Smith you do not mean it to be supposed that it is a metaphorical contact. I have not had such an experience and therefore find no necessity for any explanation. Freud had a good deal to say about the psycho-analysis of religion; he seemed to think there was no need to seek any other than a psycho-analytical explanation.

ROBIN In other words, he did not believe in God.

P.A. That could be one conclusion. I do not know if he had any other views.

PRIEST Whether he had or not, I cannot see that any one man's views, however impressive, can be regarded as relevant to someone who is not Freud. Freud spoke of a psycho-analysis of religion; if I had time I could write a book about the religion of psycho-analysis.

P.A. Could you give us a rough idea of what your book would contain?

PRIEST I think I could write an introductory volume or two about the many "religions" that have existed, been discarded for another, been in turn replaced as more in conformity with the needs of time. For all its apparatus of erudition I see Psycho-analysis as yet one more religion—not the True religion—destined to flourish for its day and then be heard no more.

P.A. Why categorize it as a religion? Most of us try to be scientific; this is tantamount to claiming only one standard—the Truth. It is not incompatible with the religious stress on truth, but that does not make it a religion.

PRIEST The fact that people who have claimed to be God-fearing show little respect for the truth does not make all religion false, or God only a fiction spawned by a fevered imagination. Is that not more likely to be true of psycho-analysis? After all, who are the originators in psycho-analysis? Is it not generated by neurotics and worse?

P.A. I think it likely, but the revolt against neurosis and psychosis is also generated from amongst these same people. If you gather together a group of neurotics, psychotics, hypochondriacs and other disturbed people they soon rebel against themselves and their troubles.

ROBIN Is that any more than what people do who want to escape the consequences of a mistaken choice?

P.A. I think so. I doubt if individuals make a choice; they cannot know what the "choice" is. The first requisite of a choice is that the person making it knows what the alternatives are from which he or she is to choose. But assuming that they have had a choice and made the wrong one, ought we not to attempt to correct it? If the belief in a almighty spirit is mistaken, if experience leads us to suppose that there is no such spirit, we should cease behaving as if there were.

PRIEST I agree. But does your experience support the idea that people give it any serious thought? From what I see of psycho-analysts they do not know what religion is; they simply transfer their allegiance from one undisciplined, desire-ridden system of emotion and ideas to another. I have heard psycho-analysts discussing; their discussion itself betrays all the characteristics which I have recognized as pathognomonic of religion of a primitive, undisciplined, intellectually unstructured kind. They argue heatedly, adducing national, racial, aesthetic and other emotionally coloured motivations in support of their particular brand of activity.

P.A. I would not deny that we do all these things, but we do in fact continue to question ourselves and our motives in a disciplined manner. We may not succeed; neither do we give up the attempt.

PRIEST I hate to appear to sit in judgement but I have to judge, to appraise such evidence as I have as it touches my private life and my responsibility for my own thoughts and actions. You have as many sects of psycho-analysts as there are in any religion I know. You have as many psycho-analytic "saints" with their individual following of devotees.

P.A. We are human and show all the weaknesses of that biological category. We do not cease to worship and adore because adoration and worship are basic, fundamental and therefore unalterable, inalienable characteristics; we try to allow for that fact.

PRIEST Ought you not then to make room for the capacity to worship and adore—even to depend on something worthy of dependence, adoration and worship? Otherwise such capacities either "fust in us unused", or become debased by the object worshipped.

P.A. True. The individual who adores a particular nation, or drug—such as alcohol—may be debased by that fact and unable to release himself from a loyalty which has become debasing and dangerous. Loyalties that are health-giving and growth-fostering at one stage become a barrier when the individual cannot transcend them. The barrier can be anything from the limitations imposed by our animal nature, to something temporary that has become hardened, calcified, rigid—I borrow the terms from medical descriptions of arterial degeneration; there is reason to suppose some spiritual counterpart, some unwillingness to entertain new ideas, which is inseparable from advancing physical age.

ROBIN Cannot the "religion" of psycho-analysis, or the investigation of psycho-analysis by theologians, teach psycho-analysts something valuable, as the psycho-analysis of religion could teach theologians something valuable for theology? Why should be any difficulty?

P.A. There **is** a difficulty: the very efficacy of teaching is a matter for caution because we do not know what those taught will learn. Children often learn to emulate their parent's faults. Even the good intentions of parents and teachers can be nullified by that fact.

PRIEST What man professes is not so important as what man is. [AMF, III, 542–6]

The religion of the psycho-analytic movement

Taking into account that as occurs in most of Freud's legacy, Bion uses them in agreement and had nothing to add or to expand, the same seems to occur with the psycho-analysis of religion. What he expanded was the scrutiny of the religion of psycho-analysis. Perhaps his own development allows us to state the issue more precisely: the religion of the psycho-analytic movement.

The following dialogue may be better grasped if read in conjunction with the entry, "Kleinian". It follows the dialogue where a sense of illumination appears that Bion refers to as having experienced when undergoing an analysis with Mrs. Klein. Bion's view about the place occupied by literature as an "ancestral psycho-analysis" is also valid to religion.

The reader must remember that the character "Rosemary's mother" represents a whore.

ROBIN I appreciate the point, but I would like to know more about the "illumination".

P.A. Had you not better ask yourself to whom you owe such illu-mination as has saved your journey from being plunged in ever-lasting night, or, worse still, in the blaze of everlasting certainty and good fortune?

PRIEST May I introduce a note of pity for the unfortunates who have been plunged in the everlasting gloom and self-satisfaction of scientific knowledge—a fate which has deterred many from the joys of devotion to God and respect for His truth.

ALICE Surely scientists devote themselves in all modesty to the truth. Even women have been known to wish to bear children in whom a love of truth can germinate; we are not only ambitious to be sexually satisfied.

ROSEMARY Most of the men my mother knew behaved as if that was the only thing in life.

ROLAND Good God!

PRIEST Poor God! Can you imagine what it would be like to be worshipped by men and women? Even Socrates is said to have been tried and condemned to death by his betters. Some of you may remember the story of the Garden of Gethsemane.

ROBIN God Almighty first planted a garden and indeed, said Bacon, it is the purest of all pleasures.

P.A. One of the purest of human pleasures appears to be the plea-sure of cruelty. Could Priest enlighten us about this?

PRIEST Perhaps I can do so by reminding you of a religious doctrine of the Immaculate Conception; that is in contrast to "human pleasures". It seems to me that psycho-analysts' discoveries may be something which has been known to the Church for a long time.

P.A. Psycho-analysts who respect the truth have done and still try to do just that—respect the truth. But we do not put it in the terms you use.

PRIEST But what you say and the way you say it matter. For this reason the Catholic Church is particular about what it says and how it says it. We are often accused of narrow-mindedness and bigotry for being particular and not co-operating with people who believe themselves to be our allies.

P.A. We have been deflected from our problem, namely, to account for facts that lead us to think that the existing theories are inadequate but too true to be discarded without loss. Maybe it is significant that the discussion that obtrudes centres on ownership, on who created or owned the idea.

PRIEST Or rather, who owned the owner—God or man? But let us debate the idea further tomorrow . . .

PRIEST What is the psycho-analytic view of original sin? Do you deny there is such a thing?

P.A. I hesitate to say I believe or disbelieve in something reported as a fact by someone else. I have been convinced that certain observations could be more easily explained if there were such a thing as original guilt. [AMF, III, 560–2]

BION I get the idea—thanks to the bi-lingual description achieved by Alice and Rosemary co-operating to describe the . . . the . . . er

ALICE {Bitch.

ROSEMARY {Lady.

BION Your happy combination and clarification you achieve by your joint efforts encourages me to draw attention to another union not unlike the one I was describing between our two enemies Soma and Psyche. Sometimes the two characters do not share the same body; each contributes a real physical and imaginary component. They tend to be over-simply described as 'homosexual' or "heterosexual", or "married", or "in partnership". In those situations in which the disguise—the conventional costume—excites psychiatric attention, they are liable to be described as participating in a *folie-à-deux*. If they excite the attention of the Board of Trade they may become known as a famous business venture, although the dividing line—caesura?—between that and a bankruptcy, or criminal association, or un-happy-marriage, may not be so easy to determine in close investigation as it is in a purely literary or grammatical scrutiny. Words and articulate speech are wonderful inventions—still in their infancy.

ROLAND Yet you psycho-analysts talk as if you were learned people.

P.A. True; and that often leads the cognoscenti—amongst whose prophetic community perhaps I should include Roland—to suppose that we know nothing whatever.

PRIEST It is often assumed that theologians, priests, prophets—as P.A.'s intonation just suggested—also know nothing, that God is a figment of the imagination. There is truth in the criticism because the gods most people believe in *are* figments created by such imaginative capacity as is available.

P.A. Some religions could be described as *folies-à-deux*; that is, relationships between the individual and a god created by the individual. These realities are fundamentally real, but are made to appear unreal by verbal dependence on splitting as the basis of articulate speech. For example, we speak of "religious melancholia". A poor labourer I knew was in a state of profound depression because he *believed* that the cow on which he depended to earn a living had tuberculosis.

BION Who or what had tuberculosis? His cow? His wife? Or daughter? Or the society he had to serve? These questions cannot be investigated here—only in contact with the patient.

P.A. There is always the risk the investigator will catch the complaint—a risk he may not want to run. The analogy in the mental sphere of activity is the psychiatrist's fear that he himself will "catch the complaint"—or find he has already caught it—if he allows himself to have a close contact. [AMF, III, 565–6]

Recommended cross-references: Kleinian, Mystic, Truth.
Suggested cross-references: Atonement, Intuition, Real Psycho-analysis.

Scientific deductive system: The contributions of independently-minded epistemologists such as Bradley, Prichard and Braithwaite, as well as short sections of Popper's work, seem to have influenced

Bion to consider the scientific deductive systems as an important analogy to psycho-analysis. He includes a category in the Grid with this name, as the step ahead after the formation of concepts, and leading, according to Braithwaite and Bradley, to calculus.

The scientific deductive system starts from purely empirical, lower level data and from them attempts to make a generalization. Even though the flaws of the deductive systems, which never go ahead from the premises, were not specifically criticized by Bion, he was able to scrutinize some limitations of the method. He abandons the attempt at a purely deductive system from 1965 onwards.

Misuses and misunderstandings: Many think Bion was a neo-positivist because of his references to this model. He respected them but this idea conflates positivists and neo-positivists. Bion's courting of neo-positivism centres on his attempt at a syntax of psycho-analytical propositions and resulted in the Grid (q.v.)

Recommended cross-references: Mathematization of psycho-analysis, Scientific Method

Suggested cross-reference: Grid.

Scientific method:

> I am convinced of the strength of the scientific position of psycho-analytic practice. I believe that the practice of psycho-analysis in making psycho-analysis an essential training experience deals with the fundamental difficulties for the time being because it makes conscious and unconscious available for correlation; but I do not consider the need less pressing than to investigate the weaknesses that spring form faulty theory construction, lack of notation and failure of methodical care and maintenance of psycho-analytical equipment. [LE, 77–8]

> The scientific law is closely related to, and an epitome of, experience. [C, 8]

The validation of psycho-analytic theories, intra-session interpretations, and their scientific status was an omnipresent feature of Bion's contributions to psycho-analysis and of his daily work. It becomes clear that he had preoccupations with unwarranted flights of imagination disguised as analytic theories, the proliferation of descriptions dealing with the same underlying configuration that lingers unobserved.

In regard to a faulty apprehension of reality Bion notices that the problems of the schizophrenic were similar to the problems posed by the mathematician, the scientist, and the philosopher.

He had a *psycho-analytical* interest in the attempts of philosophers, mainly Plato, Aristotle, Bacon, Pascal, Locke, Hume, Kant, Poincaré and eminent British independents of his own lifetime. Namely, Prichard—from whose work Bion uses the seminal study *Knowledge and Perception*; Bradley (*The Principles of Logic*) and Braithwaite (*Scientific Explanation*).

Bion's copy of Popper's flawed, but nevertheless best-seller and trend-setter, *The Logic of Scientific Discovery* is full of critical side comments. He was able to see that the prevailing views of science in his epoch were mainly of positivist inspiration and were of no use to analysts. He uses the concepts of common sense (Aristotle, Locke) and constant conjunction (Hume). Bion inserts himself explicitly in the platonic tradition. His hypotheses hint at the fact that psycho-analysis may contribute to the positivist's limitations. Bion's earliest studies display that common sense must be used when dealing with psychotics, who have lost it (please refer to the entry, Common Sense).

Very early in his works he resorted to quantum physics, probability, model-making (including the use of myths) and mathematical analogies in order to enhance the analyst's scientific clout, in line with Freud's original project for analysis.

His earlier confrontation of analysis with positivist science appears in an extended form in *Cogitations*. Bion was fully aware of the serious criticisms of positivist science. They were raised before the advent of the positivist religion by Comte. That is, Bion started from Hume's critical view of science. To back this view, it will suffice to quote Bion himself in a paper written as early as 1959. This paper states firmly an attempt at real knowledge and a respect toward reality. His later writings, at the end of his life, were expansions, collecting of data and more information that perfected the same view. He does not label the current prevailing view about science as positivism, something we may, thanks to the efforts of many researchers—including Bion's—do more freely now:

> In spite of the advances of science in recent years, the methods employed in scientific work are under critical scrutiny . . .

In philosophy the question is not new though it is unnecessary to go back earlier than Hume to find the origins of the present controversies. The problem as it appears to the philosopher has been stated by Prichard. He says,

"Though we are aware that any knowledge at which we arrive is the result of a process on our part, we do not reflect on the nature of the process—at any rate in any systematic way—and make it the object of a special study. But sooner or later knowledge of our mistakes and the desire to be sure that we are getting the genuine article, i.e., something which is really knowledge, lead us to reflect on the process . . . in the end we find ourselves having to ask whether we are capable of knowing at all and are not merely under the illusion of thinking we can know". [C,84]

The importance of this quotation of Prichard in the whole of Bion's work since then, in shaping and vectoring its direction as a kind of compass, cannot be stressed enough. Until then, Bion examined the state of the minds of patients and observed the psychotic's problems in dealing with reality and with phantasy. From then on he would resolutely attack the problem trying to examine the analyst's state of mind, beyond the issues of counter-transference or of personal analysis. This does not mean that he skipped these issues—he simply knew that they could only be dealt with experientially, in the analyst's analysis, rather than in written texts. It is just the "processes" by which one gets knowledge, which Bion would focus on through the analytic experience. In doing this, as did Freud, he had at his behest the processes through which one does *not* get knowledge.

This echoes Kant's critique of pure reason, a method of noticing the obstacles to getting knowledge. Kant, Freud and Bion therefore focused not only on the *object* of study but also on the *methods* of studying it. These methods included particularities of the mental equipment of the observer and the interference that the observer makes on the object observed.

Taking into account that Bradley, Prichard and Braithwaite's works never attained the popularity of Popper and latecomers such as Kuhn and Lakatos, perhaps we should remember who they were. In the opinion of the author, the lack of secular or worldly popularity among contemporaries is not a reliable index of the value of the contributions, as vouched for by innumerable examples ranging from Van Gogh to Nietzsche, to name just two.

Harold Arthur Prichard was born in 1871 and died in 1947. He founded the so-called English school of intuitionism; he was an acknowledged Oxford scholar, a specialist in Kant. According to him, direct perception of concrete objects allows knowledge of universals and their connections; his essays, published posthumously in 1950, form the work that Bion read: *Knowledge and Perception*. Richard Bevan Braithwaite was younger than Bion, born in 1900 and dying in 1990. He was educated in physics and mathematics and became a scholar at Cambridge. He made a seminal, but unfortunately little recognized, contribution on the nature of scientific reasoning named induction; his use of models, and of probabilistic models in particular, led him to basic work in the field of the game theory (which was made famous in recent days due to the film *A Beautiful Mind* from 2001, which is a version of John Nash's life). Perhaps the study that will remain a classic from Braithwaite is from 1953: *Scientific Explanation: a Study of Theory, Probability and Law in Science*, which was used by Bion. Francis Herbert Bradley was the oldest of the trio, born in 1846 and dying in 1924—a long life, despite many physical disabilities that included a difficult kidney disease. Also an Oxford scholar as were Prichard and Bion, he had perhaps the broader formation and outlook, being a sensible critic of Shakespeare. His work *The Principles of Logic* is quoted by Bion, and was published in 1883. In this book, he furnishes a description of thought. From him Bion used the concept of judgements having contents, called by Bradley, "ideas". Let us remember that Bion called the instrument, Grid, "Idea". These ideas "represent reality", and are universals, and so represent kinds of things, even though the things in themselves are all individual. This seems to be a problem, the old problem of science since at least Bacon. Bradley resolves this issue distinguishing forms of judgement in a way that profits from Kant and above all, in the opinion of the author, from Hegel.

This discrimination is between grammatical and logical forms of a judgement. The logical form is always that of conditionals that assert that *"universal connections between qualities obtaining in reality"*. These qualities are universals—putting him firmly in the Plato-Kant tradition—but the connections are conditional, while reality is a "whole" (in Hegel's sense). We, human beings, can have contact with this "whole" through immediate experience. Judgements are abstractions from immediate experiences too, but these are non-relational experiences.

It is from here that Bion developed his hypothesis that an emotional experience is not divisible from a relationship and also his theory of Links (please refer to these specific entries). But judgements are inescapably relational, and therefore they cannot represent non-relational reality accurately, which means, they fail to reach truth. Bion uses Hegel but does not fall into Hegel's extreme idealism, because Bion states that thought is never identical to the reality it purports to apprehend and therefore it is never more than an approximation.

There are other seminal works from Bradley, such as *Appearance and Reality*, published in 1893, where he states that reality is never self-contradictory; its appearance is. Bertrand Russell's work can be seen as a direct consequence of Bradley's efforts.

> Braithwaite favours the view that the scientific hypothesis consists of a generalization and nothing else. He admits that Hume's formulation of the theory of constant conjunction is open to grave criticism and that it has done much to obscure the value of the view that he (Braithwaite) puts forward, though with important modifications. In particular he stresses the close connection that exists between Hume's view of constant conjunction, and Hume's view that there is no element beyond a generalization in a scientific hypothesis except a psychological fact about the association of ideas or beliefs in the mind of the person believing the law. It is evident to Braithwaite that there is a desire ... to believe that a scientific law asserts, in addition to the generalization, that there exists some kind of relationship between the facts about which the generalization is made which is analogous to the logical relation holding between premise and conclusion in a deductive inference. [C, 13]

Modern physics

Bion was also fully aware that *"in spite of the advances of science in recent years, the methods employed in scientific work are under critical scrutiny"* (C, 84)—which means, he was well informed about the advancements made by quantum physicists. *"In the natural sciences the quantum mechanical theories have disturbed the classical concept of an objective world of facts which is studied objectively"* (C, 84).

Bion has noted that the observer interferes with the object observed. He used Werner Heisenberg and Niels Bohr's contributions in this sense; he does not specifically quote Freud about this observation. From Hume he draws the concept of constant conjunctions, and with it, the notion that reason is the slave of passions. From Poincaré Bion uses the notion that man's methods of measurement of space—which play a part in the very concept of space—are related to man's awareness of his own body. That is, it has an emotional basis. From Riemann he was able to use the fact that our ideas of space can well be dispensed with: *"No psycho-analyst would be surprised at the attribution of the origins of mensuration to the experiences of infancy and childhood"* (C, 85).

Repeatedly he introduces the suggestion that psycho-analysis could improve our insights about the origins of that which became known under the denomination, "science". This would be a useful tool for those who, due to forgetfulness, are lost in the maze that awaits anyone who tries to implant self-advertised scientific methods (in fact, pseudo-scientific methods) into psycho-analysis.

Bion did not emphasize in an explicit way that five years before the quantum and relativistic physicists, Freud was able to elicit the interference of the observer in the phenomena observed. Nevertheless, he was able to put due weight on the psycho-analytic way that this finding from Freud was contemporary with the modern tendencies in science, which are still valid. After all, a few years are negligible in the scale of time that measures human achievements. These methods in many aspects ran counter to positivist religion:

> In the natural sciences the quantum mechanical theories have disturbed the classical concept of an objective world of facts which is studied objectively. And the work of Freud has at the same time excited criticism that it is unscientific because it does not conform to the standards associated with classical physics and chemistry; it constitutes an attack on the pretensions of the human being to possess a capacity for objective observation and judgement by showing how often the manifestations of human beliefs and attitudes are remarkable for their efficacy as a disguise for unconscious impulses rather than for their contribution to knowledge of the subjects they purport to discuss. [C, 84–5]

During his time, psycho-analysis was—as it is, again, in the ever-occurring cycles of ignorance and unawareness of previous achievements—under heavy criticism on the basis that it was not scientific.

Anti-scientific fashions

Personalities who gained contemporary influence and power such as Eysenck and Popper in the fifties and sixties, to quote just two, without grasping what analysis is, tried to criticize it using positivistic criteria. Their names and most of their work have vanished now—fashion being *"the cunning livery of hell"* (Shakespeare, *Measure for Measure*). There were relatively isolated attempts to examine the scientific status of psycho-analysis, in a continuous trend towards legitimating it extra-psycho-analytically. This occurred via transplanted models that tried to lead psycho-analysis towards fashion-approved science or fashion-approved philosophy.

From there were born the many attempts to reduce it to behaviorism (during the forties), to existentialism (during the fifties), to neurological models (the fifties and sixties), to structuralism (in the seventies). During the eighties and nineties, this trend continued unabated: post-modernism, heideggerianism, and positivism.

The same lack of grasp of analysis lingers on, now within the psycho-analytic movement. The earlier critics had at their favour the excuse of ignorance; as outsiders, they perhaps did not feel obliged to know what psycho-analysis was all about. Surprisingly, some members of the analytic movement began to level the same kind of criticism against analysis. Many of them—as did Eysenck in the fifties and early sixties, and perhaps unwittingly inspired by him—try to use methods that had very limited success in academic psychology, the field where they obtained their graduate or postgraduate training. Taking into account that they do not refer to their historic forebears, one wonders what kind of analysis they had and what kind of historical information about philosophy of science they have. The comment is not intended to attack anyone; it is linked to a basic distrust of psycho-analysis that emerges when one notices the attempts to transplant models that were superseded by psycho-analysis itself since Freud. It is a well known fact that analysts tend to repeat their analysts' models. If the training analyst distrusts analysis, overtly or unconsciously—this can be seen, even if roughly, in the attacks towards the frequency of sessions—the trainee will tend to distrust it too. Many among the exponents of the adaptation of extraneous positivist models of research and evaluation of analytic results are overcritical in their accusations of colleagues who imitate their analysts and supervisors. Is it not high time for them to scrutinize this posture in themselves, with no projection or projective identification? This would display their remaining trust—if any—in analysis.

A similar issue was detected by Sokal and Brickmont, noting the post-modernist fashionable expropriation of physics due to little learning (1997).

Unconscious and the numinous realm

Perhaps alone in his time, Bion was able to see that psycho-analysis was not exactly un-scientific. If it had some problems with regard to the undistorted apprehension of reality, all other so-called scientific disciplines suffered from the same problem.

> The mathematician can investigate invariants common to circular object and ellipse, that represents it, by algebraic projective geometry ... though they are part of Euclidean geometry; therefore psycho-analysts need not be dismayed if it can be shown that there is no place in their theories for measurement and other entities that are a commonplace of disciplines accepted as scientific. Just as there are geometrical properties invariant under projection, and others that are not, so there are properties that are invariant under psycho-analysis and others that are not. [T, 2]

> How can something people "feel" be measured? By postulating temperature after ridding oneself of prejudice of pairs of opposites. Then it is found that things, inanimate objects, are sensitive to temperature though they do not feel "heat and cold". What about love and hate? Are they not "prejudices"? Should it not simply be "x"—the amount of x, like the amount of temperature? Then one might be able to measure x even if one cannot measure love and hate, or heat and cold. [C, 2]

In doing this, Bion proposes that it is possible to have the most scientific posture of all, that of lack of prejudices. In addition, he is able to respect the Plato-Kantian perception that one deals with phenomena and may intuit their correspondent noumena without "owning them" and much less naming them. He also adopted—at least after 1959—the posture that accepts pairs of opposites without trying to resolve the opposition through splitting.

This would help him to see something that was to be published three years later (in *Elements of Psycho-analysis*)—one of the main inner features of Klein's theory about the positions: PS and D in a non-splitting, but rather dynamic process of balance/imbalance between the two.

Instead of trying to fit psycho-analysis into a Procrustean bed of pseudo-scientific technicalities—such as statistical studies that try to legitimate unwarranted, imaginative cause–effect relationships, reproducibility of data, statistically controlled, grossly homogenized control groups, falsifiability, etc.—he resorted to the philosophy of science. As we saw, he used different authors, from Hume and Kant to the physicists.

He attempted to integrate—rather than to transplant—the philosopher of science's observations with observations from psycho-analysis. He was able to see that the psychotic is perforce a bad scientist. Alternatively, in his own words, that the problems that the mathematician, the scientist and the philosopher of science faced were the same problems that the analyst faced.

> What is not so easily appreciated is the immediacy of the impingement of the problems with which the philosopher of science is familiar on the mental phenomena that modern psycho-analytic methods make overt. [C, 9]

These attempts dealt with Melanie Klein's theory and had three definite moments:

(i)   The first one related to the concept of common sense, the ability to symbolize and the concept of cause according to Braithwaite, as well as their analogies with Klein's theory of the positions. This attempt was halted after the advent of Bion's application of Sylvester and Cayley's theory of transformations and invariances to psycho-analysis.

(ii) The second one was made at the same time and related to the positions. It used the concept of selected fact, from Poincaré (please refer to this specific entry).

(iii) The third one related to the ability to think in the absence of the concrete object, and led to the expansion of the study of the relationship of the baby with the breast and the concept of point. He expanded this point with mathematical analogies; they are covered mainly in the entries, Atonement, Analytic View, Mathematization of psycho-analysis and Real psycho-analysis.

The idea of cause is dealt with in a specific entry, "Cause". The latter phase is dealt with in the specific entries, "Circle, Point, line, and Mathematization of psycho-analysis".

The first two led to the formulations contained in the books *Learning from Experience* and *Elements of Psycho-analysis*. They can reasonably be seen as preparatory papers to both books by endowing them with a scientific basis. The empirical approach was the study of clinical cases and trained psycho-analytic observation.

This first phase can be subsumed with the aid of the following quotation:

> The fact that I here equate with what Bradley calls "the actual element" is in a sense in no way different from the facts or actual elements that are the objects of curiosity, elucidation, and study in any science whatever, although this fact may be obscured because it is a "fact" or "actual element" of the kind that the analyst is inviting the patient to study—namely, the patient's own.
>
> It will be observed that in the theory I am putting forward I am postulating a phenomenon with three facets:
>
> (1)   what Bradley would call "actual elements in an actual union", which is identical with what the scientist would call "observable data" in a relationship with each other that is equally observable,
>
> (2)   an ideational counterpart of the above, which is dependent upon the individual's ability to translate an "actual element" into an idea. (The psychotic fails to do this, and even when he verbalizes still thinks that words are things.) This operation depends on the individual's capacity to tolerate the depression of the depressive position and therefore to achieve symbol formation. This phase is identical with the scientist's ability to produce a scientific deductive system and the representation of this, which is called calculus [Braithwaite, p. 23],

(3)   a mental development that is associated with an ability "to see facts as they really are" [Samuel Johnson to Bennett Langton ...] and internally with a sense of well-being that has an instantaneous ephemeral effect and a lasting sense of permanently increased mental stability. [C, 5–6] The notes in brackets are Mrs. Bion's when she published the paper in *Cogitations*).

What is meant by item (2)? It means that the "correspondent" theory of science, that of Plato, Kant and Spinoza, among others, is being put to use. One cannot access the numinous realm directly but one may glimpse it, intuit it, through its phenomenal manifestations. The problem of the scientist, or of the scientific ability of any person is to translate the "raw empirical material" that was apprehended from the senses, the things-in-themselves (that two years later Bion would call beta-elements) into "thinkable", "symbolizable" data.

This equates the psychotic's problem with that of the analyst who cannot deal with Oedipus on levels of sophistication that surpass its sexual meaning. For example, those who cannot grasp the hallucinatory nature of transference phenomena and take the psycho-analytic theories as things in themselves turn psycho-analysis into a manipulation of symbols.

Please refer to the specific entries, "Kleinian", "Manipulations of symbols", "Oedipus" to scrutinize the issue further. Bion would turn the criticisms of scientists towards **psycho-analysis** into warnings to members of the **psycho-analytic movement**, who in his view behaved like the *"erudite"* who *"remains blind to the thing described"* (AMF, I, 5).

What is meant by (3)? It means Freud's love of truth as the scientific *Weltanschauung* of psycho-analysis. It may be seen as a kind of declaration of principles. It also embodies the description of PS to D and the obverse, later to be represented through the quasi-mathematical notation, PS⟺D.

It also means that Braithwaite's work is behind Bion's attempts that would occupy many years of his life. Namely, to endow psycho-analytic theories with a level of sophistication that could qualify them to jump from "lower level data", raw empirical material drawn from the clinical and subjective descriptions, to the more general level of abstraction that characterizes a valid scientific law.

Elements of Psycho-analysis would embody the development of this attempt. The categories of deductive system and algebraic calculus that were included in the Grid are not to be seen as goals of analysis. They are seen rather as classifications that mark this degree of generalization—something that began in our era with Sir Francis Bacon's attempts.

> The question that arises now is this: how far is the scientific outlook, the attempt to understand, a compromise between the necessity, imposed by the compulsion to survive the "reality principle", of knowing the facts of external reality, and the necessity, imposed by the psyche's intolerance of the paranoid–schizoid position or the depressive position, to move freely from one position to the other and back without depressively coloured persecutory feelings on the one hand, and depressive feelings untinged with feelings of persecution on the other?

> The quotations on scientific method which I have cited from Poincaré and on causation from Bradley are open to the objection that they are expressions of the inner tensions of the personalities of their authors, and in view of the subject matter of this paper cannot be taken as valid descriptions of scientific method. Since it is my objective to show that scientific method itself lacks the "objectivity" that is widely attributed to it, and may indeed spring from very deep-seated elements in the personality which seek fulfilment, it is obvious that the very thesis of this paper may be taken as a refutation of its premises. [C, 7]

The philosophically-informed reader will notice some resemblance of this observation to Rousseau's views of certain branches of science.

The study ends with a clinical example of a patient who sees *"blood everywhere"*. He expresses this through a series of acted-out, seemingly disjointed and unimportant physical manifestations. Bion seemed to have been an intuitive person with an uncanny ability to grasp the messages conveyed by patients who resorted to seemingly irrational talk and seemingly minor acting-out. In the paper published posthumously about Scientific Method, which contains the description of the patient who says *"blood everywhere"*, Bion shows a psycho-analytic application of the concept. He differentiates between a kind of *"lost common sense"* that characterizes the patient under a superficial view and another kind of *"common sense"* which is non-rational. The latter emerges in analysis (C, 9).

Common sense is often confused with commonplace and good sense (see the entry, "Common sense").

The clinical example is of a patient who notices the couch in some disorder and proceeds to tidy it up in a subdued way. *"In due course evidence from his associations indicates that at this particular juncture, and taken with sundry other facts not germane to this discussion, he is experiencing an increase in anxiety and, furthermore, that the anxiety has as its ideational content the disordered couch as part of the furniture of a scene of parental intercourse"* (C, 9).

This phrase seems to demand from the reader a minimum of psycho-analytic experience. If it is not available the phrase becomes incomprehensible and arbitrary. The psycho-analytic experience means, in the final instance, the analyst's experience with his or her own Oedipus. Phrases such as *"furniture of dreams"*, that Bion used earlier in his works ("Development of schizophrenic thought" and "The difference between the psychotic and the non-psychotic personalities") demand the ability to grasp, that is, the perception of the psychotic phenomena. Here the "scientific approach" satisfies one of Popper's criteria to tell if a practice is scientific—namely, that of the reproducibility of phenomena. This criterion is the empirical practice in analysis itself. Freud had already stated it, but there are resistances to realizing that this can only be obtained through the analyst's training analysis. As with the discovery of penicillin or the theory of relativity, there are new intuitive discoveries in any analysis which are non-rational, outside the realm of that which is understandable. It is rather "livable" in the purest sense of the empirically observed fact.

Let us follow Bion: *"This conclusion, and the interpretation that is the psycho-analytic act by which it is expressed, is arrived at on the basis of observed facts seen in the light of a psycho-analytic hypothesis"* (C, 9). Later Bion would call it the "intuitive psycho-analytic approach" (see the entries, Intuition, Oedipus).

Common sense enters here: *"But common sense tells this patient that he is lying on an ordinary couch and that ordinary people, as he himself might say, would know that that is what it is and that its disorder was due to the movements of the previous patient upon it"* (C, 9).

Bion states that the patient resorts to that which Kant called "naïve realism": "*Common sense, the highest common factor of sense, so to speak would support his view of what the senses convey*" (C, 10). A patient acting under this aegis will level against his analyst the idea that the analyst is crazy, in the same way that many onlookers, reading texts written by great analysts, thought that the authors were crazy. Many years later, Bion would point out that no analyst can tolerate his work unless he is prepared to tolerate this kind of accusation:

> The fiction can be so rhetorical as to be incomprehensible; or so realistic that the dialogue becomes audible to others. There is thus a double fear: that of the conversation being so theoretical that the thoughts might be taken for meaningless jargon; and that of the seeming reality. Having two sets of feelings about the same facts is felt as madness and disliked accordingly. This is one reason why it is felt necessary to have an analyst; another reason is the wish for me to be available to be regarded as mad and used to being regarded as mad. There is a fear that you might be called an analysand, or reciprocally, that you may be accused of insanity. Should I then be tough and resilient enough to be regarded and treated as insane while being sane? If so, it is not surprising that psycho-analysts are, almost as a function of being analysts, supposed to qualify for being insane and called such. It is part of the price they have to pay for being psycho-analysts. [AMF, I, 113]

This view of common sense is a social one: "*I propose that we may now say that common sense is a term commonly employed to cover experiences in which the speaker feels that his contemporaries, individuals whom he knows, would without hesitation hold the view he has put forward in common with each other*" (C, 9–10).

But there is more than common sense: Bion adopts (without mentioning the source) Locke's view; common sense refers to the conjoined use of more than one of the five basic human senses. This has many advantages, such as the fact that it is biological; it is linked to survival and hence to the demands of the reality principle; it is independent of social conventions and prejudices. It returns the issue to the private, intra-psychic sphere, the realm of real psycho-analysis that differentiates it from philosophy, anthropology, sociology, poetry, and mythology:

... he has a feeling of certitude, of confidence, associated with a belief that all his senses are in harmony and support each on the evidence of the rest. In this sense also, private to the individual himself, the term, "common sense", is felt to be an adequate description covering an experience felt to be supported by all the senses without disharmony. As contrast, I may cite the experience in which a tactile impression, of, say, fur—sudden and unpredicted—gives rise to the idea of an animal, which then has to be confirmed or refuted visually; and so, it is hoped, the common-sense view is achieved.

But there is a difficulty. So far one might say that the patient's view is essentially at one with the strictly scientific view that Braithwaite investigates after limiting the scope of his survey ... The analyst, however, is also able to claim that his interpretation is based on common sense: but it is common only to some psycho-analysts who may be presumed to witness the same events and make the same deductions.

The analyst's problem is not associated with the objection that the phenomenologist might raise, although it can be argued that an awareness of the phenomenological philosopher's criticisms of scientific theory is implicitly supported by the analyst's view that all analysts should be psycho-analysed. [C, 10]

The issue at stake is to attain "*a sphere concerned with the transformation of private knowledge to public knowledge*" (C, 10). This problem obtrudes in the psychotic's way, in the phenomenologist's task, the scientist's task, and the psycho-analyst's task. General laws of science allow the public-action. Bion emphasizes an important component in making observations obtained primarily from the senses, lower level empirical data, into public, general laws: this component "*is dependent on the mental equipment of the observer. The philosopher of science concerns himself, as is already apparent from the brief survey I have made of Braithwaite's demarcation of the area that he wishes to discuss, with a limited aspect of the observer's mental equipment. Even the phenomenological philosopher of scientific method intends to restrict his field, though it is doubtful whether he means to restrict it so severely as in fact it is—thanks to the lack of the psycho-analytic discoveries that could have given greater freedom. The psycho-analyst, as is to be expected, excludes no part of the mental equipment from his survey except in so far as his knowledge and capacity by their own limitations forbid automatically the fullness of inquiry he would desire. His investigation of scientific technique has been imposed on him first by Freud's impulsion to investigate the human mind scientifically, and second by Freud's realization that his discoveries compelled suspicions of the mental equipment of the investigator—Freud himself in the first instance.* [C, 11–12]

Bion is proposing to regard psycho-analysis as the scientific activity *par excellence*—the diminishing of: (i) dogma, (ii) prejudices, (iii) unwillingness for data gathering, (iii) lowering the personal factor in order to apprehend reality. This is indicated in the following passage:

> I am persuaded that much psycho-analytic work done has been an investigation of the scientific technique or mental component, but not under that name. One has only to consider Freud's Theory of the Reality Principle and its dominance to appreciate that he is describing a development that must include in its more sophisticated manifestations the elaboration of what we now call scientific techniques of—or techniques known to science as—deduction, induction, hypothesis. [C, 12]

This text belongs to a period when Bion had a hypothesis about the state of mind that characterized the scientist—not at all different from the psychotic—that tends to dismiss the emotional feature in constant conjunctions. This hypothesis would be maintained, but the so-called scientific method would be regarded differently after 1965, when Bion abandoned his attempts that resembled the neopositivist approach of Schlick, Carnap and others. This is expanded in other entries in this dictionary (Grid).

> Although I expressly disclaim anything new in what I have to say here—precisely because in my view psycho-analysis has all along concerned itself with and elucidated these problems—yet I believe that there may be something novel in the juxtaposition of the facts which will serve to focus psycho-analytic attention more directly and purposively on elements that have still not been sufficiently regarded.

> This brings me to the difficulty that I have had to approach through this long digression. The individual whose development has allowed the establishment of the reality principle to take place has

established—with varying degrees of sophistication—a vast mass
of hypotheses in the course of his life. [C, 12]

The same statement would appear in more concise terms in the
end of his life:

> P.A. Even theories and theoretical terms are supposed to remind us
> of a reality. I have no doubt that one "talks to" an experienced
> person; the matter of psycho-analysis is such that analyst and
> analysand cannot afford to neglect the total sophisticated capacities
> of which both are capable. The psycho-analyst has a lifetime of
> experience, including the experience of technical psycho-analytic
> training; the analysand, even if only a young child, has a consider-
> able body of experience to fall back on. It is certain that the psycho-
> analysis will fail if the analysand does not respect the knowledge,
> character and wisdom of the analyst—and vice-versa. [AMF, 496]

In other words: there is a kind of "scientific function of the
mind" that is linked to survival, which tries to meet the demands
of the reality principle. Science is a new method for trying to apprehend reality as it is. Let us return to Bion's text from 1959:

> Most of these have some degree of justification both in the external
> circumstances of the period in which the formulation occurred, and
> in the quality and the degree of mental equipment available to the
> individual at the time. In other words, we do not need to assume
> that they were unjustified, although, as with the case I have
> mentioned, the patient is not slow to say that the *analyst's* recon-
> struction of what he believes to be the patient's original but still
> current hypothetical formulation is unjustified. So it is—on the
> level of mind on which the patient is at his most adult, most sophis-
> ticated, most scientific . . .

> The point to which I would draw attention is the scientist's view
> that the scientific hypothesis is a generalization abstracted from the
> fact that certain facts have been found to be constantly conjoined—
> the constant conjunction theory. The complication is that clinical
> experience shows how strong is the desire to formulate a hypothesis
> that will state that certain events are constantly conjoined and that
> therefore we must regard the relationship to the facts from which it
> is supposed to be educed as a generalization, as being two-way; that
> is to say that the hypothesis may be regarded as (a) educed from

constantly conjoined facts, and (b) designed, however it may be derived, to affirm that certain facts are constantly conjoined. It will be observed that the latter view is quite compatible with the former—incompatibility of the two views is not the point. [C, 12–14]

Bion proposes to assume that "*both views are correct*"; this being the case, the scientific hypothesis fulfils three functions: (i) a private experience is "*transmuted*" into a public communication; (b) the memory that allows us to state that some facts are "*agglomerated, articulated or integrated*" is linked to reality and reality-testing; (c) the meeting of the various elements and facts of the ideational counterpart of a given reality (which means that the elements do not need to meet in external reality) "*begin a process that issues in the change we call effect*" (Bion uses Braithwaite's formulation), in the same sense as Poincaré's "*selected fact*" (please see the entry, "Selected Fact") (C, 14–15).

This means that, at this time, Bion accepts it as scientifically sound to state that common sense "*may be, and should be, accepted as the arbiter that decides what are the facts in external reality to which these mental activities relate*". He was fully able to realize, during an epoch when there are no other records of any analyst having realized— with the possible exception of Freud, in 1936, in "The question of a *Weltanschauung*", that "*The philosopher of science has always been brought to a standstill at this point, caught between the logic of the idealist philosopher on the one hand, and the feeling of unreality to which an acceptance of such logic would expose him on the other. There is essentially no difference between the reactions of Braithwaite and Doctor Johnson to the demands of the idealist.*

It is possible that the scientist's dilemma, and therefore our own, may be seen differently if we now return to clinical psycho-analysis for the light it may throw on common sense and on that particular instance of scientific hypothesis and deduction known to us as a psycho-analytic interpretation" (C, 15)

Experto credite (Aenid, xi, 283; or, Credit one who has proved)

"*Where is the patient's common sense? What has happened to it?*" (C, 17).

Fresh problems await the scientifically-minded psycho-analyst. Was the situation complicated enough in cases where seemingly commonsensical ideas were just made to appear as this, due to the fact that they are socially shared? They were, in reality, just rationalized adult views, as in the case of that patient who tidied up the couch and was given an interpretation based on "witnessing" the parental intercourse. What happens with a patient labelled right from the start as psychotic?

Let us remember that the paper we are relying on to depict Bion's views on the scientific approach was written two years after his decisive step in displaying the universality of psychosis, with the paper on "Psychotic and non-psychotic personalities" (q.v.). The patient in question is used to lying down but on a certain day *"looks apprehensively and cautiously about him, finally seating himself precariously on the very edge of the couch"*. After displaying unequivocal—at least, unequivocal under Bion's commonsensical view that he expects to be shared by the reader—of anxiety, a posture of confirming preconceptions through perfunctory surveys, the patient immerses himself in deep and prolonged verbal silence, denoting a lessening of anxiety, which is replaced by dejection. Bion draws his attention to this behaviour, which seems to indicate that the patient is only vaguely aware of the presence of another person in the room. He emphasizes an observable fact:

Dr. Bion: "You are not lying down today"

Patient: "There is blood everywhere" [C, 15]

Due to the fact that Bion feels that the tone expresses distaste, the reply *"carries the suggestion that it is the presence of blood everywhere that makes him unwilling to lie down"* (C, 15).

It was already stated that the publication and attempt to share data depends on shareable psycho-analytic experience, meaning, personal analysis of the observers who try to communicate with each other. But a report of data that were not observed by the reader always stumbles on the fact that make-believe is called on. Common sense is impossible, for the reader did not use his senses with an experience he did not observe factually first hand. The living first-hand experience is the exclusive domain of analyst and analysand. *"Unfortunately, in this instance the reader can have no impression of the episode of which I speak other than that conveyed by me. But he can have impressions of what he may regard as similar experiences*

of his own. It therefore seems fair to say that I have given him an oppor-
tunity for the exercise of his common sense so that he can decide for himself
whether or not his common sense tells him that an event such as I describe
actually took place or not. In short, I am saying that it is common sense
to say and believe that the facts were what I said they were" (C, 16).

To state this is not too different from modern communications accepted as scientific. How many, among the readers of prestigious medical journals, for example, *The Lancet*, are actually able to "repro-duce" the experiences reported by a given scientist? And if they reproduce *a posteriori* or recognize the writing as mirroring their past successful (or better still, unsuccessful) experiences, is there any difference from that which Bion states? Common sense is the basis here: "... *the nature of the common sense to which I appeal and to which, in conformity with the views of a powerful school of philosophers to which I adhere, I accord an extremely important role"* (C, 16). He says that he contents himself *"with a partial limitation of the term to cover that aspect of the personality which is a compact of a component of the senses, common to two or more of the senses, and which in my belief has a social component analogous to that which Freud supposed might be the case with the sexual impulses, and which appears to me to be true of all emotional drives"* [Freud, "Instincts and their vicissitudes", 1915c, *SE* 14].

Returning to the patient: *"Where is the patient's common sense? What has happened to it? ... Is there any reason to doubt that the patient's judgement that there is blood everywhere is in his opinion a common-sense view?"*. After all, there exists in the patient's answer a kind of commonsensical communication. It is "rational"; it has a cause and effect relationship in Bion's inference of his rationale. For who with common sense would be willing to lie down on a couch where blood is everywhere?

Bion enumerates some reasons *"for doubting"* that the patient in fact expresses a common sense view. *"He has shown in previous simi-lar situations that he does not believe I share his view; the readiness with which he volunteered his explanation for not lying on the couch is an expression of confidence that I shall tolerate his opinion, not that I shall share it ... he knows that **his** view is not the 'common' sense one, and he prefers that the difference in outlook should not become public. He may be supposed, therefore, to feel that his sense of 'blood everywhere' is not common sense, is not in accord with the 'common' view demanded of him as a price of his membership of the group"* (C, 17).

The reader may gather that Bion stays within the boundaries of his observational experience within the session. There is a conjunction of the previous experience with the patient, with what happens in the session; the monitoring of the patient's views—rather than the analyst's possible views or prejudices—is focused. If the common sense of the scientifically-minded reader and of the scientifically-minded writer—meaning, a repertoire of commonly shared clinical experiences—is called upon, one may notice that the patient's answer—perhaps too readily given—carries a paradoxical non-commonsensical aspect. Namely, it seems not to be coherent with the observation ("You are not lying down today"). It is, to any mildly psychiatrically experienced reader, linked to hallucination. The same kind of reader will perceive without much difficulty that 'trained' psychiatric patients domesticate themselves and try to hide their delusional and/or hallucinatory activity—which seems to have happened at the beginning of the session and with the rational answer.

"One answer to the question, 'Where is his common sense?' is therefore that it is where it always has been; it is still a part of that non-psychotic part of the personality which I believe ... always to remain in existence" (C, 17). If the patient manages to survive, there is always a non-disturbed part that remains respectful to some aspects of reality or truth.

Now begins the truly psycho-analytical stage in Bion's writing. It is a kind of respectful attitude towards the manifest content of the patient's wording. It nevertheless may seem strange to some audiences since the time of Freud. This respect "sees" that truth, like beauty, is more than skin deep. Words carry some hidden, underlying truth. One fails to apprehend this truth if one takes the words at their face value. One must realize the paradox that words both hide **and** betray an inner truth:

> But now I think I see the answers to my two questions. Where is the patient's common sense? Obviously, it is "everywhere". What has happened to it? Equally obviously, it has been turned into blood—"blood everywhere". [C, 18]

Moreover, this statement is purely psycho-analytical in the sense that symptoms can be regarded as the last bastions of attempts at health, a paradox that was elicited by Freud (see for example, 'The paths to symptom formation', *Introductory Lectures on Psycho-analysis*, XXIII, *SE*, *XVI*).

One is reminded that Bion had argued that in the first interpretation there was common sense in some ways—one would not lie down on a couch "with blood everywhere"; one would not be willing to display openly one's own hallucinations. The second interpretation, stemming from a new hypothesis in the light of which he now regards the episode, has a common sense to him and his patient, "*in the limited field of that which is common to the patient and me*" (C, 18).

He now asks if he can maintain that this description "*is a common-sense description in a wider, extra-analytic context, and if so, in what way?. . .*

It is evident that even in this limited respect the interpretation of the patient's behaviour that I have proposed cannot, on the facts I have given so far, be regarded as a 'sense' common to the patient and myself" (C, 18).

And now Bion resorts to another among his preferred philosophical models, that of Poincaré, to which we referred at the beginning of this entry, which would be valid at least up to 1965. The purely psycho-analytical dealing with the manifest wording is "*an idea selected or accepted in a penumbra of circumstances for which Poincaré says the mathematician seeks—'the link that unites facts which have a deep but hidden analogy'* [*Science and Method*, p. 27]. *For if it is indeed a fact that the blood which the patient describes as being everywhere is the transmuted common sense for which I am looking, then this fact does link a number of other facts in a way that demonstrates a deep but hidden analogy. Thus the patient, as I know, believes he is mad and has always felt himself to be unlike others, to have a feeling compatible with that of having no 'sense' felt in common with others, and no senses that appear to have a factor common to each other*" (C, 18).

Free-floating attention and alert attention to seemingly minor experiential facts, analogically comparable to that which allowed Fleming to discover penicillin, are main compounds of the non-stop scientific activity of the analyst during the session:

I know, furthermore, that this patient considers the sight of blood to be significant; it is felt to be something that has been lost, and the loss is felt to be associated with disaster for the object that has lost it. In the episode I have recounted, its presence was associated with feelings of depression and persecution (these last being observations of my common sense). I know the patient's hatred of reality is strongly coloured by the feeling that a sense of reality carries with it a stimulation of the socially polarized aspect of his emotional drives, and that this stimulation is felt to menace the ego-centric aspect of his emotional drives and therefore his narcissism, thus increasing his fear of annihilation. [C, 19]

Bion makes clear that he is not arguing that his interpretation is based on previous observations alone; that it is not a scientific hypothesis in the sense that the term *"is used by those who consider a hypothesis to be a generalization from a number of particular observations of fact"*. This view *"still seems"* to him to *"have substance"*, but what he says is not a challenge or rejection of experience, but rather, in his characteristic way, a valuing of the multifarious experiential situations that may become part of the unconscious repertoire and therefore cannot be said to be controlled: *"I do not wish to exclude from debate the influence exerted by numerous stimuli, subliminal or overt, which are received over a period of psycho-analytic experience"* (C, 19).

For this reason he says that *"it would be misleading"* (C, 19) to state that a specific interpretation *"owes nothing to the stream of stimuli which I as analyst, have received"*. In Bion's illustration, the interpretation was that *"blood is everywhere"* is the patient's common sense influenced by projective identification everywhere (C, 17–19). The reader may remember that this interpretation was qualified by the author as purely psycho-analytical. It is a psycho-analytic appreciation of the patient's wording, without being enslaved by its manifest, overt meaning. This apparent meaning constitutes commonplace and not common sense. It is commonplace travestied as common sense, as appeared in the first interpretation, that illuminates to the patient **his** "social-istic" meaning, namely, that he, as anyone with his senses functioning **obviously** could not lie down on a couch stained with "blood everywhere". It is also commonsensical to a seasoned, certified madman that he could not communicate the idea freely, fearing the accusation of having been hallucinating. Anyway, to emphasize, as Bion does, that the second interpretation is linked to experience, does not imply that it is *"based on experience"* alone (C, 19); it would be *"equally misleading to* say" this. Here we see Bion as the practitioner who does not jump to hasty conclusions, or, as he would quote years later, does not look irritably for fact and reason in a way that Keats warned us not to do. Using the terms he would coin six years later, he already actively practised, both intra-session and dealing with his experience after it, discipline on memory, understanding and desire. One may recall that Freud perhaps did not do this. For this reason he had to renounce both cocaine and trauma theory years later. Both seemed to be based on experience. They might have been linked to some experience, but they were not based on experience in an exclusive way. Further observation demanded a change in Freud's views about the experiences, which included more data than before. There is a paradox that demands to be tolerated. He qualifies his second interpretation as a "description", that *"should be reserved for beliefs, interpretations, hypotheses, which have demonstrably undergone what common sense would recognize as reality-testing … I, as individual, need to consider what the 'group' will accept as reality-testing before I can feel that my view has the sanction of 'my' common sense"* (C, 19–20).

In analysis, the analyst depends on the patient's response and the analytic couple forms a group. This is exactly what Freud said at the beginning of his paper, "Constructions in analysis" (SE, XXIII), and the issue was and continues to be the validation of interpretations in the work of Bion. Truth and insight emerge through a creative emotional experience, which depends on a relationship (see the entry, "Emotional experience"). This does not differ too much from experiments in the inanimate realm and especially where the frontiers between inanimate and animate, or matter or energy, are not clear, such as in the great Universe and in the quanta universe—the scientist "dialogues" with "something". This "something" has special properties, which "answer" to his experiment. The scientific experiment is a continuous interference of the observer and his methods and a measuring of the results of these interferences. In the words of Bion, he "shall therefore suggest" that the second interpretation *"has, as one of the components to which it owes its emergence, the influence of external events on the analyst's psyche both in shaping the form the interpretation takes as a crystallization of experience, the memory component, and as a compendium facilitating prediction, and by virtue of that, reality-testing"* (C, 20). The word "prediction" must be taken with due care: it is linked, obviously, to the repertoire of experiences that allow one to learn unconsciously from them.

In 1963 (*Elements of Psycho-analysis*), he would call it, "premonition", which is linked to Kant's "sensible intuition". [See these entries in this dictionary, where all relevant quotations in Bion's work are included.]

Even though, as we shall soon see, he explicitly says that he adheres to Kant, it would take him four additional years to quote Kant's dictum about blind intuitions and empty concepts (which he does in *Transformations*). Therefore, "*there remains the element whose existence was suspected by Hume and classified by him as 'psychological'. This element is most obtrusive before the point at which the common-sense synthesis of experience becomes a scientific ordering in a scientific system*"(C, 20). The issue at stake is when in the history of the individual, or in the human race, or in the history of a science, is the point where "*there were no generalizations believed . . . rarely any one historical date at which it is possible to say that the first hypothesis was adumbrated?*". In this quote from Braithwaite (C, 20), Bion paraphrases him, "*To this I would add that the same holds true of the history of an analysis—there is rarely a precise moment at which it can be said that a particular interpretation was first enunciated.*" Does this means that everything stems from the individual psyche, the troubling conundrum that blinds the philosopher in the no-man's land of the warring parties, realists versus idealists? By no means:

"*Nevertheless, even though it is in fact difficult to say that a given moment is* **the** *moment, we may yet suppose such a moment to exist, and it is before this point is reached that the so-called psychological factors are suspected of playing a dominant role in the scientific activity.*" In other words, "*there is a reason to look to the mentality of the analyst himself for the major contribution of elements in the totality of elements which issues in the interpretation . . . that the patient feels his common sense not as an integral part of his personality but as blood, dangerous and persecuting, lying about him everywhere*" (C, 20). The mentality of the analyst includes his personal analysis and experience with analysis.

His last use of the phrase was in *A Memoir of the Future*. The character Roland, a foolhardy man who does not think and endangers his own life closely, resembles Bion's experiences as a soldier, when he jeopardized his survival (WM, 106). At one moment, Roland "endangers" himself by not paying attention to the way he could escape from bullets and repeats the phrase, *"Blood every-where"* (AMF, I, 58). In the end, his seemingly commonsensical view that a post-Nazi conqueror, "Man", armed just with a bar of chocolate, leads him to pay no attention to the fact that it has real bullets and is "shot" (AMF, II, 370).

Bion rates highly Hume's insistence that there is nothing in a scientific hypothesis but a generalization; that the added elements drawn from experience do not belong to the scientific generalization properly speaking, but are continuous expressions of the psychological factor in the observer. Hume recognized a tendency in the human mind for certain ideas to be associated together. He rescued the Platonic realm. Before Hume, no philosopher of science was prepared to admit that this something extra (the added elements to generalization) did not exist at all, or that its existence lay in the personality of the human being.

After Hume, even Kant took many years to recognize the realism included in Hume's seemingly unrealistic denunciation of the "scandal of philosophy" (in Kant's terms). Kant might have been more permeable to Hume's contribution had he followed the steps of his own master, Hamann. This "something extra" was supposed to be analogous to the logic of the human mind, rather than a function of external reality. In this sense it could not exist to the extent that it could well just be a product of the mind. If this sounds perilously idealistic, let us keep firmly in mind that Bion's criticism of the neutrality of the observer is linked to the ultimate impossibility to grab, master or "own" the numinous realm. To master "O", the noumena, or ultimate reality, is what the psychotic thinks he (or she) is able to do. The naïve realist and the naïve idealist make precisely the same mistake. To defend the possible non-existence, or unknowability of the "something extra" (the added elements drawn from experience and external to scientific generalization) is **not** a solipsistic or idealistic denial of external reality. On the contrary, to defend this posture is reverence and awe towards the numinous realm, in other words, it means recognizing the limitations of our realizations and schemes.

> My view diverges from the view that the scientific hypothesis or law includes more than a generalization and that that something is a function of external reality. It approximates to the views of those epistemologists—Kant, Whewell, Mill, Peirce, Poincaré, Russell and

Popper—who tend to the beliefs compatible with the idea that scientific knowledge is the result of the growth of common-sense knowledge. [C, 21]

Bion approximates his views to those of a certain current without blindly adhering to it. This current sees what is known by the name of "scientific knowledge" as the result of a growth of common-sense knowledge. But this does not mean that the object of knowledge is itself common sense. Also, this phrase cannot be identified with Thomas Kuhn's mistake. Namely, that peer groups decide the issue to be researched. In Kuhn's case, peer review groups arbitrarily choose something according to an agreement that is purely political; paradigms are not derived from nature, empirical data, or real needs, Summing up, Bion's posture cannot be seen as if it had a relativistic overtone or a denial of experience. From 1962 onwards Bion would make more explicit his criticism to Popper.

There is no denial of the intuitive approach to that which is real and natural. This means that due to accretions of commonsensical knowledge one could well be nearer the noumena than one previously was. This is displayed, for example, by the perennial insights on the transmutation of matter and energy, or on Oedipus.

This posture would be expanded through the theory of transformations and invariances (q.v.). Following suit, Bion resorts to the kind of insight, or contact with "O", which seems to be open to the so-called "mystics". Although Bion would only put forth this theory four years later, it seems fair to state that he was opening a door for it in 1959, with *Cogitations*, by avoiding partisan adhesion to either positivism or relativist idealism.

For now, Bion proposes a method for not being entrapped by the realist/idealist conundrum. He elicits a paradox and simultaneously stresses that psycho-analysis may contribute as much to science as the other way round. There is no preponderance, no tutelage of either approach:

My agreements—and disagreements—with these epistemologists are a direct consequence of a psyco-analytic investigation of the phenomena known to all of them under various synonyms for scientific common sense. It is my view that the impasse in which the scientists and philosophers of science find themselves is not capable

of further adumbration, let alone resolution, without the employment of psycho-analytic research, and more precisely research into
the phenomena collectively called common sense which are the
main theme of this inquiry. I say the main theme, but in fact I
propose to make it so only because its data, elusive though they are,
are none the less more accessible to preliminary investigation than
phenomena associated with intuition, the first hypothesis, the inspiration (Karl Popper, *The Logic of Scientific Discovery*, pp. 31, 32). If I
do not elucidate this last, it will be because I cannot. In fact I do not
consider the elaboration of a deductive system from facts declared
by common sense to be so can be separated from the earlier
phenomenon which is a precondition for the elaboration of a deductive system, namely the inspiration. I propose, therefore, to make no
strenuous effort to separate the phenomena from each other. [C, 21]

Bion eventually left aside his pretensions towards a scientific
deductive system within the psycho-analytic realm. This coincided
with a general abandonment of these systems by authors from
other branches of advanced science such as physics. This abandonment began with the book *Transformations*. He would not become an
"intuitivist" either. Bion would never polarize his views, but would
rather propose, from this paper on, a posture that would persist
into his later works, in a more accentuated and explicit way. For the
lack of a better name, it would not be put of place to name this
posture "tolerance of paradoxes", meaning the consideration of
antithetical pairs and their resulting synthesis. This posture would
be expounded in consummated form in the trilogy *A Memoir of the
Future*. It was clearly prefigured in 1959. In the excerpt from *Cogitations* that I will quote below, one may notice the following aspects:

(i)   Poincaré's influence, which is reviewed under the entry,
       "Selected fact".
(ii)   The heavy usage of the psycho-analytic posture and practice,
       expressed by looking for hidden aspects of anything. In this
       case, it is the detection of an affirmative ethos, albeit non-
       apparent and less material, in phrases constructed with the
       negative word, "no".
(iii) The illumination through (i) and (ii) of what "in effect" is being
       said, beyond what is being *uttered* (whose immateriality would
       later be defined as "ultra-" and "infra-sensuous" (q.v.).

(iv) Lack of judgement, authority or superiority, either from the analyst over the patient or the obverse.

This is the first time that Bion uses the double arrow that later would be used to illuminate further: (i) Klein's theory of positions; (ii) the relationship between container and contained; (iii) and the pair narcissism and social-ism.

> I shall first consider the opposite of the hunch. "I don't know why", says the patient. "I don't understand", replies the patient to a particularly clear interpretation I have just given him. By "particularly clear" I mean one that has, in my opinion, drawn together a number of apparently unrelated facts in a way that demonstrates their relationship, and does so in terms so precise that the expression of the interpretation does not vitiate the deduction that is intrinsically dependent on its mode of expression. These two statements, "I don't know why", and "I don't understand", are as active, as affirmative as "I know", or, "I understand". In effect my interpretation has said, "This is why . . .", and, "Listen to what I am telling you, and you will find I have made you understand . . ." Both statements are implicit declarations by me that the relationship between the patient and myself is an analogue of the relationship that might exist between his capacity for inspiration, whatever that is, and the ideational counterpart of apparently unrelated elements scattered and apparently foreign to one another. I have in effect said, "I know why . . .", i.e. I unite elements. The patient has in effect said, "I, unlike you, do *not* know why . . ." My point is that this statement is a declaration of equality with me; not simply rivalry, but equality of status. "I unite" is one statement. "I disunite . . ." is the antiphonal reply. I propose to clarify my point in a series of formulas thus:
>
> (1) I unite ⇔ I disunite;
>
> (2) I synthesize ⇔ I analyse;
>
> (3) I metabolize ⇔ I katabolize;
>
> (4) I analyse violently ⇔ I split;
>
> (5) I synthesize violently ⇔ I fuse.
>
> Analysis and synthesis are both involved in understanding. If the act is carried out lovingly it leads to understanding; if carried out violently, i.e. violently with hate, then it leads to splitting and cruel juxtaposition or fusion. [C, 21–2]

His considerations about the possibility of discriminating whether a given statement is true or false were always empirical. This possibility was made following Spinoza and Kant's criterion of 'correspondence'. That is, a statement must necessarily have a counterpart in reality to be considered an expression of truth. Bion immersed himself in the study of contemporary philosophers of science in his quest to validate interpretations. One of the results of this research was the Grid (q.v.), which displays a kind of courtship with neo-positivism. Another result was the adoption of analogies with physics and mathematics. These disciplines are usually regarded as the height of science in terms of the precision of their formulations (to get as near as possible to reality as it is) and also in terms of successes in realistic intervention both in material and immaterial reality. Bion's aid comes from non-positivist physics.

The problem *"is inherent in psycho-analytic work and confronts the analyst at every turn . . . [it] is not new to the philosopher, but the analyst's position is more difficult because he is concerned with the practice of psycho-analysis, that is, he has to apply his theories in an empirical setting. Even so, this might amount to no more than the difficulties confronting the scientist who has to express his theories in terms of empirically verifiable data before subjecting them to experimental test, were it not for the fact that the experimental test of psycho-analysis and its theories differs in important respects from the experiments of the physicist whose procedures were marked for their rigour and commended on that account even by Kant. The physicist has, or used to have, his laboratory: the analytic situation that the analyst seeks to preserve is only similar because, I suspect, we attempt to establish an identity with the known which in fact is inadmissible in any but the most superficial way. The tribulations of the physicist since the quantum mechanical physicists have shown that their lowest-level hypotheses, their empirically verifiable data, are statistical hypotheses, may help the analyst to feel that the gap dividing him from the most rigorous scientific discipline of all has become less wide, but it does nothing to bring his subject nearer to being scientifically impeccable. Still less does it contribute to the elaboration of a method or, failing that, an understanding of the need for a method that will place all science, his own included, on a firmer basis. Furthermore, Heisenberg's exposition of the philosophy of quantum mechanics shows that the dependence of the physicist's observed facts on a relationship with facts that are not and can never be known has abolished the limiting walls of his laboratory, and therefore the laboratory itself, so that the physicist has difficulties with his laboratory analogous to the analyst's difficulty with his consulting room and analytic situation. But it does not help psycho-analysts to help themselves, or the physicists to know this, unless through knowing it we can make a breakthrough on the psycho-analytic front. Hence the need for investigating the nature of our own abstractions to a scientific view.* [C, 262–263]

The expanded use of these considerations resulted in his three first books, *Learning from Experience, Elements of Psycho-analysis* and *Transformations*. His later posture reached its most developed form in the trilogy *A Memoir of the Future*. There are literally dozens of formulations of it, especially in volume I. Some of them appear in the "recommended cross-entries". To select one that illustrates the posture:

> P.A. According to Heisenberg the fact of *observing* the play of minute physical factors influences the play being observed. I do not know if he is saying that what I have been used to regard as a *mental* phenomenon has an effect on what I call a *physical* fact; I may have been in error in discriminating between "mental" phenomena and "physical" facts. Such an "idea" is perhaps a flaw in the mental apparatus. As a human I have a prejudice in favour of regarding my thoughts as "superior" to the apparently random movements of infinitely minute particles of matter?
>
> ROLAND Are you prejudiced against the random movements of minute particles of matter?
>
> ROBIN The whole of psycho-analytic theory seems to be vitiated— as shown by the structured nature of the system itself—by favouring only those phenomena which appear to conform to classical logic, the sort of logic with which we are already familiar. [AMF, II, 265]

About scientific validation

Lest any doubts remain about Bion's posture, it may be opportune to make clear that experience, empirical data and raw lower level data were sources that gave life to his observations. But he did not expect that these data would "validate" the theories or hypotheses. In his "second thoughts" about more than fifteen years of continuous practice he felt the need to state:

I would warn against the phrase "empirically verifiable data" which I employ ... I do not mean that experience "verifies" or "validates" anything. This belief as I have come across it in the literature of the philosophy of science relates to an experience which enables the scientist to achieve a feeling of security to offset and neutralize the sense of insecurity on the discovery that discovery has exposed further vistas of unsolved problems—"thoughts" in search of a thinker. [ST, 166]

Recommended Cross-References: Analytic View, Analogy, Cause, Common sense, Dispositions, Facts, Intuition, Judgmental values, Mathematization of psycho-analysis, Mental Space, Models, Oedipus, Real psycho-analysis, Thoughts without a thinker, Truth, Ultra-sensuous, Real psycho-analysis.

&; The author, starting from these texts of Bion, proposed to summarize the psycho-analytic approach of tolerance of paradoxes since Freud—an approach enhanced by Klein and Bion—in a series of papers and books (mainly volumes VIII, *Hegel and Klein* and IX, *Hegel and Bion*, of the eleven-volume series, *A Apreensão da Realidade Psíquica*). These works address the origins of this posture, and draw comparisons and analogies with modern science. Theses include the fallacy of notions such as innate preconceptions of space and time as separate, absolute entities; the coincidence of Bion's approach to space and Hamilton and other physicists' approach to space-time and multi-dimension space; and the timelessness of the unconscious. In this series of books the term "tolerance of paradoxes" is proposed.

Selected fact: *"The term, 'selected fact', I reserve for use in emotional experiences of thought about phenomena in which time is excluded, and in all scientific deductive systems and the corresponding calculi which are constructed to represent such phenomena"* (C, 278)

"Selected fact" is a term borrowed from the philosophy of mathematics. Jules-Henri Poincaré, who was both a practising mathematician and a gifted philosopher of mathematics, coined it. He was able to reach the relativity theory one year later than Einstein using different mathematical tools. His writings about science, method and mathematical creation can be regarded as classics.

Poincaré says *"if a new result is to have any value, it must unite elements long since known, but till then scattered and seemingly foreign*

726   THE LANGUAGE OF BION

to each other, and suddenly introduce order where the appearance of disorder reigned. Then it enables us to see at a glance each of these elements in the place it occupies in the whole" (LE, 72).

Bion adds: *"The name of one element is used to particularize the selected fact, that is to say the name of that element in the realization that appears to link together elements not hitherto seen to be connected . . . The selected facts, together with the selected fact that appears to give coherence to a number of selected facts, emerge from a psycho-analytic object or series of such objects . . . The selected fact is the name of an emotional experience, the emotional experience of a sense of discovery of coherence; its significance is therefore epistemological and the relationships of selected facts must not be assumed to be logical"* (LE, 72–3).

Bion sees the concept as equivalent to the transition between PS and D in a process of synthesis. It seems that a trans-disciplinary truth has been reached, formulating perhaps a way in which the mind functions. Both "mathematical creation" and D seem to be expressions of real thought. Bion uses the term "selected fact" to describe that which the psycho-analyst must experience in the process of synthesis (LE, 72). It is difficult to find such trans-disciplinary research in any field.

> Since the philosophy of modern physics—the most successful and most rigorous of scientific disciplines—can be seen here to be quite compatible with a philosophical view of unco-ordinated and incoherent elements similar to the mental domain of isolated elements from which Poincaré describes the mathematician as attempting to escape by his discovery of the selected "fact", and since moreover the mental state described by Poincaré is quite compatible or even identical with that described by Melanie Klein in her discussion of the paranoid–schizoid and depressive positions, it is quite reasonable to suppose that the investigation and explanation of these unco-ordinated elements will be dictated by the impulse described by Poincaré and investigated in detail psycho-analytically by Melanie Klein and her co-workers, and limited by the mental capacity which in the final analysis is the tool by which the investigation is carried out. [C, 85]

The selected fact precipitates Models (q.v.). They can be the psychotic's concretization and perform the role of ejected objects; they can be ideas and emotions (EP, 39, 83).

⊕ The formulation was central in aiding Bion to build a scientific approach to psycho-analysis that was implicit in Freud's work. Nevertheless it was not couched in epistemological terms. Even though the term was used in his published works from 1962 onwards, the justifications for such a use are made more clear in his unpublished drafts dating from 1959 (please refer to the entry, "Scientific method").

From 1965 onwards Bion does not use the term "selected fact" any more. One may conclude that the use of the theory of transformations superseded it. The concept of a tool that detects underlying realities amidst seemingly disjointed material, that is, the theory of selected fact, seems to have been replaced by a more developed one, that of Invariance. The latter assumes an observational role and is increasingly seen (as it was in *Elements of Psychoanalysis*) as something that the mind does.

In 1965, the selected fact is used for the last time. It is seen as being expressed by hyperbole (q.v.). Or, hyperbole *"has. . . a wide spectrum, is flexible and lends itself easily for use by the analyst as a 'selected fact' to aid in displaying coherence which, without it, may not be apparent"* (T, 162).

The coherence of the selected fact was in the beginning seen in its Humean sense of constant conjunction. That is, giving coherence that makes sense to the observer; in the end run, the coherence already existed, waiting to be intuited.

Suggested cross-references: Models, Invariances, Scientific method.

Sensations, feelings, affects, emotions: Bion considered that for the time being there were no conditions for discriminating the counterparts in reality that some terms—instincts, emotions and impulses—try to depict (T, 67). In stating this, he avoids the decades-old discussion around the translations of the German terms, such as *Trieb* and *Instinkt*, among others. This discussion, as a matter of fact, still lingers on, unresolved.

Bion's posture implies that he made no attempt to define these terms rigorously, with the possible exception of the term "feelings", which he sees as inner sensual stimulations (see the entry "Alpha-function"). Bion also defines in a clear-cut way the phrase "emotional experience" (q.v.).

The terms "sensations", "feelings" and "emotions" are linked together in Bion's work. They were emanations of a given ultimate human reality. Therefore they were classifiable as phenomena that could be *"objects of sense"* (LE, 6). In doing this he adopted—but not exclusively—Freud's theory of consciousness as the sense organ for the perception of psychic qualities. Sensations, feelings, affects and emotions are the phenomena that manifest themselves during an analytic session. As late as 1978, when Bion wrote the third volume of *A Memoir of the Future*, he continued with this same posture: *"The nearest that the psychoanalytic couple comes to a 'fact' is when one or the other has a feeling"* (AMF, III, 536).

There are at least five issues that must be taken into consideration with regard to feelings and analysis. All of them are linked to the necessity to name feelings, affects and emotions.

1. **Unconscious feelings and splitting**—even though it may sound a contradiction in terms, feelings are many times regarded as unconscious. Perhaps one day in the future we will reach a more precise classification that discriminates feelings, affects, emotions and emotional experiences. Nowadays, it is necessary to respect that the present psycho-analytic movement uses the idea of unconscious feelings. Resistances such as splitting, denial and repression: keep emotional life at bay, ensconced into the darkness of the repressed unconscious.

2. **Naming feelings**—the patient cannot name properly what he feels because of the situation described in 1, above.

3. **The outsider's view of feelings**—even though this view can be accurate, how can we communicate it in such a way that the patient does not simply learn about the view but "becomes" it through acquiring insight?

4. **Nature/nurture**—the bodily origin of instincts, the existence of primary envy and narcissism, create a problem in deciding the possibilities and ways of dealing with feelings, affects and emotions.

5. **Hallucination**—feelings (but not emotions and affects) can be hallucinated.

One of the obstacles in naming feelings and emotions and defining them either theoretically as concepts or practically, in life and during an analytic session, seems to be the prevalence of value and moral judgements:

P.A. You may not envy the kind of eminence which stimulates my envy, but you nevertheless have feelings of envy. The fact that I may not be able to define feelings, either yours, mine or those of others which are neither yours nor mine, does not mean that they do not, did not, or may not in future exist. They may at some stage become so obtrusive that it is possible to attach a name to them.

ROBIN Although I have been aware of the pressure of what I can now call sexual or envious feelings, I would have been outraged had I been told that I was sexual or envious.

ROLAND What other people can verbalize about my feelings, especially if I can't, is particularly exasperating.

P.A. That is one component of the practice of psycho-analysis which is constant even if not constantly perceived. Guilty feelings are unwelcome and even in infants easily evoked. It is difficult to give an interpretation which is distinguished from a moral accusation.

ROLAND Surely this is a defect of psycho-analysis?

P.A. Certainly; but when I agree you and others are therefore liable to assume that it is psycho-analysis only that suffers from that weakness, whereas I believe that this is a fundamental experience. It is this fundamental experience that underlies Plato's dialogue between Socrates and Phaedrus which is being revived here—a few hundred years later—in this discussion. [AMF, III, 480]

Bion resorts to fiction in order to be more real than lifeless "real" persons. In this, he follows Shelley's opinion about Shakespeare reproduced in *A Memoir of The Future*, Prologue, page 4. The posture conveyed by the dialogue reproduced above is that feelings also emanate from bodily occurrences. Mental life is an expression of what we name "instincts". These instincts are species-dependent, basically animal, genetic, innate, inherited. They are the soil, the earth upon which social experiences (mother in the first instance) will be sown:

EM Now you have muddled me. I shall be *body*; for ever I shall gird at your mind.

MIND Hullo! Where have you sprung from?

BODY What—you again? I am Body; you can call me Soma if you like. Who are you?

MIND Call me Psyche—Psyche-Soma.

BODY Soma-Psyche.

MIND We must be related.

BODY Never—not if I can help it.

MIND Oh, come. Not as bad as that, is it?

BODY Worse. You got us into this air. Luckily I brought some liquid with me. What are you doing?

MIND Nothing; it must be my phrenes, that diaphragm going up and down. I'm breathing in air—fluid, not liquid. What did you bring that wet stuff for? Beautiful odour.

BODY You could not know about the odour if I had not the liquid to hold your atoms with. Typical of Mind—all words and no content. Where did you find them?

MIND Borrowed from the future—you are borrowing them from me; do you get them through the diaphragm?

BODY *They* penetrate *it*. But the meaning does not get through. Where did you get your pains from?

MIND Borrowed—from the past. The meaning does not get through the barrier though. Funny—the meaning does not not get through whether it is from you to me, or from me to you.

BODY It is the meaning of pain that I am sending to you; the words get through—which I have not—but the meaning is lost.

MIND What is that amusing little affair sticking out? I like it. It has a mind of its own—just like me.

BODY It's just like me—has a body of its own. That's why it is so erect. Your mind—no evidence for it at all.

MIND Don't be ridiculous. I suffer anxiety as much as you have pain. In fact I have pain about which you know nothing. I suffered intensely when we were rejected. I asked you to call me Psyche and promised to call you Soma.

SOMA All right Psyche; I don't admit that there is any such person other than a figment of my digestion.

PSYCHE Who are you talking to then?

SOMA I'm talking to myself and the sound is reflected back by one of my fetal membranes.

PSYCHE Your feetal membranes! Ha, ha! Very good! Is that your pun or mine?

SOMA It's the only language you understand.

PSYCHE It's the only language you hear. All you talk is pain.

SOMA All you respect is pain or lack of it. The only time I can get anything over to you is pain-talk from the hills.

PSYCHE Plain talk through your stoma. Excuse me if I borrow to talk to this idiotic nipple a moment—there! An erection at once!

SOMA Thanks to my liquid evacuations. Who is that?

PSYCHE I bit it.

SOMA It had just bitten me. Bite it again! That's *me*—not *it*.

PSYCHE It can't be. I put my foot in it—was it your stoma? You have confused me again. Pain, Feet—all mixed up. Why can't you take your choice?

SOMA I do. If you had any respect for my "feelings" and did what I feel, you wouldn't be in this mess.

PSYCHE I am in this mess because I was squeezed into it. Who is responsible—your feelings or your ideas? All that has me is yours—amniotic fluid, light, smell, taste, noise, I'm wrapped up in it. Look out! I am getting absorbed!

SOMA I'll pi you out when I've absorbed you. All piss, shit, and piety. You can idea-lize it—get a good price for it no doubt! Bless me—I'm getting absorbed too. Help!

PSYCHE That's what comes of penetrating in or out. I'm confused.

SOMA That's what comes of not penetrating—you break up or down. [AMF, III, 433–435]

Sense of truth: Shakespeare often "used" lesser characters to convey some of his most profound and insightful truths about mankind and the behaviour of humanity/inhumanity. This Shakespearian device has been noted by Frank Kermode, among others. One example is found in *Macbeth*, where a murderer (a secondary character) provides insight into the nature of contempt for life. Macbeth sends murderers to kill his own best friend. Macbeth warns the assassins that his friend is a gallant and fiery knight. The murderers retort by saying that this information, and even the knight's name, is of no importance whatsoever:

> "Ay, in the catalogue ye go for men,
> As hounds and greyhounds, mongrels, spaniels, curs,
> Shoughs, water-rugs, and demi-wolves are clipt
> All by the name of dogs." (Ill, i, 91)

This excerpt reveals that for a murderer, or for anyone displaying contempt and disregard for life, it does not matter who is being killed.

The same device seems to apply to a special concept of Bion's, that of the sense of truth. It occupies a strikingly small part in his work. It was stated in one of his earliest writings. This writing must be seen, nevertheless, as a harbinger, as the shape of things to come.

Perhaps his definition of "sense of truth" is as important to the practising analyst who strives to keep a non-judgmental posture, as it is overlooked in the literature about his work hitherto available:

Definition. *"We may now consider further the relationship of rudimentary consciousness to psychic quality. The emotions fulfil a similar function for the psyche to that of the senses in relation to objects in space and time. That is to say the counterpart of the common-sense view in private knowledge is the common emotional view: a sense of truth is experienced if the view of an object which is hated can be conjoined to a view of the same object when it is loved and the conjunction confirms that the object experienced by different emotions is the same object"* (ST, 119).

It is first and foremost a practical application of Melanie Klein's notion of the integration of a whole object and the inception of depressive position. This notion, in turn, takes to its last consequences Freud's insights into the splitting of the ego in the processes of defence.

It is also one of Bion's more clear-cut definitions that allow the analyst to cope with paradoxes without a hasty attempt to solve them; or without being prey to memory, desire and understanding.

Suggested cross-references: Absolute truth, Analytic view, Atonement, Becoming, Binocular view, Commonsense,

Compassion, Correlation, Disturbed personality, Enforced splitting, O, Jargon, Judgmental Values, Mystic, Philosophy, Real psycho-analysis, Reality Sensuous and Psychic, Sense of Truth, Thinking, Truth-Function, Ultra-sensuous, Unknowable, Unknown.

📖 Sir Isaiah Berlin's *The Sense of Reality*

Sensuous: This term always has the meaning of something that can be apprehended through the sensuous apparatus. It corresponds to the philosophical term, "sensible". With the possible exception of a few dialogues in *A Memoir of the Future*, some of them stated in the negative sense (for example, AMF, I, 14: "*Both girls were ignorant of sensuous pleasure*"), more often than not the term has no sexual implications in the work of Bion.

Recommended cross-reference: Non-sensuous.

Sensuous apparatus: Bion uses this term in its neurological and neurophysiological sense, namely, the five basic human senses, and others such as the proprioceptives. He uses it as Kant and Freud used it. The term refers to the harbour of whatever stimulus it is. The senses are transducers; they are the advanced posts that allow an apprehension, albeit imperfect, of transient and partial aspects of reality—internal and external.

Freud considered consciousness as a sensuous organ—that of apprehension of psychic reality; Bion, after critically scrutinizing such a concept, came to accept it.

Sex:

> P.A. People of different sex find it easier to resolve their anatomi-cal and physiological differences than their differences in outlook. After all, the physical can be subjected to tactile and visual and olfactory investigation and resolution. [AMF, II, 389]

It is a well-known fact that painting, sculpture, prose, theatre, opera and films which appear to display "explicit sex scenes" more often than not have nothing to do with real sexual relationships. If those works are seen *vis-à-vis* painting, sculpture, prose, theatre, opera and films that have no sensuously apprehensible references to the issue, a striking fact is elicited. Real sex emerges as more living and often is more respectful to its unspoken but noticeable immaterial reality.

Sex and sexuality are a central issue in Bion's work. Many fail to perceive it; many prefer actual mentioning—just like in the situation quoted above. This is for reasons that are amenable to be seen exclusively in the realm of personal analysis. Bion commented that if a book does not contain explicit references to these issues it is not regarded as a proper psycho-analytic book or paper.

Bion suggests focusing on Oedipus under vertexes other than the sexual; the theory of container and contained has a sexual ethos clearly indicated by the genetic symbols chosen to represent it: ♀ ♂. Sexuality envelops reality "sensuous and psychic".

> Freud said infants were sexual; this was denied and re-buried. [AMF, Prologue, 5]

Sex is an issue whose concretization, both in real life and in the psycho-analytic movement, and above all in the analytic session, proved to be frequent and, with equal frequency, damaging.

> ROBIN Do you make a distinction between individuals—precise, particular men and women—and their minds?

> P.A. Sometimes that distinction is relevant. Increasingly I am aware that there is something more than that which presents itself to my senses—sound, sight, hearing, touch. I have feelings that are aroused by something that I do not smell or touch or hear or see. My perceptions are not fine enough—blunted by the constant battering of sensuous reality. I shall not live long enough to reach *those* facts except in rudimentary degree.

> ALICE If it is rudimentary: perhaps it is something you could and did experience when you yourself were a rudimentary character—in the womb.

> P.A. Were you aware in pregnancy of a "character" in your body?

> ALICE Emphatically. One kick in the belly is not the same as another.

> ROBIN I should be interested to know what P.A. thinks of maternal intuition. Do you think that paternally gifted psycho-analysts would be capable of such fine discriminations?

> P.A. I am a prey to my prejudices. There may be contributions which paternal genes confer and others which derive from both parents.

ROLAND You seem to suggest that as a psycho-analyst you are compacted of the best of both sexes. [AMF, III, 514–515]

ROLAND I saw a horrible photograph of a duel between two people armed with sabres in which one had decapitated his opponent in one stroke. I was not really claiming to have been so completely separated from my central nervous system, or the seat of my intelligence.

ALICE You often talk as if, because I am a woman, I can't ever have had an intelligence from which to be separated.

P.A. Perhaps that is because he has never been completely separated from his primordial mind and is still dominated by a belief that as a woman has not got a penis she cannot have a capacity for masculine thinking.

ALICE Does the caesura connect or separate? He often behaves as if he were not a male sexual animal.

ROLAND That's not fair! You're behaving like a female sexual animal, and I can hardly be blamed if I am cautious—sometimes.

PAUL This is not an occasion for display of the matrimonial experience. But if I say so, it will be assumed that I and my nominally saintly predecessor are opposed to sex. The biological creator does not appear to be on good terms with the creator of morals. Verbal intercourse is not granted the freedom that sociologically we are supposed to have.

P.A. Freedom often seems to be driven "underground"—or should I say "subterrane"?

ALICE: Please yourself; but suppose both the dictator and liberator go underground and meet there. [AMF, II, 248–249]

ALICE I agree. It sounds like a clever man demonstrating his superiority to the simple folk who believe in God.

P.A. I am not sure about your "simple folk". "Fundamentals" are often simple; "folk" are not. It is true that it may be difficult to distinguish between the "simplicity", say, of genius, and the "simplicity" of the fraud who has learned to simulate the characteristics of genius. The garb of the great is often used to clothe the nakedness of the fraud; money is used to cover the bankruptcy of the poor; a beautiful girl instinctively wraps an ugly soul in her looks.

ALICE I have known men fall for the divinity of a beautiful nit-wit.

P.A. Why restrict it to the male? Physical sex often masquerades as passionate love.

ROBIN The beauty of a handsome man or woman is easily and quickly "perceived". The reality behind may require more investigation than the greedy swallower of mental bait has achieved.

ROLAND There are many "glittering" prizes offered for the greedy soul. [AMF, II, 268–9]

ROBIN I thought psycho-analysis was all sex.

P.A. Since psycho-analysis is a human interest you would naturally assume, without having to be told by a psycho-analyst, that it was sure to be sexual—"all sex", as you call it. As psycho-analytic theories are about, or purport to be about, human beings, you would feel they should resemble real life, real people. If so, sex ought to appear somewhere in the theories. [AMF, II, 303]

SCHOOLBOY At school I wrote some articles for the magazine labelled "Sex on the Games Field"—a long and pretty accurate account of the biology master's lesson on the reproductive process of dandelions, both sexual and vegetative. I had an imaginary interview with the groundsman whom I asked about sex. He replied, "I know nothing about sex, but them perky dandelions will certainly be the death of me". Anyway, funny or not, that was the death of me. It was the title that did it, even though there had been a lot about Richard Coeur de Lion. The Head asked for me to be removed. My poor mother was broken-hearted; my dear Dad was furious but secretly thought it funny. In the end, as I was due to go into the army, they let me stay to the end of term; that was more respectable and it was hoped I would get bumped off, so all were satisfied . . . [AMF, II, 377]

Reality sensuous and psychic: feelings

"Alice" and "Rosemary", respectively, represent a former wife of a landowner and a former whore-skivvy. These two characters represent the formation of a non-reproductive, pleasure-oriented sexualized pair, full of sadistic phantasies of triumph and domination. "Rosemary" "humiliates" Alice after years of "being humiliated" by her; she also "makes sex" with "Roland" and is trying to "marry" a post-Nazi all-mighty conqueror, "Man":

> ROSEMARY ... Scientific bunkum. What do *you* know about the waves emitted by my feet when I chose to make them twinkle, twinkle on the hard, hard slum pavements of my street? I have seen the natural, unspoilt louts and blackguards of my slum follow my heels, threads of invisible steel hooking their eyes and dragging them helpless at my feet till I chose to release them. Love! You don't know what it is—none of you.
>
> P.A. Your beliefs are expressions of great confidence in your powers; how you come to such "beliefs" and what evidence has convinced you they are "facts"; I don't know.
>
> . . .
>
> ROSEMARY I feel it; I know it.
>
> P.A. Your feelings are one kind of evidence. But don't make the mistake of acting as if you had a different sort of evidence. Alice *feels* you love her, but the feeling leads her to suppose facts. She thinks she can depend on you; she can't. If she cannot depend on herself she would be unwise to depend on anyone else.
>
> ROSEMARY Me, for example.
>
> P.A. For example, yes.
>
> ROSEMARY I agree. My principles would not allow me to think otherwise: the same principle which would not allow either loving or being loved by Man. I depend on my hooks—
>
> P.A. And on his eyes to provide you with "material" into which you can insert those same "hooks". In other terms—my psychoanalytic terms—sex.
>
> ROSEMARY (yawning) How interesting.
>
> P.A. Not in the least. Usually sex interest has died by puberty, leaving only a mental vestige which cannot be relied on any more than you could rely on your vestigial tail to support you if you tried to hang by it from the branch of a tree.
>
> ALICE How ridiculous!
>
> P.A. I gave a ridiculous example to illustrate ridiculous dependence.

SHERLOCK I thought the whole of psycho-analysis depended on sex.

P.A. In the practice of psycho-analysis I depend on ideas. [AMF, II, 400–401]

Suggested cross-references: Container/Contained, Facts, Oedipus, Real psycho-analysis.

Social-ism: See the entry, Narcissism and Social-ism

Stammer, stammerer: It seems that Bion paid **special** attention to this symptom. As it frequently occurs in his work as in the contributions of great psycho-analysts such as Freud, Klein and Winnicott, seemingly minor features point to important mental mechanisms and functions. Stammer is related to psychosis and to fear of annihilation, to the extent that it seems to be linked to feelings of being unable to breathe and to tolerate reality itself.

☺ In 1959, a clinical observation on stammering was that "*intolerance of frustration leads to intolerance of stimulation*". Therefore stammering becomes a recalcitrant symptom (C, 48).

This intolerance of stimulation can be so marked that it comes to encompass any stimulation and all kinds of stimulation. However, how can one live in a world in which stimuli are absent? Sensuous stimuli are the port-of-entry of everything; without them, there is no life, no alpha-function, no dreams, no unconscious and no conscious. Bion suggests that "*the stammer is a repudiation of awareness, evacuation of awareness of what is currently taking place; it is the antithesis of α. It is therefore incompatible with a state of self consciousness*" (C, 77). He asks if the stammerer has no personality; his own guess is that the stammerer has "*a marked personality, often irascible*".

One year later (1960), apparently having to deal with the same patient, Bion suggests that the stammer corresponds to a kind of oral flatus. It also points to the eruption of the psychotic personality. "*The session increasingly gave me the feeling that he was having, or was about to have, a psychotic breakdown. Everything pointed to the idea that he felt as if he could not breathe, that some man was refusing to let him get air in; and he was swearing and attacking the man with his oral flatus—the stammer. His attitude was euphoric, perhaps megalomanic. I drew attention to what seemed to be evidence that he felt unable to learn from the experience he was having with me"* (C, 142). To be unable to learn from experience means, again, starvation of reality. Psychosis erupts because *"The need to know the truth then becomes a matter of psychic need"* (C, 143).

Bion's latest development on stammer is to be found in *Attention and Interpretation*, from 1970. He adjoins to the issue the imbalance of container and contained:

> The following will serve as a model for a theoretical formulation of this kind of link: a man speaking of an emotional experience in which he was closely involved began to stammer badly as the memory became increasingly vivid to him. The aspects of the model that are significant are these: . . . he was trying to contain himself, as one sometimes says of someone about to lose control of himself; he was trying to "contain" his emotions within a form of words, as one might speak of a general attempting to "contain" enemy forces within a given zone.

> The words that should have represented the meaning the man wanted to express were fragmented by the emotional forces to which he wished to give only verbal expression; the verbal formulation could not "contain" his emotions, which broke through and dispersed it as enemy forces might break through the forces that strove to contain them.

> The stammerer, in his attempt to avoid the contingency I have described, resorted to modes of expression so boring that they failed to express the meaning he wished to convey . . . His verbal formulation could be described as like to the military forces that are worn by the attrition to which they are subjected by the contained forces. The meaning he was striving to express was denuded of meaning. His attempts to use his tongue for verbal expression failed to "contain" his wish to use his tongue for masturbatory movement in his mouth.

> Sometimes the stammerer could be reduced to silence. This situation can be represented by a visual image of a man who talked so much that any meaning he wished to express was drowned by his flood of words. [AI, 93–4]

&⍭ Bion's own suggestions and his further developments in the observation of the here and now of the session lead to the hypothesis that, at the exact moment when the stammerer stammers, the stammerer renounces, out of hate towards reality, to his personality. Therefore, the question Bion addresses about the lack of personality would have some grounds. In that moment, and only that moment, the very moment of an intense dedication to the stammer-in-itself, the stammerer may be conceived of as having no personality. Through projective identification, he tries to divest the analyst of his personality too. The sexualization of thought processes, described by Freud (in the case of Little Hans, and in *Totem and taboo*) is made due to hate of frustration and reality. The language is masturbatory and the act of talking is masturbatory too.

Stupidity: Please refer to the entries Arrogance and Curiosity.

Successful analysis: *"If analysis has been successful in restoring the personality of the patient he will approximate to being the person he was when his development became compromised"* (T, 143).

Suggested cross-references: Analytic view, Atonement, Real Psycho-analysis.

Symbiotic: A term introduced in Bion's second theory of links, 1970 (please refer to the entry "Links").

Note

1. Number 34 corresponds in Bion's *Second Thoughts* to the first two paragraphs of "Notes on the theory of schizophrenia", 1953 (ST).

T

T: A quasi-mathematical symbol used to represent **Transformation** (q.v.) (T, 10).

Tα: α quasi-mathematical symbol used to represent the *process* of **Transformation** (q.v.) (T, 10).

Inaccuracy As far as the research of the author goes, here the student of Bion's contributions to psycho-analysis finds one of only four points in his whole work where an imprecise definition obtrudes. In *Attention and Interpretation* Bion attributes to the sign Tα the value of *"the point from which the transformation starts"* (AI, 4). One may safely dismiss this definition as incomplete. Even though the processes of transformation will include the point from which they start, they encompass more than this.

Recommended cross-reference: Transformation.

Tβ: A quasi-mathematical symbol used to represent the *end-product* of a transformation (q.v.) (T, 10).

Theories: Bion states that an analyst must have few theories to work with (LE, 42). He names the theories that he personally works with in *Elements of Psycho-analysis*: (i) Freud's two principles of mental functioning, (ii) Klein's positions, (iii) Oedipus, (iv) and his own contribution to the theory of psycho-analysis, the theory of container/contained. He stresses that the grasp of a few theories is more useful than a myriad of theories poorly understood.

Later he would stress that the analyst needs to know the vocabulary he uses precisely, so he can compare how the patient hears it (in "Evidence", 1976). The vast majority of Bion's contributions to psycho-analysis were observational theories, rather than theories of psycho-analysis. The exceptions are: a theory of thinking, the theory of container and contained and the posthumously published "metatheory". The latter is no more than a preliminary draft.

The issue with theories was the unnecessary multiplication of *ad hoc* explanations that are always encircling the same basic configuration—which are doomed, this way, to remain unnoticed.

Theories and fashion

> ROBIN . . . Surely "unconscious" claims are far more open to misinterpretation.
>
> P.A. Agreed—I do not wish to decry the events of which I know nothing. But I have been compelled to notice that "fashions" in beliefs, in theories, in varieties of psycho-analysis and in psycho-analysts are as plentiful as fashions in cosmetics. I suspect that the fundamental source of fashion, whether in people, religions, "scientific" theories or holiday resorts is, or ought to be, one goal of our curiosity. As individuals we cannot hope to do more than reach some outlying, peripheral goal and please ourselves by claiming that it is ultimate truth; or alternatively fall into despair at discovering our insignificance.
>
> ROLAND Most people with common sense know that.
>
> P.A. Most people with any common sense are, in my experience, very few people indeed. Common sense is only rarely in fashion. "Real" common sense, in contrast to cosmetic common sense, tells too many uncomfortable things. [AMF, III, 525]

In talking about the great authors, including Milton and Virgil, Bion warns about readings and solipsistic relativism:

... The reader, the beholder, if "he hath ears to hear" and permits himself to listen, may still catch its echo that may grow "faint at last". Our thinking is prodigal; the cost is mental pollution, a by-product of mental combustion liable to become the most significant creation. [AMF, 2, 234]

Need for theories

Theories are also theories that a patient has about himself. The limit of any theory is commented on:

ROBIN . . . I take it you do not talk to the id, because that is only a theoretical term.

P.A. Even theories and theoretical terms are supposed to remind us of a reality. I have no doubt that one "talks to" an experienced person; the matter of psycho-analysis is such that analyst and analysand cannot afford to neglect the total sophisticated capacities of which both are capable. The psycho-analyst has a lifetime of experience, including the experience of technical psycho-analytical training; the analysand, even if only a young child, has a consider-able body of experience to fall back on. [MF, III, 496]

Thinking, theory of: One of Bion's epistemological contributions to psycho-analysis was to discern a "system of psycho-analytical the-ory" from a "system of theories of observation" in psycho-analysis.

One of the comparatively few contributions of Bion to the "system of psycho-analytical theory" was his theory of thinking. It was first proposed in 1961, at the International Psycho-analytical Congress held in Edinburgh. It was published as a paper—"A theory of thinking" in the *IJPA* and re-published as the first chapter of the book, *Learning from Experience*. This book is wholly based on the paper.

The paper in turn is based on Freud's "Formulations on the two principles of mental functioning", enriched by Bion's extensive experience with patients labelled as psychotics. This experience indicated the usefulness of Freud's observations on the deleterious effects of the prevalence of the principle of pleasure/unpleasure when primary narcissism and envy exist. It also showed the exis-tence of a precocious hallucinatory activity linked to allegiance to this principle.

The paper helps to dispel paradisiacal views that fuelled ideas of pathology and parental guilt, such as attacks against weaning. In a way not dissimilar from Winnicott's, Bion shows the formative function of the absence of a wished breast, or idealized breast. It is in line with the perception that development without resistance does not exist—here understood as an opposing force. This realization seems easy to achieve in the physical, concrete reality. No living system, such as for example the human osteo-muscular system, grows without a resistance. It was a realization that would be unaltered throughout the whole of Bion's work.

This realization also includes pain; its importance seems to be seminal, to the point that Bion included it as one of the elements of psycho-analysis (please refer to this specific entry).

The initial formulation was that the infant has an innate pre-conception of a breast. It looks for a breast. It has a "disposition" to it (C, 262). If the child is to survive, it unavoidably finds a breast. This breast is unavoidably different from the infant's pre-conception, but a coupling occurs. This coupling means that a realization of the breast occurred. The difference between the real breast and the wished-for breast corresponds to a seminal experience, that Bion calls, "No-Breast". If and when the "No-Breast" is tolerated, there occurs the obtrusion of thinking processes. The infant is enabled to symbolize the breast; the infant is enabled to think the "No-Breast". The concept of a breast emerges when the pre-conception mates with the realization. In early times Bion called this concept a thought.

This theory allowed a more precise view of the origins of thinking processes. It is not a brainy or rational activity, but an activity dependent on emotional experiences. There was a loosely stated dependence of thinking on emotions, but its functioning was not properly described.

The same paper includes an important differentiation between a sense of truth, and judgmental ideas of right or wrong. The sense of truth precludes judgement; it obtrudes when the person achieves the realization that the object that is loved and the object that is hated are one and the same object. Ideas of right or wrong emerge when the discrimination between true and false is not possible. The "basic falsity", so to say, is the hallucination of a breast, or the idea that the No-Breast is "wrong". This means, nature itself, or the principle of reality, is wrong in that it brings pain and frustration of desire.

In 1965 the theory of thinking was formulated in the following terms:

> On the interplay between the no-thing and the realization that is felt to approximate to it depends the development of thought, and by thought I mean, in this context, that which enables problems to be solved in the absence of the object. [T, 106–7]

The theory of thinking evolved to the theory of Links (q.v.)

Recommended cross-references: Breast, Conception, Link, Preconception.

Thoughts without a thinker: In the *Discours sur le Méthode* René Descartes formulated the idea of a thought without a thinker. He formulates it in its negative sense in order to discard it. It was a time when the seeds of positivism were being laid down and the realm of the Platonic forms, a negative realm, was subjected to oblivion and denial. Therefore, "negation" was all that remained from the perception of this realm. To negate was used as a kind of scientific tool. In this sense Descartes "proved" that a thought without a thinker had to be regarded as an absurdity. It would not constitute an exaggeration to say that Descartes acted as if Fleming had thrown out the mould—instead of discovering the penicillin.

Bion retakes this discharged hypothesis and investigates the possibility of treating it in a Darwinian sense. He creates a working hypothesis drawn from the experience with psychotic phenomena in analysis. He does the same that Freud did in his own time with dreams—to quote but one example. Bion and Freud used something that was seen as disposable or not meriting the respect of scientists.

Bion proposes that thoughts may be considered as epistemologically precedent to the thinker. Thoughts may be imposed on the human being from the necessity of survival. Indeed, this seems to be a reasonable basis of the earliest thought of all, namely, the thought of a breast. The term "reasonable" is here used as mirroring a root, rather than a rationalized thought; it also means something that stems from observation.

The primeval thought of a breast is imposed by the reality of the no-breast. The inception of this thought stems from the necessity to deal with an object in its absence. The development of thinking processes would be that of an increasing degree of sophistication in dealing with increased complex frustrations, expectations and needs.

This proposal is coherent with—and seems to have originated from—the hypothesis of inborn pre-conceptions first proposed by Kant, which survived at least until Hegel. Pre-conceptions are still not thoughts. "Thoughts without a thinker" are an unavoidable consequence of Bion's theory of thinking first adumbrated in 1961.

If the pre-conceptions can mate with realizations it is easy to see that the realization is a real, outside world event. The realizations are ready before the mind is born at all and impose the very need to think about them—as well as imposing the limits of satisfaction. Freud's model of consciousness represents it as a sense organ for the perception of the psychic quality; his observation of evading reality as different from attempts to modify it further endows Bion's hypothesis about thoughts without a thinker with an empirical basis.

The allegiance to something that can be named the "transcendent tradition" in both western and eastern thought, a tradition that has regard to the numinous realm (Platonic Forms) is coherent with this hypothesis. The hypothesis does not deny the fact that the mind may produce thoughts. Is this the realm of hallucination and delusion? It remains to be elucidated if the creative genius, as it is called, produces the ideas or if the creative genius is that man or woman who is able to apprehend inner truths that already exist.

The hypothesis seems to be backed by the fact that the true work of art or of science can be recognized quite independently of culture, time and space. It can be "discovered" by independent people who sometimes never meet each other. For example: the phenomenon of relativity first described by Einstein was described by Poincaré too, a little later and in a different way.

This suggests an independence of thought with regard to the thinker. Perhaps the thinker is important in furnishing a form to the thought, and the form is personal. However, it is perhaps of secondary importance. In the Trilogy *A Memoir of the Future*, Bion suggests that the book is not his, even though he wrote it. Francis

Bacon once argued that any novelty is just oblivion ("On the vicis-situdes of things", one of his *Essays*).

⊕ The first time that Bion introduces this hypothesis is in the beginning of "A theory of thinking". "*It is convenient to regard think-ing as dependent on the successful outcome of two main mental develop-ments. The first is the development of thoughts. They require an apparatus to cope with them. The second development therefore, is of this apparatus that I shall provisionally call thinking. I repeat—thinking has to be called into existence to cope with thoughts.*

It will be noted that this differs from any theory of thought as a prod-uct of thinking, in that thinking is a development forced on the psyche by the pressure of thoughts and not the other way round" (ST, 110–111).

The issue appeared when Bion tackled the treatment of patients with disorders of thought that were reducible to disorders in their apprehension of reality. One year later the issue was further expanded, in his book *Learning from Experience*—which is, anyway, the detailed building up of "A theory of thinking" (that for educa-tional purposes may well be regarded as the first chapter of *Learning from Experience*).

Bion had to tackle patients who dealt with the apparatus of perception and apparatus of thought as "undigested facts', as some-thing that demanded to be expelled. This was the core of Melanie Klein's concept of projective identification; Bion investigated in these patients, who treated their mental apparatus as if they were faeces or flatus or urine, "*what their model*" of thinking was (LE, 82). In doing this, Bion proposed that a widespread model is to regard "*the emotional experience of the digestive system*" (LE, 82) as a model of thinking. It is common sense to talk about "undigested facts", or facts that were not amenable to be thought. In psychotic function-ing, the need for a breast, the frustration that is inescapable due to the fact that no breast can wholly satisfy the pre-conception, dictates the need to expel that which is felt as a bad breast. The absent breast, in the personality that abhors frustration, is equated to the bad breast. This was the clinical origin of the theory.

Many persons resort heavily or often to projective identification, and try to get rid of their thinking apparatus. They create a problem for the researcher to find a suitable model of thinking that applies to them. This problem. "*is simplified if 'thoughts' are regarded as epistemo-logically prior to thinking and that thinking has to be developed as a method or apparatus for dealing with 'thoughts'. If this is the case then much will depend on whether the 'thoughts' are to be evaded or modified or used as part of an attempt to evade or modify something else . . .*

An apparatus has to be produced to make it possible to think the already existent thought" (LE, 83).

> The division into two classes and the attribution of priority to "thoughts" is subject to the limitations peculiar to the relationship existing in all scientific work between the realization and the representative theory to which it is believed to approximate. The division and priority are epistemologically and logically necessary, that is to say the theory that thought is prior to thinking is itself prior, in the hierarchy of hypotheses in the scientific deductive system, to the hypothesis of thinking. A corresponding priority is epistemologically necessary in the realization corresponding to the theory of thinking I have adumbrated. [LE, 85–6]

This step allowed a successful approach to the evolution of thinking in moments that were not connected to innate pre-conceptions. However, what were the pre-conceptions? What was their status with regard to thinking? Had they, for example, visual images attached, as occurs with dreams?

One year later, *Elements of Psycho-analysis* would re-state the same hypothesis trying to cover this question. He also does this without incurring the risk, exacerbated by readers who tend to be more royalists than the king, of splitting reality or of creating warring factions in science. Bion, in the opinion of the writer of this dictionary, was able to tolerate paradoxes. The issue of thinking contains some paradoxes to be tolerated, and one of them is the existence of at least two kinds of "thinking":

> It will be observed that in the course of the discussion, commenced by making a distinction between thoughts and the apparatus for using them and then according them priority in time so that they could be studied separately from thinking, it has been necessary to reintroduce a primitive mechanics of thinking, or something very like it, to explain the development of the thoughts. In fact it is easier to believe that this spontaneous development in discussion represents the facts with a greater approximation to the truth than is the case if the accord of priority to thoughts, convenient epistemologically, is to be taken as an accurate representation of the reality of

thinking. Nevertheless there are grounds for supposing that a primitive "thinking", active in the development of a thought, should be distinguished from the thinking that is required for the use of thoughts. The thinking used in the development of thoughts differs from the thinking required to use the thoughts when developed. The latter is derived from the Ps⇔D mechanism . . . When thoughts have to be used under the exigencies of reality, be it psychic reality or external reality, the primitive mechanisms have to be endowed with capacities for precision demanded by the need for survival. We have therefore to consider the part played by the life and death instincts as well as reason, which in its embryonic form under the dominance of the pleasure principle is designed to serve as the slave of the passions, has forced it to assume a function resembling that of a master of passions and the parent of logic. [EP, 35–36]

The last phrase is seminal; Bion introduces here the suggestion, backed by clinical experience, that man learned to cheat and evade, and one of his main tools is so-called rational thinking. He is in line with thinkers such as Hume, Voltaire and Freud, to quote a few. Freud had already pointed out that "rationalization" was typical of schizophrenic thinking, having introduced the term in his study of Judge Schreber's memoirs.

In this sense, a factory of lying thinking, quite independent of thoughts that already exist, is typical of the human being who cannot tolerate frustration. *"For the search, for satisfaction of incompatible desires, would lead to frustration. Successful surmounting of the problem of frustration involves being reasonable and a phrase such as 'the dictates of reason' may enshrine the expression of primitive emotional reaction to a function intended to satisfy not frustrate. The axioms of logic therefore have their roots in the experience of a reason that fails in its primary function to satisfy the passions just as the existence of a powerful reason may reflect a capacity in that function to resist the assaults of its frustrated and outraged masters. These matters will have to be considered in so far as dominance of the reality principle stimulates the development of thought and thinking, reason, and awareness of psychic and environmental reality"* (EP, 36).

He would develop this investigation with the introduction of the interaction between container and contained and the movement between the paranoid–schizoid position and depressive position (chapter 18 of *Elements of Psycho-analysis*).

Three years later, in *Transformations*, one of the implications of the concept is mentioned, albeit briefly: *"It may at first seem strange to suggest that groups or the infinite should be regarded as epistemologically prior to all else, but less so if we consider that only when a problem is intractable, or seems to be so, will it be felt to engage, and demand, our most powerful efforts. Reciprocally the more we feel ourselves deeply engaged the more likely we are to suppose the problem **must** be intractable and that it is so intrinsically"* (T, 152).

The demands of reality, with its ultimate "intrinsic intractability" in whatever it is, are highlighted.

In 1967, that is, six years after the formulation of the hypothesis, in his commentaries that constitutes his second thoughts about his clinical experiences, he focuses on the phenomenon of hallucination. This text is a continuation of the formulations contained in *Transformations* that resorted to the mystics to gain, from the void and formless infinite, partial and transient glances of reality as it is. Bion considers a patient who says to the analyst, *"'I see what you mean' when he has a hallucination, say, of being sexually assaulted; what he means is that the **meaning** of what the psycho-analyst said appeared to him in a visual form and **not** that he understood an interpretation. This is the kind of problem to which the . . . paper, On Thinking, is an introduction.*

The fact that thinking and talking play such an important part in psycho-analysis is so obvious that it is liable to escape attention. It does not, however, escape the attention of the patient who is concentrating his attacks on linking and in particular the link between himself and the analyst; such a patient makes destructive attacks on the capacity of both analyst and himself to talk or think. If these attacks are to be properly understood, the psycho-analyst needs to be aware of the nature of the targets being attacked . . . With my present experience I would lay more stress . . . on the importance of doubting that a thinker is necessary because thoughts exist. For a proper understanding of the situation when attacks on linking are being delivered it is useful to postulate thoughts that have no thinker . . . Thoughts exist without a thinker. The idea of infinitude is prior to any idea of the finite. The finite is 'won from the dark and formless infinite' . . .

In practice, I have found this formulation, or something like it, a helpful approximation to psycho-analytical realizations. The patient who suffers from what used to be known as disturbances of thought will provide instances showing that every interpretation the psycho-analyst gives is really a thought of his. He will betray his belief that papers or books written by others, including of course his psycho-analyst, were really filched from him" (ST, 165).

This issue expresses the supreme hate that the paranoid-minded person has of the parental intercourse. The person cannot conceive that he was a product of a couple. Therefore, to deny thoughts without a thinker equals saying that one creates thoughts as an expression of the more basic statement, "I alone created myself":

> This belief extends to what in more usual patients appears as the Oedipal situation. In so far as he or she admits the facts of parental intercourse, or verbal intercourse between the psycho-analyst and himself, he is simply a lump of faeces, the product of a couple. In so far as he regards himself as his creator he has evolved out of the infinite. His human qualities (limitations) are due to the parents, by their intercourse, stealing him from himself (equated with God). The ramifications of this attitude, more clearly discerned if the psycho-analyst postulates "thoughts without a thinker", are so considerable that I require another book to attempt elucidation. Inadequate though this formulation is, I hope it will help the reader to find the continuation of the developments which I have tried to sketch out in these papers. [ST, 165–6]

The issue has consequences to science: *"I would warn against the phrase 'empirically verifiable data' which I employ ... I do not mean that experience 'verifies' or 'validates' anything. This belief as I have come across it in the literature of the philosophy of science relates to an experience which enables the scientist to achieve a feeling of security to offset and neutralize the sense of insecurity following on the discovery that discovery has exposed further vistas of unsolved problems—'thoughts' in search of a thinker"* (ST, 166).

This phrase seems to have evoked severe reactions from the establishment (see below, misuses and misunderstandings). Bion states that thoughts produced by thinkers may be indistinguishable from hallucinations. Bion seemed to need five years more to present a kind of more explicit formulation, linking thoughts without a thinker to truth, and thoughts with a thinker to lies:

> Provisionally, we may consider that the difference between a true thought and a lie consists in the fact that a thinker is logically

necessary for the lie but not for the true thought. Nobody need think the true thought: it awaits the advent of the thinker who achieves significance through the true thought. The lie and its thinker are inseparable. The thinker is of no consequence to the truth, but the truth is logically necessary to the thinker. His significance depends on whether or not he will entertain the thought, but the thought remains unaltered.

In contrast, the lie gains existence by virtue of the epistemologically prior existence of the liar. The only thoughts to which a thinker is absolutely essential are lies. Descartes's tacit assumption that thoughts presuppose a thinker is valid only for the lie. [AI, 102–3]

As a matter of consequence, one may state that if one gets a true analysis, the person of the analyst is of no importance whatsoever— provided he or she is a true analyst. Bion specifically mentions Descartes, thus confirming this writer's detection of the source of his hypothesis. Namely, that Bion provides a counterpart to the French thinker's idea that the human mind produces thoughts— period.

From 1975 to 1979 the concept would be elevated to its highest pitch. Bion's verbal formulations leave no doubt about its nature. These formulations are scattered in the Trilogy *A Memoir of the Future* and were part of his "lectures" (if this denomination really applies) all around the world. Because of limitations of space, in part, perhaps it will suffice to quote a representative, selected text.

This text makes use of all earlier developments, from philosophy to the mystic tradition, and above all, a firm use of the immaterial facts belonging to the realm of psychic reality. Real life, human feebleness, the limits of sensuous perception, human omnipotence and omniscience, attempts to apprehend reality exclusively through sense-based media—that is, not considering its "brokerage" function, as a step, meaning an intermediate, necessary action which nevertheless is not enough to apprehend reality as it is.

It is clear in the following text, as it is in many others in the Trilogy, that it seems to be so trivial that it is more often than not overlooked and dismissed even before being seriously considered by the vast majority of people, analysts included. This continues happening (as is witnessed by the pushes towards so-called "empirical research" in our field)—despite the contributions of Freud, Klein, Winnicott and Bion. The perception of the manifestation of Oedipus, the two principles of mental functioning, the positions, and the transitional phenomena—all of them belong to the realm of immaterial thoughts without a thinker.

The limitation of apprehension to the human sensuous apparatus is twofold:

(i) Each of our sensuous organs has a remarkably limited range of apprehension. Our eyes cannot go beyond the violet or the red in the spectrum of electromagnetic waves of light. Perhaps consciousness—the sensuous organ to the apprehension of psychic quality—is even more limited. As with our kidneys and our brain—and in the so-called consumerist, material-comfort–oriented civilized word—our muscle-skeletal system, it seems to be under-used. Biological beings other than humans have much wider and powerful ranges of apprehension—the sight of insects and the hearing of dogs; even though our senses can be trained and developed, like the ear of a musician or of an Native American, the limits are clear-cut. They are genetically, species-determined.

(ii) The senses are unable to apprehend immateriality, even aided by manufactured extending devices like the optical or electronic micro- and telescopes, ultra-sound and magnetic resonance. The last two were not available during Bion's time but he, like Freud before him, was fully able to realize that this was not the way. Plato, Kant and the mystics perceived this limitation in a clear way.

These considerations mark a limitation that proves to be resiliently hidden from view through the centuries. It was called "secularism" by the theologians; "materialism", "consumerism", and "technocracy" by social scientists in our century and in the previous one. This does not mean that other methods, such as psycho-analysis, music, or the Cabbalist tradition are wholly effective to the task. They are simply less ineffectual. The text displays the tolerance of paradoxes, the nature of relativity and the inadequacy of judgmental values (q.v.)

ROLAND'S VOICE (the enunciation is clear and precise. He is himself not visible and as he talks he becomes progressively more a disembodied thinker and finally pure thought without a thinker) Krishna makes the point quite clearly: he shows Arjuna that his depression is part of feelings of compassion which are unworthy of thought, still less of God-head. That kind of thing may be appropriate to reception and emission in the range of sensuous perception whether perceived directly or mechanically by constructs like radio-receivers, X-ray, films, musical instruments and, in their very crude and gross manifestations, by animals and creatures in the biological range. Very sensitive animal organisms may then be able to interpret or transform the disturbances in the waves which render them opaque and obstructive. St John of the Cross was even able to point out that an analogy can be found which may be serviceable in the process of vulgarization intended to make the grosser crudities even grosser, till they impinge on elements which are still within the spectrum of the infra-sensuous and ultra-sensuous, though not outside that very narrow and limited band. He uses, it will be remembered, the analogy of dust particles which can render perceptible a ray of light that traverses it. Recently, by mechanical means, it has been possible in the biological range (human sub-category) to detect disturbances of great violence which have completely escaped detection by animals dependent on sight, even when sight is augmented by instruments such as telescopes, spectrographs, cameras and preparations of film coated with fine grain receptors—all macroscopic. Yet these perturbations are matters of the greatest crudity and violence!

Though extremely rare and scattered over a huge range of temporal space, they only appear to be extremely rare because of the crudity and triviality of recorded time as an instrument of measurement. Time as a concept is as inadequate as topological space to provide a domain for the play of such enormous thoughts as those liberated by the freedom from dependence on a thinker. The breakdown is as trivial, though made to appear vast by the inadequacy of the framework as, to take a very gross but simple analogy, that which occurs if a simple operation such as the subtraction of five from three is attempted with sensuous objects or even a relatively sophisticated mathematics best limited by being exclusive of negative numbers though well stocked with real numbers.

The failure to grasp the trivial range of the biological spectrum, even when the field of the living is extended by the dead, the animate by the inanimate, has been matched with the vastness of the extent of the relatively minute. This is due, in part, to the failure to grasp the nature of relativity, in particular the fact that it includes paradox. The restriction imposed by limitation of thought to thoughts with thinkers implies the polarization "truth" and "falsehood", complicated further by morals, uninvestigated "moral" systems, and extensions of Plato's thought to moral views of the function of poets and artists. A similar seepage from the domain of religion may likewise be traced to the inability to respect the "thought without a thinker" and, by extension, the "relationship without related objects". How this affected even so-called practical thinking is seen in the difficulty of the "public" to grasp that an analogy is an attempt to vulgarize a relationship and *not* the objects related. The psycho-analytic approach, though valuable in having extended the conscious by the unconscious, has been vitiated by the failure to understand the practical application of doubt by the failure to understand the function of "breast", "mouth", "penis", "vagina", "container", "contained", as analogies. Even if I write it, the sensuous dominance of penis, vagina, mouth, anus, obscures the element signified by analogy . . .

ROSEMARY (yawning) Oh my God!

VOICE Why drag me in?

ROSEMARY (imperiously) Alice! Come here at once.

ALICE (submissively) Yes, Miss.

ROSEMARY Why can't you keep that crashing bore in order? Why did you marry him if you didn't know how to keep him on a lead? You at least should have learned that the factual exercise of a relationship is not the two objects related, like the cunt and the prick, but keeping one thing inside another. (Laughs contemptuously) The container and the contained! My God, I believe he has driven me mad as he is! I'm even talking this crazy non-sense. I'll get locked up if this thing goes on much longer! [AMF, 69–71]

In the opinion of the writer of this dictionary's author, the text quoted above is better read if the reader frees her or himself from preconceived opinions on the topic, and keeps and unprejudiced mind towards what he or she is about to read. Even those who are acquainted with *A Memoir of the Future*—something that may prove helpful in reviewing the excerpt quoted here—might also find it productive to approach the text anew.. The readers who have not read this work may be aided if they keep in mind that the character Roland depicts some experiences of Dr Bion. The character is a foolhardy person prone to act impulsively. "Roland" depicts someone who always tried to do the "right" thing and ended up always being "wrong". The attempt to explain, which typifies the text, is also typical of this. Anyway, this attempt may betray an insight about truth, even though truth itself is ineffable. Another way to read this text is to consider that "Roland" is a kind of "part-object" of Bion. It is easy to see that he utters some of Bion's theories of psycho-analysis, especially that of container and contained. He does this with a sense of humour, even mocking himself. The characters "Rosemary" and "Alice" try to depict a real woman and a weak woman, who change places continuously due to the action of crossed projective identifications. The text may be useful at least to the unwitting protagonists of a frequent situation. There are many "married" couples where both members are professional psycho-analysts. In addition, often analysts tend to try to analyse their relatives and husbands/wives. Why slot into technical talk that which should remain a human relationship? This problem has been made tragically clear to the psycho-analytic establishment by the paradigmatic case of Hermine Hug-Helmuth and her nephew. It seems an un-learned experience. The final part of the text addresses this issue.

Another way to read it could take into account that the text tries to embody a kind of theoretical-practical experience accumulated during approximately 80 years of life, two marriages, two daughters and one son, medical training, 50 years of psycho-analytic experience, coupled with Victorian–Edwardian schooling and non-conformist religious education, as well as multiple war experiences.

Usefulness The clinical usefulness of this suggestion cannot be over-emphasized. It is perhaps the stuff that analytic sessions are made of. The supposition is that thoughts are already existing as free floating immaterial realities, waiting for a thinker to think them. This situation can be analogically compared to the oxygen one inhales, which is already there, waiting for a breather to breathe it. If this is true, the analyst must try to apprehend these thoughts— as must the patient. Free associations would be exactly this: free floating "entities" stemming from the innermost parts of one's own self, waiting for a thinker to think them. Free floating attention would be the ability to intuit and grasp these "thoughts" which display aspects of the patient's unconscious and are formed despite the thinker.

Misuses and Misconceptions: One may notice the many asides, "it seems strange . . .", which Bion appends to the definitions. Is it because he felt the weight of incomprehension of readers or audiences? It is part of the experience of this writer that the hypothesis of thoughts without a thinker proved to be bewildering to people who nourish their Cartesian habits of mind. Moreover, it proved to be offensive to those who cannot tolerate Freud's suggestion that many scientific achievements are taken as offences to human omnipotence, such as the so-called Copernican apprehension of the universe. The idea that the mind produces thoughts, exalted by Descartes, is clearly linked to omnipotence and is perhaps one of the manifestations assumed by the not-too-hidden idea that man is the centre of the universe.

The author, when translating the later writings of Bion into the Portuguese language, turned his attention to *A Memoir of the Future* and had a special interest in the concept of thoughts without a thinker. He looked for advice from well-known and acknowledged thinkers in the forefront of psycho-analysis. Among the letters received, it may be opportune to quote Hanna Segal's answer. She stated that this hypothesis made only "sociological sense" to her, but was of no use to analysts; she added that she appreciated Bion's contributions to psycho-analysis, but she excluded the works written after 1962 from them.

Recommended cross-references: Analytic View, Atonement, Binocular view, Jargon, Judgmental values, Mystic, O, Real psychoanalysis, Scientific method, Transformations in Psycho-analysis, Truth, Ultra-sensuous.

Tool-making animal: *"Psycho-analysis tells you nothing; it is an instrument, like the blind man's stick, that extends the power to gather information"* (C, 361).

Bion hypothesizes that the constant conjunction of two abilities, namely, the ability to rationalize and the ability to make tools, due to the biological (probabilistic) variation of opposed thumbs, in the end improved mankind's primitive drive to self- and hetero-destruction.

This hypothesis was developed with the aid of a kind of metaphor, which turned into a myth in his later work: that of the stegosaurus and tyrannosaurus and the known fact that they sank under their own weight. These two gigantic reptilians excited more than any other primitive being the imagination of humans for centuries and seem to provide a concise way to convey the hypothesis.

The roots of this metaphor seem to be Bion's experiences of war. Bion fought in the First World War, where two million young Europeans died for nothing, where he perceived the insensitivity of brainy intelligence officers who talked about the "cretaceous" or lunar aspect of the battle-fields of Flanders, and where he had close contact with the deadly trap that became known as the "tank". As a psychiatrist treating traumatic neuroses and shell-shock in a hospital, Bion witnessed the events of the Second World War and the Nazi phenomenon, as well as local wars that he named *"wars of Psycho-analysis"* (AMF, II, 273). These observations further allowed him to question whether the rational functioning of the mind and the so-called developments of the civilized world were just delusional wishful thinking. This questioning is contemporary to that made by playwrights such as Friedrich Dürenmatt. It was already present in the work of the early Romantics, some of them Bion's forebears, such as William Wordsworth, John Keats, John Ruskin (who fought a vain battle against the railways), and, above all, Freud in his so-called "sociological works", which gave rise to today's "ecological movement". The issue also is relevant to the formation of ossified establishments (see the entry, "Establishment").

In 1959, Bion, in a comment about Heisenberg's *Physics and Philosophy*, advances a hypothesis for the first time that would remain unchanged until his last work. *"Man's tool-making capacity is hypertrophying as the defensive armour of stegosaurs hypertrophied and led to its extinction"* (C, 60).

In 1975 this idea was elevated to the status of a quasi-myth:

I am the discoverer of and inventor of homo alalu. I and my fellow homines with our opposable thumbs learned how to give birth and life by opposing penis to penis, vulva to vulva, till one of us began to swell up and up till the whole earth and sky was filled with the swelling and the roaring. [AMF, I, 41]

I knew a delightful old stegosaurus who thought he had found *the* answer to the tyrannosaurus. But the "answer" was so successful that it turned into a kind of tyrannosaurus itself and loaded him with such fame—not to mention exoskeleton—that he sank under its own weight. In fact, he was so loaded that the only trace of him left was his skeleton. Yes, but those same dead bones gave birth to a mind. Because while all eyes were fixed on the conflict between Fate and armour (there is *no* armour against Fate) the attacker got through disguised as a bomber . . .

The tyrannosaurus provoked intrinsically an equal + opposite reaction—the stegosaurus. The stegosaurus sinks under its own "maginot line", its defensive armour which is its own weakness and makes its own armament, its own weight, under which it sinks. The self-destructive elaboration is blind to the quality which is to lead to its own destruction. [AMF, I, 60]

The same is valid for potent scientific and psycho-analytic theories, those that get nearer "O":

If the Oedipus story is the weapon that reveals homo, it is also the story that conceals, but does not reveal, that by which it will destroy itself. What happened to Delphi? And Socrates? If man is a tool-making animal he will not observe that that same capacity will be more than he can protect himself against. Superficially it may become clear that he is a clever monkey who can produce an atomic bomb that is a potential menace to his existence. While his gaze physiological is directed to observation and "detoxication" of the menace *represented* by the atomic bomb, it will, by the same token, be directed away from the growing annihilating force, the "helpless infant". "Too much learning will make thee mad . . ." Too much "tyranny"-freedom, food, armour, defensiveness; the list can be extended—but the only reality that matters is that which is denoted by "too much". Quantity, + and −, requires awareness. In the language suitable for communicating, it would be called a capacity for discrimination of quantity and quality. But in the domain that concerns us there is nothing that lends itself to the exercise of discrimination; there is no quality, no quantity to be discerned. Relativity is relationship, transference, the psycho-analytic term and its corresponding approximate realization. [AMF, I, 61]

Bion composes a quasi-myth about the drawbacks of a developed mind, while avoiding a romanticized adhesion to irrationalism.

In other words, he takes into account the human irrational instinctual basis, but he does not confuse it with irrationality for its own sake. Bion's quasi-myth assumes the form of a dialogue between two unexpected characters, Adolf Tyrranosaurus and Albert Stegosaurus. The resemblance with the British Empire and Germany is more than passing. In a Shakespearean way, Bion resorts to a historically imprecise but effective metaphor, reminding the reader of two iconic characters, Albert (Queen Victoria's husband) and Adolf Hitler. Moreover, both the British and the German empires were ruled, at given points in time, by the same family, the "House of Hanover".

"Full stop. Sleep. There appear: ALBERT STEGOSAURUS and his close relative ADOLF TYRANNOSAURUS

ADOLF What the devil have you got all this armour plate for?

ALBERT Call me Albert. I've got it *for* the Devil. What the devil do you s'pose? I'm resting; it's my spore stage.

ADOLF But I got these teeth for spores. Your vegetative existence is an offence. It's provocative, blast you! It's a resistance! You put ideas into my head. I was all right before you stirred up the ten commandments. Since then I have not been able to sleep for the itch to commit adultery. It's all your fault.

ALBERT There you go! Now you are making *me* feel guilty. Why can't you keep your conscience to yourself? Now I am filled with the gnawing of conscience and re-conscience and remorse. World without end—Amen.

ADOLF Keep your religion to yourself! Now you make *me* want to attend mass. All right, serves you right if I *do* eat you!

ALBERT You have wak'd me too soon. I must slumber again.

ADOLF Do wake me—in a few thousand years' time.

ALBERT By that time I shall have reached your anus.

ADOLF The right place for anyone's remorse—keep right away from my mouth and teeth! Right up to the other end of my alimentary canal.

ALBERT Don't blame me if you have digestive pains. You mustn't blame me if you devour me. My armour plate, my resistances, my spores are pretty tough. Are you sure your anus can take it?

ADOLF I've got a pretty tough unconscious. I don't let my right hand know what I'm up to. It will take a few thousand years till your concepts cease to be blind and your thoughts without content are discovered by a thinker without thoughts who has room for a few thoughts who can't find a thinker to give them a home.

ALBERT You give me a headache.

ADOLF I told you to keep your thoughts in their proper place! If you let them get above themselves no wonder your head aches! Take my advice—keep your head for your thoughts. What's that tiny little thing you've got up there?

ALBERT A rudimentary brain.

ADOLF Hmmm ... I don't like it. Mark my words, it will burst your head open! Chacun a son goût. Ow! What's that? You've shoved your thoughts into me, vile creature.

ALBERT You shouldn't want to taste what you eat. Why don't you remain satisfied with eating everything without discrimination? Keep your head away from my arse! And if I were you I'd keep your arse away from your head too! Or you'll end up by being anal-erotic!

ADOLF At least I shan't know about it. If this fool Albert thinks I can't chew up his armour! . . .

ALBERT If this fool Adolf thinks my armour can't wear down his teeth! . . .

BOTH . . . he's got something coming to him!

BOTH (out loud) Thank God we agree. [AMF, I, 83–4]

Besides the embodiment of the concept of the tool-making animal, there are living references to:

(i)   he basics of psycho-analysis, such as projective identification, and its attendant damage to one's own authority and self-responsibility; unending guilt, related to basic human issues dealt with by religion—albeit largely unsuccessfully; splitting; the transit between conscious and unconscious; the principle of pleasure being challenged by the presence of pain (headache).

(ii) Other basics as well: of biology, such as malignant spore forms of existence. This was already adumbrated through the metaphor of the restricted life in a "disused part of a pigeon-cote", meaning, autism and delusion (AMF, I, 29; also, AMF, I, 75; it was equated to envy as well), moral judgement (the ten commandments).

Recommended cross-references: Establishment, Mind, Real psycho-analysis, Violence of feelings.

&; The author proposed, as a development of these hypotheses adumbrated by Bion, the concept of "tolerance of paradoxes" as the basic psycho-analytic posture (for example, Sandler, 1997–2003).

Transference: Bion uses Freud's original definitions throughout his work. See, for example, his clinical studies (ST, 44, 55), when devising an observational theory that could endow psycho-analysis with firmer scientific grounds, that is, when Bion applied the theory of transformations and invariances to psycho-analysis. He tried to unify the two main theories that investigated the unconscious: transference and projective identification. Transference is seen as a special kind of transformation, which he calls "transformation in rigid motion". This means that the patient transfers "en bloc" a set of feelings from one subject (parental figures) to another subject (the analyst and other people). There the hallucinated nature of transference is made clearer when he realizes that it has hallucinosis as its medium (T, 133).

One may gauge his "pure Freud" use of the concept in a later work, from 1977. It contrasts strongly with the trends of those days (that persist, heightened, to the present) in two important ways:

(i) Bion's use of "transference" keeps itself respectful towards Freud's original definition, not debasing it, or replacing it with an alleged superiority. Many replacements were offered by others but they were devoid of empirical evidence that could support them. The exceptions were some extensions made by Klein, namely, the observation of the origins of transference that occurred earlier than hitherto suspected, as well as the *clinical* formulation of the "total situation". But they were thereafter repeated mechanically and turned into empty theorization that expanded the concept so much until it, like an old coin, lost its face value. In fact those deviations were emphasized by Bion many times, as for example in his paper *Evidence*.

(ii) Bion's understanding of "transference" was defined with a simplicity that keeps fit the fundamental ethos of the concept.

> P.A. My problem is the relationship when two minds, persons, characters, meet. Freud drew attention to one aspect of that relationship which he called "transference". I think he meant that when a man meets his analyst he transfers to him characteristics which were probably once consciously, and not unreasonably, thought to inhere in some member of the parental family. These characteristics are inappropriate when felt about a stranger—the analyst.
>
> PAUL Why the analyst? Why not other people?
>
> P.A. The analyst is typical of these "other people". In analysis these characteristic "transfers" can be discussed.
>
> ROBIN *Only* by the patient?
>
> P.A. No; the analyst also reacts to the patient. But in so far as he is unconscious of it, it is known as the counter-transference. You can read all about this in the literature, or better still, find out for yourself by having a psycho-analysis. I do not want to go into that because here, at best, we can only talk "about it"—not experience it. [AMF, II, 249–50]

> Desire and memory are discernible as elements in transference— that is, supposing we can recognize the reality for which Freud coined the term transference. [BLI, 51]

Misreadings and misunderstandings: The discrimination of transformations in rigid motion as a way to examine transference phenomena and the qualification "classical analysis" led some readers to hastily conclude that Bion's analysis became obsolete or surpassed the analysis of transference.

Transformation; transformations and invariances (concept): Transformations and Invariances are part of the same *concept*, which forms an *observational theory* (q.v.) (T, 7 and T, 34, respectively).

The concept is duly defined by Bion: a transformation is a *total* analytic experience being subjected to interpretation (T, 13). He suggests in the book *Transformations* a *"method of critical approach to psycho-analytic practice and not new psycho-analytical theories"* (T, 6). It is a practical concept that enables the psycho-analyst to observe the psycho-analytical endeavour; it partakes with the **Grid** (q.v.) the qualities of a veritable epistemological tool that evaluates the 'Truth-value' of the analyst and patient's statements as well as approximations to that which they are really doing (see **Analytic View**).

To state that the theory of transformations is a theory of psycho-analytical observation means that it is different from the psycho-analytic observation itself as well as from theories of psychoanalysis. It is intended to enhance the communication between analysts as a development of the Grid (q.v.). But now the attempt includes standardized, communicable generalizing symbols, which carry on limited semantic (meaning) fields. This diminishes the penumbra of associations of definitions and verbal statements. It was created in the wake of the attempts towards unified linguistic systems that characterized the work of some neo-positivists, mainly Schlick, Wittgenstein and Carnap. Nevertheless, Bion's concept contains some criticism of those attempts, as becomes clear in some preparatory papers (such as "Scientific method", 1959) published posthumously in *Cogitations*.

Even though it relates to the improvement of the analyst's communication within the community of analysts, the theory of transformations originates in the communication with the patient as well as of the analyst with himself, as attempted with the Grid: *"The psycho-analyst tries to help the patient to transform that part of an emotional experience of which he is unconscious into an emotional experience of which he is conscious"* (T, 32). This equals saying that Bion saw the psycho-analyst's task exactly as Freud viewed it.

He provides a fresh **formulation**, rather than any different theory, of Freud's earlier formulations, which became psycho-analytic aphorisms, such as *"turning the unconscious, conscious"*, or *"where the Id was, the Ego shall be"*.

Perhaps Bion's formulation has a built-in bent towards the clinical here-and-now living experience. *"But since scientific work demands communication of discovery to other workers the psycho-analyst must transform **his** private experience of psycho-analysis so that it becomes a public experience"* (T, 32).

Being an *observational* theory of psycho-analytic *observation* rather than a psycho-analytical theory, the *"theory of transformations and its development does not relate to the main body of psycho-analytic theory, but to the practice of psycho-analytic* **observation.** *Psycho-analytic theories, patient's or analyst's statements are representations of an emotional experience* (q.v.). *If we can understand the process of representation it helps us to understand the representation and what is being represented. The theory of transformations is intended to illuminate a chain of phenomena in which the understanding of one link, or aspect of it, helps in the understanding of others. The emphasis of this enquiry is on the nature of the transformation in a psycho-analytic session"* (T, 34).

The theory of transformations aims at that which Bion then called 'correct analysis' and 'correct interpretations' (q.v.). Later, in *A Memoir of the Future,* he reformulated those terms and integrated them into one that is a little less amenable to be confused with a penumbra of judgmental associations: *'real analysis'* (q.v.). It gives to the reader who is not prone to make hasty value judgements, a chance to see that the question is whether to apprehend or not to apprehend reality as it is, to the maximum possible extent—psycho-analysis as a scientific activity.

He states that all psycho-analysts would agree that *"correct analysis"* demands that the analyst's verbal formulations obey a need, namely, to *"formulate what the patient's behaviour reveals"* (T, 35). Therefore, transformations are not a matter of the analyst's mere individual opinion. The latter falls outside the realm of scientific activity. They are often the origin of the confusion between psycho-analysis and post-modernist tendencies.

Correct analysis means that the analyst maintains a respect for truth—the truth that the *"analysand's behaviour reveals"*. The analysand's behaviour is of no importance *per se* in the analytical setting except as a pointer that hides and simultaneously betrays that which is a matter of significance—the unknown, the unconscious. Other disciplines may well attach importance to it—as for example behaviourism, and academic psychology based on phenomenal appearances.

Bion does not discuss transformation in scientific communication *"except to illustrate transformation in analytic practice"* (T, 34). This does not mean that his observational theory cannot find transdisciplinary applications. Perhaps it is the one and only development hitherto available of Moritz Schlick's, Ludwig Wittgenstein's and Rudolph Carnap's attempts towards improving the truth-value of scientific statements.

What matters is to gauge if psycho-analysis is really occurring. Being a practical device, its definition relies on a practical depiction. To allow for a didactical description one must consider a starting-point even though it is arbitrarily defined. "Something" (there is no need for this 'something' to be a material thing; it may be an immaterial fact, like psychic facts) has an initial form (this form does not necessarily have to be material either) that is subjected to observation. In a certain sense, the "some" is as important as the "thing".

With this theory Bion borrows a philosophical concept from mathematics for the third time. The first time was the borrowing of Frege's theory of numbers (in "A theory of thinking"); the second time was the borrowing of the theory of factors and functions (in *Learning from Experience*).

Origins Our research indicates that the concept was developed by two mathematicians: James Joseph Sylvester and Arthur Cayley. They lived in London and Baltimore. Sylvester died in 1897; Cayley, in 1895. Besides being a distinguished mathematician, Sylvester was a professor of natural philosophy (a field first created by Goethe and seemingly one of the roots of psycho-analysis; Sandler, 2000) and law; he worked in the United Kingdom (London) and in the United States (Baltimore), teaching at University College and at Johns Hopkins University. One of his pupils was Florence Nightingale. Arthur Cayley had in some respects a strikingly similar career, first working at Trinity College. During this time in England, both Sylvester and Cayley worked using intuition and insight; together they created the *theory of algebraic forms and invariants*. Later, the friends and former contributors met by chance at Johns Hopkins University, and again struck a very amiable, fruitful collaboration. Both are regarded as founding the British school of pure Mathematics.

The first version of the theory of invariances and transformations by the good friends Sylvester and Cayley described algebraic equation coefficients that are unaltered when their coordinates are submitted to variations—in their mathematical observation, when the coordinates are rotated or translated. Cayley later observed that the order of points formed by intersecting lines is always invariant.

This opened up the possibility of studying the relationships of space and time in physics. Cayley developed the geometry of spaces of any number of dimensions, thus escaping from the visual fetters imposed by the tridimensional Euclidean scheme. He developed the algebra of matrixes, and thanks to these developments, geometry did not depend on points or lines to construct a geometrical space any more. Hamilton came from him and displayed the six-dimensional space; both Hamilton's and Cayley's work were the immediate forerunners of Einstein, who used their achievements to discover the theory of relativity. This was done in the absence of the concrete objects—the stars and the atom—and could be useful to analysts as an example of the feasibility of a non-sensuous work.

Let us emphasize the foundation of the concept of transformation and invariance. The first transformation is linked to the act of observation about "something" (whatever it is); the observation itself creates an impression in the mind of the observer that produces a transformation. Transformation means a change in form; for the form acquired in the "brain and mind" is not the "something" any more; the prefix "trans" already indicates that there is a transience here, operating in the original situation.

All the authors who have dealt with transformations and invariants until now, their explicit or conscious use of the concept notwithstanding, took into account that there is an interference of the observer in the fact observed (Kant, 1781; Freud, 1900, 1901, 1912; Heisenberg, 1958). The trans-formation, *the alteration in the apprehensible form*, appertaining to the realm of phenomena (Kant, 1781) *also implies a conservation of seminal features of the material or immaterial fact, object or person* observed, that is, subjected to an attempt at communication. This is a paradox that demands tolerance. Those seminal features are not given directly to the sense apparatus and are called **invariances** (q.v.) in the way that Sylvester and Cayley observed in mathematics. They appertain to the realm of the noumena, or '**O**' (q.v.) as Bion calls it. Invariances are a Siamese twin of the concept of Transformations. It is a necessary antithetical pair that calls to be observed through a **binocular vision** (q.v.). A tolerance of paradoxes is necessary to deal with both simultaneously.

As far as this author's research into the history of ideas goes, even though Freud, Planck and Einstein implicitly used the concept of transformations and invariances in the science of mind and in the science of energy and matter respectively, it was a quantum physicist, Paul Dirac, who was able to bring it to the fore in an explicit way. He used the concepts of Transformations and Invariances to assert that nature works on certain fundamental laws, which are permanent and invariant. In Dirac's own words, the invariants or fundamental laws *"do not govern the world as it appears in our mental picture in any very direct way, but instead they control a substratum of which we cannot form a mental picture without introducing irrelevancies. The formulation of these laws requires the use of the mathematics of transformations. The important things in the world appear as the invariants (or more generally the nearly invariants, or quantities with simple transformation properties) of these transformations"* (Dirac, 1930, vii).

Paul Dirac was a Frenchman who settled in Britain. He was perhaps the most successful professor of quantum mechanics ever to appear, having chosen a special method of teaching that resulted in the most widely accepted textbook of Quantum mechanics to this date. This method is called by him the "symbolic method" (Dirac, 1930, p. ix), *"which deals directly in an abstract way with the quantities of fundamental importance (the invariances, etc., of the transformations)"*. He left aside the method most familiar to mathematics of his time and of today, the method of coordinates or representations. This method deals with sets of numbers corresponding to those quantities, involving complicated matrix calculus developed by authors such as Planck, Bohr, Heisenberg, Schrödinger and others. Dirac states that *"the symbolic method, however, seems to go more deeply into the nature of things"*.

It is not difficult to see that Freud implicitly used the concept in psycho-analysis to elicit just the fundamental key-concepts of our field: the manifest and latent content of dreams translates into, respectively, transformations (he uses this name to depict daytime residues that provide forms to dreams) and invariances, for reality material and psychic; transference is a concept where invariances flow back and forth in different forms, or transform themselves: past psychic experiences are transplanted to present day persons (see for example *The Interpretation of Dreams*, 1900; "The dynamics of transference", 1912; "On transience", 1915).

Bion does not deal with Transformations and Invariances just as a theoretical concept, but as a *dynamic activity* by no means restricted to psycho-analysis. Transformations and invariances are performed by human beings in many endeavours. Many of them are human tasks that endeavour to go more than skin-deep—he calls them a "group of transformations" and chooses as paradigmatic the following activities: painting, mathematics and psycho-analysis. *"For my present purpose it is convenient to regard psycho-analysis as belonging to the group of transformations. The original experience, the realization, in the instance of the painter the subject that he paints, and in the instance of the psycho-analyst the experience of analysing his patient, are* **transformed** *by painting in the one and analysis in the other into a painting and a psycho-analytic description respectively* (T, 3–4)."

An interpretation is a transformation: *"The psycho-analytic interpretation given in the course of an analysis can be seen to belong to this same group of transformations. An interpretation is a transformation; to display the invariants, an experience, felt and described in one way, is described in another"* (T, 4).

In introducing the term, Bion states that he uses *"borrowed philosophical and other terms for psycho-analytical purposes because the meaning with which they are already invested comes near to the meaning I seek to convey"* (T, 6). Also, he stresses the necessity to keep in mind the specificity of the psycho-analytic use of theory: *". . . the theory of transformations itself must be freed from existing associations if it is to be fitted for its psycho-analytic tasks. The suggestion of projective transformations differentiated from rigid motion transformations is but one step to indicate the possibilities"* (T, 140–141). The apparent contradiction is made less contradictory if one is reminded of his own warning: *"Since psycho-analysis will continue to develop we cannot speak of invariants under psycho-analysis as if psycho-analysis were a static condition"* (T, 4). Bion also has to steer his way as he construes the theory; one is reminded of Otto von Neurath's metaphor on science. Neurath was part of the neo-positivist movement (also known as the Vienna Philosophical Circle) in the first quarter of the twentieth century, along with philosophers such as Moritz Schlick, Ludwig Wittgenstein, and Karl Popper, among others. In *Anti-Spengler,* von Neurath formulated a metaphorical account of scientific work. He asked the reader to imagine sailors in a primitive, circular-shaped boat in the middle of the ocean. Because they are in high seas, they must change the original non-hydrodynamic circular form into a more fish-shaped, funnelled one. In order to transform the boat the sailors use floating pieces of wood found in the water, as well as the wood that composed the original structure. They cannot disembark and set the boat on firm soil, something that would enable them to reconstruct it right from the start and with more ease. Instead, they must work while keeping themselves in the old boat, struggling stormy waves and violent tempests. "This is our fate, as scientists", Neurath adds.

The main modification in Sylvester and Cayley's original concept is always to take two vertexes into account—that of the analyst and that of the patient. This kind of adaptation takes into consideration a pair and an emotional experience, which cannot be conceived of without a couple—in other words, that which typifies analysis.

It is easy to see that psycho-analysis realized the fact that psychic reality and the unconscious are not sensuously apprehensible in a direct way (making them the legitimate inheritors of Plato and Kant's numinous realm). There is an underlying "substratum", the same referred to in the field of physics by Paul Dirac, and observed as the constant of Planck and the constant of Einstein .In our field, it is the unconscious itself, which cannot be know in its entirety, but can be intuited, subsumed and inferred from free associations, dreams and many other manifestations. Freud observed that *"The unconscious is the true psychical reality; in its innermost nature it is at much unknown to us as the reality of the external world, and it is as incompletely presented by the data of consciousness as is the external world by the communications of our sense organs"* (Freud, 1900, *The Interpretation of Dreams*, p.613).

Both Freud and Bion respected Kant's discoveries about the unknowable stuff of the numinous realm—as did the physicists Planck, Einstein, Dirac, Schrodinger, Bohr and Heisenberg, among others. The application of the concepts of transformations and invariances seemed almost natural to the psycho-analytic endeavour and to a theory of observation in psycho-analysis that intended to enhance its scientific status, especially the scientific accurateness or soundness of the analytic interpretations—its truth-value.

Bion makes his borrowing explicit: *"By analogy with the artist and the mathematician I propose that the work of the psycho-analyst should be regarded as transformation of a realization (the actual psycho-analytic experience) into an interpretation or series of interpretations. Two concepts have been introduced, transformation and invariance. The book will be devoted to these concepts and their application to the problems of psycho-analytical practice. I use borrowed philosophical and other terms for psycho-analytical purposes because the meaning with which they are already invested comes near to the meaning I seek to convey. When I write 'transformation' or 'invariance' I leave it to be understood that I am discussing psycho-analysis"* (T, 6).

Despite a perusal in Bion's library it remains unknown to the author why Bion did not quote Sylvester and Cayley's formulation of the concept and Dirac's application of their perception. The wording is important: it is a *perception*, that is, the product of observation rather than an idea. This perhaps accounts for the low acceptance of this formulation, which depends on realization and experience. In general, Sylvester's insights, as those of Freud and many others such as Klein and Bion in psycho-analysis, face resistances due to this demand for experience. Usually one tries to understand that which appertains to the numinous realm of "O"; but this is unknowable, not amenable to be understood. Dirac, who at least as far as my research goes applied it for the first time to physics, does not quote Sylvester and Cayley either. Was it, perhaps, too pervasive an idea during those times to be brought up explicitly? Or was the formation of people like Dirac and Bion so much more encompassing than it is today that they took for granted that any educated person knew of the concept of transformations and invariances? Bion does quote Heisenberg in connection with an important offshoot of Dirac's famous lectures, concerning the interference of the observer in the phenomenon under observation. Bion applied the concept of transformations and invariants for the second time in the history of *applied* science; Dirac was the first to apply it in physics. In 2001, R. Nozik, the distinguished American philosopher, just before his early death, applied it to philosophy—without mentioning Sylvester or Bion, but paying homage to Dirac.

Let us return to Bion's wording and his pioneering application to fields other than physics after this brief detour on the origins of the term. The concept caused quite a stir in the psycho-analytic movement. At any rate, not only does it provide a firmer scientific foundation for the validation of interpretations, but it also offers an integrating approach to the Babel of theories that have occurred since.

> For my present purpose it is helpful to regard psycho-analytical theories as belonging to the category of groups of transformations, a technique analogous to that of a painter, by which the facts of an analytic experience (the realization) are transformed into an interpretation (the representation). Any interpretation belongs to the class of statements embodying invariants under one particular psycho-analytic theory; thus an interpretation could be comprehensible because of its embodiment of 'invariants under the theory of the Oedipus situation . . . [T, 4]

> The analyst's main concern must be with the material of which he has direct evidence, namely, the emotional experience of the analytic sessions themselves. It is in his approach to this that the concepts of transformation and invariance can play an illuminating role. [T, 7]

Misuses and Misconceptions: The misconceptions that seem to have appeared are linked to at least five factors:

i.   Superficial readings that use the term "transformations" in a banal, commonplace way.
ii. An early splitting of "transformations" from the inescapable other side, "invariances".
iii. Lack of knowledge about the mathematical origins of the term.
iv. A dismissal both of the scientific ethos of mathematics, and of Bion's psycho-analytic hypothesis about it. Mathematics is an early human attempt to apprehend reality as it is; in *Transformations,* Bion suggests that mathematics is also an attempt to deal with psychosis.
v.   Finally, a persistent misreading that regards Bion's contributions as if they were intended to replace the psychoanalytic theories hitherto available, despite Bion's continuous warnings against this kind of distortion. For example: *"the theory of transformations is to be developed, not as an addition to or alteration of psycho-analytic observation"* (T, 36).

All those factors led to a precocious dismissal of the whole attempt of Bion by the psycho-analytic establishment. Few contributions within the psycho-analytical establishment have caused such a contradictory reaction; established authorities displayed an early abhorrence that persists to this day but more seasoned practitioners accepted it early on.

It seems that colloquial usage, so typical of little learning, soon contaminated the readings. In other words, the misreading due to less than careful reading of the book seems to be the hallmark of those who present themselves as detractors and defenders, who display a superficial approach to the concept and at the same time exceedingly complicate it. The following quotations might help make this clearer:

> The danger that the colloquial sense of a "transformation of the analysis" will infect the meaning I wish to reserve for the theory of transformation is one against which I wish to guard by using the sign T.

> The "transformation of the analysis" refers to a change of "uses" as set out on the horizontal axis of the grid. [T, 25]

The theory of transformations and invariances, when oversimplified, lends itself to misinterpretation. This is especially the case with the approach that underscores "transformations" at the expense of "invariances". Such an approach tends to approximate Bion's contribution to Lavoisier's definition of energy conservation, namely: in nature, nothing is created and nothing is destroyed; everything is transformed. Had Lavoisier known relativistic and quantum physics, he might have entertained second thoughts about his dictum. The approximation of Bion to Lavoisier banalizes and oversimplifies Bion's formulations, reducing his detailed understanding of transformations and invariances to simplistic statements such as "All that happens in the world are transformations". This reading ignores the inseparable, if paradoxical relationship between transformations and invariances. In doing so, such a reading betrays Bion's fundamental contribution, which lies not merely in each of the two elements, but as importantly in their connection.

The misconception was further complicated by the idea that Bion was "mathematicizing" psycho-analysis and that he was a mystic. When Bion abandons the neo-positivistic approach that characterizes the first chapters of *Transformations* to show the limitations of such an approach, coinciding with his increasing abandonment of the mathematical notation, he also resorts to the ability that mystics seem to have to intuit reality. This was also precociously distorted into mysticism. Some of Bion's defenders try to endow him and his oeuvre with an esoteric tone, while his detractors see it as the work of a senile man. Both kinds of reading prevailed during the sixties and seventies. Comparatively few people in the world paid attention to *Transformations*.

The early and persistent splitting of the concept, concealing its "invariant" part, coupled with and dependent on the previously existent superficial, colloquial reading, was fated, in the eighties, to be mixed with the tradition of the idealistic (or subjectivist) and hermeneutic schools of philosophy. In the wake of this mixing, some have tried to tie Bion's work to Lacan's.

Perhaps more dangerous is the authoritarian view that splits some parts of Bion's writings concerning the opinion of the analyst. This splitting may be used to serve a preconceived idealistic tendency, which reflects paranoid–schizoid traits of the reader. The first part of chapter four (page 37) is very clear in stressing the need to respect truth and on the sincerity of the analyst, as well as the impossibility to "own" ultimate truth. Nonetheless, this text is used to deny truth and reality, unwittingly unearthing the old subjectivism/idealism that plagued philosophy and worried Kant, among many others. In this distorted reading of Bion's text, the psychoanalytic endeavour would be very simple, for it would suffice for the analyst to issue his personal opinions; no allegiance to "O", or to "O(patient)" as Bion calls it, would be necessary.

Again and again the denial of the built-in feature of invariance in the concept of transformations was rampant. The invariance, clearly stated in the first page of the book, puts it firmly outside the idealistic trend. The reader who understands this work as idealistic not only denies a great deal of the book, but also many other papers from Bion. Among them, the study "On arrogance" (q.v.), which warns about patients who see the analyst as the most important person in the room. Unfortunately, this view is not exclusive to patients: there are many analysts who, despite Bion's warning, also imbue themselves with this importance. The danger of such a position is, as mentioned above, idealism, that is, the predominance of the analyst's ideas over the apprehension of psychic reality. Idealism and self-importance in analysis are also related to desire (the desire to achieve "fame", for instance). Bion's admonition about the need to discipline desire is therefore also relevant to ensure the truth-value of the process of analysis. In 1947, Bion wrote the paper "Psychiatry at a time of crisis" (C, 336), where he addressed these issues by making explicit his opinion on a distorted or debased current of the Romantic Movement, which falls back on idealism by stating that any apprehension of reality is a chimera. What is left to us, this extremism states, are just the fabrications of the mind. Idealists dismiss those who do not share their views as simpletons, ignoramuses or blind technicians. The idealistic/relativistic view denies the existence of reality and truth at all. Other hard science theories such as quantum mechanics were similarly distorted for more than twenty years and the term "transformations" seemed to be amenable to be used under a blind relativism (Norris, 1999; Sandler, 2001) that threatened it with losing its scientific status. This use serves well the authoritarian professional who prefers to see his personal opinions reigning above the patient's reality.

Among Bion's warnings about idealism and relativism, which we regard as responsible for denying invariances, one may quote still another one: *"The term 'transformation' may mislead unless the limitations of the implications of 'form' are recognized"* (T, 12). Perhaps the reader can see the definition of transformations: something trans-forms itself but something remains the same. The differences between the initial and final forms of a process of trans-formation are epiphenomena that demand recognition but are not the important part of the whole process. The important part is the tolerance of the paradox transformations–invariances, an antithetical pair. The transformations that divorce themselves from invariances—thus introducing an idiosyncrasy, a hallucinated individualistic bias—imply *deformation*—Bion's term for it (T, 12).

The idealistic reading of Bion's theory meets its realization in the severe pathology of thought. One finds many references to this, for example: *"From the analytic treatment as a whole I hope to discover from the invariants in this material what O is, what he **does** to transform O (that is to say, the nature of T(patient)α) and, consequently, the nature of T(patient)"* (T, 15).

Bion seemed to be fully aware of this idealistic danger that encircled his contribution as one may gather from the number of warnings he issued about this. One finds them scattered in the book:

*"This may seem to introduce a dangerous doctrine opening the way for the analyst who theorizes unhampered by the facts of practice, but the theory of transformations is inapplicable to any situation to which observation is not an essential. Observation is to be made and recorded in a form suitable for working **with** but inimical to wayward and undisciplined fabrications. As grid categories show; any scientific theory can be used in accordance with the categories of column 2 [that is, falsities; q.v. specific entry and Grid] but it may be possible to prevent unpredictable changes from the uses of one grid column to the uses of another. In short, the theory is to aid observation and recording in terms suitable for scientific manipulation without the presence of the objects"* (T, 39–40). Or in other terms, exactly that which any baby must do with the no-breast in order to symbolize—think—a real breast; it is that which Aristotle did when he formulated the mathematical objects; it is that which the infant makes when he or she introjects the internal object (see entry "Psycho-analytical object"); and, finally it is that which Minkowsky and Einstein did with spaces of n-dimensions (see Sandler, 1997). Let us follow Bion's warnings:

What psycho-analytic thinking requires is a method of notation and rules for its employment that will enable work to be done in the *absence* of the object, to facilitate further work in the *presence* of the object. The barrier to this is presented by unfettered play of an analyst's phantasies has long been recognized: pedantic statement on the one hand and verbalization loaded with unobserved implications on the other mean that the potential for misunderstanding and erroneous deduction is so high as to vitiate the value of the work done with such defective tools. [T, 44]

The reading of the continuation of this part of the book furnishes the reader with the sense of truth that emanates from a scientifically precise formulation. Nevertheless it is highly debatable, forty years later, whether Bion's warnings were read, grasped and taken seriously.

One can notice that from its inception the concept of Transformation(s) encompasses the two complementary matching poles. I borrow the double arrow that Bion used to represent the ever changing living movement in tandem between the positions: transformations⇔invariance. These positions seem to be inescapable. But the equally inescapable resort to single words, which is necessary in written communication (as Bion formulates more fully in *A Memoir of the Future*), is always doomed to the failure of this same communication. The cumbersome verbal formulation transformations⇔invariance would not resolve the problem.

As occurs in some of Bion's concepts (as well as in Freud's and Klein's), the solution to the misunderstanding is to be found in the ability of the reader to tolerate the built-in paradox of the counterpart of the concept in reality. This ability depends on the reader working through his paranoid and/or schizoid nuclei. The loss of perception to one of the poles of the antithetical (dialectical) pair that composes the ethos of the concept, echoing that which occurs in the concept of caesura (q.v.), has the unavoidable consequences of either damaging the concept or making the reader blind to its counterpart in reality. The unbridled and disordered "transformations"—the "eternal change" pole of the pair—will prevail if the reader denies the other pole, that which un-changes. This appeals to the narcissistic and omnipotent reader, who fancies imposing his personal ideas on reality as it is.

Either prevailing pole debases the concept. A stultified paralysis in the "invariance" pole appeals to the naïve realist who fancies an immovable, unchanging world. The idealist cannot perceive that which transcends, unchanged; conversely, the realist cannot perceive that which changes. Both cling to immanence and lose perception of reality. In using the theory of transformations, attention must be paid to that which changes (usually linked to illusory appearances) in order to detect emanations of "O", that which un-changes. Both occur simultaneously and none should be felt by the analyst as dazzling, at the cost of an unavoidable splitting.

A final example

Even though Bion furnishes many case histories in the book *Transformations*, the author thinks that the most illuminating writings about "Transformations and Invariants" as an observational tool to analytical work, are to be found in the Trilogy *A Memoir of the Future*. It seems to be a "practical demo" in scientific-artistic and empirical-intuitive terms, of many theoretical-observational issues raised by the text *Transformations*. There, as we shall soon see, Bion had partially formulated the issues in the guise of quasi-mathematical representations.

In the Trilogy he abandons this mode and tries psycho-analytically-oriented artistic formulations (drawn from poetry and prose) and improves his method of using *metaphorical analogies.* In the same vein, but in a different form, much more akin to prose, Bion does something that Freud had done with analogies, in so far as they encompass a striking amount of western civilization's achievements in the area of knowledge. To construct the analogies Bion spares no philosophical, epistemological, mystical (not to be confused with mysticism), physical, mathematical, medical and psycho-analytical achievements.

Clinical, practical examples of transformations abound in his work. Due to the scope of this dictionary, only one example can be quoted here. However, because all of these instances are always so deep and illuminating, this one single excerpt will suffice. The excerpt has been taken from *A Memoir of the Future.* In this work, Bion takes a fresh approach and makes almost-living formulations on transformations and invariances. If the book *Transformations* contains the theory, the trilogy *A Memoir of the Future* contains the practice of the concept. This is directly illustrated by the following example:

PSYCHIATRIST You'll wake the whole place, you fool. Nurse, give him a shot—morphia, and quick!

NURSE That is nearly a lethal dose isn't it?

PSYCHIATRIST My job here is to keep order. If it's his life or mine, it's OK by me if it's *his*! What is a lethal dose of morphia for him is a soporific for the boss. What is a soporific for the boss is bread and butter for me.

BION What that man What's-his-name calls "Transformations", isn't it?

STATE PSYCHIATRIST Why, even *I* am transformed. Not a bad little job is it? I'm surprised Newton found it wiser to be master of the mind till he found it safer to be master of the mint. That chap—

Jesus—is still a nuisance though. "We have scotch'd the snake not kill'd it" as Shakespeare, as he called himself, has it. "Canst thou not minister to a mind diseased?" It's no good driving them underground. Only palliative. Stone death had no fellow. Ah, here they are—stout fellows, both. First murderer and second murderer. They look a bit rough, but hearts of gold really. Fine family these Cains. Best of the bunch! You there, don't you play the flute or something? And you? Poet aren't you? Homer? All Greek to me, but . . . say, you! Can't you turn out something good with fighting and murder in it? Oh, I'll get it translated, never you fear! We've a top notch translation department in the F.B.I. What's that?— Fucking Bloody Infantry. *That* doesn't sound quite right surely? Anyway—stout fellows all. Nurse—no, not you—the male nurse. Ah, here you are. Fetch up a bucket full of decorations. We shall need them shortly. Put in a few guaranteed hero brand. That usually sends them to sleep quietly. 'An army marches on its belly'. So does Satan though. *He's* a fine reliable chap now! Suffer the little children to come unto me with gently smiling jaws. I love little children—especially if they are young enough and tender enough. What, are they *still* sleeping? They sleep, with their eyes of stone, without sense, without life, beneath the rosy hues which stain the white radiance of eternity. These wretched poets—"ante Agamemnona multi"—why can't you let them sleep in their graves unwept, unhonoured and unsung? "What"? they smile, "our names, our deeds—so soon erases Time upon his tablet? Where life's glory lies enrolled? Their name liveth for ever more". Now, thank God, we can go to sleep.

ALICE What a night! Roland, what on earth were you up to? Tossing and turning and shouting! I could hardly get a wink of sleep.

ROLAND What are *you* up to?. [AMF, I, 81–2]

The invariances and unfolding transformations, the stuff that dreams and life and hallucination are made of, are presented. The state psychiatrist displays that the transformation and the invariance, with all their transcendent irradiance, begins to be formulated. The state psychiatrist seems to be delirious but its oneiric nature is increasingly clear. The reference to Sir Isaac Newton is a special kind of unkind transformation: the fear before the unknown leading to disaster and decay. Newton lost his mind; he was thereafter designated manager of the Mint by the government of

England, after having been declared unable to carry on research in physics. Bion makes a pun with the fact. Other invariances appear with Jesus and Shakespeare (in *Hamlet*); the invariance we name "death" is now confronted with life and some of its achievements, in the perennial transformations linked to the fusion and defusion of life and death instincts. The dream turns into a nightmare.

Usefulness The theory of transformations and invariances tries to resolve problems of communication between an analyst and his (or her) colleagues. It also attempts to improve the scientific value of interpretations (in the sense that they may be more approximate to truth, and apprehend reality as nearly as possible in a given context), as well as make explicit the points of view used to make statements. The theory strives to make explicit states of mind of the analyst (especially those under the unobserved aegis of memory, desire and understanding), and to get closer to the hallucinated nature of the patient's communication. Finally, Bion himself states that *"The theory of transformations must serve to illuminate and solve problems that lie unsolved at the heart of certain forms of mental disturbance; and to do the same for problems inherent to the psychoanalysis of such disturbances"* (T, 39).

📖 It would be advisable to see the interchange between the character "P.A." and "Priest", from which both emerge transformed without losing their respective invariances; and the interchange of Alice and Roland with lower class people, from which they emerge un-transformed in their invariant lack of contact with themselves. To indicate a few more passages:

Book I (The Dream): In pages 3–50, to see Projective Transformations at work, see the characters "Alice" and "Rosemary" and the dealing with feelings of hopelessness. To see Transformations in hallucinosis, note the false English farm, the false marriage between "Alice" and "Roland", the false status of employee/employer of "Alice" and "Rosemary", the false safety acquired by the character "Robin" in a pigeon house and by the character "Roland" in foolhardiness and contemptuous behaviour. Also, social environments based on erudition and social honours (pp. 4–5, 75–82, 92–100, 105, 171–178). For Transformations in K, see pages 53, 55, 76–77, 111–112, 117; for Transformations in "O", pages 33–46, 54–55, 105, 118, 201–202 (on this last page, see the talk of the character "Myself").

Book II (The Past Presented): pages 261–302, especially pages 300–301 (about "O"), 361–381. For Transformations in psycho-analysis, see the talks between the characters "P.A." and "Priest"; on hallucinosis, the "marriage" of the characters "Rosemary" and "Man".

Book III (The Dawn of Oblivion): see the "talks" between "somites" and children (from pp. 4–18), for examples of Transformations in rigid motion and hallucinosis; for Transformations in psycho-analysis and its differentiation of anything, all the "talks" and interchanges between the characters "P.A." and "Priest".

Two points to ponder It still remains unknown to the author the possible reasons why Bion, who was almost invariably careful in quoting his forebears, let in a more vague way (see T, 6) the origin of the term transformations and invariances. He does not quote Sylvester, Cayley or Dirac. Interestingly enough, Paul Dirac, when applying the concepts in physics, did not quote Sylvester and Cayley either! And Robert Nozik, the one and only author who after Bion in analysis and Dirac in physics uses the concept in philosophy, quotes just Dirac. The sense in which they all use the concept is the same except for Bion's inclusion of the binocular view (two vertexes).

Did Bion and Dirac before him take for granted that the educated reader would instantly be reminded of the distinguished nineteenth-century mathematicians? Francesca Bion's research into Bion's library did not produce any evidence that he knew Dirac's use of the concept. The question may interest future researchers.

At the risk of being pretentious, one might suggest another title for *Transformations*, using Sylvester's and Cayley's formulation: *Transformations and Invariances*. This might remind us of Eliott Jaques' suggestion for Melanie Klein to name her book *Envy and Gratitude* instead of simply *Envy* as was her original intention. Obviously, she accepted the suggestion.

Suggested cross-references: Transformations in Hallucinosis, Transformations in −K, Transformations: Symbols, Transformations, theory of, Transformations, Types of.

Transformations in hallucinosis: The term "hallucinosis" was taken from psychiatry. No wonder, for Bion had a solid foundation in this field. Psychiatric foundation proves to be an asset when coupled with clinical experience in psycho-analysis, not only in the case of Bion, but also that of Klein, Freud, Fairbairn, the brothers Menninger, and more recently Wallerstein and Green.

In the case of hallucinosis as well as with that which occurred with hallucination (q.v.) proper, Bion maintains the ethos of the original formulation as it existed in psychiatry. It has a powerful descriptive (phenomenal) quality. Characteristically, as it seems to occur when psycho-analysis used previous psychiatric experience, psychiatry described phenomena that up to that point had only been seen under the vertex of pathology.

Psycho-analysis shows that those phenomena correspond to quantitative rather than qualitative variations of some features of mental functioning. Therefore those features can be seen anytime, anywhere in any living person, provided one has some specific conditions of observation. Those conditions demand intimacy and time, as they are found in analysis.

The psychiatric concepts were thus refined and made more observable by psycho-analysis; its "microscopic" features, so to say, are made visible. Hallucinosis in psycho-analysis corresponds exactly to hallucinosis in psychiatry, except for two important differences, namely, (i.) under the psycho-analytic vertex, as evidenced by direct participant observation in the analytic session, it is seen as a manifestation of the psychosis of everyday life. In contrast, the psychiatric vertex sees it as a pathological condition; (ii.) participant observation means that the concept is seen as an event associated with a couple; an emotional experience that depends on a relationship (LE, 42).

As usual Bion does not go to lengths in defining hallucinosis. Instead, he furnishes abundant data about its features as they unfold in the analytic session. From other moments of his work one may hypothesize that he took for granted that the reader would grasp the implicit definitions through exercising his capacity to recall his (the reader's) own experience and join it with the approach that Bion is proposing. I also surmise that Bion hoped that the reader could count on psychiatric knowledge and experience. Therefore the basic definition of hallucinosis as it is used in psychiatry and by Freud himself would pose no problem to the reader. But experience shows that this has not always been the case. Therefore, we include in this text the psychiatric definition of hallucinosis taken from the classic dictionaries (Campbell) and textbooks from

America (Freedman & Kaplan, Arieti); Europe (Mayer-Gross & Slater, Ey, Jaspers, Spoerry) and Brazil (Doyle).

Definition. Hallucinosis, psychiatrically speaking, corresponds to a state where hallucinations and delusions exist in an otherwise seemingly normal personality. It is classically defined as the acute or recurring obtruding of hallucinations (q.v. objectless perceptions) in persons who otherwise maintain their intellectual capacities. There is neither mental confusion nor other signs of intellectual decay. Hallucinations were first described as linked to exogenous intoxication, the most typical being alcoholic hallucinosis and bromide intoxication. In the former, paranoid phenomena usually accompany auditory hallucinations. Some patients exhibit violent behaviour. It is relevant to analysts that in those cases, when the pathogenic exogenous stimulus is long gone, the symptoms of intoxication persist; the acute turns into chronic. The idea of using the term in the psycho-analytic practice seems to display ingenuity so typical of Bion's observations. The main features of hallucinosis are thus namely: (i.) hallucinations in tandem with conserved intellectual activity, (ii.) an acutely intoxicated mental state, chronically maintained; (iii.) violence of feelings; (iv)an external trigger that, like Lewis Carroll's Cheshire cat in *Alice in Wonderland*, is discarded but its effect remains (in the case of *Alice*, the cat disappears but the smile remains). These features can be observed in multifarious ways during the evolution and involution of a single session, or moments in the session. In psycho-analysis, hallucinosis corresponds to the appearance of hallucination and delusion as elicited in emotional experiences existent as the relationship of analyst and analysand unfolds. One must remember Freud's and Bion's emphasis that analysis consists of verbal communications; transformations (q.v.) are conveyed through this medium. A state of hallucinosis during an analytic session indicates that special care must be taken to detect seemingly "normal" features in the verbal intercourse and to allow for the psycho-analytic approach to seemingly bizarre or disconnected verbal statements. The feeling that everything is "normal" must be taken as a warning that a state of hallucinosis is prevailing. Avoidance of experiencing pain as well as feelings of superiority—in the end, over pain itself—are prevalent. The operation of *"envy, greed, rivalry, "moral" and scientific superiority"* is suggestive of the presence of hallucinosis (T, 133).

The normalcy of the intra-session verbal intercourse must be suspected. Characteristically, there is a prevalence of rational dialogue. Authoritarian, pedagogic, moral postures are observable in the patient and he or she tries to evoke them in the analyst; suggestive or supportive therapy procedures can be elicited under a careful scrutiny. It is not an exaggeration to state that hallucinosis is a travesty of reality; as with any hallucinated or delirious production, it bears parentage to lies and stems from hate towards truth. It forms the basis of collusion and socially shared feelings of well-being (ill-founded, anyway). In the same book, *Transformations*, in which Bion proposes the concept, he states that the group extracts its sense of well-being from lies, from evasion of reality. The issue is, as Bion clearly states just after introducing the concept, that the supposition that *all* transformations (analyst's and analysand's) are expressed verbally *"cannot be legitimately maintained"* with patients who make transformations in hallucinosis or any other unknown realm (T, 67). One must bear in mind that there is no overt aggressive behaviour; the violence of feelings is intra-session and makes its presence felt through the use of projective identification and attempts to evoke counter-transference reactions.

The first time that Bion uses the term, in *Transformations*, p. 63, he states that the mother's relative inability to accept the infant's projective identification and the association of such a failure with intellectual disturbances corresponds to the very same complications aroused by the existence of an extremely understanding mother, because of her capacity to *accept* projective identification. One must bear this paradox, in order to be able to grasp that which Bion is trying to convey. In both cases there is a hope, a desirous hope, of an ever-fulfilling situation. There prevails a "greed for satisfaction". This is the origin of hallucination and hallucinosis, as we shall see. Let us continue with Bion's text. He states that an associated reaction to this state of affairs is akin to character disturbances: there is an inability to face the loss of an *"idyllic state"* and it is accompanied by an attempt to replace it by a new phase; the new phase is instantly suppressed to the extent that it involves pain. *"It is against this background of hallucinosis, projective identification, splitting and persecution, accepted as if it were the ideally happy state, that I want to consider the domain of verbal communication. The sense of well-being engendered by a belief in the existence of the perfectly understanding mother (or analyst) adds force to the fear and hatred of thoughts, which are closely associated with, and therefore may be indistinguishable from, the 'no breast'. A painful state of mind is clung to, including depression, because the alternative is felt to be worse, namely that thought and thinking mean that a near perfect breast has been destroyed"* (T, 63).

The "whole issue" of the origin of hallucinosis is stressed again and again and one sees it as an integration and development of Bion's earlier research in the fifties, about the psychotic non-thought ("Schizophrenic Thinking", q.v.): *"Intolerance of a no-thing, taken together with the conviction that any object capable of a representative function is . . . not a representation at all but a no-thing itself, precludes the possibility of words . . . Thus actual murder is to be sought instead of the thought represented by the word 'murder', an actual breast or penis rather than the thought represented by those words, and so on until quite complex actions and real objects are elaborated as part of acting-out. Such procedures do not produce the results ordinarily achieved by thought, but contribute to states approximating to stupor, fear of stupor, hallucinosis, fear of hallucinosis, megalomania and fear of megalomania."* Or, that which fails to be an analytic session turns into an activity in which *"quite complex actions and real objects are elaborated as part of acting-out"* (T, 82).

If the state of hallucinosis is not perceived, the acting-out and an acted-out session remain unobserved, taken as if it were a real session. The overt manifestations must not necessarily be florid, such as demonstrations of rage, depression or the like. (This, Bion describes as "propaganda"—chapter IV of *Transformations*, and "hyperbole", q.v.). Let us consider a professional who is unable to detect the presence of hallucinosis. He or she will fail to see that some patients are able, so to speak, to "do the trick": to utter words, to imitate a rationally-oriented colloquial discourse. This professional will not realize the occurrence of a bizarre reaction to his or her interpretations, because this reaction is clothed in wording familiar to the professional. At the base of this there is a failure to realize that what is going on may in fact be in a mental state that *"precludes the possibility of words."* The description of the "key/milkman" case at chapter 10 of *Transformations*(page 131) furnishes an illustration of the clinical situation and its handling.

Function

What is the utility of bringing the situation of hallucinosis to the fore? Bion uses an analogy drawn from geometry: *"The simple example I have taken of a straight line that may cut a circle in two points that are (i) real and distinct, or, (ii) real and coincident (if the line is a tangent), or (iii) conjugate complex (if the line lies entirely 'outside the circle') poses a problem that the mathematician has been able to solve by taking a mathematical point of view, but I use it to illustrate the nature of the psychological problem. I shall state this as follows: in the domain of thought where a straight line can be regarded as lying within, or touching, or wholly outside, a circle, a transformation has been effected whereby certain characteristics, lending themselves to mathematical manipulation, have been manipulated mathematically to adumbrate and then solve a mathematical problem. The residual characteristics however retain their problem, un-named (un-bound) and so uninvestigated. Hallucinosis is a domain, analogous to that of mathematics, in which their solution is sought. The mathematical problem resembles a psycho-analytic problem in that it is necessary that the solution should have a wide degree of applicability and acceptance and so avoid the need to apply different arguments to different cases when the different cases appear to have essentially the same configuration"* (T, 83).

Therefore the concept is useful intra-session, to aid the analyst in rescuing the analytic vertex, in observing hitherto unrecognized disturbances of thought, collusion and fakery (rational, rationalized "analysis"). Another utility is that it can address a persistent problem in the psycho-analytic establishment, that was variously stated, for example in the idea of "one psycho-analysis or many" (Wallerstein, 1996). The obverse is also existent, as Bion often emphasized, that many times people use different terms to describe the same situations. The scientific status of psycho-analysis is dependent on the fact that analysts must be able to converse with each other:

> Any analyst will recognize the confusion that is caused, or at best the sense of dissatisfaction that prevails, when a discussion by members makes it quite clear that the configuration of the case is apprehended by all, but the arguments formulated in its elucidation vary from member to member and from case to case. It is essential that such a state of affairs should be made unnecessary if progress is to take place. [T, 83]

The usefulness of the concept cannot be overstressed. Many phenomena that until Bion's observation appeared as "normal" must necessarily be regarded as meriting psycho-analytical attention. One may be enabled—through one's personal analysis—to deal with elements of the statements as if they appertain to category A6. That means, dealing with them as if they were acted-out β-**elements** (q.v.) or acted-out **definitory hypotheses** (q.v.). *"As a result of treating the elements of the statement as A6 certain factors peripheral to A6 elements can be seen to be activated and can be detected in analysis"* (T, 132). Its observation and accounting helps to make the analysis more profound, careful and probably useful to the patient, to the extent that it marks and elicits the extent he (she) is wasting his or her life in unreal deeds and actions disguised as real. The observation of it diminishes considerably the risks of shared hallucination and collusion of the analytical pair.

Factors and rules of hallucinosis

Bion describes (T, 132, 133) six factors that are not usually detected or are detected without realization of their hallucinated nature, namely:

i.   Hallucination as a mode of acquiring independence, wherein independence is regarded as superior to psycho-analysis, which is a form of interdependence (as is marriage, parental relations and any meaningful relationship).
ii.   The failure of hallucination (an unavoidable outcome) is *"attributed to the rivalry, envy and thieving propensities of the analyst"*.
iii. Rivalry, envy, greed, thieving, the sense of being blameless: all those manifestations deserve closer scrutiny as *"***invariants*** (q.v.) under hallucinosis"*.
iv.   It is worthwhile to widen the concept of hallucinosis in order to realize that many configurations *"at present are not recognized as being the same"*.
v.   Hallucinosis is one of the media of transformations in rigid motion (q.v.) and projective transformations (q.v.).
vi.   There are rules of transformations in hallucinosis *"that must be established by clinical observation"* (T, 132–133).

How to detect it clinically

He proposes, *provisionally*, the following rules of transformations in hallucinosis:

> A. If an object is "top", it dictates "action"; it is superior in all respects to all other objects and is self-sufficient and independent of them.
>
> B. Objects that can occupy such a position include (a) Father, (b) Mother, (c) Analyst, (d) Aim, object or ambition, (e) Interpretation, (f) Ideas, whether moral or scientific.
>
> C. The only relationship between two objects is that of superior to inferior.
>
> D. To receive is better than to give. [T, 133]

The basic mental state of the patient is an inability to tolerate frustration. Bion looks for Shelley's help to state this verbally: "*that state of mind in which ideas may be supposed to assume the force of sensations through the confusion of thought with the objects of thought, and the excess of passion animating the creations of imagination*". Shelley formulates his poetic intuition in this way. Before jumping to any conclusion that Bion would be endorsing an "idealistic" view (in the philosophical sense of the world; see for example Sandler, 2001) view, one must be reminded that Shelley, for all his humanity and generosity, was a kind of flawed poet if compared for example with Keats or Wordsworth, due to his excess of romanticism.

Clinically, one must try to respect free associations and the interplay between manifest content and the eliciting of latent contents in day dreaming activity. This means Bion's extensions and rescuing of Freud's ethos: a respect for Freud's fundamental rules of not being fooled by external appearances of phenomena, taken to its last consequences in the here and now of the session. The hallucinatory character of transference, for example (**transformations in rigid motions**, q.v.) was stated by Freud himself (Freud, 1912). The issue at stake is to rescue the oneiric nature of human communication and to discern it from the hallucinatory character of human communication—exactly in the same sense that Freud attempted to do in the interpretation of dreams. Special care must be taken not to mistake (as occurs with many who try to use the concept) the presence of theatrical, hysterical and overt concrete manifestations as well as hallucination and delusion for examples of hallucinosis. The equilibrium between seemingly normal attitudes and covert "madness" (something that a layman would notice, but the psychologically and psycho-analytically trained ear fails to), is what matters.

A kind of "naïveté" (in the sense used by Schiller and, later, by Isaiah Berlin when he wrote about Verdi) is called for, from the analyst. In later writings, Bion stated that this "naïveté" is achieved through a discipline of memory and desire, and, above all understanding. To recognize hallucinosis, one must be able to get rid of the memories of one's own prejudiced values, judgements and ideas of normality; of desire to the extent that desire is the main fuel of hallucinosis; and understanding, for understanding throws one into Cartesian, rational, cause–effect and judgmental cages. Using this state of mind, in the first instance obtainable through the experiencing of hallucination in one's own analysis (as Bion would develop later, in *Attention and Interpretation*), one will realize more fully that reason is a slave of passion, composing beliefs felt psychologically as necessary (T, 73 and 137).

Transformations in hallucinosis have factual counterparts built in the external milieu thanks to the human capacity to make tools and to furnish forms to their delusions (Sandler, 1997a). Hyperbolic emotional climates may be created, more or less subtly (T, 34 and 141; see below), which are eminently hallucinated; people *do things* in a manic fashion, giving preference to acting-out where no thinking interpolates between impulse and action, *"full of sound and fury, signifying nothing"* (*Macbeth*, V,v,19). They are made especially visible in the analytic session—provided that the analyst can "blind himself artificially" and "hear with the third ear" (Reik, 1948) in order to reach the *"ultra and infra sensuous"* (please refer to this specific entry).

Patients usually look for analysis because they feel the existence of obstacles to the free exercising of hallucinosis, stemming from reality, or the facts as they are. Hallucinosis is a social fact to the same extent that projective identification is: both need "adequate receptors" to collude with them. It prevails when intolerance of pain and frustration is also prevalent.

The outcome of hallucinosis in the session and the posture of the analyst

Bion observed that he could not continue investigating the issue if he did not scrutinize the relationship of the transformations of the patient *vis-à-vis* the transformations of the analyst (T, 141). One may see that any relationship based on rivalry of superiority is indicative of hallucinosis. There is no evidence that human beings can be superior to each other. Macro-socially speaking, the Two Great Collective Murders of the twentieth century, Nazism and Stalinism, were based on the idea of superiority (in the first case, of a race—in fact, a false one—and in the second, of a given social stratum).

    *"The patient whose transformations are effected in the medium of hallucinosis might almost have as his motto 'actions speak louder than words' with its hint of rivalry as an essential feature of the relationship. The analyst appears to be offered the choice of abandoning his technique, which is an admission of surrender to the superior wisdom and technique of the analysand, or, keeping to analysis and thereby showing by **his** actions that **he** consider **his** technique superior; either course would fit in with an acting out of rivalry"* (T, 136). He emphasizes, *"What matters . . . is not rivalry so much as rivalry under transformations in hallucinosis"* (T, 137). This would be the crux of the whole issue, for the patient thinks that he can resolve a problem through the use of transformations in hallucinosis; it is further complicated by a secondary problem, namely, the one caused by the method employed for its solution. The secondary problem is especially serious in analysis, due to the fact that the patient uses a method to resolve it—a basically lying one—and the analyst uses another one—basically, one that respects truth as it is. The basic disagreement will almost unavoidably turn into a war between truth and lie, and both members of the couple are liable to resort to a kind of wrestling to prove the *"respective virtues of a transformation in hallucinosis and a transformation in psychoanalysis"* (T, 142). The patient feels, and the analyst must resist, through discipline in memory and desire, that *'the disagreement between patient and analyst is a disagreement between rivals and that it concerns rival methods of approach'* (T, 142). In fact a method that nourishes respect to truth cannot rival a method that resorts to lies due to the simple fact that the second one is hallucinated—that is, nonexistent. *"Unless this point is made clear, no progress can be made"*

(T, 142). The issue is exemplified by an idea that Bion quotes a number of times (for example, *Cogitations*, pp. 6 and 114). Dr Johnson, in a letter to Bennet Langton, says that he does not know if the consolation derived from truth—if any—is superior to that stemming from lies, but he is sure that the former is durable and the latter, due to its very nature, is *"fallacious and fugitive"*. The recuperation of the psycho-analytic vertex that was lost, and this means, an allegiance to Freud's ethos, with no nodding to the then (and now) fashionable way to evade analysis, namely, the relational or inter-subjective approach, is clear in the next phrase: *"When it* [it: the point mentioned above] *has been made clear the disagreement still continues but it becomes endopsychic: the rival methods struggle for supremacy within the patient"* (T, 142). The problem is serious, because it is analysis itself that is at stake—that analysis and the whole psycho-analytic movement. The "within the patient" concept means that one must deal with projective identification and must take responsibility for oneself. This differentiates analysis from authoritarian, pedagogical, charismatic and suggestive methods. *"The characteristics of the conflict are easier to discern when externalized as a conflict between analyst and patient and this can lead to a collusion between the two for the patient finds it more tolerable and the analysis easier"* (T, 142). The analyst who feels he is superior, wise, goodness-in-itself will be easy prey to the environment full of projective identification that ensues. Then, no analysis can follow—again, this stresses the fundamental function of the analyst's analysis (T, 142).

If one remembers the rules of hallucinosis mentioned above, it is easy to see that the patient feels that he does not need analysis or an analyst, because he can provide, through imagination and rationalization, all that he "needs" for a cure, and he knows better than the analyst how to obtain cure from this kind of material he himself produced. He feels he is the "top" now. "Cure" and "pleasure" mark the rivalry, and hallucinosis is seen as superior to psycho-analysis. Getting a cure is equated with "winning". It is a catch-22 situation to the analyst, for the beneficial results of a real analysis are always seen as the "defect" of the analysand. Therefore the analyst will always be liable to be blamed for collecting "proofs" of the superiority of analysis over hallucinosis. If the analyst displays compassion, he will be admired and therefore he will be the object of a renewed cycle of greed and envy. Bion also considers (T, 144) that the issue is further complicated by innate propensities towards narcissism. *"The impression such patients give of suffering from a character disorder derives from the sense that their well-being and vitality spring from the same characteristics which give trouble"* (T, 144). Therefore, *"although the analyst is under an obligation to speak with as little ambiguity as possible, in fact his aims are limited to the analysand who is free to receive interpretations in whatever way he chooses"* (T, 145). Or in other terms, stated in *A Memoir of the Future*, the analyst tells the patient his characteristics; whether they are debits or credits, it is up for the patient to decide.

Hallucinosis and rivalry under hallucinosis lead to a difficult situation: it is almost impossible, without the analyst having a real analysis himself, without disciplining or minimally controlling his own possible desires to be "the top" too, to *"conduct himself in such a manner that his association with the analysand is beneficial to the analysand. The exercise, in the patient's view, is the establishment of the superiority of rivalry, envy and hate over compassion, complementation and generosity"* (T, 143). The patient will try to evoke in the analyst the idea that the analyst is wise, good, serene, and compassionate; and will provoke him to host his rivalry and hate. Unless the issue is returned to the intrapsychic problem, the outcome will be destructive to both. This can be seen especially in "successful analysis" but also in cases of abandonment with feelings that the "analyst is hard, incompetent". This stresses the analyst's necessity to look for an analysis himself that ought to be as extensive and profound as possible. The ambience is not necessarily irrational or grossly abnormal; the patient's ideas and discourse are similar to the analyst's; the values, too. Obtrusion of judgmental values indicates the presence of hallucinosis.

The mathematics of hallucinosis

A most misunderstood point of Bion's attempts to reach a common ground of communication between analysts is its expression as a scientific basis for analysis. This means isolating and describing fundamental elements of psycho-analysis. Equally misunderstood are his mathematical analogies. They are taken, even by people who were interested in his earlier work, in a concrete way, as if he were trying to "mathematicize" psycho-analysis—a seriously distorted way to attack his work, in my view. His statements in this area are made explicit in the entry, **Mathematization of psycho-analysis** (q.v.). For now, we may note that Bion only resorts to mathematical *analogies* in parts of his work where he dwells on hallucinosis. It is a "Lewis Carroll" maths for psycho-analysis—or a philosophy of mathematics as a counterpart to the human attempt to deal with the mind.

Bion proposes a "mathematics of hallucinosis", in terms of a relationship with the breast that is felt as non-existent if the breast is frustrating in any way (T, 133). The analyst must experience hallucinosis in order to perceive it in the patient (T, 36 and 40). He explores how the human being deals or does not deal with frustration. Many cannot tolerate it and turn it into "nothingness", meaning, zero breast. He proposes a quasi-mathematical representation or notation of hallucinosis: Zero breast plus one real breast equals one hallucinated breast (or 1 breast + 0 breast = 1 breast). Mathematically, we have this, $1 + 0 = 1$, or "*memory of satisfaction is used to deny the absence of satisfaction*" (T, 134). One cannot put up with the fact that $1 + 0 = ?$—? being an unknown. The problem is, to use 1 to "*remove the noughtness of 0*". So Bion concludes: "*in the domain of hallucinosis, $0 - 0 = 1$*". He wonders what would be the result of adding 0 to 0. In the domain of reality, it would be zero but in the realm of hallucinosis it would be an unbearable O^0. Stating it verbally and not quasi-mathematically: "*. . . if noughtness is added to noughtness the noughtness is multiplied by itself. The emotional state that might provide a background realization approximating to this is the state of complete freedom from the restriction imposed by contact with realizations of any kind*" (T, 134).

Again, the importance of this cannot be overstressed. It means that paranoid–schizoid phenomena and malignant endogenous narcissism know no restraints. The idealistic thought that the breast that is desired or needed must coincide with the real breast that is available ends up signifying that the world is a product of one's mind. Freedom is confused with libertinism. There grows a mental cancer: "*The ability of 0 [meaning, zero] to increase thus by parthenogenesis corresponds to the characteristics of greed which is also able to grow and flourish exceedingly by supplying itself with unrestricted supplies of nothing*" (T, 134). The final result seems to be "*a raging inferno of greedy non-existence*".

This special kind of transformation is often the medium through which transformations in rigid motion or projective transformations come into being (T, 133). The observation of its occurrence may sharpen and attune observation of psycho-analytically relevant facts during an actual session.

In the Trilogy *A Memoir of the Future* there are perhaps the best examples of transformations in hallucinosis available. They are put into colloquial terms and depictions of real life—better to say, unreal non-life—of the hallucinosis of everyday life. Book I begins with a kind of unmasking of a hallucinosis of master and servant of the British empire, of the superiority of schooling over practical life as it is, of superiority of any kind, among many other instances of hallucinosis.

Suggested cross-references: Atonement, Dream, Dream-work-alpha, Hyperbole, −K, Projective Transformations, Transformation (concept), Transformations, types of, Transformations, theory of, Transformations in Rigid Motions, Transformations in Psycho-Analysis (in K and O), Real psycho-analysis.

Transformations in K: This is one of the types of transformations one is bound to make when trying to apprehend reality. The concept expands the earlier one, of K link (in *Learning from Experience*), and is presented in the book, *Transformations*. It is typical of science, and is a first step for analysts who aim at Transformations in O. They may or may not eventuate in the latter.

The concept puts that which was a link, and an expression of the instincts, into a finer observation with regard to its role in the thought processes and especially the analyst's thought processes . It is one of the modes of "transformations in psycho-analysis", together with transformations in O (q.v.).

Suggested cross references: Atonement; Real psycho-analysis; O; Transformations; Ultimate reality.

Transformations in −K: −K refers to a belief that to misunderstand is superior to understanding. When it was introduced, in the last chapter of *Learning from Experience*, it was not so well characterized as a link—as the K link which inspired it—and opened up the perception to some practical problems that were seen more clearly only when Bion was able to discern the realm of "minus". Therefore the mechanisms of Hallucinosis, Catastrophic Change and Transformations in "O" could be integrated into the theory of Minus K, "upgrading", so to speak, the concept into the framework of Transformations and Invariances.

Transformations in O: Please refer to the entries, "O" and "Transformations in psycho-analysis".

Transformations in psycho-analysis: This concept is made explicit in the work *Transformations* but has not gained widespread use. It encompasses two modalities. One of them has to do with "knowledge"; the other with ultimate reality, the numinous realm, "O". To get a clearer picture of Bion's idea on the semantic field of these words, one may refer to the entries, "K-link" and "O".

Transformations in psycho-analysis have two sub-types: transformations in K and transformations in O (T, 144). They function in an interlinked way:

In K (knowledge)—those are performed by processes of knowledge, thoughts-with-a-thinker (EP, 35; 1965, 141ff.). They include rational elements, that is, elements from the secondary process. If one regards the analytic situation as a relationship where patient and analyst are linked, K has been seen (since 1962) as an intrinsic and necessary link in the act of interpretation. This means that K is preferable to Hate and Love links that introduce an erratic bias in the views of the analyst.

Three years later a development of this theory occurred. In the exact measure that the issues of truth and its apprehension were increasingly dominating Bion's preoccupations about the quality of the analytic work, limitations of K come to the fore. It is no longer a goal—not in an exclusive way. K seems to be necessary rather than sufficient.

In O—transient glimpses stemming from intuitions of part aspects of the *existence* of the numinous realm (T, 147, 156), thoughts-with-a-thinker (Bion, 1962a, 1962b, 83) are performed by processes of being (in contrast with "talking about", "understanding").

Transformations in K and O have to do with truth. They are aided by the experience of epistemological errors as preliminary steps in the apprehension of reality. Therefore, the three kinds of transformations—in rigid motion (or transference), projective transformations (projective identification), in hallucinosis—as well as statements belonging to category 2 of the Grid (q.v.) are possible pathways towards O.

Bion emphasizes some problems linked to transformations in O. One of them is that some people nourish a conscious belief that illusion is essential to the survival of humanity. He thinks, *"the remainder of us believe it unconsciously but, no less tenaciously for that"* (T, 147). But even the many who consider truth essential also state, *"the gap cannot be bridged because the nature of the human being precludes knowledge of anything beyond phenomena save conjecture"*. Bion calls it "the inaccessibility of O" and regards it as a phenomenon familiar to analysts under the *"guise of resistance"*. There is a *"gap between O and knowledge"*.

Is Bion supporting the relativist/idealist cause? Hardly. He leaves an alternative open: *"From this conviction of the inaccessibility of absolute reality the mystics must be exempted"*. By mystics, he surmises that the reader will know that he is referring to the Cabbalists—both Jewish and Catholic—and other thinkers and theologians such as Dante, Meister Eckhart, St John of the Cross, John Milton, Ruysbroek, and William Blake. They looked for and attained a mental state in which the experience of that which is ineffable is possible. This is a remarkable statement. It has some consequences in the analytic room and the analyst's assessment of each patient's psychic reality at a given moment (T, 147).

Bion furnishes us with a simple statement, constructed in colloquial language, that throws new light on something that Freud had discovered, but perhaps was not so explicit about: *"Resistance is only manifest when the threat is contact with what is believed to be real. There is no resistance to anything because it is believed to be false"* (T, 147).

All of this encircles the nature of the difficulties to be disposed of in order to apprehend reality: *"Resistance operates because it is feared that the reality of the object is imminent. O represents this dimension of anything whatever—its reality"* (T, 147).

The task of the analyst would be to get as near to O as possible. He must transform his perceptions of what is going on in the session, including lies, into something that intuits the nature of O and expresses it in terms more attainable to both analyst and patient. These demand to be experienced, a step further from knowledge (K).

"*It is not knowledge of reality that is at stake, nor yet the human equipment for knowing. The belief that reality is or could be known is mistaken because reality is not something which lends itself to being known. It is impossible to know reality for the same reason that makes it impossible to sing potatoes; they may be grown, or pulled, or eaten, but not sung. Reality has to be 'been': there should be a transitive verb 'to be' expressly for use with the term 'reality'. . .*

The point at issue is how to pass from 'knowing' 'phenomena' to 'being' that which is 'real'" (T, 148). Alternatively, from K towards O.

Comparing Transformations in K and Transformations in O: new views on a known phenomenon, resistance

K is seemingly a first step, and more akin to classical psycho-analysis as Bion describes it. The name "classical" is a respectful way of describing something that transcends time and space. However, it may be enriched by renewed views of it (see the entry, Classical analysis). Therefore, transformations in K are mandatory.

The intuitive act of insight demands something more. In the following text, one may remember that Bion used a quasi-mathematical system of notations. To talk about the journey from Knowing to Being means getting transiently nearer that which is intuitable. It is just like the "potatoeness"—its apprehension that allows one to use potatoes without knowing its ultimate reality. The system of notation describes the journey towards "O" with the aid of an arrow whose sense is from Knowledge toward the numinous realm ("O").

Also, to read the following text correctly, one must bear in mind that column 2 is the deposit of lies, which is the contrasting necessary paradox to ultimate truth or ultimate reality.

In this same text, $T\alpha$ means processes of transformations.

$T\beta$ means final products of a transformation.

K means knowing or knowledge as a process.

O means ultimate reality.

→ means a vector that gives a sense.

Interpretations are part of K. The anxiety lest transformation in K leads to transformations in O is responsible for the form of resistance in which interpretations appear to be accepted but in fact the

> acceptance is with the intention of "knowing about" rather than "becoming". In other terms, it is an acceptance to preserve the K link as a col. 2 element against transformation in O. By agreeing with the interpretation it is hoped that the analyst will be inveigled into a collusive relationship to preserve K without being aware that he is doing so. If the manoeuvre is successful transformations in K fulfil an F_2 role preventing the inception of $T\alpha \rightarrow T\beta = K \rightarrow O$. [T, 160]

This matters to an analysis because there is a hiatus between "knowing phenomena" and "being a reality". It is a flash between two dark nights, but this flash is all, to use a quotation of Poincaré's that is very dear to Bion. It seems to involve a peremptory and uncritical adhesion to column 2 (lies) statements. Statements known to be false form a barrier against statements believed to be true.

An interpretation must, therefore, favour a transition: between *"knowing about"* reality to *"becoming real"* (T, 153) this difference could account for patients who "know" many things about themselves, are able to talk psycho-analytically about their personalities but remain virgin of analysis.

With the aid of an artificially constructed fable, which nevertheless uses real facts, Bishop Berkeley argued with Sir Isaac Newton about their difficulties with the theory of "fluxions" and of "departed quantities". Berkeley launched a series of attacks against a beleaguered Newton, with a polemical tone. The polemical tone confers to Berkeley's statements the status of *"column 2 category, denying though he acknowledges the truth of Newton's result, the validity of the method"* (the reading of the diatribe and of the historical facts is recommended; however a summary would be out of place here. T, 157–8).

To the practising analyst, where truth matters in his work, one may see the difficulties involved in the way between K and O through the aid of some mystics. Bion chooses St John of the Cross and his descriptions of the "three nights of the soul": *"transformations in K are feared when they threaten the emergence of transformations in O. This can be restated as fear when $T\alpha \rightarrow T\beta = K \rightarrow O$. Resistance to an interpretation is resistance against change from K to O. Change from K to O is a special case of Transformation; it is of particular concern to the analyst in his function of aiding maturation of the personalities of his patients . . .*

transformation in O, or . . . from K→O – that involves 'becoming' – is felt as inseparable from becoming God, ultimate reality, the First Cause. The 'dark night' pain is fear of megalomania. This fear inhibits acceptance of being responsible, that is mature, because it appears to involve **being** *God, being the First Cause, being ultimate reality with a pain that can be, though inadequately, expressed by 'megalomania'"* (T, 158–9).

This can be illustrated by the difference between being an armchair cook, footballer, or driver, or music buff or critic, or analyst, or patient, and facing a hot stove, the loneliness and sweat of a football camp in a match, or race track, or a performer on stage, or the experiencing of real analysis. This involves the skills needed for them, the intuition and experience and the "megalomania" of throwing oneself into the unknown waters of experience. Bion states this in terms of Transformations in K and O: *". . . resistances, though apparently K phenomena, derive from Transformations in O. Hatred and fear derive from the fact that transformations in K threaten the further transformation"* [towards O] . . .

The resistance based on hatred and fear of T K → T O manifests itself as preference for knowing about something to becoming something" (T, 163).

Misuses and misunderstandings: When an analyst tries to apprehend a given personality's reality, he is not restricted to the philosophical and theological *"know thyself, accept thyself, be thyself".* The use of philosophical concepts such as "ultimate reality" as well as theological concepts as "mystic" must not be taken literally. This apprehension of Bion's work misled persons to conclude that he is just a theoretician (Edward Joseph). Others stated that he tried to mathematize psycho-analysis (q.v.) It is Bion himself who warns against this pedagogical, authoritarian, religious downgrading of his work and of psycho-analysis itself: *"implicit in psycho-analytic procedure is the idea that this exhortation cannot be put into practice without the psycho-analytic experience"* (T, 148).

Personal responsibility to be and to become oneself and the "sense of solitude" as described by Klein in another context are at stake:

Any interpretation may be accepted in K but rejected in O; acceptance in O means that acceptance of an interpretation enabling the patient to "know" that part of himself to which attention has been drawn is felt to involve "being" or "becoming" that person. For many interpretations this price is paid. But some are felt to involve too high a price, notably those which the patient regards as involving him in "going mad" or committing murder of himself or someone else, or becoming "responsible" and therefore guilty. There is one class of interpretations, which seem to illuminate good qualities, to which the objection is not easy to understand. The extreme example, interpretations which involve "becoming O" are dreaded as inseparable from megalomania, or what the psychiatrists or public might name delusions of grandeur or other diagnosis implying grave pathological disorder . . .

In O the falsity of the statement is secondary to the fact that it is known to be so for it is the latter that inhibits growth whereas the former is part of human inadequacy. In K the fact that the statement is known to be false is secondary to the fact that it is so for it is the latter that inhibits the establishment of meaning whereas the former is part of individual maladjustment. [T, 164, 168]

Suggested cross-references: Atonement, Classical analysis, Correct Interpretation, Types of transformations, Real psychoanalysis.

Transformations in rigid motion: These correspond *exactly* to Freud's original definition of Transference (ideas, emotions, feelings that can be or cannot be realistic in their origin, dedicated to meaningful persons during the patient's infancy that are "transferred" to the analyst, in a hallucinated way; Freud, 1912; T, pp. 19 and 27; 1977, p. 44).
Cross-references: Projective Transformations, Transformations in Hallucinosis and Transformations in Psycho-Analysis (in K and O), Transformation (concept), Transformations, types of; Transformations theory of, Transformations in −K.

Transformations: symbols: Bion tried to construe quasi-mathematical symbols in order to synthesize the ethos of the concept of Transformations and Invariances. He made this alongside his attempt to provide examples, which are sometimes highly practical and sometimes analogical and metaphorical, in order to convey what Transformation and Invariance are all about. The symbols also seemed to facilitate the classification of some kinds of transformations he observed.

We will resort to a compacted synopsis in order to present the concept and each kind of transformation he elicited. They are also presented in specific entries. See Transformations, Types of; see also Analytic view; Transformations in Rigid Motion: Projective Transformations; Transformations in Hallucinosis; Transformations in Psycho-Analysis (in K and in O); Transformations, Theory of; Transformations in −K.

Synoptic presentation of a cycle of transformations: (Table 3)

Table 3

Symbol	Definition (the references allow the reader to scrutinize the original definitions as contained in the original printed edition of Bion's book Transformations)	Practical examples
"O"	Represents the numinous realm: ultimate reality, the thing in itself (T, 31). In "O" one may find the invariances	"Poppyishness" (T, 1), or "Spoonerism" (LE, 1)
T	Cycles of trans-formations: changes in *form* (presentation) of events in the realm of *phenomena* (Kant, 1781); counterparts of "O"	Consider two persons who observe a field of poppies. One is a painter (pi) and the other (t), a drug-addict.
Tα	Processes through which a given Transformation occurs. Tα is the process, employing α-elements, by which the individual arrives at Tβ (T, 152)	Both painter and addict are aware of sensuous impressions. The painter couples those impressions with some emotional experiences and paints on a canvas; the drug addict also couples the sensuous impressions with emotional experiences that differ significantly in their nature from the painter's. He thinks of opium.

(*continued*}

Table 3 (*continued*)

Symbol	Definition (the references allow the reader to scrutinize the original definitions as contained in the original printed edition of Bion's book *Transformations*)	Practical examples
Tβ	End product of a Transformation	A picture depicting a field of poppies.
Ta	A given analyst's cycle of Transformations	**Ta** (analyst's Transformations) **Taα** = mental processes through which an analyst furnishes an interpretation (T,17). **Taβ** = the interpretation (or construction; Freud, 1937; T, p. 25) In our example: **Tpi** (painter's Transformations)—**Tpiα** = impressions, emotions, painting technique **Tpiβ** = the picture
Tp	The patient's Transformations	**Tp** (painter's Transformations)—**Tpα** = dream work **pβ** = a dream, the talk during a session, the painting. **Tt** (drug-addict's Transformations)—**Ttα** = impressions, desire; **Ttβ** = he makes opium.

Transformations, types of: Bion describes four types of positive transformations and one type of negative transformation.

The description qualifies as a real typology:

Positive:

Transformations in Rigid Motion—corresponding to transference as described by Freud.

Projective Transformations—corresponding to projective identification as described by Klein.

Transformations in Hallucinosis.

Transformations in Psycho-Analysis: in K and in O.

Negative:

Transformations in −K.

He hoped future researchers would describe other types.

Usefulness The seeming advantage of putting transference and projective identification as different types of a same general mechanism, transformation, is above all scientific and could be seen as a step towards a unified theory of psycho-analysis.

Recommended cross-references: this dictionary contains expanded comments about each type.

Tropisms: The concept of tropisms refers to one of Bion's rare attempts to formulate a theory of psycho-analysis. It is included in this dictionary for historical reasons, as it was almost entirely abandoned. It gave rise to manifold different contributions belonging both to the main body of theories of psycho-analysis and to Bion's remarkably original contribution to psycho-analysis, the theories of observation.

It can be stated that it was replaced or superseded by the following theories, which are reviewed in detail in specific entries in this dictionary:

(i)   The model of thinking based on pre-conceptions which mate with realizations.
(ii) The theory of reverie.
(iii) The theory of violent emotions.
(iv) The theory of container–contained.
(v)   The observational theory of the triad of arrogance, stupidity and curiosity.
(vi) The observational theory of the links (both the first theory, about L, K and H and the second one, about parasitism, commensalism and symbiosis).

Bion borrows the term from biology, where the concept is well-known. His leitmotif is Melanie Klein's theory of projective identification. The paper "On arrogance", written two years earlier, seems to contain the seeds of this concept; taking into account that this paper was published again in 1967 and the development of the idea of Tropisms was not, one may conclude that the former was accepted as a vehicle to Bion's second thoughts and the latter, as a sketch to express and reflect his thoughts.

The theory seems to have some daringly imaginative features, perhaps more pretentious than usually seen in the work of Bion, concerning its all-encompassing scope: *"The tropisms are the matrix from which all mental life springs"* (C, 35).

Was he not comfortable with Freud's theory of instincts that covers roughly the same area? Even though it starts from clinical features it is a theory that also at this point differs from other attempts of Bion, broader scopes of study were the rule. It would not be misplaced to conjecture that those features contributed to its replacement by more partial and narrowly-focused theories. Obviously both suggestions are the responsibility of the author; unfortunately Bion is no longer alive. These are questions that are fated to remain unanswered.

In the formulation of theory, which is contemporary to his attempts at a replacement of Freud's theory of consciousness and a development of Freud's theory of dream work (see the entry, dream-work-α), Bion saw the tropisms as basically an **action:** *"the action appropriate to the tropisms in the patient who comes for treatment is a seeking for an object with which projective identification is possible"* (C, 35).

In considering the tropisms individually he hypothesized three goals that were sought by tropisms: (1) an object to murder or to be murdered by; (2) a parasite or a host; (3) an object to create or by which to be created.

He stated that patients who looked for treatment were inescapably looking for an object with which projective identification was possible. In that epoch he believed in causes: *"This is due to the fact that in such a patient the tropism of creation is stronger than the tropism of murder"* (C, 35).

He also made explicit some factors that affected the tropisms and the aftermath of this movement of seeking, when these factors were prevalent. The theory is also remarkably different from other theories that he developed about the belief in causes as well as in traumas and popular over-simplifications of the kind, "weak personality":

The tropisms may be communicated. In certain circumstances they are too powerful for the modes of communication available to the personality. This, presumably, may be because the personality is too weak or ill-developed if the traumatic situation arrives prematurely. [C, 34]

What seems to rescue Bion from these more simplistic relations of cause and effect is Melanie Klein's and Freud's psycho-analytic vertex. The first can be seen in this quotation: "*But when this situation* [the traumatic situation] *does arise, all the future development of the personality depends in whether an object, the breast, exists into which the tropisms can be projected*" (C, 34). And the second, in this quotation: "*Associated with the strength of the tropisms, but probably secondary to it, is an intolerance of frustration*" (C, 34).

The outcome is dependent on the strength of the tropisms. It is described in three forms: (i) in terms of the patient; (ii) in terms of the object into which projective identifications are made; (iii) and in terms of seminal features of the psycho-analytic method.

With regard to the patient's characteristics, the absence of a breast coupled with violent seeking results in disaster "*which ultimately takes the form of loss of contact with reality, apathy, or mania . . . agitated melancholia . . . obsessive depression . . . its essential quality is aggressiveness and hate*" (C, 34).

With regard to the object, if such a welcoming object exists it must be a breast capable of receiving projective identification. The outcome is more favourable. He is intrinsically talking about something that three years later he would name "reverie" (q.v.).

With regard to the analytic method, the strength of tropisms is not seen as "*psychopathologically*" important. Nevertheless, "*it presents a grave problem as it jeopardizes the analytic approach since frustration is essential to it [the analytic approach]—not extrinsic*" (C, 34).

The original paper includes some comments about the introjection and re-introjection of tropisms that are ill-accepted by an unwelcoming breast; something that later would be seen as nameless dread (q.v.). He considers that the infant's cry, tactile and visual senses are "*engaged not only to communicate but also to control the tropism*" (C, 35).

The concept would resurface in *Transformations*. It is not a matter of stubbornness or insistence. Bion was trying to investigate the mysterious nature of movements towards life itself and their obverse. He seemed to resort to any means at his disposal.

The attempt now will be stated with the aid of quasi-mathematical symbols, devised to facilitate communication, around the Grid and using the concept of saturation (q.v.). To follow Bion's argument here it is necessary to keep in mind the following nomenclature:

↑← This double arrow where two arrows, one pointing "above" and one pointing "left" are constantly conjoined, means, *"in search of existence"* (T, 107).

It is not small talk—it can be visualized by an infant looking for a breast, for example, or the act of birth, or the birth of a thought. It is a symbol that purports to discover some realization that approximates to it. It may be seen as the discovery of some constant conjunction. It reunites psychic reality and material reality. It belongs to the realm of sense-perception. In this sense it is previous to awareness, and differs from, as Bion clearly emphasizes, Freud's hypothesis about consciousness as the sensuous organ that apprehends the psychic quality. This double arrow symbol is a β-element. It may or may not transform itself into an α-element.

If one keeps in mind that the symbol stands for *"in search of existence"*, it is necessary to remember, as the analytic practice shows, that *"stupor and violent greedy ambition to possess all the qualities of existence"* must be included in something that searches for existence. The symbol can be represented both in its positive, life-seeking form, and destructive, greedy form, that is, something that can be seen as negative. Therefore Bion proposes the symbol:

± ↑←

Or, decomposed into its two parts, + ↑←

And − ↑←

In terms of the Grid, one may imagine a dynamic movement in the direction of the definitory hypothesis and actions, that is, the category of the Grid named A1. If you feel any difficulty in following this nomenclature, please consult the entry, "Grid", in this dictionary. A familiarity with it will make it easier to follow the argument.

"It is necessary to suppose that there is awareness of a constant conjunction" (T, 108).

As a *"temporary measure"* (C, 108) Bion uses the symbol, *"Cs, as a sign for 'awareness'"*. Cs is not separable from "plus and minus search for existence", or, stated in graphic terms,

Cs is not separable from ± ↑←

Therefore one may have Cs (A1), which means, a "definitory hypothesis in search of existence". It is an action and it is a dynamic movement. *"Cs(A1) is the nature of a tropism"*. With this dry phrase Bion brings the term back, after six years. *"This 'consciousness' is an awareness of a lack of existence that demands an existence, a thought in search of a meaning, a definitory hypothesis in search of a realization approximating to it, a psyche seeking for a physical habitation to give it existence, ? seeking ?"* (T, 109). Intuition is seen as a function of it (q.v.).

🕐 The term starts from an all-encompassing theory and comes to have the nature of an ancillary description of a fact linked to the unconscious, to life and to thinking processes.

Truth:

> ... "truth" is the name I give to the quality that I attribute to any statement that is a hypothesis relating to phenomena with which I have an "I know ..." relationship. [C, 270—written between 1961–1967]

> The failure to bring about ... a commonsense view induces a mental state of debility in the patient as if starvation of truth was somehow analogous to alimentary starvation. [ST, 119—written circa 1966]

> ... healthy mental growth seems to depend on truth as the living organism depends on food. [T, 38]

> By definition and by the tradition of all scientific discipline, the psycho-analytic movement is committed to the truth as the central aim. [AI, 99—written circa 1968]

Bion's earliest posture would be maintained up to the end of his life. In some aspects of his work he changed, but this is not one of them. Quite the contrary: this view was polished like a piece of jewellery.

In the beginning, from clinical experience he makes an analogy of truth and nourishment. Right from the start such a posture differs from ideas of attaining absolute truth, to the extent that Bion's stance depends on common sense. Common sense (q.v.) in turn relates this posture unequivocally with reality. The way that the psycho-analytic movement seems to have dealt with truth and reality in the last century echoes the way that the encircling social milieu dealt with it: abhorrence, denial, and contempt. The issue has turned itself into a taboo in the last forty years. Terms such as "psychic reality" are increasingly left aside.

The fact that science in general, and Freud, Klein and Bion in particular, made explicit their allegiance to the scientific endeavour, namely, to get nearer reality *as it is*, seems to have ignited a contrary reaction of the same intensity.

Any mention of truth is too often subjected to prejudice. Anyone who merely utters the word, or expresses an inclination to pursue it, is misunderstood as having the pretension to *own* the truth, to know it in its entirety in a static way. The doubt about the very existence of truth and reality proves to be popular both among the intelligentsia and laymen. There is no equivalent interest in the work of individuals who strive to get near "reality as it is" (a phrase uttered by Socrates, Plato, Browne, Bacon, Kant, Johnson, to quote a few, who may be considered Bion's forerunners). The demagogue and the quack are more loved than a politician who promises to do that which is possible or the physician who tells the patient the truth about a serious illness.

Nowadays whoever is interested in reality or truth runs the risk of being seen as a misguided simpleton, or a pretentious positivist. Solipsists, as they were called in Freud's time, or post-modernists as they like to be called today, advertise themselves and have an image of themselves as not interested in issues such as truth; they regard it as illusory and non-existent. They see themselves as safe from falling prey to essentialism and absolute truth. But in fact their posture betrays a hidden fact: they operate just like one who is overwhelmed by feelings of having "attained" the ultimate truth, namely, that truth does not exist. Are they trying to get rid of the fact that this real, hidden posture runs against their outwardly advertised posture? Is it a case of projective identification? In other words, the outward idealist shelters an inner power of absolute truth. But this truth itself is unbearable, and, in trying to get rid of it, the "idealist" is left with trying to put his own abhorred truth in someone else (above all, the scientist).

Truth in analysis is not truth in general except as an ethical posture. Truth in analysis is linked to self-knowledge: "*Since self-knowledge is an aim of psycho-analytic procedure . . .*" (EP, 91).

Truth in analysis and in science is not just a philosopher of science's theoretical problem: *"Herein lies one advantage that the psycho-analyst possesses over the philosopher; his statements can be related to realizations and realizations to a psycho-analytic theory"* (T, 44). Five years later Bion would put it in simpler terms: *". . . the psycho-analyst is concerned **practically** with a problem that the philosopher approaches **theoretically**"* (AI, 97).

> Psycho-analytic procedure pre-supposes that the welfare of the patient demands a constant supply of truth as inevitably as his physical survival demands food. It further presupposes that the discovery of the truth about himself is a pre-condition of an ability to learn the truth, or at least to seek it in his relationship with himself and others. It is supposed at first that he cannot discover the truth about himself without assistance from the analyst and others. [C, 99]

> I assume that the permanently therapeutic effect of a psycho-analysis, if any, depends on the extent to which the analysand has been able to use the experience to see one aspect of his life, namely himself as he is. It is the function of the psycho-analyst to use the experience of such facilities for contact as the patient is able to extend to him, to elucidate the truth about the patient's personality and mental characteristics, and to exhibit them to the patient in a way that makes it possible to him to entertain a reasonable conviction that the statements (propositions) made about himself represent facts.

> It follows that a psycho-analysis is a joint activity of analyst and analysand to determine the truth; that being so, the two are engaged—no matter how imperfectly—on what is in intention a scientific activity. [C, 114]

Bion pointed out that *"The truth of a statement does not imply that there is a realization approximating to the true statement"* (ST, 119). The mathematician did realize this long ago. Bion saw that the mathematician's insight could be helped by the insight obtained in later times by the psycho-analyst, Freud, albeit in different terms: that psychic reality has an intrinsic immaterialness that turns it into a different form of existence *vis-à-vis* material reality. But the reality itself, or "existence" (which appears at least in two forms or transformations) does exist and is real. *"O does not fall in the domain of knowledge or learning save incidentally; it can 'become', but it cannot be 'known'"* (AI, 27). The words "save incidentally" must not be negated.

Fear of truth seems to be related to primitive states of love and hate. Both lead to idealization, to quote just an example of a distortion of reality in the area of the onlooker's perception. The issue illustrates the basic psycho-analytic view to the extent that reality presents itself in the form of paradoxical pairs which cannot be forced into over-simplification: instincts of death and life, two principles of mental functioning, and PS and D are a few examples of it.

Analysis deals with paradoxical pairs, any time. In the decisive moment of the session the words uttered and what they really mean function as beauty, which is more than skin deep. Both form a pair, as manifest and latent contents. Bion starts from these pairs described by Freud and Klein. In discussing the obstructions that inhibit an infant's impulse to obtain sustenance from the breast, even—or especially—from a good breast, Bion states that *"Love in infant or mother or both increases rather than decreases the obstruction partly because love is inseparable from envy of the object so loved, partly because it is felt to arouse envy and jealousy in a third object that is excluded. The part played by love may escape notice because envy, rivalry and hate obscure it, although hate would not exist if love were not present. Violence of emotion compels reinforcement of the obstruction because violence is not distinguished from destructiveness and subsequent guilt and depression"* (LE, 10).

Hiram Jackson, an American politician, observed during the course of the First World War that in war the first casualty is truth. Violence of emotions can be seen as an evolving internal war in each mind that suffers from it (probably an innate trait). Therefore truth probably is felt as unbearable to the personality that hates frustration. The narcissistic patient usually displays violent emotions. He is prone to regard anything relating to him as acquiring an unrealistic, disproportionate importance. He cannot tolerate his own imperfections or anything other than his own idealized view of him (her) self. Therefore, violence of emotions can preclude the search for truth.

"Violence, attributed to emotions by me here, is not intended to imply only quantity of feeling. I shall consider only love and hate because I

regard them as comprising all others. I do not separate love and life instincts, or hate and death instincts, nor shall I consider whether the violence implies an origin in the instinctual endowment or is secondary to an external environment stimulus. It may on occasion be due to a deficiency in a capacity for thought, or some other function proper to the onset of the reality principle ... Violence, then, though related to quantity or degree, contributes to a qualitative change in the emotion. The qualitative change makes love and hate possess appreciably cruel strains together with diminishing concern for the object, Both love and hate thus become more easily associated with a lack of concern for truth and life" (C, 249–250)—which stems from Klein's observation that it is not only hate that destroys the object, but the intensity of love too, to the extent that it carries with it greed and envy (Klein, 1936).

This means that truth as it is cannot be perceived any more: materialness gets the upper hand. A hallucinated breast full of non-nourishing immaterialness flourishes in autism. In the first case it produces that which Kant named "naïve realism"; it manifests itself as schizoid phenomena; in the second case, it produces that which the author once proposed to call, "naïve idealism", and manifests itself through paranoid phenomena. This seems to be linked to the relationship of the baby with the breast, in the sense of an envious situation that precludes concern for truth and life (please refer to the entries, Sense of Truth; Compassion; Thinking; also, Misuses and misunderstandings, below).

> The most important characteristic is its hatred of any new development in the personality as if the new development were a rival to be destroyed. The emergence therefore of any tendency to search for the truth, to establish contact with reality and in short to be scientific in no matter how rudimentary a fashion is met by destructive attacks on the tendency and the reassertion of the "moral" superiority. This implies an assertion of what in sophisticated terms would be called a moral law and a moral system superior to scientific law and a scientific system. [LE, 98]

The issue of truth in the session is pressing and serious to the analyst, to the patient and to the future of psycho-analysis within the psycho-analytic movement. Concern for truth and life marks one of the very rare attempts by Bion to construe a psycho-analytical theory *per se* and seems to constitute its main frame. It was doomed to remain unpublished during his lifetime. Parts of it emerged, albeit forming more a theory of observation in psycho-analysis than of psycho-analysis proper, in *Transformations, Attention and Interpretation*, and *A Memoir of the Future*.

> I must make clear my choice not only of these terms, but also of the realities they represent . . . No single word can adequately express the ideas to which I want to draw attention. By "concern" I mean something that has in it feelings of consideration for the object, or sympathy with it, of value for it . . .
>
> A concern for truth may seem to be so closely related to impulses that operate under the dominance of the reality principle as to make it scarcely worth while to distinguish it from them by singling it our for special mention . . .
>
> The concern for truth must be distinguished from a capacity for establishing contact with reality. A man may have little capacity for that through lack of intelligence . . . or might be defective in one or more of his senses . . . Yet . . . can have an active yearning for, and respect for, truth. Conversely, a highly gifted and well-equipped person may have little concern for truth . . . Such unconcern will clearly be a matter for attention by the analyst for whom the psycho-analysis of the patient had truth as its criterion . . .
>
> A lack of concern for life means regarding a living object as indistinguishable from, or being unworthy of being distinguished from, a machine, a thing or a place . . .
>
> Lack of concern means a lack of respect for himself and, *a fortiori*, of others, which is fundamental and of proportionately grave import for analysis. It is clear that lack of such respect means lack also of a safeguard against murderous or suicidal impulses . . .
>
> The patient who has no regard for truth, for himself, or for his analyst achieves a kind of freedom arising from the fact that so much destructive activity is open to him for so long. He can behave in a way that destroys his respect for himself and his analyst, provided he always retains enough contact with reality to feel that there is some respect to destroy; and this he can always assume if his analyst continues to see him . . . But destruction of the analysis is to be avoided, for it entails loss of freedom—at least till a new object is found—thus introducing a need for moderation that is apparent at other points in the closed system the patient strives to

produce. An obvious instance of this is the need to avoid successful suicide or murder. In brief, it is necessary for the patient to
avoid any step calculated to effect change, and yet to change
enough to ensure more analysis either for the reason that he has
temporarily become a greater liability and needs more care, or
because he shows such promise that it would be wrong to stop just
when affairs have reached so happy a posture. But it is clear that
the limitations on freedom, and the subsequent frustration, are
associated with the patient's sensitiveness to reality. He must therefore lose some of this freedom by keeping analysis going. [C,
247–49]

🕑 The view on truth was more expanded in *Brazilian Lectures, A
Memoir of the Future* and *Seminari Italiani*. Final posture, from *A
Memoir of the Future*:

ROLAND Do you think there is any kind of prayer that is not an
outrage on one's common sense? Obviously, the athletic "knees
bend" exercise could not satisfy any person of integrity. What does
P.A. think?

P.A. It is not my department. I have ideas about it like any other
man, but I would not like it supposed that because I set up as an
expert in psycho-analysis my expertise extended to religion and
other disciplines—painting, music, literature.

PRIEST Is that not somewhat cowardly?

P.A. You and others might think so, but I do not. Even in my
limited field I am not unfamiliar with a cowardly shrinking from
expressing a truth that I know will be unwelcome. One takes flight
into doubt— "What is truth?" said jesting Pilate; Bacon himself did
not wait for an answer because he knew he might be killed if he
did. Physical death is a hard price to pay—especially for those of us
who, from training and observation, believe in the obliteration of
the body. I believe also in the obliteration of one's respect for the
truth; it is not simply by physical methods—alcohol for example—
that one can destroy one's capacity for discerning or proclaiming
the Truth.

PRIEST I believe in moral, religious death. Truth can be nourished;
it can be allowed to die of neglect or be poisoned by seductions,
cowardice, too often repeated. But Truth is robust; "facts" cannot
be killed even if we do not know what they are. The fragile human

respect for the truth cannot be as easily disposed of as often appears.

P.A. I hope you are right. I cannot, however, say that my knowledge of myself or others provides me with food for hope. Religion itself gives evidence of the great force of power, bigotry, ignorance; and psycho-analysis is shot through with error and the defects of us humans who try to practise it.

PRIEST You are being extremely self-contradictory in claiming that it is a science *and* is true. It must have a point of reference outside itself. You cannot believe in Truth any more than you can "believe in God". God is—

ROLAND —or is not.

P.A. No, "God is; or is not" is only a human formulation in conformity with human principles of thinking. It has nothing to do with the reality. The only "reality" we *know about* is the various hopes, dreams, phantasies, memories and desires which are a part of us. The other reality exists, **is**, whether we like it or not. A child may want to punish a table for hurting him when he suffers a contusion. But he may desire to punish himself for "suffering" a contusion. He may ultimately be compelled to believe that, in addition to these facts, there is a table that is neither good or bad, like it or not, forgive it or punish it. We may decide to punish our god, punish ourselves for believing in "it" or "him" or "her". It will not affect the reality which will continue to be real no matter how unsearchable, un-knowable, beyond the grasp of human capacity it is/not is. After all, we do not know much about the world we live on, or the minds we are.

ALICE I thought you psycho-analysts were supposed to have discovered all about us. [AMF, III, 498–500]

Truth and Naïve Realism (the fallacy of the apprehension of reality through the senses)

MAN I believe in God anyway; I have evidence of his goodness.

ROLAND I believe in the Devil; I have evidence of his cruelty and wickedness.

P.A. I differ. Evidence is a function of the senses; they cannot lead logically to the "truth" of God—only to the truth of the reality that is *not* God. [AMF, II, 351]

Misuses and misunderstandings: Truth, or truth-O, is usually mistaken for absolute truth. Attempts to get insight, transient glimpses of aspects and emanations of truth are mistaken for feelings of ownership of absolute truth. Lest the statements in the quotations be used as some kind of puritan authority or judgement, the scientific appreciation of reality as it is can be seen when the realm of minus, of the numinous negative realm of "O" is elicited.

Absolute truth is sometimes referred to by Bion as "objective reality". In talking about the relationship between two people and the vicissitudes of its observation:

> I shall suppose that the relationship is a "constant conjunction", that is to say, that the relationship has an element in the mind of the observer and may or may not have a counterpart in reality. I make no claim for objective reality, as far as I understand the meaning usually attributed to the term, but for me, a factual situation (conjectured) an emotional state (say hate, also conjectured), a representation (Tpâ) are constantly conjoined and I record ... or bind ... it by the term "transformation". [T, 68]

> The postulate is that ... designated by O. To qualify O ... I list the following negatives: Its existence as indwelling has no significance whether it is supposed to dwell in an individual person or in God or Devil; it is not good or evil; it cannot be known, loved or hated. It can be represented by terms such as ultimate reality or truth. The most, and the least that the individual can do is to be it. Being identified with it is a measure of distance from it. The beauty of a rose is a phenomenon betraying the ugliness of O just as ugliness betrays or reveals the existence of O ... The rose *is* itself whatever it may be *said* to be. [T, 139–40]

Or, as he would put it some ten years later:

> MYSELF Perhaps I can illustrate by an example from something you *do* know. Imagine a piece of sculpture which is easier to comprehend if the structure is intended to act as a trap for light. The meaning is revealed by the pattern formed by the light thus trapped—not the structure, the carved work itself. I suggest that if I could learn how to talk to you in such a way that my words "trapped" the meaning which they neither do nor could express, I *could* communicate to you in a way that is not at present possible.

BION Like the "rests" in a musical composition?

MYSELF A musician would certainly not deny the importance of those parts of a composition in which no notes were sounding, but more has to be done than can be achieved in existent art and its well-established procedure of silences, pauses, blank spaces, rests. The "art" of conversation, as carried on as part of the conversational intercourse of psycho-analysis, requires and demands an extension in the realm of non-conversation . . .

I have suggested a "trick" by which one could manipulate things which have no meaning—the use of sounds like α and β. These are sounds analogous, as Kant said, to "thoughts without concepts", but the principle, and a reality approximating to it is also extensible to words in common use. The realizations which approximate to words such as "memory"and "desire" are opaque. . . . I suggest this quality of opacity inheres in many O's and their verbal counterparts, and the phenomena which it is usually supposed to express. If, by experiment, we discovered the verbal forms, we could also discover the thoughts to which the observation applied specifically. Thus we achieve a situation in which these could be used deliberately to obscure specific thoughts.

BION Is there anything new in this? You must often have heard, as I have, people say they don't know what you are talking about and that you are being deliberately obscure.

MYSELF They are flattering me. I am suggesting an aim, an ambition, which, if I could achieve, would enable me to be deliberately and *precisely* obscure; in which I could use certain words which could activate precisely and instantaneously, in the mind of the listener, a thought or train of thought that came between him and the thoughts and ideas already accessible and available to him.

ROSEMARY Oh, my God! [AMF, I, 189–191]

Therefore correct interpretation is couched in terms that *"The interpretation should be such that the transition from **knowing about** reality to **becoming real** is furthered"* (T, 155).

The pursuit of truth also brings forth some clinical problems, related to the stimulus it represents to some patients who use it to create a war against that which is seen as a superiority of analysis and of the analyst. Bion was aware of this from early on:

Briefly, it appears that overwhelming emotions are associated with the assumption by the patient or analyst of the qualities required to pursue the truth, and in particular a capacity to tolerate the stresses associated with the introjection of another person's projective identifications. Put into other terms, the implicit aim of psycho-analysis to pursue the truth at no matter what cost is felt to be synonymous with a claim to a capacity for containing the discarded, split-off aspects of other personalities while retaining a balanced outlook. This would appear to be the immediate signal for outbreaks of envy and hatred. [ST, 89–9]

To see in more detail the clinical use of this observation, see the entries Cure, Compassion, and Transformations in Hallucinosis.

Since Antiquity, the philosopher of science has been divided into schizoid naïve realism and paranoid naïve idealism. This occurs in the realist's confusion of animate with inanimate and in the idealist's enthroning of the products of the mind (the belief that the universe is an idea of the human being). In analysis and in science, the term "reality" is interchangeable with truth, due to its firm natural origins. Had the philosopher of science profited from the epistemological contributions of psycho-analysis, he would have had a chance not to be thrown into the darkness of ignorance disguised as the supreme and only wisdom.

Recommended cross-references: Mystic, Science versus Religion.

Suggested cross-references: Absolute truth, Analytic view, Atonement, Becoming, Common sense, Compassion, Correlation, Disturbed personality, Enforced splitting, O, Jargon, Lies, Manipulation of Symbols, Mystic, Philosophy, Real Psycho-analysis, Reality Sensuous and Psychic, Sense of Truth, Thinking, Truth-Function, Ultra-sensuous, Unknowable, Unknown.

Truth-function of the mind: Its existence was hypothesized:

Put to the test of a reality situation, it is difficult to believe that there is any technique, whatever its name, which could reveal that I am anything—remembering at the same time that I have already said what I am thinking. Assuming that there is some standard by which one could distinguish what is true and what is not, namely, that there is a sort of truth function, it is difficult to believe that I, as the object of investigation, am likely to give you a correct (truthful) answer as to what it is that I am or contain. [BL, 37]

Suggested cross-references: Absolute truth, Analytic view, Atonement, Becoming, Commonsense, Compassion, Correlation, Disturbed personality, Enforced splitting, O, Jargon, Mystic, Philosophy, Real psycho-analysis, Reality Sensuous and Psychic, Sense of Truth, Thinking, Truth-Function, Ultra-sensuous, Unknowable, Unknown.

Two-body psychology: The reader may find it weird that I include a term coined by another analyst, John Rickman, in this dictionary dedicated to Bion's terms. Nevertheless it seems to the author of this text that the ethos of this concept was enlivened by Bion without modifying it essentially; moreover, perhaps an attempt to pay homage to Bion's long-time friend, former analyst and collaborator, as an inspiration, would not be misplaced.

Bion's insistence on links and relationships seem to have been born here.

📖 *Selected Papers of John Rickman*, edited by W. Clifford-Scott. London: The Hogarth Press and the Institute of Psycho-analysis, 1951. (New Edition published by Karnac Books, 2003.)

U

Ultra-sensuous, infra-sensuous, ultra-human, infra-human, ultra-logic, infra-logic, infra-conceptual, infra-intellectual, infra-visual: *"Non-sensuous phenomena form the totality of what is commonly regarded as mental or spiritual experience"* (AI, 91).

> MAN When the mind ± has been mapped, the investigations may reveal variations in the various patterns which it displays. The important thing may not be, as the psycho-analysts suppose, only revelations in illness or diseases of the mind, but patterns indiscernible in the domain in which Bio ± exist (life and death; animate and inanimate) because the mind spans too inadequate a spectrum of reality. Who can free mathematics from the fetters exposed by its genetical links with sense? Who can find a Cartesian system which will again transform mathematics in ways analogous to the expansion of arithmetic effected by imaginary numbers, irrational numbers, Cartesian coordinates freeing geometry from Euclid by opening up the domain of algebraic deductive systems; the fumbling infancy of psycho-analysis from the domain of sensuality-based mind? [AMF, I, 130]

These terms should be read in conjunction with the terms "Mind", "Real psycho-analysis" and "Thoughts without a thinker".

It was a term created at the end of Bion's life. Perhaps it is his last onslaught on the resistances to analysis stemming from the psycho-analytic movement.

The terms were created by Bion around 1973. They were first used in his Brazilian lectures and thereafter in all volumes of *A Memoir of the Future*. They were analogies taken from the spectrum of electro-magnetic waves of light. They try to tackle a problem that was unsuccessfully dealt with through the use of terms such as "mind", "personality", "unconscious", "spirit", "soul", "character" and many others.

These terms (ultra-sensuous, infra-sensuous etc) were intended to express a posture necessary to the analyst in face of the unknown, and an attempt to grasp something beyond that which the senses can grasp; not only in terms of range but also in terms of something of a different nature. That is, the "some" in the thing. In Bion's own terms, the realm of "O" (q.v.)

To be a psycho-analyst

The analytic posture, which differentiates analysis from anything else, is covered in other entries of this dictionary (Analytic View, Atonement, Real psycho-analysis). Anyway, when discussing this new term, Bion links it with the analytic posture:

> BION You could say that if being a psycho-analyst was wearing a mental suit of clothes, one could choose whatever fictitious character one liked to be and dress up in the appropriate uniform. The trouble is if one has to *be* a psycho-analyst and not simply learn the part for purposes of acting.
>
> ROSEMARY I don't play-act; that is why I don't give you a kiss.
>
> BION Some kisses have become famous. One kiss is called a "Judas kiss" after a character who became famous and notorious. Kisses, like other actions, speak louder than words
>
> MYSELF Interpretation likewise depends on quality as well as quantity as do the things interpreted. "Loudness", expressing quantity, is not enough even in the domain of physical senses and other phenomena; all to which the term "phenomena" applies are by definition a part of the domain of the senses. We, in common with many who purport to exist or are reported to have existed and

still to exist, believe there is something "more" which can be called "ultra-" or "infra-" sensuous. It is this something more, or "something +", which we suppose to be significant for refinement by psycho-analysis in practice. [AMF, I, 203]

They are not terms to be taken as things-in-themselves; nor are they to be used as living entities or technical terms, as perhaps may be clear in the following quotation:

P.A. I shall avail myself of your permission to say "infra-conceptual".

PAUL Well, *that* is horrible enough to escape durability as an artistic expression. The world of thought shrinks its boundaries in inverse proportion to the length of the verbal weapons it uses; the shorter the "bayonet" the wider the empire it sways. [AMF, II, 249]

The issue of the limits of the apprehension of reality and facts through the senses was dealt with by Plato, Luria, Kant and Freud, among many others too numerous to list.

It became clear that the spectrum of reality that could be apprehended by the human sensuous apparatus was extremely limited. Moreover, the apprehension itself was both limited and modified by the device used to apprehend it, namely, the sensuous apparatus itself. The limitation was due to the narrow range of each sensory organ. For example, the human eye cannot apprehend electromagnetic waves below red or above violet. To those who could not realize this limitation, Kant attributed the qualification "naïve realist".

The romantics, deeply inspired by Hume, to an extent by Rousseau, and epitomized by Hamann, Maimon, von Herder and Goethe, among others, added an observation to this realization. Namely, that it was not only the fact that the senses modified the apprehension of reality that had to be taken into consideration. There are other factors that implied that modification could be so broad and deep as to entail distortion. They sometimes reached a point of no-return. Those factors were the passions and emotions. Even reason, which was seen by many people such as Descartes as a sound method to apprehend reality, came to be seen—by Hume initially—as a slave of the passions. Paradoxically, the emotions were also seen as *the* reliable tool to apprehend reality as it is.

These insights, when focused on individuals and with the posture of "to care", led to the formulation of psycho-analysis. Real reality (to borrow a term from Locke) could be unconscious, immaterial and ultimately unreachable. In Freud's terms: *"The unconscious is the true psychical reality;* **in its innermost nature it is as much unknown to us as the reality of the external world, and it is as incompletely presented by the data of consciousness as is the external world by the communications of our sense organs"** (Freud, 1900, p. 613; Freud's italics). Later, with his formulation about unconscious phantasies, it became more clear how emotions could be both reliable and unreliable tools for apprehending reality. In Shakespeare's (and Descartes') terms: *"By indirection, find the direction out"* (Hamlet). Melanie Klein would furnish copious clinical evidence for that finding.

Concrete, sensuously apprehensible, inanimate, and É

The situation and issue is not philosophical, even though philosophers and perhaps above all some mystics tried to deal with it—or had to. The situation is: life itself is at stake. Not just survival, but living.

Bion had real living experiences that showed him that to many human beings the differentiation between the animate and inanimate is problematic. The so-called psychotics or certified schizophrenics dealt with the animate with methods more applicable to the inanimate. This is depicted in Bion's clinical studies and in *Learning from Experience.* His experience in war also indicated this. This was his main base, coupled with that which was described above. Why should the human mind have such remarkable difficulties in realizing its own immaterial nature?

He attributed to the sensuous apparatus the same importance that Freud attributed to it, especially in the *Project for a Scientific Psychology* and in *The Interpretation of Dreams.* Freud focused on: (i) the sensuous apparatus as the port of entry of everything; (ii) the nature of that which calls to be perceived; (iii) the post-sensuous stage, or what happens in the mind of the dreamer and of the speaker; (iv) the return to a sensuous impression that construes the dream.

Bion's first attempts were the theories that resulted in the formulation of alpha-function. The terms that are the subject of this entry came later. They try to deal with those issues: the nature of that which is apprehended—mind's nature—the function of that which is known as CNS and ANS, the limits of our range of apprehension.

Bion coined some novel terms; the phrases infra- and ultra-sensual are part of the final evolution of an attempt to tackle the impossibility that many have to integrate material and psychic reality without mixing them.

> There seems to be something to be said for the "use" to which "things" are put. If, then, one considers the accumulation of experience and then the use which is made of these "possessions", one is using the vocabulary which has been forged for and from the world of sensuous experience. That, indeed, is the vocabulary and procedure which I am trying to use in this very communication. It is not likely to be adequate, but there is also the possibility, almost certainty perhaps, that the "use" which I am able to make of it is as widely exercised only in those respects in which it has a past and forgotten history. It is also an equipment which is peculiar to that part of the spectrum of thought-without-a-thinker which is peculiar to the biological range, from what could be called the infra-sensual to the ultra-sensual. Even so, the range is perhaps more correctly defined as infra-human (sympathetic) to ultra-human (algebraic)—in other words, a limited range of animal life. At the same time, the range is microscopic from one vertex and yet too enormous to be likely to be bridged by anything so trifling, so trivial as the products of the human animal. [AMF, I, 56]

That which seemed at first a problem of psychotics only revealed itself as a feature of the human mind—which always has a psychotic stratum.

> Krishna makes the point quite clearly; he shows Arjuna that his depression is part of feelings of compassion which are unworthy of thought, still less of God-head. That kind of thing may be appropriate to reception and emission in the range of sensuous perception whether perceived directly or mechanically by constructs like radio receivers, X-ray films, musical instruments and, in their very crude and gross manifestations, by animals and creatures in the biological range. Very sensitive animal organisms may then be able to interpret or transform the disturbances in the waves which render them

opaque and obstructive. St. John of the Cross was even able to point out that an analogy can be found which may be serviceable in the process if vulgarization intended to make the grosser crudities even grosser, till they impinge on elements which are still within the spectrum of the infra-sensuous and ultra-sensuous, though not outside that very narrow and limited band. [AMF, I, 69]

MAN Let me suggest that the state of mind of the men of Ur six thousand years ago is so intensely distant that it is hardly possible for us to know what it was. We may suppose, as an hypothesis, that there could be men separated from us by an interval of time equal and opposite, that is to say, six thousand years in the future. Their state of mind could be equally impossible for us to know. Yet we may imagine the span from -6000 to $+6000$ is immeasurably small; so small, indeed, that it lies within the compass of our minds in much the same way, or more correctly, "analogous" way, that the span from the infra-red to the ultra-violet measures the spectrum of the "visible" part of the total range of electromagnetic waves (or quanta). The range to which I have arbitrarily ascribed numerical range, -6000 to $+6000$, I shall further arbitrarily describe as extending (not in numerical terms) from infra-sensual to ultra-sensual. The whole of the range is what I shall describe as lying within the domain of the human mind. I shall now assume mind to extend as far "beyond" human mentality as life extends "beyond" what our limited apparatus can conceive of as "mind". I shall suppose a bio+ and bio−, that is, something beyond even animate and inanimate. [AMF, I, 127]

MYSELF As psychological preparation I shall borrow verbal or alphabetical formulations like O, or zero, or infinity. For some centuries the visual imagery of Euclidean space limited rather than freed thought. Cartesian coordinates made, in combination with the theorem of Pythagoras, a possibility of relating points to each other without the visual aids of lines and circles. These visual aids introduced powerful, undetected, forces which distorted the balance of probability. That distortion is still incalculable. Growth, + or −, remained inaccessible to thought, if unmistakable to feeling. Conceptual thought and passionate feeling are impossible to relate within the confines of existent universes of discourse. The problem could be stated by analogy; numbers suffered repeated extensions to carry an increased load—rational numbers, irrational numbers and, latterly, complex conjugate points. In the emotional domain, persecution by passion grows to depression. The relation of the one to the other requires an extension whereby quantity transforms to quality. "Very great", "very small" intervals of time, space, probability, involve quality in a manner analogous to growth from quantity to quality. Thus, quantitative terms such as 'excessive', "inadequate", "too little", "too much", may signify a change in kind or quality; conversely, change in quality, for example, love or hate, may imply a change in quantity. This is *not* a crudity such as the difference between one German "hating" and the entire German nation "hating"; that may be "symptomatic", "significant" of a method of lateral communication. The change can be formulated in language, music, mathematics; it is, in fact, something "infra" or "ultra-" human, animate, living or bio-logical. Comparison between animate and inanimate reveals need for discrimination; the "Russians" send a mechanical probe to the moon and retain a mechanically-aided, computer-wise and otherwise, animate being on earth. By contrast, the "Americans" favour sending "animate beings" sufficiently well disciplined to be machines.

Bernardino Sahagun describes the debate between those who favour gods formed artificially, by human art, out of wood and stone which "appear" to be controllable, and those, like the Roman Catholics, who favour an independent and uncontrollable God. Jesus Christ is a compromise between the verbally articulate human Jesus who prays "Thy will be done on earth as it is in Heaven" and the Messiah. Some degree of independence is conceded to "God", although, after creation or "belief creating operation", both end products are still, from human vertex, unpredicted. The idol made out of inanimate material shows unmistakable characteristics of a kind usually attributed to animals, usually human; reciprocally, the god created out of materials, ultra- or infra-sensuous, displays characteristics usually regarded as the prerogative of idols. In other terms, ("borrowed" from the lunar illustration), the machine, regardless of race, time, space, is e- and pro-vocatively animate and the animate object similarly pro- and e-vocatively inhuman and inanimate. If we now increase the dimension, using "time" as an instrument with which to measure, we find a stability about the objects discerned and recorded by animate human animals such as saints, philosophers, scientists, artists, and (borrowing from Socrates) artisans. Socrates knew that he was not wise, yet could not mobilize facts to indicate anyone or anything, god or idol, who could plausibly be said to contest the title. In the domain of the human senses there is evidence of violence and murder from the Death Pit at Ur to Hiroshima and beyond. [AMF, I, 138–140]

ROBIN Why do you not fall back on art, or religion, or mathematics?

P.A. I have told you, I do not know any of those languages to speak them in a way which is not a gross *mis*-representation.

ROLAND You are being modest.

ROBIN I don't think he is—I think he is being a humbug.

P.A. It has often been said, and I should be claiming to be less than human if I said there was no truth in the accusation. But you will miss something if you feel that the ulterior motive is the only one; just as I think it fallacious to assume that scientific truth, or religious truth, or aesthetic truth, or musical truth or rational truth is the only truth. Even what psycho-analysts call rationalizations have to be rational. Because I think we should be aware of the ultra- or infra-sensuous, or the super-ego and id, I do not think therefore that one should deny the rest. [AMF, II, 232]

Ultra-logic, plausibility

The prefix was used to warn about the attempts to use Euclidean–Cartesian logic too:

But suppose reality does not obey any of the laws laid down by the human animal—not even the "logic" to which not only human thought, but also the universe *not* included in human thought, is supposed to conform. Is there an ultra or infra logic which does not fall within the spectrum of human logic, the logical spectrum analogous to the visual portion of the spectrum of electro-magnetic waves? [AMF, II, 395]

This kind of warning corresponds to Kant's criticism of pure reason and to Freud's insights about the illogical nature of the unconscious. Bion got further than Kant in his categories of time and space, much like Freud, Planck and Einstein:

BION The experience of physical, sensuous space was not abandoned. It was clung to with such tenacity that it prevented the loss of security involved if pictorial sense were lost. It obscured realizations that Euclidean proofs depended on their being visually obvious. Euclidean geometry thus remained for centuries without a rival. There was no rival in the sphere of education since communication of what is known, by those who know it, to those who are ignorant of it, depends on visual sense. The "obvious" was evidence and proof of the truth of what was asserted. "Time" was as unquestioned as "space". Events are supposed to occur at a particular time and in a particular place; the "past" and "future" depend upon sensuous experience, but there is no more recognition of that than of the dependence of Euclidean geometry on the sense of sight. Theories about "mental life" are taken for granted, as was the background to the theories of Euclidean geometry; similar assumptions about "mental time and space" imperil growth of mental life. Theories of causation, commonly adumbrated in the context of the physical world, are based on the undiscussed and unquestioned foundation of ideas about time and space. Newton accepted that foundation. What he applied to the physical world is applicable to the mental or psychical or spiritual world. Should these assumptions be accepted by psycho-analysts or philosophers? Descartes has no doubt about the value of philosophical Doubt and yet did not doubt the validity of "cogito ergo sum"; although he came so near he did not take the final step. The psycho-analytical theory, first formulated by Melanie Klein, I propose to extend to areas not in fact included by her in the therapeutic domain for which she proposed it. The extension involves supposing that not only does the individual harbour omnipotent phantasies of destruction and dispersal, but that there is an omnipotent being or force that destroys the whole object and disperses the fragments widely.

MYSELF I can see that in the sphere of astronomy, where so much depends on the sense of sight either directly or at a remove—as in the examinations and comparison of photographs—it may be possible, by putting together the "facts" of many hundreds of photographs, to draw a sequence which could be supposed to represent a "moving picture": of events like the development of our own sun as if in a few moments one could scrutinize an event which may have taken many centuries. But I do not see what useful purpose is served by such a fictitious construction.

MAN It gives immediacy and reality to something which might otherwise be hard to understand.

BION Is it not just there that the danger lies? One more plausible theory is created to swell the enormous supply of plausible theories.

MAN Of course. But fear of what might happen is a bad master.

BION So is plausibility. I wonder how many plausible theories have been used and bewildered the human race. I would like to know. I am not sure of the ease with which "plausible" theories are produced. In this context of "plausible theories" about which we are talking, the plausible theory (or "convincing interpretation" may be hard to come by. It is plausible and false. Witness the idea that "the sun rises"—what trouble that has caused! We do not know the cost in suffering caused by the belief in a Christian God, or the god of Abraham's Ur, or Hitler's Germany, or peyotism—or god of any kind. [AMF, I, 171–2]

⊕ Even though the concept carries with it the bulk of recommendations to analysts about achieving a practice that could be named "real psycho-analysis", it must be read carefully in order to avoid judgmental values (q.v.):

MYSELF Not quite. I don't mean to be advocating anything. I suggest that somehow functions can be handed over to machines or mechanical methods. We ourselves learnt to walk "mechanically" at some point and this was, and still is, a very useful skill; but even now it is useful to resort from time to time to specific, skilled movement. I do not exclude the value of "mechanical thinking" or "mechanical interpretation", but I don't want *that* progress to take the place of, or to preclude the development of, the ultra- or infra-sensuous even though I may not know what that is or even if it exists. The pathology laboratory should not be substituted for clinical observation, or vice-versa. [AMF, I, 204]

The concept was carried much further and more clearly to encompass a picture, albeit of a whole lifetime of perceptions and too late for processing of those perceptions. This time the analogy—which was to be repeated throughout his latest conferences in New York (1977) and São Paulo (1978)—hypothesized a certain stimulus that could hit the pre-natal being. Taking into account that the brain, the eye and ear are ready in the fourth month of pregnancy, the hypothesis has a sound neurophysiological basis. He carried it further, suggesting that fear—"sub-thalamic fear"—may be a basic structuring emotion of man. The model of a pre-natal life is used to hint at the "stellar" or "quantum" dimension of the psycho-analytic issue, that is, how much is unknown. It suggests the huge, perhaps immeasurable complexity of possible variables encompassed by the events we try, as analysts, to study.

The following text encircles the analytic endeavour and the analytic view more and more. One should give special importance, in the view of this dictionary's author, to the phrases that depict the tolerance Bion had toward paradoxes (such as physical and mental) and also the phrase that says, "It is intended to". Analysis does not germinate in the air but is the product of learning, attention and effort linked to caring.

> SEVEN WEEKS EMBRYO If I had thought I would turn out like Helen of Troy I would have drowned myself in amniotic fluid. Luckily Six Weeks appreciated the difference and passed it on to his mesonephros. No wonder Rosemary was tired of people who could only see the progeny of her ectoderm. I'm not sure I want to be jammed up with Six Weeks though.
>
> P.A. Beauty is in the eye of ectoderm—as soon as the shell has developed it wants to become permanent. No wonder we are all insects at heart—just as well some of us developed an endo-skeleton.
>
> ROLAND What is wonderful about that? I have always had a spine and even my penis was often erect, but I can't see that I am better for it.
>
> DOCTOR You would if your lack of spine got you into a prisoner of war camp or a flabby penis had kept you out of marriage.
>
> ALICE I never discouraged an erection of nipple, clitoris or penis.
>
> P.A. Hmmmm ... nor do I, though I see plenty who do. Sexual maturity is often thought to be the end of the journey when in fact it is another beginning.
>
> DOCTOR What more is there besides sexual maturity?
>
> P.A. Terms like "sexual maturity" ought to be used precisely for physical maturity as in adolescence. By being allowed to spread, it disguises the absence of passionate love that is not only physical or mental, but a development of the fusion of both.
>
> ROSEMARY Sounds interesting.
>
> P.A. It is intended to. If you are right about it the sound may travel through the liquid medium and reach the auditory apparatus within you.

ALICE What about the pits?

P.A. Whether it is the pressure of sound waves which are sub-sonic or infra-visual they could reach the auditory and optic pits. Unfortunately Doctor may be so blinded by his psychiatric training that he would not interpret them correctly when they bounce back to his mind. So many won't see or listen because they say they are visual or auditory hallucinations, or chemically generated feelings of pugnacity or fear born of the adrenals—as if that made them unworthy of attention. Freud listened to and quoted his great teacher Charcot. If others did likewise they would repeat their observations, however compulsively repetitive they seemed to be, until a pattern became discernible in the chaos of chance. Look at your facts. Respect them even if you do not like them. The mists may clear and reveal a pattern which is so disagreeable—

PRIEST Or so blindingly brilliant, as Arjuna and others found—

P.A. Or so deep a void, so black, so astronomical a hole that you regret the price you have to pay.

VOICE What price is that?

ALICE What echo was that?

ROSEMARY It makes me shudder.

DOCTOR It bounces back from the hole and its sides.

P.A. We probably learn the price too late.

ALICE Too late for what?

P.A. For us to mend our course. Too "late" or "early", as measured against a scale of time which is relevant only to our ephemeral existence, not the millennia of millennia needed to plumb the nearest confines of reality.

ALICE Shall we get together?

SOMITE THREE Delighted—but let me remind you that the rest of you have spent all your energies trying to get rid of me. Were it not for my persistence—

GERM PLASM *Your* persistence! *Mine* you mean.

SOMITE THREE I nourished you and provided the conditions for your survival.

ALL (ante-natal) SOULS Had it not been for our parental care and your capacity to make the best of it, which we learnt from you, none of the post-natal crowd would exist.

ALL (post-natal) SOULS Let us agree that there are certain basic fundamentals of character and environment—Choice and Chance, as Yeats put it—which cannot be extinguished without our own extinction.

SOMITE THREE All I say is—

SEVEN WEEKS All we say is—

P.A. All I say is, do not forget what we owe to all of us—though I do not find a belly-ache or strabismus helpful.

ALL (ante-natal) SOULS We do not find it helpful to have to choose "pains" as our only method of drawing attention to our existence. We do not find Depression or Paranoia helpful to our struggles.

P.A. If I may speak for All Post-Natal Souls, we don't find it helpful to have to be depressed or mad before we get attention. [AMF, III, 471–3]

Misuses and misunderstandings: At the time of the writing of this dictionary, thirty years after the introduction of the term, it still has not been really noticed by the analytic movement. Therefore there seems to be no misuse of it yet—as far as this author's research goes.

This seems justified because many misunderstandings already encircle many of Bion's terms and definitions—echoing that which occurred with other great authors' contributions. The fate of the terms may reflect the mythical prohibition of knowledge.

The conjectural part of this warning is the optimistic idea that the term will ever gain attention. This being the case, it is very probable that it will be subjected to sensuous-concretization. That is, readers may lose sight of its analogical value. Perhaps some will try to "measure" infra- or ultra-sensuous quantities. Or use the term in the quantitative, albeit literal sense, such as "too much ultra-sensual".

Many environments already exist that call themselves—despite Bion's pleas against it—"bionians". In these circles it is already a commonplace jargon, "this is sensorial" or "this is too sensorial"; meaning, something worthy of contempt.

The term that means a real fact, namely, something that occurs beyond and before the human capacity of sensuous apprehension, may more probably than not be used to describe a hallucinated fact within the sensuous capacities. One may see that no theory is safe from concretization. It was Bion himself who observed it in the last-but-one year of his life:

> These primitive elements of thought are difficult to represent by any verbal formulation, because we have to rely on language which was elaborated later for other purposes. When I tried to employ meaningless terms—alpha and beta were typical—I found that "concepts without intuition which are empty and intuitions without concepts which are blind" rapidly became "black holes into which turbulence had seeped and empty concepts flooded with riotous meaning". [AMF, II, 229]

For now to misunderstand is merely a conjecture for the future. The conjecture is based on experience. Nevertheless, its shadow seems already to be cast. Whiffs of this hallucinated concretization are already being felt. Some groups believe that Bion said that a morula or an embryo or spermatozoa has a mind—and that they can study it.

Perhaps a good prevention, if any exists, would be to follow Bion's advice, as given first in the Introduction to *Learning from Experience* and thereafter in other texts: the writings of good authors should be read and forgotten. Their use in practice depends on experience in the here and now of the session.

Suggested cross-references: Analytic view, Atonement, Controversy, Mind, O, Real Psycho-analysis, Reality Psychic and Sensuous, Thoughts-without-a-thinker, Transformations in O, Vertex.

📖 Suggested further readings: the Jewish and Christian Cabbala; Goethe's *Faust*, especially the last part; William Blake's *Book of Urizen*, Freud's *The Interpretation of Dreams*, *The Question of a Weltanschauung*, *Analysis Terminable and Interminable*; Lewis Carroll's *Through the Looking Glass*; Machado de Assis' *Memórias Póstumas de Braz Cubas*; James Joyce's *Finnegan's Wake*; Nietzsche's *Also sprach Zarathustra*.

Understanding: Please refer to the entry, **Discipline on Memory, Desire and Understanding.**

University: *"P.A. By 'university' I think you mean a number of individuals gathered together and self-endowed with the privilege of declaring who is, and who is not, worthy of joining their association"* (AMF, II, 247).

Unknowable, unknown: By resorting to a not yet widely used colloquial verbal formulation, Bion rescues the ethos of Freud's most fundamental observations, those regarding the nature of the unconscious, the realm of the id. Interestingly enough, the colloquial expression in English corresponds exactly to the meaning of the word in German—*unbewußt*—not known. One may find this in many quotations from Freud, such as *"The unconscious is the true psychical reality; **in its innermost nature it is as most unknown to us as the reality of the external world, and it is as incompletely presented by the data of consciousness as is the external world by the communications of our sense organs**"* (Freud, 1900, p.613; Freud's bold).

Many who adhere to Bion's contributions remain aloof from this. The Kantian origin of Freud, which is clear in the quotation above, continues unabated in Bion's work

Many felt it strange that an analyst would base himself so heavily on Kant to construe his theories in the way Bion did. Perhaps no one before or after him used Kant in such an explicit way: it is implicit in Freud but it requires an attentive and informed reader. Bion used it from the notion of the innate pre-conceptions (q.v.) to the heavy usage of the numinous realm; from the relationships of concepts with intuitions to the full profiting of the concepts of primary and secondary characteristics of anything. The ethos of Freud stemmed from Kant; other analysts, such as Reik, brought Kant's contributions to the consideration of the psycho-analytical movement before Bion did so.

Many do not notice that Freud's concept of the unconscious was a current one in German romanticism; it corresponds to Bion's insistence about the unknown. Psycho-analysis was from its inception a research into the unknown. This is made with unconscious, analytically-trained intuitive tools: the patient's free associations and dreams that evolve from the unknown and the analyst's free floating attention and experience stored in his capacity to dream and intuit from it (or play, in Klein and Winnicott's extensions of it). All of this emanates from the unknown in the decisive moment of the here and now of the session.

The concept of "O", the quasi-mathematical symbol for the numinous realm, the unknown and ultimately unknowable, rescued Freud's discovery of psycho-analysis from the gilded tombstone of self-aware adoration of consciousness clothed in psycho-analytical wording. The latter is built with rigid a priori reasoning, pre-patterned theorizing—which turned psycho-analysis into a clever, erudite manipulation of symbols.

"Ultimately unknowable" is a restrained attitude if compared with pretensions more typical of an alchemist or of an esoteric mystic to achieve ownership or conscious knowledge of essences. Ultimately unknowable refers to the fact that reality does not let itself be known, but lets it be perceived, used, in the same sense, as Bion puts it, that potatoes cannot be sung but can be eaten, planted, fried, etc. Reality demands to be intuited and can become so.

> Pascal's phrase, "Le silence de ces espaces infinies m'effraie" can serve as an expression of intolerance and fear of the "unknowable" and hence of the unconscious in the sense of the undiscovered or the un-evolved. [T, 171]

Misuses and misconceptions: The misuses seem to stem from people who cannot have Pascal's humility, reverence and awe coupled with Pascal's fortitude and refusal to submit to authority. To shun the experiencing of the unknown is a pretension to total knowledge and a denial of any possibility of steps or stages of knowing; ultimately it equals a profound distrust of the existence of truth itself. *"Psycho-analysis itself is just a stripe on the coat of the Tiger. Ultimately it may meet the Tiger—The Thing-Itself—O"* (AMF, I, 112). The naive idealist or solipsistic reader, prey to paranoid anxieties, denies the last phrase. The naive realist reader, prey to schizoid anxieties, mistakes the stripe on the coat for the Tiger; he takes it concretely.

Ultimately unknowable is often mistaken for non-existent, non-intuitable, non-usable. The uncertainty principle is often turned into a principle of ignorance. Knowledge belongs to the conscious realm; evolving and becoming, emanations of "O" and to be at-one (see Atonement) belong to the realm of the ultimately unknowable, but "be-able"—that is, existent. Freud's metaphor of the unconscious as an onion and its many layers is still valid. The "onion-ness" can be intuited.

&; The author, starting from *Transformations* and *A Memoir of the Future*, tries to assess the difficult relationship of the Western thinking tradition and science with the unknown, and the birth of psycho-analysis in a series of books and some papers published elsewhere (see the third part of the Bibliography) . These texts explore the psychic mechanisms that define the term, "naïve idealism" and Kant's term "naïve realism".

See also, Absolute truth, Analytic view, Atonement, Becoming, Disturbed personality, O, Jargon, Real analysis, Reality Sensuous and Psychic, Truth.

V

Verbalized thoughts: Bion considers the environment in which the analyst works in the same way that Freud considered it. Nothing more than a talk occurs when these two persons, who are functioning as analyst and patient, meet. That is, using Bion's words, the analyst works through an environment constituted by *"verbalized thoughts"*.

It seemed a logical step to him to obtain an assessment, in terms of the truth-value, of the verbalizations—either the analyst's or the patient's verbalizations.

In Bion's time, epistemologists considered a non-plus-ultra attempt to achieve this. It consisted of a kind of scrutiny of the grammatical consistency of scientific statements. They allegedly could turn them into statements amenable to verification. This was the project of neo-positivists since Moritz Schlick, from the twenties. It survived in England up to the sixties due to the work of some German émigrés. Outstanding among these was Rudolph Carnap.

Bion seemed to be influenced by this trend. His attempt in this direction was materialized by the Grid (q.v.). It was used to categorize verbalized thoughts in a *"more precise"* way. He states that verbalized thoughts must *"be truthful"* and must be included in the categories that belonged to the two axes of the Grid: functions of thinking and genetics of thinking (please refer to the entry, Grid, in this dictionary, for a detailed account of the two axes and categories). More specifically, he stated that the truthful statements uttered by the analyst should be included in the genetic categories of conceptions and concepts; possibly, also, pre-conceptions and scientific systems. The functions of the analyst's truthful statements should belong to the categories of definitory hypotheses, notation, attention and inquiry. In terms of the Grid, rows E, F and possibly D and G; and columns 1, 3, 4 and 5. He assessed that rows corresponding to deductive scientific systems and algebraic calculus (G and H) applied to phenomena far more sophisticated and precise than those that could be achieved by psycho-analysis as he knew it.

This account synthesizes his idea on verbalized thoughts and the analyst's verbalized thoughts. They can be found in this way in *Transformations*, pages 4 and 38.

Suggested cross-references: Analytic view, Grid.

Verbal thoughts: Please refer to the entries: Grid, Schizophrenia, Verbalized Thoughts.

Vertex: *"I hope that there will be evolved a method of designating the vertex with brevity and precision"* (AI, 55).

Vertex is a mathematical (geometric) term used by Bion as an aid to formulate the conditions under which an observation is made. The clear statement of these conditions is in itself a condition—it is **the** scientific condition *par excellence*.

The first time Bion uses the term is connected with the mathematical analogies with circles, points and lines. He proposed an exercise in order to help the reader to familiarize himself with the concept:

"We may start with a mental image of a line in front of us. We can suppose that the two ends of the line are joined to our eye or that our eye projects the line outwards to a point where we want it. In both instances the eye is the vertex of a configuration of lines. We can rotate the line so that it is end-on to our 'line of sight' and so appears as a point" (T, 89). The exercise goes on, considering the point as being projected outward while remaining attached to the eye and other situations.

He follows on considering the popular and colloquial expressions that display a change of vertex or the adoption of more than one vertex to solve problems or to get nearer reality. Namely, "hot on the scent", "smelling a rat" (T, 90), which constantly conjoin tactile with olfactory senses and olfactory with sight senses, respectively. Also, *"Musical methods of notation are in their adequacy reminiscent of algebraic methods of geometrical notation"*, emphasizing that the visual vertex has a superior power to illuminate a problem, over all other mental counterparts of the senses. This was a fact already noticed by Freud and can be seen in dreams, which are predominantly visual.

Vertexes can be seen as an evolution of Bion's earlier considerations about common sense. They also help in furthering the study of hallucination. *"Reversal of direction in the system of which the vertex is a part is associated with what are ordinarily known as hallucinations"* (T, 91).

Bion preferred to use the term "vertex", rather than the term "point of view":

"I am unwilling to use a term such as 'point-of-view' because I do not wish to be reduced to writing 'from the point of view of digestion' or 'from the point of the view of a sense of smell' when the distinctions between metaphorical and literal usages are fine yet difficult to preserve. I can describe my use of the term 'vertex' as an example taking a mathematical term . . . and using it as a model" (T, 91). The mathematical term is regarded as a scientific term and the model is akin to myths and dreams.

The issue also touches in the problems of communication:

BION I was speaking conversationally.

SHERLOCK Ah! In my kind of work you have to be precise.

MYSELF So you have in ours. Unfortunately we have to talk conversational English and that is not a language intended to be used for the purposes for which we have to use it.

SHERLOCK I, alas, have to use the language my author puts at *my* disposal.

MYSELF You—meaning both of you—don't do badly. My characters are not fictional and they are very dissatisfied with such means of communication as I put at their disposal.

SHERLOCK "Means of communication"! Do you mean English? If not—

MYSELF No, I don't. If it is English, that is *not* enough. I am aware that conversational English is inadequate; but you should hear what they say about anything else.

BION Jargon, for example.

SHERLOCK HOLMES Why not paint or draw or compose music, or—

BION —play the violin. Did you ever try your violin playing on your clients or criminals or courts of law? [AMF, I, 202]

ROBIN Well, I have a mind, of course.

ROLAND That is what we are discussing.

ROBIN If we could talk the language of mathematics . . .

PAUL If we could speak the language of religion . . .

ALICE If we could only learn to look at what artists paint . . .

ROLAND What is wrong with not talking at all and listening to the music?

EDMUND Once it would have been understood when we were exhorted to hear the music of the spheres.

ROBIN I wouldn't object if I could speak the "mathematics" of the spheres.

P.A. There may be something to be said for the language of the psycho-analyst.

ROLAND He hasn't got a language—only "jargon".

P.A. That is not so. I try to talk English because it is the best I know. But I do not know it well enough to speak it for the purpose of what I want to convey. I do not talk Jargonese any more than Paul talks Journalese . . . This is my lack and your misfortune in so far as you want me to talk a language *you* can "understand" and I want you to meet me at least half-way by talking a language *I* can understand. [AMF, II, 230–1]

It will be remembered that the term "vertex" can be understood as similar to "point of view" except in certain special conditions. There is a psychological or mental specificity analogous to the specificity associated with the relationship of sense organs to sense impressions. To allow for this specificity it is necessary to discard the term "point of view" and replace it by a more abstract term such as "vertex". [AI, 126]

His latest formulation of the use of vertexes is perhaps the simplest he achieved:

P.A. . . . . We are concerned not with what the individual *means* to say so much as with what he does *not* intend to say, but does in fact say.

ROLAND This depends on your interpretation of *what* he says— not what he *says*.

P.A. I am concerned with what he says and what it is about. My interpretation is my attempt to formulate *what* he says so that he can compare it with his other ideas.

ROLAND If I say I am going to Munden I mean just that; I don't mean I am going to have a sexual orgy.

P.A. If, as is the case, I am having a social intercourse with you, I am concerned only with the fact that you intend to go to Munden. If you were coming to me for medical advice I would be concerned with your physical fitness to go, or would expect to hear and observe for myself what medical matters were involved in your journey from here to there. If you said you wanted mental help I would regard the intention "to go to Munden" as "peripheral" to what is involved. If I considered that I had your permission to find out what was involved in coming to me and in "going to Munden", I would direct my response to the area signalized by the words "sexual orgy". [AMF, II, 269]

Some years earlier he already had a quasi-colloquial formulation on vertex, in discussing controversies among analysts:

. . . many difficulties could be obviated by more precise definition of the point of view (vertex). It is permissible for an observer to say that he has no evidence of infantile sexuality provided he also adds that he is an aeronautical engineer and does not take anything but a cursory view of children. What is *not* permissible is that he should say that he has no evidence of infantile sexuality without mentioning his vertex. [AI, 55]

Another explanation of the use of the term is given in the same book:

> The vertex of the dreamer is not that of the dreamer awake; the vertex of the artist is not that of the interpreter of the work of art. Similarly, the vertex of the psycho-analyst, and changes of vertex corresponding to moment-to-moment changes in a session, effect the transformations made manifest in associations and interpretations. [AI, 93]

The opening chapter, a "pro-knowledge" (Bion called it "Prologue") introduction to *A Memoir of the Future* synthesizes and reunites his previous observations contained in *Transformations* and *Attention and Interpretation* in straightforward language:

> The advantage of falling back on borrowing a mathematical term like "vertex" is that it can make it possible to talk to lunatics who are thrown into confusion if you say things like "from the point of view of smell". It is very exasperating to find a man who interrupts by saying, "My eyes don't smell", or, "My smell can't see any view". My exasperation doesn't help either. Now I remember a bit of a dream about violence and murder. Something about Albert and Victoria, I think. Suppose these vertices are separate and distinct, the two vertices could contribute to a harmonization rather like binocular vision. Suppose I used my alimentary canal as a sort of telescope. I could get down to the arse and look up at the mouth full of teeth and tonsils and tongue. Or rush up to the top end of the alimentary canal and watch what my arse-hole was up to . . .
>
> Suppose the vertices were separate and coincident. This would do if one of the points which was separate and distinct rushed down the arc to meet the other; but, judging by what it felt like last night, it was more like sound travelling in bent tubes. [AMF, I, 3–4]

Bion shows how the evolutions from a vertex must be taken into consideration (chapter 8, *Attention and Interpretation*)—even the messianic expectation, *"formulated and institutionalized in the Christian religion, may represent the evolved aspect of an element which is represented also at its evolved stage by the Oedipus myth"* (AI, 84).

The psycho-analytic vertex

The vertexes of the analyst, of the patient and of the public are stated in the first chapter of *Transformations*. The vertexes are just the starting point from where transformations are made; the differences of vertexes help, through comparison, to detect the invariance that generated the transformations.

> ... although the analyst is under an obligation to speak with as little ambiguity as possible, in fact his aims are limited by the analysand who is free to receive interpretations in whatever way he chooses. In a sense it can seem that the analyst is hoist with his own petard: he is free to interpret the statements of the analysand how he will; the analysand retorts in kind. The analyst is not free except in the sense that when the patient comes to him for analysis he is obliged to speak in a way which would not be tolerable in any other frame of reference and then only from a particular vertex.

> The patient's response would also be intolerable if there were no psycho-analytic indulgence to excuse it, or, if it were not for a psycho-analytic vertex. [T, 145]

Suggested cross-references: Analytic view, Catastrophic Change, Controversy, Mathematization of psycho-analysis (especially the sub-item, **Vertex and frustration**), Ultra-sensuous.

Violent emotions: The concept of violent emotions is a part of Bion's third attempt at a purely psycho-analytic theory, as different from almost all his earlier attempts, with the sole exceptions of his theory on thinking and the theory of container and contained. It is his first attempt to integrate Freud and Klein. Prior to this and thereafter he also made extensions based on Freud and Klein's theories. These acute and minute observations came to constitute theories of observation in psycho-analysis. A pure psycho-analytical theory appeared no more—the theory of alpha-function, beta-elements, bizarre objects, reverie, the links, enforced splitting, the realm of minus, all were either *"working tools"* (LE, 89) or observational theories. They helped observation in the here and now of the session.

Violent emotions are part of a "Metatheory". This attempt was doomed to remain unpublished until 1992; it was due to Francesca

Bion's fortitude that we can study it today. It served as a preparation for subdued formulation of it, or better to say, a use of this psycho-analytic theory to build a theory of observation in psycho-analysis, in *Transformations* (pp. 8, 9, 51ff., see Hyperbole).

Violent emotions are the jumping board to acting-out. They are an expression of the paranoid–schizoid position. They do not exclusively express, as the verbal formulation may indicate, "*quantity of feeling*". In dealing with it Bion does not "*consider whether the violence implies an origin in the individual endowment or is secondary to an external environment*"; but the fact that it is perhaps innate does not preclude observing that it may on occasion be due to "*a deficiency in a capacity for thought . . . proper to the onset of the reality principle which tends to produce arrest at a stage where action is a method of unburdening the psyche of accretions of stimuli, and so contributes to the physical expression of love or hate which can be characteristic of violence. Violence, then, though related to quantity or degree, contributes to a qualitative change in the emotion. The qualitative changes make love and hate possess appreciably cruel strains together with diminishing concern for the object. Both love and hate thus become more easily associated with a lack of concern for truth and life*" (C, 249–250).

The person feigns, through exaggeration, the love he/she lacks. Perhaps this perception stems from Klein's observation that it is not only hate but the intensity of love that destroys the object (Klein, 1934).

Y

Y: A quasi-mathematical sign used to denote development of the psycho-analytical object (LE, 69–70).

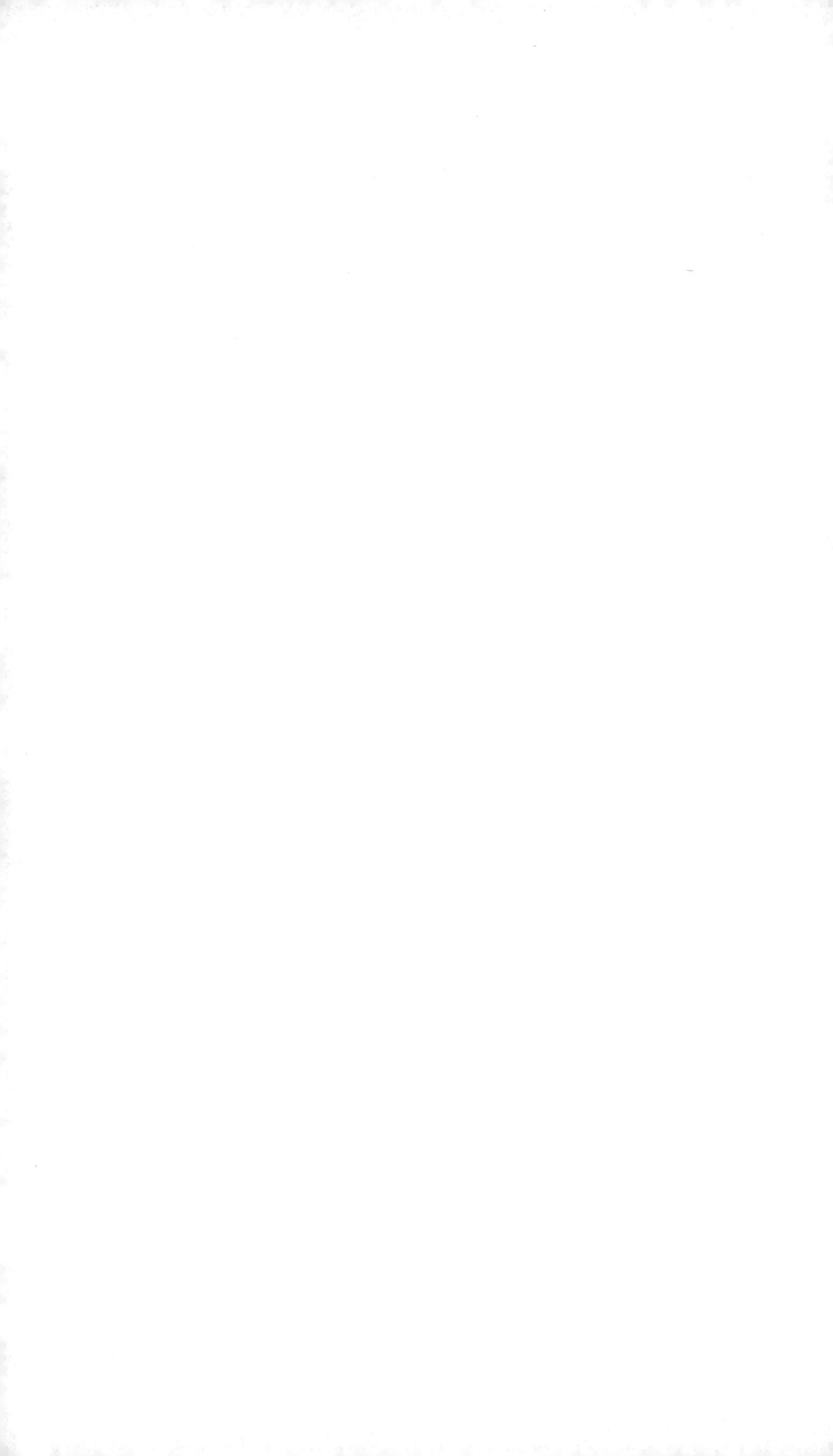

BIBLIOGRAPHY

Works of Bion used to build the text:

1. Short papers

1940 The war of nerves. In: E. Miller & H. Crichton-Miller (Eds.), *The Neuroses in War*. London: Macmillan.

1943 Intra-group tensions in therapy. *The Lancet*, 27 November 1943.

1946 The leaderless group project. *Bulletin of the Menninger Clinic, 10* (May).

1948 Psychiatry at a time of crisis. *British Journal of Medical Psychology, 21*.

1966 Catastrophic Change *Bulletin 5*, British Psycho-Analytic Society.

1967 Notes on memory and desire. *The Psycho-analytic Forum, 2*. Re-published in: F. Bion (Ed.), *Cogitations*. London: Karnac, 1992.

1976 Emotional turbulence. In: *Borderline Disorders* by P. Hartocollis. New York: International Universities Press. Re-published in: F. Bion (Ed.), *Clinical Seminars and Other Works*. London: Karnac, 1994.

1976 On a quotation from Freud. In: *Borderline Disorders* by P. Hartocollis, New York, International Universities Press. Re-published in: F. Bion (Ed.), *Clinical Seminars and Other Works*. London: Karnac, 1994.

1976 Evidence. *Bulletin 8*, British Psycho-Analytic Society. Re-published in: F. Bion (Ed.), *Clinical Seminars and Other Works*. London: Karnac, 1994.

1977 *Two Papers: The Grid and Caesura*. Rio de Janeiro: Imago.

1979 Making the best from a bad job. *Bulletin 10*, British Psycho-Analytic Society.

2. Books

1961 *Experience in Groups*. London: Tavistock.

1962 *Learning from Experience*. London: Heinemann Medical Books.

1963 *Elements of Psycho-analysis*. London: Heinemann Medical Books.

1965 *Transformations*. London: Heinemann Medical Books.

1967 *Second Thoughts*. London: Heinemann Medical Books.

1970 *Attention and Interpretation*. Tavistock.

1975 The dream. In *A Memoir of The Future*. London: Karnac, 1990.

c. 1975 *Taming Wild Thoughts*. F. Bion & P. Bion Talamo (Eds.). London: Karnac, 1997.

1977 The past presented. In: *A Memoir of The Future*. London: Karnac, 1990.

1979 The dawn of oblivion. In: *A Memoir of The Future*. London: Karnac, 1990.

1982 *The Long Week-End* volume I. F. Bion (Ed.). Oxford: Fleetwood Press. Re-published London: Karnac, 1982.

1985 *All My Sins Remembered: Another Part of a Life and The Other Side of Genius*. F. Bion (Ed.). Oxford: Fleetwood Press. Re-published London: Karnac, 1991.

1991 *Cogitations*. F. Bion (Ed.). London: Karnac, 1992.

3. Conferences and seminars

1973 *Brazilian Lectures I*. London: Karnac, 1992.

1974 *Brazilian Lectures II*. London: Karnac, 1992.

1978 *Four Discussions with W. R. Bion*. Perthshire: Clunie Press.

1979 *Bion in New York and Sao Paulo*. Perthshire: Clunie Press.

1987 *Clinical Seminars and Four Papers*. Oxford: Fleetwood Press.

1978 *Taming Wild Thoughts and The Grid 2*. Karnac, 1997.

1978 *Seminari Italiani*. Rome: Bolatti Boringhieri, 1990.

4. Partnerships

1980 *A Key to A Memoir of the Future* (with Francesca Bion). Perthshire: Clunie Press; re-published in *A Memoir of The Future*. London: Karnac, 1990.

General bibliography

Alves, D. B. (1989). Sobre o sentimento de soledade: Paidéa II. *Rev. Bras. Psicanal.* 23: 209.

Anscombe, G. E. M. (1959). *An Introduction to Wittgenstein's* Tractacus. London: Hutchinson.

Bachelard, G. (1938). *A Formação do Espírito Científico (contribuição para uma psicanálise do conhecimento)*. Vers‹o brasileira, por E.S.Abreu. S‹o Paulo: Contraponto, 1996.

Berlin, I. (1996). *The Sense of Reality: Studies in Ideas and Their History.* London: Chatto & Windus.

Bicudo, V. L. (1996). Personal communication.

Bion, W. R.(1977). Introduction. In *Seven Servants*. New York: Jason Aronson, 1977.

Chuster, A. (1997). "The myth of Satan". Presented at the W. R. Bion Centennial held at Turin.

Ferenczi, S. (1928). The elasticity of psycho-analytic technique. In: M. Balint (Ed.)., *Final Contributions to the Problems and Methods of Psycho-analysis*, E. Mosbacher (Trans.), pp. 87–102. London: The Hogarth Press and the Institute of Psycho-analysis (1955).

Freud, S. (1895). Project for a scientific psychology. *S.E.*, I.

Freud, S. (1900). The interpretation of dreams. *S.E.*, IV & V.

Freud, S. (1912). The dynamics of transference. *S.E.*, XII.

Freud, S. (1915). Instincts and their vicissitudes. *S.E.*, XIV.

Freud, S. (1925). Negation. *S.E.*, XIX

Freud, S. (1926). Inhibitions, symptoms and anxiety. *S.E.*, XX.

Freud, S. (1933). New introductory letters in psycho-analysis. *S.E.*, XXII.

Freud, S. (1937). Constructions in analysis. *S.E.*, XXIII.

Freud, S. (1938a). Analysis terminable and interminable. *S.E.*, XXIII.

Freud, S. (1938b). Splitting of the ego in the process of defence. *S.E.*, XXIII.

Freud, S. (1938c). An outline of psycho-analysis. *S.E.*, XXIII.

Freud, S. (1939). Findings, ideas, problems. *S.E.*, XXIII.

Ferro, A. (1999). Narrative derivatives of alpha-elements. Presented at the meeting, "Bion's Readers around the World", Non-official session at IPAC, Santiago de Chile.

Fromm-Reichmann, F. (1950). *Principles of Intensive Psychotherapy.* Chicago: The University of Chicago Press.

Green, A. (1992). Book Review, *Cogitations. International Journal of Psycho-Analysis*, 73: 585.

Green, A. (1995). Has sexuality anything to do with psychoanalysis? *International Journal of Psycho-Analysis, 76*: 871.

Green, A. (2000). The central phobic position: a new formulation of the free association method. *International Journal of Psycho-Analysis, 81*: 429.

Green, A. (2001). *4 questions pour André Green*. São Paulo: Departamento de Publicações da Sociedade Brasileira de Psicanálise de São Paulo.

Hartmann, N. (1960). *A Filosofia do Idealismo Alemão*. Portuguese version, by J. G. Belo. Lisboa: Fundação Calouste Gulbekian, 1983.

Hempel, C. G. (1962). Explanation in science and in history. In: R. G. Colodny (Ed.), *Frontiers of Science and Philosophy*, pp. 7-33. London: Allen & Unwin.

Hume, D. (1748). *An Enquiry Concerning Human Understanding*. In: L. A. Selby-Biggs (Ed.), *The Great Books of the Western World*. Chicago: Encyclopaedia Britannica Inc., 1994.

Jones, E. (1937). Rationalism and psycho-analysis. In: *Essays in Applied Psycho-Analysis*. London: The Hogarth Press and the Institute of Psycho-Analysis, 1951.

Jones, E. (1955). *Sigmund Freud: Life and Work*. Vol. II. *Years of Maturity*. London: The Hogarth Press and the Institute of Psycho-Analysis, 1956.

Jones, E. (1956). *Sigmund Freud: Life and Work*. Vol. III. *The Last Phase*. London: The Hogarth Press and the Institute of Psycho-Analysis, 1957.

Joseph, B. (2002). Public supervision held at Sociedade Brasileira de Psicanálise de São Paulo, tape-recorded.

Joseph, E. (1980). Interview .IDE: vol. III

Kant, I. (1781). *Critique of Pure Reason*. M. T.Miklejohn (Trans.). In: *The Great Books of the Western World*. Chicago: Encyclopaedia Britannica, 1994.

Kant, I. (1783). Prolegômenos. Brazilian version, by T.M.Bernkopf. In *Os Pensadores*. São Paulo: Abril Cultural, 1980.

Kleene, S. C. (1959). *Introduction to Metamathematics*. Amsterdam: North Holland Publishing Company.

Klein, M. (1928). Early stages of the Oedipus conflict. In: *Contributions to Psycho-Analysis*. London: The Hogarth Press and the Institute of Psycho-Analysis, 1950.

Klein, M. (1930). The importance of symbol-formation in the development of the ego. In: *Contributions to Psycho-Analysis*. London: The Hogarth Press and the Institute of Psycho-Analysis, 1950.

Klein, M. (1932). *The Psycho-Analysis of Children*. London: The Hogarth Press and the Institute of Psycho-Analysis, 1959.

Klein, M. (1945). The Oedipus complex in the light of early anxieties. In: *Contributions to Psycho-Analysis*. London: The Hogarth Press and the Institute of Psycho-Analysis, 1950.

Klein, M. (1946). Notes on some schizoid mechanisms. In: M. Klein, P. Heimann, S. Isaacs, & J. Riviere (Ed.), *Developments in Psycho-Analysis*. London: The Hogarth Press and the Institute of Psycho-Analysis, 1952

Klein, M. (1957). *Envy and Gratitude*. London: Tavistock.

Klein, M. (1961). On the sense of loneliness. In: *Our Adult World and Other Essays*. London: Heinemann Medical Books.

Lawrence, W. G., Bain, A., & Gould, L. (1996). The fifth basic assumption. *Free Associations*, 6: 28–55

Meltzer, D. (1983). Speech at the Memorial Meeting to W. R. Bion. *International Review of Psycho-analysis*, 8: 11.

Menninger, K. (1960).*Teoria de la Técnica Psicoanalitica*. Spanish version, por M. Gonzalez. Mexico: Editorial Pax- Mexico, 1960.

Norris, C. (1997). *Against Relativism*. London: Blackwell.

Penrose, R. (1989). *The Emperor's New Mind (concerning computers, minds and the laws of physics)*. New York: Penguin, 1991.

Pepe, D. (1989). Il circolo filosofico de Viena. In: Domenico de Masi (Ed.). *L'emozione e la regola*. Roma: Guis, Laterza & Figli Spa

Planck, M. (1949). *Scientific Autobiography*. F. Gaynor (Trans.). In: *The Great Books of the Western World*. Chicago: Encyclopaedia Britannica, 1994.

Reik, T. (1948). *Listening with the Third Ear*. Nova Iorque: Grove Press.

Rickman, J. (1950). The factor of number in individual and group dynamics. In: W. C. M. Scott & S. Payne (Ed.). *Selected Contributions to Psycho-Analysis*. London: The Hogarth Press and the Institute of Psycho-Analysis.

Rosen, J. (1953). *Direct Analysis: Selected Papers*. New York: Grunne & Stratton.

Rosenfeld, H. (1965). *Os estados psicóticos*. Brazilian version, por J. Salomão & P. D. Correa. Rio de Janeiro: Zahar, 1968.

Ruben, D. H. (1993). Introduction. In: D. H. Ruben (Ed.). *Explanation* (pp. 1–16). Oxford: Oxford University Press.

Ruskin, J. (1894). *Sesame and Lillies*. Orpington: George Allen.

Russell, B. (1925). *ABC da Relatividade*. G.Rebuá (Trans.). Rio de Janeiro: Zahar Editores, 1963.

Sanders, K. (1986). *A Matter of Interest*. Strathclyde: Clunie Press.

Sandler, E. H., Camargo, C. V., Sandler, P. C., Botelho, E. Z., Mattos, L. L., & Serebrenik, T. (1997). "The myth of Ajax". Presented at the W. R. Bion Centennial held at Turin.

Sandler, J. J. (1992). Interview. IDE: vol. 15.

Sokal, A., & Brikmont, J. (1997). *Fashionable Nonsense. Post Modern Intellectuals' Abuse of Science.* New York: Picador USA, 1999.

Symington, J., & Symington, N. (1997). *O pensamento clínico de Wilfred Bion.* Lisbon: Climiepsi Editores, 1999.

Ruben, D. H. (1993). Introduction. In: D. H. Ruben (Ed.), *Explanation* (pp. 1-16). Oxford: Oxford University Press.

Schrödinger, E. (1944). *What is Life?* In: *The Great Books of the Western World.* Chicago: Encyclopaedia Britannica, 1994.

Segal, H. (1989). Personal letter to the author

Singer, I. B. (1950). *The Family Moskat.* New York: Alfred Knopfinger.

Talamo, P. B. (1995). On alpha-function. Comment at the meeting "Bion readers around the world", non-official session at the IPAC, San Francisco

Wallerstein, R. (1988). One psycho-analysis or many? *International Journal of Psycho-Analysis,* 69: 5–21.

Wordsworth, W. (1798). Preface to *Lyrical Ballads.* In: *Wordsworth Poetry & Prose.* Oxford: Clarendon Press, 1960

Works of the author used in the text:

Sandler, P. C. (1987). Grade? *Rev. Bras. Psicanál.,* 21: 203.

Sandler, P. C. (1988). *Introdução a "Uma Memória do Futuro", de W. R. Bion.* Rio de Janeiro: Imago Editora Ltada.

Sandler, P. C. (1990). *Fatos: a tragédia do conhecimento em psicanálise.* Rio de Janeiro: Imago Editora Ltada.

Sandler, P. C. (1994). Cogitations. *Rev. Bras. Psicanal.* 28: 347.

Sandler, P. C. (1997a). The apprehension of psychic reality: extensions of Bion's theory of alpha-function. *International Journal of Psycho-Analysis,* 78: 43.

Sandler, P. C. (1997b). *A apreensᵃo da realidade psíquica (The Apprehension of Psychic Reality),* Volume I. Rio de Janeiro: Imago.

Sandler, P. C. (1999). Um desenvolvimento e aplicação clínica do instrumento de Bion, o grid. *Rev. Bras. Psicanál.,* 33: 13.

Sandler, P. C. (2000a). *As origens da psicanálise na obra de Kant (The Origins of Psychoanalysis in the Work of Kant).* Volume III in the series, *A apreensão da realidade psíquica (The Apprehension of Psychic Reality),* Rio de Janeiro: Imago.

Sandler, P. C. (2000b). Turbulência e urgência (*Turbulence and Urgency*). Volume IV in the series, *A apreensão da realidade psíquica* (*The Apprehension of Psychic Reality*). Rio de Janeiro: Imago.

Sandler, P. C. (2000c). What is thinking—an attempt at an integrated study of W. R. Bion's contributions to the processes of knowing. In: P. Bion Talamo, F. Borgogno, & S. Merciai (Eds.), *W. R. Bion: Between Past and Present*. London: Karnac.

Sandler, P. C. (2001a). *A apreensão da realidade psíquica* (*The Apprehension of Psychic Reality*), Volume V: *Goethe e a psicanálise* (*Goethe and Psychoanalysis*). Rio de Janeiro: Imago.

Sandler, P. C. (2001b). Le projet scientifique de Freud en danger un siècle plus tard? (Is Freud's scientific project in danger a century later?). *Rev Fr Psychanal*, 65:181–201 (In special issue: *Courants contemporains de la psychanalyse* (*Current Trends in Psychoanalysis*).

Sandler, P. C. (2001c). Psychoanalysis and epistemology: Relatives, friends or strangers? Official panel, 42nd IPA conference, Nice, 22–27 July 2001

Sandler, P. C. (2001d). O Quarto Pressuposto. *Rev. Bras. Psicanal.*, 35: 907.

Sandler, P. C. (2002). *O Belo é Eterno* (*A Thing of Beauty is a Joy Forever*). Volume VI in the series, *A Apreensão da Realidade Psíquica* (*The Apprehension of Psychic Reality*). Rio de Janeiro: Imago.

Sandler, P. C. (2003a). Bion's *War Memoirs*: A psychoanalytical commentary. In: R. M. Lipgar & M. Pines (Eds.), *Building on Bion: Roots*. London: Jessica Kingsley.

Sandler, P. C. (2003b). *Hegel e Klein* (*Hegel and Klein*). Vol. VII in the series, *A apreens‹o da realidade psíquica* (*The Apprehension of Psychic Reality*). Rio de Janeiro: Imago.

Sandler, P. C. (2005). The origins of the work of Bion. *International Journal of Psycho-analysis*, in press.